# Diving and Subaquatic Medicine

# DEDICATION

This book is dedicated to
the memory of Pluto who died, even though
he never left dry land.

# Diving and Subaquatic Medicine

*Third edition*

**Carl Edmonds**
**Christopher Lowry**
**and**
**John Pennefather**

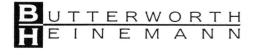

Butterworth-Heinemann
Linacre House, Jordan Hill, Oxford OX2 8DP
225 Wildwood Avenue, Woburn, MA 01801-2041
A division of Reed Educational and Professional Publishing Ltd

℞ A member of the Reed Elsevier plc group

OXFORD    BOSTON    JOHANNESBURG
MELBOURNE    NEW DELHI    SINGAPORE

First published by Diving Medical Centre, NSW, Australia 1976
Second Edition 1981
Third edition 1992
Paperback edition 1994
Reprinted 1995, 1997 (twice), 1998

**British Library Cataloguing in Publication Data**
Edmonds, Carl
  Diving and subaquatic medicine. - 3rd ed.
  I. Title  II. Pennefather, John
  III. Lowry, Christopher
  617.1

ISBN0 7506 2131 1

**Library of Congress Cataloguing in Publication Data**
Edmonds, Carl
  Diving and subaquatic medicine/Carl Edmonds, Christopher Lowry
  and John Pennefather. - 3rd ed.
  p.  cm.
  Includes bibliographical references and index.
  ISBN 07506 2131 1
  1. Submarine medicine.  I. Lowry, Christopher.  II. Pennefather,
  John.  III. Title
  RC1005.E35                                          91-4910
  616.9'8022-dc20                                        CIP

Typeset by TecSet Ltd, Wallington, Surrey
Printed and bound in Great Britain by Redwood Books, Trowbridge, Wiltshire

# Contents

# Preface to the third edition

CE: We are going to have to run a sixth printing of our *Diving and Subaquatic Medicine* text. How about doing a third edition instead?

CL: No way. I am too busy.

CE: How about if we only write on rainy days, when it should not interfere with surfing or sailboarding?

CL: I suppose I could handle that.

JP: You agreed that the second edition was to be the last.

CE: I lied.

JP: Don't you think that there are now enough diving medical books on the market?

CE: Would you really want your doctors to have to rely on the other texts to learn how to treat injured divers?

JP: OK, but under protest.

CE: Is there any other way?

*Carl Edmonds, Christopher Lowry and*
*John Pennefather*
*Sydney, Australia*
*1991*

# Preface to the first and second editions

This book is written for doctors and paramedics who are called upon to minister to the medical needs of those divers who venture on or under the sea.

The very generous praise given by reviewers to our earlier edition of *Diving and Subaquatic Medicine*, and their surprising acceptance outside the Australasian region, inspired us to prepare another edition of this text.

Diving accidents are now better defined, investigated and treated than when we commenced writing on this subject 20 years ago. It is our intent to present, as completely as possible, an advanced and informative book on clinical diving medicine. We have avoided the temptation to write either a simplistic text or a research tome.

We have in mind the diving clinician, the physician responsible for scuba divers, the diving paramedic and the exceptional diving instructor who needs a factual reference text. We have not encompassed the needs of specialized deep or saturation diving units, operational or research groups, hyperbaric oxygen or submarine physicians. But because good clinicians have a renaissance quality, refusing to accept the limitations of any speciality, we have included review chapters on these subjects. Although the purist may not relish these inclusions, they are appreciated by most clinicians.

The recent extension of diving as a sport and as a commercial activity has led to the bewildered medical practitioner being confronted with diving problems in which he has received little or no formal training. Even doctors experienced in diving may find themselves in a similar situation – without a comprehensive clinical text available.

This book encompasses the range of diving disorders exhibited by both the amateur scuba diver and the professional deep sea diver. It presents all aspects of diving medicine from the ancient history to the latest research, in a concise and authoritative manner. Each medical disorder is dealt with from an historical, aetiological, clinical, pathological, preventive and therapeutic perspective. Summaries, case histories and revision aids are interspersed throughout. For the doctor who is not familiar with the world of diving, introductory chapters on physics, physiology, equipment and the diving environments have been included.

In the second edition, we have attempted to be less insular. Instead of an Australian book for Australians, we have sought the advice and guidance of respected friends and colleagues from other countries, and from other disciplines, especially in the UK, USA, Canada, Japan and mainland Europe. This has not prevented us from being judgemental and selective when we deemed it fit. The inclusion of anecdotes and occasional humour may lessen the load on the reader, as it has on the authors.

This will almost certainly be the last edition of this text, at least in its current format. One of the physicians is more interested in diving the remote areas, than in writing about them. Another has moved into a specialist anaesthetic practice, and the scientist author is the sole survivor at the Royal Australian Navy School of Underwater Medicine.

To the speciality of diving medicine, to its courageous pioneers (many of whom are still bubbling and finning), and for the comradeship that diving has engendered, we shall be forever grateful.

*Carl Edmonds, Christopher Lowry and*
*John Pennefather*
*Sydney, Australia*
*September 1980*

# Acknowledgements

We wish to acknowledge the assistance given by the Royal Australian Navy, the Canadian Forces, the French Navy, the Royal Navy and the United States Navy, for permission to reproduce excerpts from the Diving Manuals, and to the many authors upon whose work we have so heavily drawn. Our families, who have suffered unfairly, and our underpaid secretaries also deserve acknowledgement.

Special appreciation is given to the Medical Services of the Royal Australian Navy. Approval and support from this department, and its respective directors, have allowed the development of the School of Underwater Medicine, where we met and worked together.

A number of experts have been consulted, to review and advise on specific chapters. Our gratitude is extended to these valued colleagues, but they are not to blame for the final inclusions for each chapter. They include:

Peter Bennett
Fred Bove
Ralph Brauer
Gregg Briggs
Glen Egstrom
Joe Farmer
Des Gorman
John Hayman
Bernie Hudson

Eric Kindwall
Dale Mole
Ed Murrell
Robert Pritchard
Stephen Ruff
Ed Thalmann
John Williamson
David Yount

# Authors

Carl EDMONDS, MB, BS (Sydney), MRCP (Lond), FRACP, FACOM, DPM, MRCPsych, FRANZCP, DipDHM

Director, Diving Medical Centre, Sydney. 1970–91

Formerly, Officer in Charge Royal Australian Navy School of Underwater Medicine 1967–75

Formerly, President, South Pacific Underwater Medicine Society, 1970–75

Consultant in Underwater Medicine to the Royal Australian Navy, 1975–1991

Christopher LOWRY, MB, BS (Sydney), DipDHM, FFARACS

Director, Diving Medical Centre, Sydney, 1973–91

Formerly, Deputy Medical Officer in Charge, Royal Australian Navy School of Underwater Medicine, 1973–74

Visiting Anaesthetist, Royal North Shore Hospital, Sydney 1980–1991

Lismore Base Hospital, 1991

John PENNEFATHER, BSc (Hons)

Scientific Officer at the Royal Australian Navy School of Underwater Medicine, 1972–91

# 1

# History of diving

## Breath-hold diving

The origins of breath-hold diving are lost in time. Archaeologists claim that Neanderthal man, an extinct primitive human, dived for food. By 4500 BC, underwater exploration had advanced from the first timid dive to an industry that supplied the community with shells, food and pearls.

From the ancient **Greek civilization** until today, fishermen have dived for sponges. In earlier days, sponges were used by soldiers as water canteens and wound dressings, as well as for washing. Breath-hold diving for sponges continued until the nineteenth century when helmet diving equipment was introduced, allowing the intrepid to gamble their lives in order to reach the deeper sponge beds. To the hazards of the sea were added an array of diving diseases – 'diver's palsy', 'burst lung', 'sponge fisherman's disease', 'blow-up' and more. Divers still leave from the Greek island of Kalimnos for 3-month expeditions, to search the waters off northern Africa for sponges.

The ancient Greeks laid down the first rules on the legal rights of divers in relation to the goods they salvaged. The diver was entitled to a portion of the cargo and his share increased with depth. Many divers would prefer this arrangement to that offered by modern governments and diving companies. One Greek fisherman and diver, named Glaucus, plunged into the ocean never to return, and was raised to the status of God.

In other parts of the world, industries involving breath-hold diving persist to this time. Notable examples include the **Ama**, or diving women of Japan and Korea, and the pearl divers of the Tuamoto Archipelago.

The Ama have existed as a group for over 2000 years. Originally, the male divers were fishermen and the women collected shells and plants. In more recent times, diving has been restricted to the women, with the men serving as tenders. Some attribute the change in pattern to better endurance of the women in cold water. Others pay homage to the folklore that diving reduces the virility of males. The shells and seaweeds collected by the Ama are still a prized part of Korean and Japanese cuisine.

There is a long history of the use of divers for strategic purposes. Divers were involved in military operations during the Trojan Wars from 1194 to 1184 BC. They sabotaged enemy ships by boring holes in the hull or cutting the anchor ropes. Divers were also used to construct underwater defences designed to protect ports from the attacking fleets. The attackers in their turn used divers to remove the obstructions.

By Roman times precautions were being taken against divers. The anchor cables were made of iron chain to make them difficult to cut, and special guards with diving experience were used to protect the fleet against underwater attackers.

Some Roman divers were also involved in a rather different campaign – Mark Anthony's attempt to capture the heart of Cleopatra. Mark Anthony participated in a fishing contest held in Cleopatra's presence and attempted to improve his standing by having his divers ensure a constant supply of fish on his line. The Queen showed her displeasure at this subterfuge by having one of her divers fasten a salted fish to his hook.

Marco Polo and other travellers to India and Sri Lanka saw the pearl diving on the Coromandel coast. They reported that most diving was to depths of 10–15 metres but that the divers could reach 27 metres*. They used a weight on a rope to assist descent and a net to put the oysters in; when they wished to surface they were assisted by an attendant who hauled on a rope attached to the net – they had no other equipment. They were noted to hold the nose during descent.

The most skilled of the American native divers came from Margarita Island. Travellers who observed them during the sixteenth, seventeenth and eighteenth centuries reported that the natives could descend to 30 metres and remain submerged for 15 minutes. They could dive from sunrise to sunset 7 days a week. The divers attributed their endurance to tobacco!

---

*The conversion 10 metres = 32.8 feet may assist readers whose conception of depth is derived from the anatomy of King Henry I.

They also claimed to possess a secret chemical which they rubbed over their bodies to repel sharks. The Spaniards exploited the native divers for pearling, salvage and smuggling goods past customs. The demand for divers was indicated by their value on the slave market; prices of up to 150 gold pieces were paid.

## Early equipment

The history of diving with equipment is long and complex, and in the early stages it is mixed with legend. The exploits of Jonah are described with conviction in one text, but there is a shortage of supporting evidence. Further reference is made to him later, on the technicality that he was more a submariner than a diver. As his descent was involuntary, he was at best a reluctant pioneer diver. The history of submarine escape, when the submariner may become a diver, is discussed in Chapter 38.

Some claim that Alexander the Great descended in a diving bell during the third century BC. Details of the event are vague and some of the fish stories attributed to him were spectacular. One fish was said to have taken 3 days to swim past. It is most unlikely that the artisans of the time could make glass as depicted in most of the illustrations of the 'event'. This may have been a product of artistic licence, or evidence that the incident is based more in fable than fact.

**Snorkels**, breathing tubes made from reeds and bamboos (now plastic or rubber), were developed in many parts of the world. They allow the diver to breathe with the head under water. Aristotle infers that the Greeks used them. Columbus reported that the North American Indians would swim towards wild fowl, breathing through a reed and keeping their bodies submerged. They were able to capture the birds with nets, spears or even with their bare hands. The Australian aborigine used a similar approach to hunt wild duck. Various people have 'invented' long hose snorkels. The one designed by Vegetius, dated 1511, blocked the diver's vision and imposed impossible loads on the breathing muscles.

Some have interpreted an Assyrian drawing dated 900 BC as an early diving set. The drawing shows a man with a tube in his mouth, the

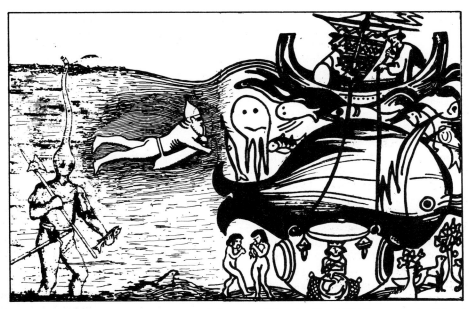

**Figure 1.1** Diving non-events: a montage of diagrams of Vegetius Hood (1511), an Assyrian Frieze (900 BC) and Alexander the Great submerged in a diving bell (third century BC)

tube being connected to some sort of bladder or bag. It is more probably a float or life jacket.

Leonardo da Vinci sketched diving sets and fins. One set was really a snorkel that had the disadvantage of a large dead space. Another of his ideas was for the diver to have a 'wine skin to contain the breath'. This was probably the first recorded design of a self-contained breathing apparatus. His drawings appear tentative so it is probably safe to assume that there was no practical diving equipment in Europe at that time. Another Italian, Borelli, in 1680, realized that Leonardo was in error and that the diver's air would have to be purified before he breathed it again. He suggested that the air could be purified and re-breathed by passing it through a copper tube cooled by the sea water. With this concept he had the basic idea of a re-breathing set. It might also be claimed that he had the basis of the experimental cryogenic diving set in which gas is carried in liquid form and purified by freezing out carbon dioxide.

**Diving bells** were the first successful method of increasing endurance underwater, apart from snorkels. They consist of a weighted chamber, open at the bottom, in which one or more people could be lowered under water. The early use of bells was limited to short periods in shallow water, but later a method of supplying fresh air was developed. The first fully documented use of diving bells dates from the sixteenth century.

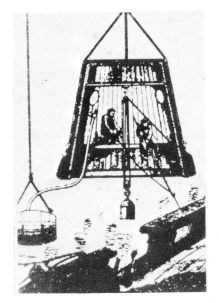

**Figure 1.2** Edmund Halley's diving bell (1691): the weighted barrels of air which were used to replenish the air can be clearly seen

In 1691, Edmund Halley, the English astronomer who predicted the orbit of the comet that bears his name, patented a diving bell which was supplied with air. With this development diving bells became more widespread. They were used for salvage, treasure recovery and general construction work. Halley's bell was supplied with air from weighted barrels, which were hauled from the surface. Dives to 20 metres for up to $1\frac{1}{2}$ hours were recorded. Halley also devised a method of supplying air to a diver from a hose connected to the bell, the length of hose restricting the diver to the area close to the bell. It is not known if this was successful. Halley was one of the earliest recorded sufferers of middle-ear barotrauma.

It is probable that Halley was not entitled to his patent. Swedish divers had devised a small bell, occupied by one person, with a gas supply similar to that later patented by Halley. Between 1659 and 1665, 50 bronze cannon, each weighing over 1000 kg, were salvaged from the '*Vasa*' – this Swedish warship had sunk in 30 metres of water in Stockholm harbour. The guns were recovered by divers working from a bell, assisted by ropes from the surface. This task would not be easy for divers even with the best modern equipment.

## Modern diving equipment

The first people to be exposed to a pressure change in a vessel on the surface were patients exposed to higher or lower pressure as a therapy for various conditions. The origins of diving medical research can be traced to these experiments. The history of hyperbaric medicine is discussed in Chapter 37.

During the second half of the eighteenth century, reliable air pumps were developed, which were able to supply air against the pressures experienced by divers. Several people had the idea of using these pumps for diving and they developed what are now called open helmets which covered the head and shoulders. Air was pumped down to the diver and the excess air escaped from the bottom of the helmet. The diver could breathe because his head and neck were in air, or at least they were until he bent over or fell. If this happened, or if the hose or pump leaked, the helmet flooded and the diver was likely to drown.

**Standard rig** or **standard diving dress** was first produced in 1837 by Augustus Siebe, a naturalized Englishman. This equipment consisted of a rigid helmet sealed to a flexible waterproof suit. Air was pumped down from the surface into the helmet, and excess air bled off through an outlet valve. The diver could control his buoyancy by adjusting the flow through his outlet valve and thus the volume of air in his suit. This type of equipment, with a few refinements, is still in use.

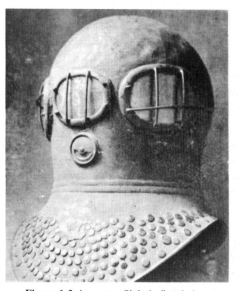

**Figure 1.3** Augustus Siebe's first helmet

There is some doubt about the origins of the Siebe closed dress. It has been suggested that it was designed by John Deane and constructed by Siebe. Deane had experimented with an old suit of armour converted into a diving suit, but Siebe certainly deserves the credit for marketing the first acceptable equipment of this type.

Several types of diving suits and a bell were used by the Royal Engineers on dives on the wreck of the '*Royal George*' which was a danger to navigation in Spithead anchorage. The Siebe suit was found to be greatly superior to the other designs. Siebe's apparatus allowed the diver to bend over, or even lie down, without the risk of flooding the helmet. Also, the diver could control his depth easily. A diver in an open helmet had to rely on his tenders to do this. In an obituary, Siebe was described as the father of diving.

Improved versions of the Siebe suit are still in use, some of them made by Siebe Gorman Ltd, the continuation of the firm started by Siebe. In more modern versions, the helmet is fitted with means of communication to allow the diver to confer with another diver or the surface.

One of the developments of the Siebe closed helmet was the United States Navy Mark 5 helmet. It probably set a record by being in service for 75 years. It has recently been replaced by the Mark 12 set. There is little difference between the two sets in operation, the main difference being in the materials used.

The first diving school was set up by the Royal Navy in 1843. Corporal Jones, who had gained his experience on the wreck of the '*Royal George*', was the instructor.

Decompression sickness was noted in divers following the development of the Siebe closed dress. This disease had already been observed in workers employed in pressurized caissons and tunnels, in which the working area is pressurized to keep the water out. The history of decompression sickness is discussed in Chapter 11.

If Siebe was the father of diving, Paul Bert and J. S. Haldane were the fathers of diving medicine. Paul Bert published a textbook *La Pression Barometrique* based on his studies of the physiological effect of changes in pressure. His book is still used as a reference text, even though it was first published in 1878. Bert showed that decompression sickness was caused by the formation of gas bubbles in the body, and suggested that gradual ascent would prevent decompression sickness. He also showed that pain could be relieved by a return to higher pressures.

J. S. Haldane, a Scottish scientist, was appointed to a Royal Navy committee to investigate the problem of decompression sickness in divers. At that time the Royal Navy had a diving depth limit of 30 metres, but deeper dives had been recorded. Greek and Swedish divers had reached 58 metres in 1904 and Alexander Lambert had recovered gold bullion from a wreck in 50 metres of water in 1885, but had developed partial paralysis from decompression sickness.

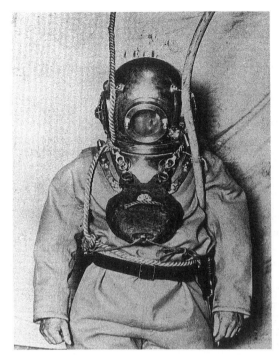

**Figure 1.4** Standard diving dress worn by a diver in Haldane's time. The hose is the air supply. The rope is the lifeline for controlling ascent and descent rates. It is also used to pass messages using an agreed code

Haldane concluded from Paul Bert's results that a diver could be hauled safely to the surface from 10 metres with no evidence of decompression sickness. He deduced from this that a diver could be surfaced from greater than 10 metres in stages, provided that time was spent at each stage to allow absorbed nitrogen to pass out of the body in a controlled manner. This theory was tested on goats, and then men in chambers. Later, practical dives were undertaken which culminated in an open water dive to 64 metres in 1906. This work led to the publication of the first acceptable set of decompression tables, as well as several practical improvements to the diving equipment used. A suit from this time is shown in Figure 1.4.

In 1914, US Navy divers reached 84 metres. The next year they raised a submarine near Hawaii from a depth of 93 metres. This was a remarkable feat considering that the salvage techniques had to be evolved by trial and error. The divers used air, so they were exposed to a dangerous degree of nitrogen narcosis, as well as decompression sickness.

## Self-contained equipment

**Self-contained underwater breathing apparatus** (**SCUBA**, but referred to as scuba throughout the text) is used to describe any diving set that allows the diver to carry his air supply with him. In workable form, it dates from the early nineteenth century. There is a brief report of an American engineer, Charles Condert, who made a type of scuba in which the air was stored in a copper pipe worn around his body. The gas was released into a hood that covered the upper half of his body. Accumulation of carbon dioxide was controlled by allowing the respired gas to escape through a small hole. It was then replaced by fresh gas from the cylinder. He died while diving with his equipment in the East River in 1831.

Another early development was the Rouquayrol and Denayrouze device of 1865 (Figure 1.5). This set was supplied with air from the surface in the same manner as the Siebe closed helmet suit, and was fitted with an air reservoir so that the diver could detach himself from the air hose for a few minutes. The endurance was limited by the amount of air in the reservoir.

The first successful equipment with an independent air supply appears to have been developed and patented in 1918 by a Japanese – Ohgushi. His system could be operated with a supply of air from the surface or as a scuba with an air supply cylinder carried on the back. The diver controlled his air supply by triggering air flow into his mask with his teeth. Another scuba was devised by Le Prieur in 1933. In this set, the diver carried a compressed air bottle on his chest and released air into his face mask by opening a tap.

In 1943, Jacques **Cousteau** and Emile **Gagnan** developed the first scuba incorporating an automatic **demand valve** to release air as the diver inhaled. This valve was triggered by the diver's breathing, so the diver was no longer required to operate a tap to obtain each breath of air. In developing this valve, which was pressure compensated so that changes in depth did not affect its function, Cousteau and Gagnan invented the scuba as we know it today. It was an adaptation of a reducing valve Gagnan had evaluated for use in gas-powered cars.

**Closed circuit oxygen sets** were developed during the same period as the modern scuba. In these re-breathing sets the diver is supplied with oxygen and the carbon dioxide is removed. These sets are often called scuba, but they should be considered separately because of the difference in principles involved. The first successful re-breathing set was designed by an Englishman, H. A. Fleuss, in 1878. This was an oxygen set in which carbon dioxide was absorbed by rope soaked in caustic potash.

As a result of the absence of lines and hoses from the diver to the surface, the set was used in flooded mines and tunnels where the extra mobility, compared to the standard rig, was needed. Great risks were taken with this set and its successors, because the work of Paul Bert on oxygen toxicity was not widely known. This equipment was the precursor of oxygen sets used in clandestine operations in both World Wars and of other sets used in submarine escape, fire fighting and mine rescue.

## Modern military diving

The military use of divers in modern warfare was, until 1918, largely restricted to the salvage of damaged ships, clearing of channels blocked by wrecks and assorted ships' husbandry duties. One significant clandestine operation conducted during World War I was the

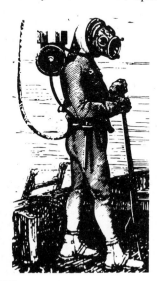

**Figure 1.5** The aerophore, devised by Rouquayrol and Denayrouze (1865): this device was widely used and was an important milestone in the development of the modern scuba

recovery of code books and minefield charts from a sunken German submarine. This was of more significance as an intelligence operation, although the diving activity was also kept secret.

During World War I, Italy developed a human torpedo or chariot that was used in 1918 to attack an Austrian battleship in Pola Harbour. The attack was a success in that the ship was sunk, but unfortunately it coincided with the fall of the Austro-Hungarian Empire and the ship was already in friendly hands! The potential of this method of attack was noted by the Italian Navy. They put it to use in World War II with divers wearing oxygen re-breathing sets as underwater pilots. In passing, it is interesting to note that the idea of the chariot was suggested to the British Admiralty in 1909 and Davis took out patents on a small submarine and human torpedo controlled by divers in 1914. This was pre-dated by a one-person submarine designed by J. P. Holland in 1875.

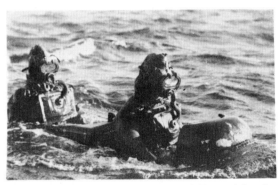

**Figure 1.6** 'Human torpedoes' successfully used by the Royal Navy against the Italian shipping during World War II. The divers riding the torpedo are wearing closed circuit re-breathing sets

Diving played a greater part in offensive operations during World War II. Exploits of note include those of the Italian Navy, who used divers, riding modified torpedos, to attack ships in Gibraltar and Alexandria. After a series of unsuccessful attempts, with loss of life, they succeeded in sinking several ships in Gibraltar harbour in mid-1941. Later that year, three teams managed to enter Alexandria harbour and damage two battleships and a tanker. Even Sir Winston Churchill, who did not often praise his enemies, said they showed 'extraordinary courage and ingenuity'. Churchill had previously been responsible for rejecting

suggestions that the Royal Navy use similar weapons.

In Gibraltar a special type of underwater war evolved. The Italians had a secret base in Spain, only 6 miles away, and launched several attacks which were opposed by a group of British divers who tried to remove the Italian mines before they exploded. On at least one occasion the British arrived before the Italians had left and an underwater battle ensued.

Divers from the allied nations made several successful attacks on enemy ships, but their most important offensive role was in the field of reconnaissance and beach clearance. In most operations the divers worked from submarines or small boats. They first surveyed the approaches to several potential landing sites and, after a choice had been made, they cleared the obstructions that could impede the landing craft. One of the more famous exploits of an American diving group was to land unofficially and leave a 'Welcome' sign on the beach to greet the US Marines spearheading the invasion of Guam.

The research back-up to these exploits was largely devoted to improvement of equipment and the investigation of the nature and onset of oxygen toxicity (see Chapter 18). This work was important because most of these offensive operations were conducted by divers wearing oxygen breathing apparatus. The subjects were the unsung heroes of the work. This group of scientists, sailors and conscientious objectors deliberately and repeatedly suffered oxygen toxicity in attempts to understand the condition.

**Oxygen/nitrogen mixtures** were first used for diving by the Royal Navy in conjunction with standard diving rig. It was based on an idea proposed by Sir Leonard Hill and developed by Siebe, Gorman and Co. Ltd. The advantage of this equipment was that, by increasing the ratio of oxygen to nitrogen in the breathing gas it was possible to reduce or eliminate decompression requirements. It is normally used with equipment in which most of the gas is breathed again after the carbon dioxide has been removed. This allows reduction of the total gas volume required by the diver.

During the war this idea was adapted to a self-contained semi-closed rebreathing apparatus. It was first used extensively by divers clearing mines. This development was conducted by the Admiralty Experimental

Diving Unit in conjunction with Siebe, Gorman and Co. Ltd. The change to a self-contained set was needed to reduce the number of people at risk from accidental explosions in mine-clearing operations. The reduction, or elimination, of decompression time was desirable in increasing the diver's chances of survival if something went wrong. The equipment was constructed from non-magnetic materials to reduce the likelihood of activating magnetic mines and was silent during operation, for work on acoustically triggered mines.

## Deep diving

The search for means to allow human beings to descend deeper has been a continuing process. By the early twentieth century, deep diving research had enabled divers to reach depths in excess of 90 metres; at this depth the narcosis induced by nitrogen incapacitated most men.

After World War I the Royal Navy diving research was designed to extend their depth capability beyond 60 metres. Equipment was improved, the submersible decompression chamber was introduced, and new decompression schedules were developed. These used periods of oxygen breathing to reduce decompression time. Dives were made to 107 metres, but nitrogen narcosis at these depths made such dives unrewarding and dangerous.

**Helium diving** resulted from a series of American developments. In 1919 a scientist, Professor Elihu Thompson, suggested that nitrogen narcosis could be avoided by replacing the nitrogen in the diver's gas supply with helium. At that stage, the idea was not practical because helium cost over $US2000 per cubic foot. Later the price dropped to about 3 cents per cubic foot, following the exploitation of natural gas supplies which contained helium.

Research into the use of helium was conducted during the 1920s and 1930s. By the end of the 1930s, divers in a compression chamber had reached a pressure equal to a depth of 150 metres and a dive to 128 metres was made in Lake Michigan. Between the two World Wars, the USA had a virtual monopoly on the supply of helium, and so dominated research into deep diving.

**Hydrogen diving**, using hydrogen in gas mixtures for deep diving, was first tried by Arne Zetterström, a Swedish engineer. His pioneering work on the use of hydrogen in a diver's gas mixture has not yet been fully developed. He demonstrated that hypoxia and risks of explosion could be avoided if the diver used air from the surface to 30 metres, changed to 4% oxygen in nitrogen and then changed to 4% or less oxygen in hydrogen. In this manner, the diver received adequate oxygen and the formation of an explosive mixture of oxygen and hydrogen was prevented.

In 1945, Zetterström dived in 160 metres in open water. Unfortunately, an error was made by the operators controlling his ascent. They hauled him up too fast and he died from hypoxia and decompression sickness. The error was accidental and was not related to his planned decompression schedule.

Interest in hydrogen for use in deep diving has not been great, but mice and monkeys have been pressurized to over 1000 metres on oxygen/hydrogen mixtures. The relative cheapness of hydrogen compared to helium, and the probability of a helium shortage in the future, may mean that hydrogen will eventually be widely used in deep dives. French workers have reported good results using a mixture of hydrogen and helium as diluting gas.

Other European workers have followed Zetterström in his radical approach to deep diving. Mention must be made of the Swiss workers, Keller and Buhlmann. Keller performed an incredible 305 metre (1000 feet) dive in the open sea in December 1962, and Buhlmann developed and tested related decompression regimes.

**Modern gas mixture sets** have evolved as the result of several pressures. The price of helium has again increased and has become a significant cost. This, combined with a desire to increase the diver's mobility, has encouraged the development of more sophisticated mixed gas sets. The most complex of these has separate cylinders of oxygen and diluting gas. The composition of the diver's inspired gas is maintained by the action of electronic control systems which regulate the release of gas from each cylinder. The first of these sets was developed in the 1950s, but they have been refined and improved since then.

**Modern air or gas mixture helmets** have several advantages compared to the older equipment. A demand system reduces the amount of gas used, compared to the standard rig. The sealing system reduces the chance of a diver drowning. The primary gas supply normally comes to the diver from the surface or a diving bell and may be combined with heating and communications. A second gas supply comes from a cylinder on the diver's back. The Americans, Bob Kirby and Bev Morgan, have led the way with a whole series of helmet systems. Their Superlite 17 is shown in Figure 4.3. It can be used with compressed air or gas mixtures. When used with gas mixtures, it can also be modified to use gas supplied from a diving bell and return the exhaled gas to the bell. This requires two pumps, called a push–pull system, to move the gas to and from the diver. These helmets can operate to depths of over 450 metres.

**Saturation diving** is probably the most important development in diving since World War II. Behnke suggested that caisson workers could be kept under pressure for long periods and decompressed slowly at the end of their job rather than undertake a series of compressions, and risk decompression sickness after each one.

The first people to spend long periods in an elevated pressure environment were patients treated in a hyperbaric chamber. Between 1921 and 1934 an American, Dr Orvil Cunningham, pressurized people to 3 ATA for up to 5 days and decompressed them in 2 days.

A US Navy Medical Officer, George Bond, and others adopted this idea for diving. The first of these dives involved tests on animals and men in chambers; then in 1962 Robert Stenuit spent 24 hours at 60 metres in the Mediterranean Sea off the coast of France.

Progress was rapid with both the French inspired '*Conshelf*' experiments and the American '*Sealab*' experiments seeking greater depths and durations of exposure. In 1965, the former astronaut Scott Carpenter spent a month at 60 metres and two divers spent 2 days at a depth equivalent to almost 200 metres. Unfortunately people paid for this progress. Lives were lost and there has been a significant incidence of bone necrosis induced by these experiments.

In most saturation diving systems, the divers either live in an underwater habitat or in a chamber on the surface. In the latter case, another chamber is needed to transfer them under pressure to and from their work site. Operations can also be conducted from small submarines or submersibles with the divers operating from a compartment that can be opened to the sea. They can either move to a separate chamber on the submarine's tender or remain in the submarine for their period of decompression. The use of this equipment offers several advantages: the submarine speeds the diver's movement around the work site, provides better lighting and carries extra equipment. Also a technical expert who is not a diver can observe and control the operation from within the submarine.

Operations involving saturation dives have become almost routine for work in deep water. The stimulus for this work is partly military and partly commercial. Divers work on the rigs and pipelines needed in the exploitation of oil and natural gas fields. The needs of the oil companies have resulted in strenuous efforts to extend the depth and efficiency of the associated diving activities. Diving firms are now prepared to sign contracts that may require them to work at over 500 metres.

Man is pursuing other avenues in his efforts to exploit the sea. **Armoured diving suits** withstand the pressure exerted by the water and allow the diver to avoid the hazards of increased and changing pressures. In effect the diver becomes a small submarine. The mobility and dexterity of divers wearing earlier armoured suits were limited and they were not widely used. The newer suits such as the British 'JIM' have become an accepted piece of diving equipment (Figure 1.7). They can be fitted with claws for manipulating equipment. JIM has a 20-hour endurance for its life support system and can allow work at 450 metres (1500 feet). A development from JIM is a diving suit called WASP, in which movement is aided by propellors. This device is a compromise between a diver and a one-person submarine.

**Liquid breathing** trials in which the lungs are flooded and the body supplied with oxygen in solution have only been conducted in laboratories and hospitals (see Chapter 3). The

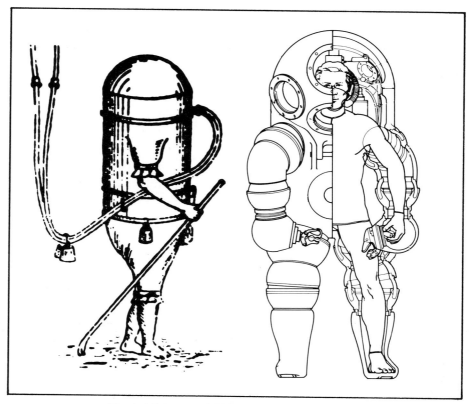

**Figure 1.7** Armoured diving suits, past and present (JIM)

potential advantages of breathing liquids are the elimination of decompression sickness as a problem, freedom to descend to virtually any depth and the possibility of the diver extracting the oxygen dissolved in the water.

# Recommended reading

BERT, P. (1878). *Barometric Pressure*, translated by Mary Alice Hitchcock and Fred A. Hitchcock (1943). College Book Co.

DAVIS, R.H. (1955). *Deep Diving and Submarine Operations*, 6th edn. London: Siebe, Gorman & Co.

DUGAN, J. (1956) *Man Explores the Sea*. London: Hamish Hamilton.

DUGAN, J. (1967). *World Beneath the Sea*. New York: National Geographic Society.

MARX, R.F. (1978). *Into the Deep*. New York: Van Nostrand Reinhold.

OHRELIUS, B. (1962). *Vasa, the King's Ship*, translated by M. Michael. London: Cassell.

PENZIAS, W. and GOODMAN, W.M. (1973). *Man Beneath the Sea*. New York: Wiley Interscience.

RAHN, H. (1965). *Breathhold Diving and the Ama of Japan*. Pub. 1341. National Academy of Sciences, Washington, USA.

SHELFORD, W.O. (1972). Ohgushi's peerless respirator. *Skin Diver* Nov., 32–34.

*US Navy Diving Manual*, Vol. 1 (1988). NAVSEA 0994-LP-001-9010.

# 2

# Physics

## Introduction

A knowledge of the physical laws and principles relating to diving is essential before there can be understanding of most of the medical problems encountered. Aspects of physics which have a wide application to diving are discussed in this chapter.

## Pressure, gases and diving

On the surface of the earth, we are exposed to the pressure exerted by the atmosphere – this is called the atmospheric or barometric pressure. Most people are happy to regard this pressure as being due to the mass of the atmosphere pressing down on them. A flaw in this argument is that the pressure remains in a bottle after it is sealed, although its contents are contained and are no longer exposed to the column of air above.

The explanation in physics books is that pressure is generated by collisions of the molecules of gas in accordance with the kinetic theory of gases. Either explanation is acceptable for the following discussion.

An observer would find that the pressure decreased as he or she moved upward through the atmosphere, and increased as he or she moved down into a mine or into the sea. At the top of Mount Everest the atmospheric pressure is about four-tenths of that at sea level. Because water is much heavier than air, the pressure changes experienced by a diver are much greater than those encountered by climbers or aviators.

Pressure is measured in a variety of units from either of two reference points. It can be expressed with respect to a vacuum, i.e. zero pressure and this reading is called an absolute pressure. The second method measures pressures above or below local pressure, and these readings are called gauge pressures. Thus, at sea level the absolute pressure is 1 atmosphere (1 ATA) and the gauge pressure is 0. These units are commonly abbreviated to ATA and ATG. Common examples are the barometric pressure used by weather forecasters, an absolute pressure and the blood pressure, a gauge pressure reading.

With descent in water pressure increases. For each 10 metres depth in sea water, the pressure increases by 1 atmosphere, starting from 1 ATA or 0 ATG at the surface. The gauge pressure remains 1 atmosphere less than the absolute pressure, e.g. at 10 metres, the pressure is 1 ATG and 2 ATA. At 90 metres, the pressure is 9 ATG and 10 ATA.

Because diving research involves facets of engineering and science, the world of diving is plagued with a multiplicity of units for expression of pressures. These include absolute and gauge atmospheres, pascals and multiples such as the kilopascal, feet of sea water, metres of sea water, pounds per square inch, bars and torrs, and several other rarer units. Table 2.1 contains conversions for the more commonly used units.

**Table 2.1 Pressure conversion factors**

| | |
|---|---|
| 1 atmosphere | = 10.08 (10) metres sea water |
| | = 33.07 (33) feet sea water |
| | = 33.90 (34) feet fresh water |
| | = 101.3 kilopascals per metre$^2$ (kPa/m$^2$) |
| | = 1.033 kg/cm$^2$ |
| | = 14.696 (14.7) lb/in$^2$ |
| | = 1.013 bars |
| | = 760 millimetres mercury (mmHg) |
| | = 1 ATA |

Commonly used approximations are shown in brackets. Actual conversions from sea water depth to ATA depends on salinity and temperature.

## Pressure and volume changes

The relationship between changes in volume of a gas and the pressure applied to it is described by **Boyle's law**. This states that, *if the temperature remains constant, the volume of a given mass of gas is inversely proportional to the absolute pressure.* This means that *absolute* pressure multiplied by volume gives a constant, the value of the constant changing with the mass of gas considered. To a mathematician this means that $PV = K$ or $P_1V_1 = P_2V_{21}$, where $P$ and $V$ are pressure and volume. For example, 10 litres of gas at sea level pressure (1 ATA) will be compressed:

to 5 litres at 2 ATA (10 metres or 33 feet)
to 2 litres at 5 ATA (40 metres or 132 feet)
to 1 litre at 10 ATA (90 metres or 297 feet).

During ascent into the atmosphere the reverse happens and the gas expands; the 10 litres of air would expand: to 20 litres at 0.5 ATA (an altitude of about 5000 metres or 18 000 feet), to 40 litres at 0.25 ATA (an altitude of about 10 300 metres or 33 400 feet).

---

*Gases volumes expand when pressure decreases and contract when pressure increases.*

---

The point is that the volume of a mass of gas in a flexible container decreases with pressure or depth increase and expands during ascent or pressure reduction (Figure 2.1). It will be

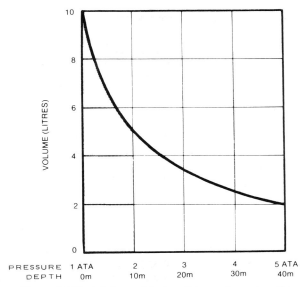

VOLUME (LITRES)

PRESSURE 1 ATA    2    3    4    5 ATA
DEPTH    0m    10m    20m    30m    40m

**Figure 2.1** Boyle's law: while breathing under water, the diver's respiratory volume is about the same as it would be if he worked at the same rate on the surface. Due to the increase in density of his breathing gas under increased pressure, he must move a greater mass of gas with each breath. In some situations, this physical effect can limit the diver's capacity to do work

noted that volume changes are greatest near the surface. Conversely, gas has to be added if the volume of a container or gas space is to remain constant as the pressure is increased. The effects of this law are important in many aspects of diving medicine.

During descent, the pressure in the water is transmitted through the body to the tissue surrounding the gas spaces. The pressure in any gas space in the body should increase to equal the surrounding pressure. In the lungs, during breath-hold dives, this is accomplished by a decrease in lung volume. Air must enter cavities with rigid walls, such as the sinuses or the middle ear. If this air entry does not take place to equalize pressures, then a pressure difference between the space and the surrounding tissue will develop. The result is tissue distortion and damage such as congestion, oedema or haemorrhage. This develops if the pressure in the vessels is greater than the pressure in a gas-filled space. Pressure changes in the middle ear can also result in rupture of the tympanic membrane.

During ascent, as the pressure decreases, gas within body spaces will expand. Unless gas is vented from the space, the expanding gas will exert pressure on the surrounding tissue and will eventually damage it. The same volume changes with pressure occur in bubbles in tissue or blood. Again, the volume changes are greatest close to the surface. An injury caused by pressure change is called barotrauma.

> *Barotrauma is the general name for an injury caused by pressure change.*

While breathing air under water, the diver's respiratory volume is about the same as it would be if he worked at the same rate on the surface. The first consequence of this is that a gas cylinder which contains enough air for a 100 minute dive at 1 ATA would last about 50 minutes at 2 ATA (10 metres), or 20 minutes at 5 ATA (40 metres) for dives with the same energy expenditure.

Because of the increase in density of breathing gas under increased pressure, the diver must move a greater mass of gas with each breath. In some situations, this physical effect can limit the capacity to do work.

### Temperature and volume changes

**Charles' law** states: *if the pressure is constant, the volume of a mass of gas is proportional to the absolute temperature.* The absolute temperature (in kelvins or K) is always 273° more than the centigrade temperature. A more useful expression of the law is

$$\frac{V_1}{T_1} = \frac{V_2}{T_2} \text{ or } \frac{V}{T} = k$$

where $V_1$ is the volume of a mass of gas at temperature $T_1$ kelvins and $V_2$ is its volume after the temperature has changed to $T_2$ kelvins. This law has much less relevance to diving medicine than Boyle's law; however, it should be remembered when considering gas volumes and how they may change. For example, a diver might have a vital capacity of 6 litres, measured at 37°C (310 K). If it was measured by exhaling into a balloon and later measuring the volume of the balloon, Charles' law must be used to correct for the changes in temperature. If the measurement is made at 17°C (290 K) then the balloon would measure 5.6 litres:

$$\frac{6}{310} = \frac{V_2}{290}$$

$$V_2 = 5.6 \text{ litres.}$$

Unless Charles' law was applied it might be thought that 5.6 litres was the true vital capacity.

Boyle's and Charles' laws may be combined and used if temperature and pressure both change – from $P_1$ and $T_1$ to $P_2$ and $T_2$ with a volume change from $V_1$ to $V_2$. The combined laws can be expressed as the universal gas equation:

$$\frac{P_1 \times V_1}{T_1} = \frac{P_2 \times V_2}{T_2}$$

For example, a 1 litre gas sample is collected at 37°C from a diver at 20 metres and is brought to the surface, at 1 ATA, at a temperature of 17°C. What will be the volume of the gas sample?

20 metres = 3 ATA; 37°C = 310 K; 17°C = 290 K.

$$\frac{P_1 \times V_1}{T_1} = \frac{P_2 \times V_2}{T_2}$$

$$\frac{3 \times 1}{310} = \frac{1 \times V_2}{290}$$

$$V_2 = 2.81 \text{ litres.}$$

Another temperature–pressure problem may cause discord. This is the effect of temperature on the pressure in a gas cylinder. A diver might pay to have his compressed air cylinder filled to 200 ATA. The gas compressor may heat the gas so the cylinder is charged with gas at 47°C. When he gets in the water at 7°C the diver is incensed to find he only has 175 ATA in his cylinder. In this case $V_1 = V_2$ because the cylinder is rigid and the pressure falls as the gas cools.

$$47°C = 320 \text{ K}, 7°C = 280 \text{ K}, V_1 = V_2 = k$$

$$\frac{200 \times k}{320} = \frac{P_2 \times k}{280}$$

$$P_2 = 175 \text{ ATA.}$$

## Pressure and the diver's body

Most people have difficulty in understanding why the pressure of the water does not crush the diver. The answer to this problem may be considered in two ways.

The solid and liquid parts of the body are virtually incompressible, so a pressure applied to them does not cause any change in volume. The pressure is transmitted through them. After immersion, the increased pressure pushes on the skin which pushes on the tissues underneath and so on through the body until the skin on the other side is pushed back against the water pressure. So the system remains in balance. Readers with a background in physics will recognize the application of **Pascal's principle**.

The effect of pressure on the gas spaces in the diver's body is more complex. The basic fact is that the applied pressure does not cause any problem if the pressure in the gas space can remain similar to that of the surrounding water. There would, for example, be no physical damage to divers' lungs if they were exposed to a pressure of 100 metres of water pressure – provided that this pressure was balanced by the pressure exerted by surrounding water acting on the walls of the lung to balance any tendency of the lungs to expand. Pressure differences between gas spaces, tissues and the surrounding water are the causes of barotrauma.

## Partial pressures in gas mixtures

**Dalton's law** states that *the total pressure exerted by a mixture of gases is the sum of the partial pressures that would be exerted by each of the gases if it alone occupied the total volume.* In air, which is approximately 80% nitrogen and 20% oxygen, the total pressure of 1 ATA is comprised of the partial pressures of nitrogen (0.8 ATA) and oxygen (0.2 ATA). At 2 ATA these partial pressures will rise to 1.6 and 0.4 ATA respectively.

The partial pressures of breathing gases can be manipulated to the diver's advantage if he breathes a gas mixture. For example, the composition of the gas breathed may be modified to reduce the chance of decompression sickness by decreasing the percentage of inert gas in the mixture.

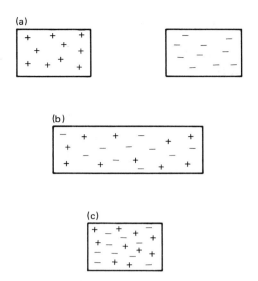

**Figure 2.2** Dalton's law: (a) two spaces each at 1 ATA; (b) total pressure 1 ATA, 0.5 ATA of each component of the mixture; (c) total pressure 2 ATA, 1 ATA of each component of the mixture

Undesirable effects can also occur. Air from an industrial area may contain over 0.3% carbon dioxide and 0.002% carbon monoxide. At high pressures, both constituents could be toxic unless measures were taken to remove these contaminants before use.

It may be necessary to combine Boyle's and Dalton's laws in calculations. For example, it may be decided that a diver should be given a mixture with a partial pressure of 0.8 ATA oxygen and 1.2 ATA nitrogen in a recompression chamber pressurized to 2 ATA. If oxygen and air are the only gases available, the gas laws can be used to calculate how to prepare a cylinder charged with the right gas mixture. The mixture is to be 40% oxygen and 60% nitrogen.

If the gas is to be prepared in a cylinder charged to 200 ATA, it should contain 120 ATA of nitrogen. If this is to be obtained from compressed air (assumed to be 80% nitrogen in this exercise), it will be necessary to put 150 ATA of compressed air into the cylinder (30 ATA of oxygen + 120 ATA of nitrogen). The mixing is generally done by putting 50 ATA of oxygen into the cylinder from another supply and then topping up with air to 200 ATA.

If an oxygen analyser is available it may be best to check the mixture before adding all the air. Most pressure gauges normally have slight errors, which may cause deviations in composition from that desired.

This mixing process cannot be used as successfully with helium mixtures. At high pressures helium does not follow the predictions of Boyle's law accurately – it is less compressible than the ideal gas described by Boyle's law.

## Solution of gases in liquids

**Henry's law** states that *at a constant temperature the amount of a gas that will dissolve in a liquid is proportional to the partial pressure of the gas over the liquid.* This law implies an equilibrium in which equal amounts of each gas are passing into and out of any solution in contact with it. At sea level (1 ATA), human body tissues contain about 1 litre of gaseous nitrogen in solution. If a man dived to 10 metres and breathed air at 2 ATA, he would eventually reach equilibrium again and have twice as much nitrogen in solution in his body. The time taken to reach a new equilibrium depends on the solubility of the gas in the tissues and the rate of gas supplied to each tissue.

When the total pressure, or the partial pressure, of a particular gas is reduced, gas must pass out of solution. If a rapid total pressure drop occurs, a tissue may contain more gas than it can hold in solution. In this situation bubbles may form and cause decompression sickness. Bubble formation is discussed later in this chapter.

The physiological effects of the solubility of gases are also relevant in nitrogen narcosis and oxygen toxicity. These reactions are explored in Chapters 15 and 18.

It should be noted that each gas has a different solubility and the amount of a gas which will dissolve in a liquid depends on the liquid. For example, carbon dioxide is very soluble in water compared to other common gases; beer aerated with compressed air would have far fewer bubbles; nitrogen is more soluble in fats and oils than in aqueous solutions.

Henry's law is also time dependent. It takes time for gases to enter and leave solution or

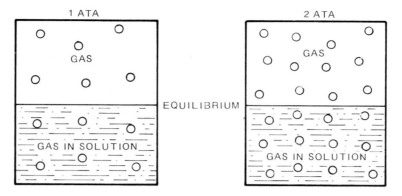

**Figure 2.3** Henry's law

form bubbles. If this was not so champagne would go flat as soon as the cork was popped. Surface decompression depends on this aspect of Henry's law. In this procedure a diver surfaces from a dive without decompressing and is quickly pressurized in a chamber on the surface. The pressure in the chamber is then slowly reduced. If the pressurization in the chamber is delayed, or the chamber pressure reduced too rapidly, gas would form bubbles in the body and the diver would develop decompression sickness.

## Gas movement in body tissues

In a permeable substance, such as body tissues, gas molecules can migrate by diffusion, i.e. gas molecules dissolve in the tissue and tend to move from one area to another until the partial pressure of the gas is the same at each point.

Gas movement is not instantaneous and equilibration can take hours. Also, gas pressures tend to equilibrate, not the number of gas molecules. If a gas is twice as soluble in one tissue compared to another, then there will be twice as many of its molecules in the first tissue to produce the same partial pressure in the tissues. This information can be calculated from the solubility coefficients of the gas in the components of the tissue.

The rate of gas movement between the two points depends on several factors. The difference in partial pressure and the distance between the two points may be combined into a concentration gradient. The other major factor

is the permeability of the tissue, an expression of the ease of gas movement. A large partial pressure between two points which are close together (a steep gradient) and a greater permeability both increase the rate of gas transfer.

During a dive, partial pressures of gas increase with descent and decrease with ascent. Partial pressures are illustrated in relation to gas movements for a hypothetical tissue in Figure 2.4. In Figure 2.4a the inert gas pressure in the tissue is in equilibrium with the blood which, in turn, is in equilibrium with the atmosphere.

If there is an increase in pressure there will be an increase in the inert gas tension in the blood. This gas gradually diffuses through the tissue until the system equilibrates at the higher pressure (Figure 2.4b–d). In diving parlance the tissue is called 'saturated' (Figure 2.4a,d). If the pressure is reduced before this time there may be a situation where some of the tissue is gaining and some is losing gas (Figure 2.4e,f). In this situation gas bubbles may form in the tissue and cause decompression sickness.

## Buoyancy

**Archimedes' principle** states that *any object, wholly or partially immersed in liquid, is buoyed up by a force equal to the weight of liquid displaced*. A diver is an object immersed in water and is therefore affected by this prin-

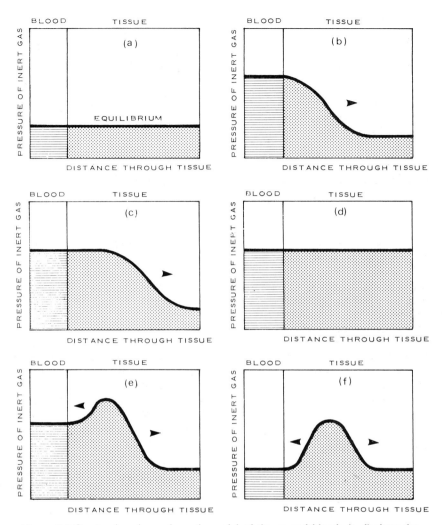

**Figure 2.4** Gas tensions in a schematic model of tissues and blood: (a–d) show the manner in which tissues become saturated when the environmental pressure is increased. (a) At surface pressure of 1 ATA; (b) at 2.5 ATA after $\frac{1}{2}$ hour; (c) at 2.5 ATA after 4 hours; (d) at 2.5 ATA after 8 hours. (a,d) Tensions when 'saturated' at the respective ambient pressures. (e) Situation after partial reduction in external pressure (tissue still gaining nitrogen); (f) situation in tissue shortly after return to normal pressure. Saturation diving is represented in (a)–(d) and conventional scuba diving is represented in (a), (b), (e) and (f)

ciple. It determines the effort he must employ to dive. If a diver weighs less than the weight of water he displaces, he will tend to float to the surface, i.e. he has positive buoyancy, which makes descent difficult. If he weighs more than the weight of water he displaces, he has negative buoyancy, which will assist descent and make ascent harder.

A diver can change buoyancy in several ways. If he wears a weight belt he increases weight by a significant amount and displaces a little more water, so he will decrease his buoyancy. If the diver displaces more water he will increase buoyancy. This can be done to a small degree by retaining more air in the lungs at the end of each breath. A wet suit also increases the diver's buoyancy. A buoyancy changing device, often called a buoyancy vest or compensator (BC), can be used. This has an inflatable air space that the diver can inflate or deflate as needed. With this buoyancy can be made positive, negative or neutral.

If a diver attains a state of neutral buoyancy, i.e. he displaces his weight of water, he neither rises nor sinks in the water and can experience a sensation similar to the weightlessness of space. In some situations this can augment any tendency to disorientation, which may be hazardous.

An interesting combination of the effects of Boyle's law and Archimedes' principle is shown by the changes in buoyancy experienced by a diver wearing an inflatable vest or a compressible unit. If slightly positively buoyant at the surface, the diver will experience some difficulty in descending. As he descends he will pass through a zone where he is neutrally buoyant and if he descends further he may reach a stage where he is negatively buoyant. The increased pressure decreases his buoyancy because the pressure changes reduce the volume of the vest or suit which reduces the volume of fluid displaced, and hence buoyancy.

The weight of the scuba cylinders decreases as gas is consumed from it, and this will lead to an increase in buoyancy.

## Altitude and saturation diving

Our conventional idea of diving is that a diver descends from the sea surface (1 ATA) and returns when the dive has finished. There is a series of variations from this. A diver might have to dive in a mountain lake where the pressure on the surface is less than 1 ATA. Another variation is where a diver starts from an environment where the pressure is greater than 1 ATA. This happens when divers operate from a pressurized compartment to reduce the decompression required during a series of dives. These conditions can cause problems that require consideration of the physics involved.

For simplicity, the following description is based on the useful, but not strictly accurate, traditional belief that the ratio of the pressure reached during the dive to the pressure after the dive determines the decompression required. If this ratio is less than 2:1 then a diver can theoretically ascend safely without pausing during ascent. This means that a diver from the sea surface (1 ATA) can dive 10 metres (2 ATA) and ascend safely.

A diver operating in a high mountain lake, surface pressure 0.5 ATA, could only dive to 5 metres (1 ATA) before he has to worry about decompression. This statement ignores the minor correction that will be required if it is a fresh water lake – fresh water is less dense than salt water.

On the same basis, a diver living in an artificial environment where the pressure is 10 ATA (90 metres) could dive to 20 ATA (190 metres) and not pause during ascent. This system is used in saturation diving, but the eventual return to the surface can take several days. The use of such environments has proved to be invaluable where deep or long dives are required (see Chapter 36).

Another pressure problem occurs when a diver, who dives in the ocean, then flies or ascends into mountains. For example, a 5 metre dive (1.5 ATA) could be followed by an immediate ascent to a pressure of 0.75 ATA, with little risk. Deeper dives or higher ascents may require the diver to pause at the surface if he is to avoid decompression sickness. This problem may seem unimportant, but it is encountered by every diver tourist who wants to fly home after his last dive. It is also encountered when it is necessary to transport a diver with decompression sickness. There may be an increase in pain when the pressure is decreased, even by a small amount.

Another aspect of the problem of diving in a high altitude lake concerns the rate at which a diver may have to exhale during ascent. A diver who ascends from 10 metres (2 ATA) to the surface (1 ATA) would find that the volume of gas in his lungs has doubled. Most divers realize this and exhale at a controlled rate during ascent. They may not realize that a similar doubling in gas volume occurs during the 5 metres of ascent to the surface, where the pressure is 0.5 ATA.

The diver's equipment can also be affected or damaged by high altitudes. Some pressure gauges only start to register when the pressure is greater than 1 ATA. These gauges (Bellows and Bourdon-tube types) would try to indicate a negative depth, perhaps bending the needle, till the diver exceeded 1 ATA. The other common depth gauge, a capillary tube, indicates the depth by an air–water boundary. The volume of gas trapped in the capillary decreases with depth. For a diver starting from 0.5 ATA, this gauge would show the diver had reached 10 metres depth when he was only at 5 metres.

Some decompression meters are damaged by exposure to altitude (e.g. as in aircraft travel) and none is applicable to altitude diving or saturation excursions.

# Bubble formation and resolution

## Causes of bubble formation

The mechanisms involved in the formation of bubbles and their behaviour are not completely understood. Some knowledge of the factors involved in their formation and behaviour is important as a background to understanding the causes and rationale of treatment of decompression sickness.

A gas bubble can only form when the concentration of a dissolved gas is greater than can be maintained in solution in the surrounding tissue. In diving it normally occurs when the pressure is reduced after a dive. The amount of gas in solution is greater than would dissolve at that pressure. This condition is termed 'supersaturation'.

Early workers suggested that a considerable degree of 'supersaturation' may be required before a bubble of sufficient size to cause any symptoms can develop. It was thought that this was caused by the surface tension forces which exert considerable hydrostatic pressure on a small bubble, tending to force it back into solution. In larger bubbles these forces are proportionately less important because of the decrease in the surface-to-volume ratio of the bubble. It is now known that there was an overestimation of the effects of surface tension on bubbles in biological systems. Some substances, e.g. the surfactants, lower surface tension in biological systems.

Later workers tend to support the theory that the body's ability to tolerate 'supersaturation' may be due to its ability to tolerate a certain number of small gas bubbles without developing any symptoms.

## Site of bubble formation

Bubbles form at sites where conditions are most favourable for their development. Two local features could be expected to promote bubble formation: the first is a region of low pressure and the second, the presence of a suitable surface.

Regions of low pressure promote the formation of bubbles by causing an increase in supersaturation and they occur in areas of turbulence in flowing liquids. This helps to explain the formation of intravascular bubbles. Shearing forces which can occur in many tissues also cause regions of low pressure; they may be the cause of formation of both intravascular bubbles and extravascular bubbles in joint spaces, tendons etc.

A gas bubble tends to cling to a hydrophobic surface and this increases its stability. The effects of surface tension are also reduced if the bubble forms in a surface irregularity. Here a bubble can grow and seed off other bubbles from the crevice into the surrounding fluid. Both hydrophobic surfaces and surface irregularities aid bubble formation by allowing the bubble to avoid some of the surface tension effects.

A special case in bubble formation is encountered when the diver is breathing one gas mixture while his body is surrounded by another. It is possible for the partial pressure gradients of gases to result in the total pressure of dissolved gas to be greater than the ambient pressure. The diffusion phenomenon is called isobaric counterdiffusion (see pages 149–150).

## Bubble behaviour

Once a bubble has formed and grown beyond the stage where its surface tension can force it back into solution, its volume will change with the relative rates of diffusion of gas into and out of the bubble. Its volume will also change in response to any changes in surrounding pressures. There is some debate on what process limits the rate of inert gas transfer to and from the bubble. It could be that the gas tensions in the bubble are in equilibrium with the surrounding tissues and that gas movement is limited by the rate of transfer from this tissue to the blood flowing past it. This will be related to the blood flow rate and is called perfusion limiting.

The alternative hypothesis is that diffusion from the bubble to the surrounding tissue is the limiting process and that the tissue surrounding the bubble is in equilibrium with the blood – this is termed 'diffusion limiting'. We have written this section as if diffusion limits gas transfer to and from a bubble. The practical conclusions would need little alteration if perfusion limited gas transfer.

The rate of diffusion of gas into and out of a bubble is influenced by a variety of physical and physiological factors. In terms of treatment of decompression sickness and air embolism, the most important of these is the difference in partial pressures between the bubble and the surrounding fluid. It can be shown that partial pressure gradients will cause the slow elimination of an air bubble from an air-breathing subject, without changes in environmental pressure or inspired gas composition. The physical principles involved are the same as those involved in the resolution of a small pneumothorax or an artificial gas cavity.

Because of the problems encountered while waiting for a gas bubble to resolve, attention has been concentrated on methods of speeding up this process. The rate of removal of inert gas from a bubble can be increased by increasing the partial pressure gradient of inert gas from the bubble to the tissues, blood and lungs. This can be achieved if the subject breathes oxygen, which reduces the inert gas tension in the lungs and increases the gradient.

Compression aids the resolution of bubbles in several ways:

1. At higher pressures the bubble will be smaller. This gives an increase in the surface-to-volume ratio and results in an increase in the relative importance of surface tension in removing the bubble.
2. After compression the partial pressure of the gas in the bubble (which obeys Boyle's and Dalton's laws) will be much greater than that existing in the tissue surrounding it, and gas will pass from the bubble to the tissue.
3. The gradient will gradually diminish as the tissue surrounding the bubble becomes equilibrated with the new partial pressures. It has been shown that, following equilibra-

tion, the partial pressure gradient from the bubble to the lungs is still greater than that existing at lower pressures. Compression also reduces the clinical effects of the bubble by reducing its size.

> *Compressing a diver and giving him oxygen-rich mixtures to breathe hastens the elimination of inert gas bubbles.*

It is possible to increase the size of a bubble by supplying the subject with an inappropriate gas mixture. If a diver has been breathing air, any bubble in his body will be composed mainly of nitrogen. If he then breathes an oxygen/helium mixture the blood will become equilibrated with helium. Initially the bubble will grow because helium, in the process of replacing the nitrogen, diffuses into the bubble more rapidly than nitrogen diffuses out.

This discussion could lead the reader to deduce that pressurization to the maximum possible pressure, combined with 100% oxygen, would be the appropriate treatment for any inert gas bubble in a physiological system. This is correct, but unfortunately there are medical constraints involved in the treatment of decompression sickness and air embolism which limit the extent to which these principles can be applied.

# Physical aspects of the marine environment

## Heat

Diving and exposure to high pressures change the heat transfer from the diver's body. In air there is some insulation from the air trapped near the body, either by the clothes or the hair and the boundary layer. In water this is lost. The water adjacent to the skin is heated, expands slightly and causes a convection current which tends to remove the layer of warmed water. The process is accelerated by any movement of the diver or the water. The net result is that an immersed diver cools (or heats up) much quicker than he would in air of the same temperature.

Heat loss is also increased in warming the inhaled air or gas. For a diver breathing air most of this heat is used to humidify the dry air used for diving. It is not sufficient to cause concern in most circumstances. The heat lost in a helium dive is more significant. Helium has a greater specific heat than nitrogen. The problem is compounded because, at depth, the mass of gas inhaled per breath is increased and so the heat loss is increased. It may be necessary to warm the inhaled gas or use other measures to reduce this heat loss. The heat transfer by conduction is also increased in a helium environment. The result of this is that a helium diver may need external heating to maintain body warmth at a water, or gas, temperature where external warming would not be required if he was in an air environment.

In warm environments, it is possible for a diver to suffer heat stress. If he is wearing a protective suit he cannot lose heat by sweating because the sweat cannot evaporate. In a chamber the atmosphere can become saturated with water and, again, cooling is prevented.

> *A diver in water or a helium-rich environment can cool or heat up at a temperature that would be comfortable in an air environment.*

## Light

Even in the cleanest ocean water, only about 20% of the incident light reaches a depth of 10 metres and only 1% reaches 85 metres. Clean water has a maximum transparency to light with a wavelength of 480 nanometres (nm) (blue). This variation of absorption with wavelength causes distortion of colours and is responsible for the blue-green hues seen at depth. Red and orange light is absorbed the most. Because of the absorption of light, the deep ocean appears black and lights are needed for observation or photography. Because of the greater absorption of reds by water, some illumination is needed to see the true colours even at shallow depths. Part of the appeal of diving at night is that objects which have a blue-green colour in natural light have a new brightness when illuminated at close range with a torch.

Coastal water, with more suspended material, has a maximum transparency in the yellow-green band, about 530 nm. Absorption and scattering of light by the suspended particles restrict vision and can tend to even out illumination. This can make the light intensity the same in all directions and is an important factor in causing loss of orientation.

When the eye focuses on an object in air, most of the refraction of light rays occurs at the air–cornea interface. In water this refractive power is lost and the eye is incapable of focusing. A face mask provides an air–cornea boundary, which restores refraction at the cornea surface to normal. Refraction also occurs at the face mask surface, mainly at the glass–air boundary. This results in an apparent size increase of about 30% and makes objects appear closer than they are. Practice and adaption of the hand–eye coordination system allows the diver to compensate for this distortion, except when describing the size of fish.

Masks also restrict vision by narrowing the peripheral fields and distorting objects that subtend large visual angles. Both absorption of light by water, which reduces apparent contrast, and scattering by suspended particles reduce visual acuity. Attempts have been made to improve the diver's vision by modification of his face mask, the use of coloured filters and contact lenses. These have been only partly successful and impose their own problems.

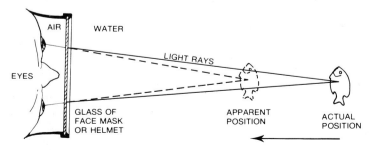

**Figure 2.5** Displacement of image in water

## Sound

Sound in water is transmitted as waves with a longitudinal mode of vibration. The speed of sound in water is about 1550 metres/second in sea water and 1410 metres/second in fresh water at 15°C. Water is a better transmitter of sound than air, so sounds travel greater distances under water. Low pitched sounds travel further than higher pitched sounds. Transmission of sound is enhanced by reflection from the surface. This reflection also enhances the transmission of sound in air over water but reduces the transmission of sounds from air to water and from water to air.

Both high pressure air and helium/oxygen mixtures causes speech distortion. Distortion is greater when breathing helium mixtures and can render speech indecipherable. Distortion in air results in the voice becoming more nasal and crisp as the pressure increases. These changes have been attributed to the increase in gas density causing greater sound transmission through the walls of the throat compared to the transmission through the mouth.

**Helium speech distortion**, the 'Donald Duck' effect, is attributed to an increase in the frequency of some of the resonant components of speech sounds. It is caused by the higher velocity of sound in helium/oxygen mixtures. There is no change in the frequency of vocal fold vibration. Electronic frequency analysis and shifting techniques can be used to transform the speech into a more understandable form.

It is often thought that verbal communication under water is denied the less well-equipped air diver. This is not necessarily so. If the diver produces an air pocket to speak into, then he may be heard by his companion, who must temporarily cease generating noise by breathing. The air pocket may be an oronasal mask, a face mask pulled over the mouth or even an air space created by cupped hands over the mouth. The resulting speech is clear, if somewhat attenuated by the air–water interface. Helmet divers can communicate easily by touching their helmets together, and using the air–copper–air pathway. Novices, who do not appreciate the width of the helmet, may also experience a characteristic 'boiiing', as the contact is made prematurely.

## Diving gases

Amateur diving is almost entirely based on the use of compressed air as a breathing gas. Commercial, military and experimental diving can involve the use of other more exotic gas mixtures, particularly in the attempts to reach greater depths in support of the offshore oil industry. For this reason, it is desirable to give the reader some salient points on the gases mentioned in this text and related literature.

**Oxygen** (atomic weight 16, molecular weight 32) is the essential constituent of all breathing mixtures. At high altitude people survive with less than 0.1 ATA in their inspired air; for diving, oxygen should be present at a partial pressure of at least 0.2 ATA to avoid hypoxia. At higher partial pressures oxygen causes oxygen toxicity. Prolonged exposure to over 0.5 ATA causes pulmonary oxygen toxicity and shorter exposures to over 2 ATA results in central nervous system effects. The risk of these problems may be acceptable in a recompression chamber where oxygen may be used at partial pressures of up to 2.8 ATA.

In the range 0.2–2.8 ATA, oxygen has little effect on the respiratory centre and minute volume will remain close to normal. Oxygen is vasoactive, high oxygen tensions causing profound vasoconstriction.

**Nitrogen** (atomic weight 14, molecule weight 28) is the major component of air – about 79%. Nitrogen is often considered to be physiologically inert. Bubbles, composed mainly of nitrogen, can cause decompression sickness if a diver who has been breathing air or an oxygen/nitrogen mixture ascends too rapidly. In solution it may cause nitrogen narcosis at depth. At partial pressures of nitrogen greater than about 2.5 ATA, there is a demonstrable fall-off in the diver's performance. At higher partial pressures, the effect is likely to cause the diver to make mistakes. The other problem that restricts the use of nitrogen is its considerable density at increased pressure. The addition of a lighter gas makes it easier to breathe at great depths.

Despite these disadvantages, nitrogen is of major importance in diving at depths less than 50 metres and as a part of more complex mixtures at greater depths.

**Helium** (atomic weight 4) is a light, inert gas. It is found in natural gas wells in several countries. These deposits will probably be exhausted by the end of the century. Helium is used to dilute oxygen for dives to depths greater than 50 metres, where nitrogen should not be used alone. The two major advantages of helium are that it does not cause narcosis and, because of its lightness, helium/oxygen mixtures are easier to breathe than most alternatives. Helium/oxygen mixtures can allow a shorter decompression time than an equivalent saturation dive with the diver breathing air, because helium diffuses more rapidly.

The use of helium can cause several problems. The speech of a diver at great depths may need electronic processing to make it understandable, because of the distortion referred to earlier. A diver in a helium atmosphere is more susceptible to heat and cold because the high thermal conductivity speeds the transfer of heat to and from the diver. The other problem with the use of helium is that it is associated with a disorder called the high-pressure neurological syndrome (see Chapter 16).

**Hydrogen** (atomic weight 1, molecular weight 2) has the advantage of being readily available at low cost. Because of its lightness it is the easiest gas to breathe. These factors may lead to its use as a replacement for helium. Hydrogen is not yet widely employed for operational diving. The reluctance to use it is due to fears of an explosion. This hazard can be prevented if the oxygen level does not exceed 4% (suitable for depths in excess of 30 metres, 100 feet). Hypoxia can be prevented by changing to another gas near the surface. Hydrogen causes similar thermal and speech distortion problems to helium.

**Neon** (atomic weight 20) in its pure form is probably too costly to consider as a gas to dilute oxygen. Crude neon – 75% neon, 25% helium – is a by-product of liquid air production. It is thought that this, mixed with oxygen, may produce a mixture that is less narcotic than air and causes less speech distortion and heat exchange problems than helium/oxygen mixtures. Because of the density of the mixture, crude neon could not be used in very deep dives.

**Argon** (atomic weight 40) is sometimes suggested as a suitable inert gas. It is denser and more narcotic than nitrogen, and may cause extra decompression requirements. It is sometimes used to study the effects of increased gas density at lower pressures than would be needed with lighter gases.

## Recommended reading

FLOOK, V. (1987). Physics and physiology in the hyperbaric environment. *Clinical Physics and Physiological Measurements* **8**, 197–230.

SCHILLING, C.W., WERTS, M.F. and SCHANDELMEIER, N.R. (Eds) (1976). *The Underwater Handbook. A Guide to Physiology and Performance for the Engineer.* New York: Plenum Press.

*US Navy Diving Manual* (1988). NAVSEA 0944-LP-001-9010.

# 3
# Physiology

## Introduction

This chapter is designed to give the reader an insight into some of the physiological effects of diving and hyperbaric exposure. It does not cover the latest and/or more complex theories; rather, it briefly discusses the effects of diving on the basic physiological systems. Particular attention has been paid to the respiratory and circulatory systems because of their changes in diving.

Little or no attention has been given to some other systems because of the paucity of in-formation, or because no serious effects have been demonstrated. Other topics have been incorporated in appropriate chapters. The sections on liquid breathing and diving mammals are included because of their general interest.

## Respiration

The basic function of the respiratory system, the supply of oxygen to and the removal of carbon dioxide from the blood, is disturbed to some extent by all types of diving. The relative importance of the changes varies with depth and equipment. In breath-hold dives, the performance of human beings is restricted by hypoxia and the ability of their lungs to tolerate volume changes. When diving with equipment, the resistance to breathing, the increased dead space and increased gas density can affect the human respiratory system.

# Background physiology

Two aspects of basic respiratory physiology need to be understood: the division of lung volumes and their relationship to the relaxation/pressure curve is important in diving with breathing apparatus and in breath-hold diving; the phenomenon of dynamic airway closure is of importance in restricting gas exchange at depth.

## Lung volumes

The components of the respiratory volumes of the lung are shown on the left-hand side of Figure 3.1.

On land, the volume of air in the lungs can range from about 1 litre to about 6 litres, at total lung capacity. The exact volumes vary with size, race, age and a genetic component. On inhalation at rest, the tidal volume increases from the functional residual capacity. The volume that can be inhaled at the end of a normal breath is the inspiratory reserve volume; the residual is the volume of air in the lungs after a maximal expiration; the volume of air that can be exhaled after a normal expiration is the expiratory reserve volume; and the functional residual volume is the sum of the residual volume and the expiratory reserve volume.

## Relaxation/pressure curves

The relaxation/pressure curve on the right-hand side of Figure 3.1 is the pressure required to inflate or deflate the lungs in an intact person. It is the result of the combined elastic properties of the chest wall and the lungs. In quiet breathing, the lung volume increases from the point marked relaxation volume; this is the lung volume when the inflation pressure is zero. The functional residual capacity is close

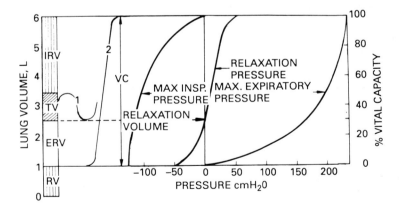

**Figure 3.1** Lung volumes and intrapulmonary pressure. The various components of lung volumes are labelled on the left. On the right the relation between lung volume, airway pressure and the maximum effort that can be made for inhalation and exhalation of air are plotted. Curve 1 is the volume change during quiet breathing and curve 2 is the volume change during a maximum inhalation starting at the residual volume. IRV = inspiratory reserve volume; TV = tidal volume; ERV = expiratory reserve volume; RV = residual volume; VC = vital capacity. (Redrawn from Lanphier and Camporesi (1982) with permission)

to the relaxation volume. This indicates that quiet breathing is mainly effected by the inspiratory muscles.

During quiet breathing, the expiratory muscles only act to force the lung volume to less than the relaxation volume. They are also used to shorten exhalation during more active breathing.

The **compliance** of the lungs is estimated from the slope of the steepest portion of the relaxation/pressure curve and it is quoted as the change in volume per unit change in pressure. When the compliance decreases, the lungs become stiffer and more force is required to bring about a given change in lung volume. This problem is encountered in several conditions in diving medicine.

The maximal inspiratory and expiratory curves indicate the force available for inhalation or exhalation of gas from the lung. The greatest inspiratory efforts can be generated when the lung volume is small, the inspiratory power available decreasing as the lungs fill. Conversely, the force available for expulsion of air is greatest when the lungs are full and it decreases as the lungs empty. The y-axis (ordinate) of this curve can shift for a diver with a snorkel or breathing apparatus.

### Dynamic airway closure

Gas density increases with depth because Boyle's law requires the volume of a mass of gas to decrease as pressure increases. This occurs even when nitrogen in the breathing mixture is replaced with the lighter helium, e.g. the density of air at 1 ATA is about 1.3 g/l, but at 10 ATA the density of air would be about 13 g/l. The use of a lighter gas helps to reduce the density, e.g. at 40 ATA the density of a 1% oxygen + helium mixture is 6.7 g/l.

As the density of a gas increases there is an increased tendency for the flow to become turbulent. As a result of this, there may be more turbulence in the gas flowing in a diver's airways at depth. More energy is needed to move gas in turbulent flow and this can cause problems when the diver exercises.

During turbulent flow the following relationships are in operation:

1. Driving pressure is proportional to the density of the gas.

2. Driving pressure is proportional to the square of the gas flow.
3. Driving pressure is inversely proportional to the fifth power of the tube radius.

Driving pressure is the physical force required to generate the gas flow; in this context it may be regarded as the respiratory work.

The first two factors in the list require an increase in driving pressure during exercise at depth. During exhalation, for reasons explained later, the diameter of the smaller airways decreases. This can lead to a further increase in driving pressure and closure of the airway.

The cause of this complication is illustrated in Figure 3.2. This series of figures uses a schematic lung and alveolus to illustrate the forces that normally keep alveoli and small airways open. The natural tendency for an isolated lung is to collapse, but in normal function it is kept inflated by the stretching forces generated by the rib cage and diaphragm.

During normal exhalation, there is a decrease in the forces inflating the lung, but

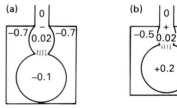

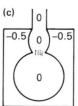 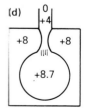

**Figure 3.2** Factors leading to airway collapse: the pressure gradient across a stylized alveolus and airway. (a) Inspiration: opening gradient 6.8 cmH$_2$O (0.68 kPa). (b) Normal expiration: opening gradient 5.2 cmH$_2$O (0.52 kPa). (c) End-expiration: opening gradient 5 cmH$_2$O (0.5 kPa). (d) Forced expiration: opening gradient 40 cmH$_2$O (4 kPa). (From Nunn (1987) with permission)

there is still a net inflating force. During forced exhalation, there will be an increase in the external pressure applied to the lungs from the action of the expiratory muscles and this may be greater than the forces that keep the small airways open.

Even when this condition has not developed fully, there will be an increase in required driving pressure during exercise with dense gas mixtures. This is because the reduced radii of small airways require an increase in driving pressure. Any increase in driving pressure can only be generated by increased respiratory effort. The consequences for deep diving are considered in the section 'Respiration in water and under pressure' (see also Figure 3.5).

Attempts have been made to implicate the phenomenon of airway collapse as a cause of **pulmonary barotrauma** of ascent, a pressure-induced injury to the lungs. It is generally attributed to either a failure to exhale or to air trapping during ascent (see Chapter 9). There is a flaw in using dynamic airway collapse to explain air trapping that leads to pulmonary barotrauma. The airway shutdown is accompanied by an elevated intrathoracic pressure, which supports the lungs and would prevent damage. External binding has been shown to protect against pulmonary barotrauma.

Barotrauma of ascent will probably occur when the pressure in all or part of the airways is greater than the surrounding pressure.

# Breath-hold diving

Human beings are comparatively poor breath-hold divers – dives longer than 2 minutes are rare and most individuals find it hard to reach depths greater than 15–20 metres. Bottle-nose dolphins can dive for 2 hours and sperm whales can reach 1000 metres. The current record depth for humans is held by Jacques Mayol, who dived to over 100 metres (with a weight to speed descent and a float to aid ascent). The maximum duration of a breath-hold dive is limited by the breakpoint, i.e. the time at which the desire to breathe cannot be resisted. This can be increased by acclimatization, reduced activity and training, which result in a decreased metabolic rate and thus a fall in oxygen consumption and carbon dioxide production. The breakpoint may also be delayed by prior hyperventilation; the risk of subsequent hypoxia and unconsciousness is discussed later.

**Depth limits** for a breath-hold diver are affected by several factors. The ratio of the total lung volume to the residual volume affects the maximum depth that can be reached without lung collapse or blood pooling in the thorax. This situation is reached when the increased pressure has compressed the initial lung volume to the residual volume. So a diver with a total lung capacity of 6 litres and a residual volume of 1.5 litres should be able to breath-hold dive to 30 metres (4 ATA) where the total lung volume would be compressed to 1.5 litres (Boyle's law).

Other factors which affect this limit include the rate of gas uptake, mainly oxygen, during the descent. This will reduce the depth reached. Carbon dioxide production will not balance the effect of oxygen consumption because the partial pressure of carbon dioxide in the lungs is buffered by arterial blood. As a result of this, the carbon dioxide tension in the lungs does not increase as much as the oxygen decreases.

In the laboratory, residual volume measurements are made after a maximal exhalation. In diving, the conditions are slightly different in that there is an external compression of the thorax by water pressure. This compression can cause the development of a greater force than the respiratory muscles can produce, forcing the lung volume to decrease to below the residual volume. This then acts as a partial vacuum in the chest. The force is also transmitted to the pulmonary circulation so there is a pressure gradient causing pooling of blood in the thorax. This blood collects in the lung vasculature and great veins, involving a volume of up to 1 litre. This pooling of blood allows a reduction in lung volume below normal residual volume and significantly increases the maximum depth that can be reached by trained breath-hold divers. Descent to a depth where the lungs are damaged by compression causes 'lung squeeze' which is a form of **pulmonary barotrauma**.

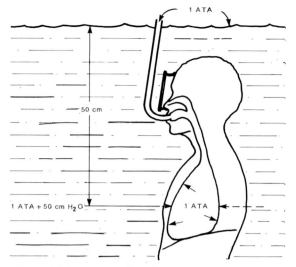

**Figure 3.3** Pressure gradient in submerged chest

The Japanese and Korean diving women, the Ama, whistle and then take a maximal inspiration prior to diving. It has been suggested that this improves their diving performance by allowing an increase in their total lung capacity. The elevated intrathoracic pressure during whistling could displace some intrathoracic blood and increase the total lung capacity if the inhalation occurred before the displaced blood had returned to the thorax. This would be the reverse of the blood pooling effect. Whistling may have value as a technique to avoid the risks of hyperventilation.

The lungs of a diver using a **snorkel** are normally below the water and so at a greater pressure than the atmosphere from which he is trying to inhale. This is equivalent to a shift of the axis to the left in Figure 3.1. The diver cannot inhale a full breath, but can exhale to less than the normal residual volume. The reduced maximal inhalation decreases the depth at which the diver would develop barotrauma and it would also decrease the oxygen stored in the lung. For these reasons, divers attempting deep dive records do not use a snorkel.

If immersed deep enough, a snorkel diver could not inhale any air. This is because the effort to inhale is greater than the pressure that can be developed on the inspiratory effort curve. The pressure difference increases with the average distance between the diver's lungs and the surface. This hydrostatic pressure, causing negative pressure breathing, limits the absolute maximum depth at which air can be inhaled through a snorkel tube to about 50 cm.

Dead space and respiratory resistance also limit the length and diameter of snorkel tubes. Any increase in diameter reduces resistance, but also increases dead space.

**Blood gases during breath-hold dives** will change with the partial pressure of the gases in the lungs (Dalton's law), as well as with changes caused by hypoxia. When the breath-hold diver descends, the partial pressures of the gases in the lungs increase and their volumes decrease. This increases the amount of oxygen that can be extracted from a breath but can lead to **hypoxia** during the ascent, especially if the diver has previously hyperventilated.

The rise in alveolar carbon dioxide tension due to descent can reverse the normal carbon dioxide gradient. This results in the passage of carbon dioxide from the lungs to the blood and accumulation in the blood and tissues. The carbon dioxide accumulated in the tissues may be exhaled between dives or retained over a series of dives, depending on the time spent on the surface between dives.

Alveolar gas tensions during a breath-hold period and breath-hold diving are presented in Figure 3.4. A very low partial pressure of oxygen occurred at the end of the dive preceded by hyperventilation. This was accompanied by confusion, loss of control and cyanosis, and the confusion could progress to unconsciousness and death. A reversed carbon dioxide gradient was maintained during the period at 10 metres (2 ATA), except for the last 20 seconds of the dive preceded by hyperventilation. This indicated continued tissue storage of carbon dioxide. During ascent the fall in alveolar oxygen tension showed that oxygen was still being extracted from the alveolar air. In the dives preceded by hyperventilation, the final oxygen tension was only slightly less than that predicted from the measurements just prior to ascent and from Dalton's law. This indicated that little oxygen was extracted during ascent.

The final alveolar carbon dioxide concentrations were greater than those predicted by Dalton's law, indicating that the normal gradient had been re-established and that

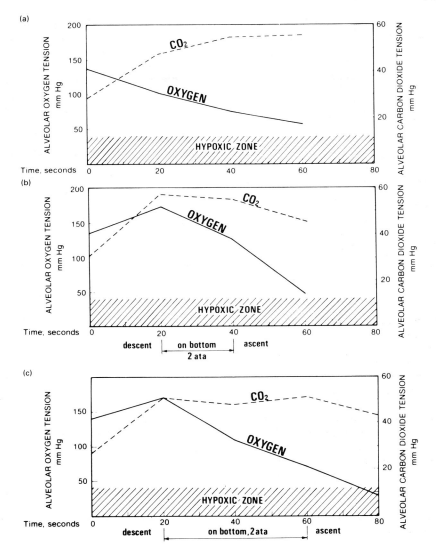

**Figure 3.4** Alveolar gas tensions during breath-holding and breath-hold dives. (a) Breath-hold on surface; (b) breath-hold dive; (c) breath-hold dive preceded by hyperventilation. These graphs are drawn from a series of breath-hold dives in a chamber to 10 metres reported by Lanphier and Rahn (1963). The dives involved a 20-second descent, 20 or 40 seconds at depth and then a 20-second ascent. These graphs show that the partial pressures of both gases increased during descent. The alveolar gas tensions did not double as might be expected from Dalton's law, indicating that oxygen was being extracted from alveolar air and carbon dioxide had passed back into the tissues from the lungs, i.e. the normal carbon dioxide gradient was reversed.

The final alveolar carbon dioxide concentrations were greater than those predicted by Dalton's law, indicating that the normal gradient had been re-established and that carbon dioxide had passed into the lungs. There would be some nitrogen absorption from the lungs during descent and during the time spent at depth. This would be followed by its release during ascent and the following period on the surface. The effects on lung volume were slight because only a small volume of nitrogen was involved, and theoretical consequences such as hypoxia caused by nitrogen release did not occur.

> *Hyperventilation is associated with uncon-sciousness in breath-hold divers.*

## Respiration in water and under pressure

When using equipment with a demand valve or a counterlung the pressure at the point from which the gas is inhaled can differ from the pressure at the chest. If upright in the water, a scuba diver shows a similar change to the snorkel diver considered above. Conversely, when swimming down, a diver can inhale to greater than normal vital capacity but cannot exhale to the normal residual volume. This results from the water pressure at this orienta-tion helping to inflate the lungs. When using a set with a counterlung, it is necessary to posi-tion the counterlung as close as possible to the lungs in order to avoid undesirable pressure differences. It is hard to inhale from a counter-lung at a lower pressure than the chest, but it is easy to inhale from but hard to exhale into a counterlung of higher pressure.

Immersion up to the neck in water reduces the vital capacity by about 10%. This is caused by hydrostatic pressure compressing the thorax and there is also a loss of gravitational effects which reduces the volume of blood in the lower (mainly leg) veins and increases thoracic blood volume. This in turn reduces the compliance of the lungs.

The maximum breathing capacity has been used to measure changes in respiratory perform-ance. It is an imperfect tool for predicting the effects of depth or gas mixtures on a diver, and it should not be used in consideration of a diver who may be expected to work for a prolonged period, because it is generally measured over a 15-second period. On the surface, when a fit subject is breathing through minimal resist-ance, the maximum ventilation which can be maintained for longer than a few minutes is about 40% of the maximum breathing capa-city.

For a diver wearing equipment that restricts his breathing capacity, the maximum ventila-tion over a period longer than a few minutes might only be 25% of his maximum breathing capacity. This has the effect of reducing his work capacity at depth. The restriction in maximum breathing capacity may be partially offset by the increased partial pressure of oxygen and the ability of some divers to tolerate elevated arterial carbon dioxide partial pressures.

The respiratory resistance in diving sets reduces maximum breathing capacity even on the surface. This problem does not occur with free flow system. Increased dead space is also a factor in reducing effective gas exchange in all sets to a varying degree. In diving operations, the increase in gas density with depth is generally a more important factor in reducing respiratory exchange. Figure 3.5 shows the reduction of maximum breathing capacity with depth. Reduction of the maximum breathing capacity to 72%, 60% and 51% of the surface values at 2, 3 and 4 ATA respectively has been found. The results from groups who have studied the work performance of divers at depth shows that work capacity decreases with increasing gas density or depth. There is also a decrease in minute volume with depth for a set work load and this reflects the development of hypercapnia.

The main cause of the decrease in respira-tory performance is probably the closure of airways discussed above. There is a tendency for the expiratory reserve volume to increase to counter the closure. So the diver breathes with almost full lungs and inhales to volumes in the zone where more effort is needed to over-come elastic forces. At high lung volumes the inspiratory muscles are less efficient. These factors can lead to fatigue of the inspiratory muscles. These effects can be reduced by creat-ing a positive pressure in the airways, which reduces airway closure and central blood pool-ing.

Replacement of nitrogen with helium or other lighter gases for deep diving reduces the density of breathing gas. This change in gases is also needed at depths greater than about 60 metres to eliminate the effects of nitrogen narcosis. The effects of breathing oxygen/helium mixtures on the maximum breathing capacity at depth is also shown in Figure 3.5.

There is evidence that continued exposure to dense gas, as is encountered in deep saturation dives, may cause an adaptive response. An increase in tidal volume and decrease in breathing rate are thought to minimize respira-tory work. There is also an increase in maxi-mum breathing capacity.

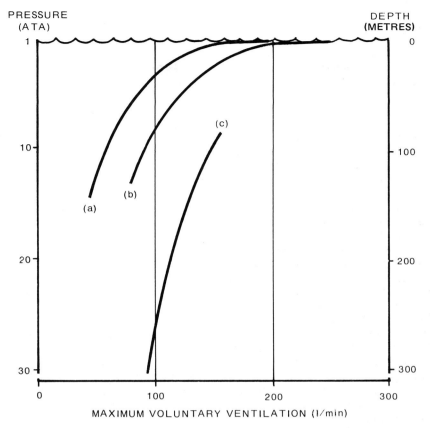

**Figure 3.5** Maximum voluntary ventilation: changes in maximum breathing capacity with a depth for a diver breathing (a) air, (b) 20% oxygen in helium, (c) predicted curve for 1% oxygen in helium. (Adapted from Lanphier, 1969)

## Metabolic gas exchange

Despite the problems discussed below, the respiratory exchange of gases in hyperbaric conditions is basically the same as at normal pressure: oxygen diffuses down a concentration gradient from the lungs to the tissues and the carbon dioxide gradient is normally in the opposite direction; the exchange of inert gases becomes important and there are changes in the finer details of metabolic gas exchange.

There is an increase in the partial pressures of the constituents of the breathing mixture with increasing depth, in accordance with Dalton's law. A diver breathing air or oxygen under pressure has higher alveolar pressures of the inhaled gases. This causes higher arterial pressures of oxygen and any other inhaled gases.

Elevated pressures of oxygen may interfere with the elimination of carbon dioxide in two ways: first, by the depression of respiration induced by high arterial oxygen tensions; secondly, by direct interference with the molecular transport of carbon dioxide. When the inspired oxygen partial pressure is elevated, there is an increase in oxygen transport in solution in the plasma. When inhaling oxygen at a partial pressure above 3 ATA, the total oxygen requirement may be carried in solution. If this happens, the haemoglobin may still be saturated with oxygen in the venous blood. This stops the transport of carbon dioxide in the form of carbaminohaemoglobin.

The overall effect of the factors discussed above is an increased carbon dioxide retention.

In some situations there may also be an increase in the inspired carbon dioxide pressure. Causes of this include the external dead space of the equipment, inadequate ventilation or failure in the absorbing system.

There is a tendency for experienced divers to be less sensitive to elevated carbon dioxide partial pressures – this reduces the total ventilation requirement during working dives. Elevated arterial carbon dioxide levels increase susceptibility to oxygen toxicity, decompression sickness and nitrogen narcosis. For these reasons, it is desirable to control the factors that cause an increased carbon dioxide retention.

With diving, there may be an increase in the alveolar-to-arterial pressure gradient. Immersion may cause mismatching of ventilation and perfusion. Divers breathing oxygen may develop areas of atelectasis.

> *Diving is associated with a tendency to retain carbon dioxide.*

### Inert gas exchange

The problem of inert gas exchange is of importance in understanding the causes and prevention of **decompression sickness** or the 'bends' (see Chapters 11 and 12). For a diver breathing air, there will be an immediate increase in the alveolar nitrogen tension, proportional to the depth of the dive. There is a concurrent increase in the arterial nitrogen tension. This gas is transported to all parts of the body, and results in an increase in tissue nitrogen tension. The rate of increase is proportional to the dive depth and the rate of blood flow to the tissue. For an equal blood flow, a tissue with more fat will show a slower increase in nitrogen tension than a tissue with a lower fat content. This is because nitrogen is more soluble in fat than other tissues. Factors that increase cardiac output, such as exercise, tend to increase gas uptake. If a diver remains at depth for sufficient time, his tissues become equilibrated with gas at that pressure.

At the end of the dive the transport mechanism is reversed. The tissues will have a higher nitrogen tension than alveolar air and there will be a movement of nitrogen from the tissues to the lungs. If the gas tension in the tissues and venous blood exceeds the ambient pressure, there will be a tendency for bubbles to form. Factors tending to oppose bubble formation include surface tension forces. In some tissues surfactant lowers surface tension and so facilitates bubble formation.

The physiology of gas uptake and elimination, and the related problem of decompression, are still not completely understood after more than 100 years of study.

Some results are not in accord with the facts outlined. For example, the concentration of radioactively labelled nitrogen in a tissue would be expected to start to fall after the subject stopped breathing the labelled gas. The results reported in a study using $^{13}N$ suggests that the level in the knee rose for at least 30 minutes after the subject stopped breathing the gas. Even the authors found the results contrary to expectations (Weathersby et al., 1986). Similar results were obtained in other studies using xenon as a marker for tissue gas. Countercurrent exchange of the labelled gas is a possible explanation of the unexpected result (Novotny et al., 1990). Dick and co-workers (1984) have shown that there are large variations in the total amount of nitrogen eliminated between similar dives.

Decompression sickness has been reported in divers who have performed a series of **deep breath-hold dives**. This developed because the average alveolar nitrogen partial pressure over the period was elevated. Enough nitrogen can be absorbed during a series of breath-hold dives to raise the tissue nitrogen partial pressure to the extent where bubble formation, and decompression sickness, occur.

The term 'Taravana' has been used for this disorder, but there is confusion in the early descriptions – with evidence of both decompression sickness and hypoxia in the Tuamotu islanders, by whom the disease was named. This is a rare event; most decompression sickness is associated with using breathing apparatus for dives to a depth greater than 10 metres.

## Cardiovascular system

There is comparatively little information available on most aspects of cardiovascular changes associated with diving. The **diving reflex**, a breath-hold bradycardia that occurs in humans and animals, has been studied extensively. It involves a fall in heart rate during breath-hold, facial immersion and diving. Its value in breath-hold diving in humans is doubtful. It is of greater significance for diving animals.

Bradycardia is also observed in response to hyperbaric exposure without immersion, e.g. in recompression chambers. Three mechanisms are thought to be responsible: an increase in vagal tone related to high oxygen pressures, a direct myocardial effect from the same cause and a nitrogen-dependent beta-blockade of the heart.

The effect of high inspired oxygen concentrations in interfering with carbon dioxide elimination was discussed above under 'Respiration'. Elevated oxygen pressures are of use in treating many diving and general medical conditions, but they also cause **oxygen toxicity** (see Chapter 18).

At the usual arterial oxygen partial pressure of 100 mmHg, haemoglobin is approximately 95% saturated and 100 ml of blood carries in the region of 19 ml oxygen combined with haemoglobin and 0.3 ml dissolved in the plasma. If the inspired oxygen partial pressure is increased, then the amount of oxygen combined with haemoglobin may increase to 20 ml% when the haemoglobin is fully saturated. The amount of oxygen carried in the plasma will increase with the oxygen partial pressure. About 4.3 ml% will be carried in this manner, when the oxygen partial pressure is 2 ATA (1520 mmHg) (Figure 3.6).

The results of this increase in arterial oxygen are that all the body's needs for oxygen may be satisfied without any reduction of oxyhaemoglobin. A high partial pressure of oxygen can be beneficial in its effect on the competitive reaction of carbon monoxide with haemoglobin and in promoting oxygen supply to hypoxic tissues.

> *In a diver breathing oxygen, the haemoglobin in venous blood may be saturated with oxygen.*

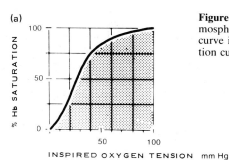

**Figure 3.6** Oxygen-carrying capacity of blood in (a) atmospheric and (b) hyperbaric oxygen environments. The curve in (a) represents the oxygen–haemoglobin dissociation curve

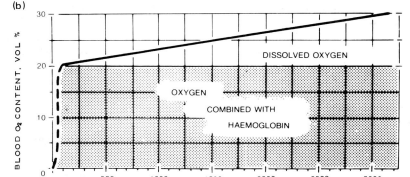

There is evidence of some **electrocardiographic changes** associated with hyperbaric exposure in chambers. The changes noted are physiologically interesting, rather than medically important. The suggested mechanisms do not appear to explain these changes completely. One suggestion is that compression reduces the volume of intestinal gas and causes blood pooling in the splanchnic circulation, resulting in the redistribution of blood flow. The electrocardiogram changes are largely attributed to changes in abdominal gas volume causing displacement of the diaphragm and movement of the heart. If this is the complete explanation, we would not expect to observe differences between exposures to oxygen/nitrogen and oxygen/helium at the same total and partial pressures.

**Immersion** creates a condition resembling the gravity-free state experienced by astronauts. The hydrostatic gradients in the circulatory system are almost exactly counterbalanced by the ambient water pressure. This reduces the volume of pooled blood in the leg veins. Also, peripheral vasoconstriction will occur in response to any cold stress. These changes result in an increase in central blood volume, leading to water diuresis, and subsequent haemoconcentration and decreased plasma volume.

Exposures to helium environments may result in hypothermia, with a consequent diuresis and a lowered blood volume, when environmental temperatures drop below 30°C.

The effect of haemoconcentration on normal dives is doubtful except that it gives divers a physiological excuse for a well-developed thirst. The rate of haemoconcentration is not great, but further concentration due to cold would increase the effect. Urine production rates of over 300 ml/hour cause problems for divers trying to keep their dry suit dry. Decompression sickness may be aggravated by haemoconcentration.

The other, more immediate, effect of increased central blood volume is on cardiac performance. In thermoneutral water, there is an increase in cardiac output as a result of increased stroke volume. In most dives this effect is increased by cold and exercise.

High partial pressures of oxygen depress **erythropoiesis**. This effect is a reverse of the changes experienced in acclimatization to altitude. In saturation exposures of sufficient length, in order for any marked erythropoietic change to develop, it is recommended practice to keep the ambient oxygen partial pressures close to normal. This is to avoid the risks of pulmonary oxygen toxicity, but also minimizes changes in red blood cell production.

A 24% decrease in erythrocyte count was reported in Sealab II which was a saturation dive where the divers were exposed to an oxygen pressure ranging from 188 to 268 mmHg.

# Endocrine system

There may not be any endocrine changes directly attributable to high environmental pressures as such. The responses noted may be due to other stimuli such as cold, stress or hyperoxia.

The Ama have been shown to have an increased basal **metabolic rate** during the colder months. This is partly due to noradrenaline; thyroid changes included an increase in thyroxine release and tissue utilization. In contrast to the Inuits (Eskimos), the specific dynamic action of increased protein intake does not appear to be a significant factor in causing the increase in basal metabolic rate.

Other endocrine changes reported in association with diving involve increased **adrenal activity**. The pattern reported suggests that the changes may be related more to anxiety and stress than to the diving itself. Increases in serum cortisol coincided with novel and potentially hazardous parts of diving training. Similar stress responses probably accompany other types of diving which entail risk and anxiety.

Adrenal responses are also involved in **oxygen toxicity**. Exposure to high pressure oxygen causes adrenal hypertrophy. This could be part of a stress reaction, but it has been shown that removal of the adrenal or thyroid glands protects against oxygen toxicity. Conversely, adrenaline or thyroxine increases oxygen toxicity, so a stress response would augment the toxicity of high pressure oxygen.

Diving can cause an increase in plasma β-endorphin levels. This may explain the 'high' felt by some divers.

**Immersion** diuresis has not been fully explained. Stimulation of cardiac atrial stretch receptors in response to increased central

**natriuretic peptide** (ANP). Other intrathoracic volume receptors have been postulated. The interactions of ANP with vasopressin and other hormones involved in diuresis in divers have not been clarified.

## Energy expenditure

Measurements of energy expenditure, while swimming on the surface and under water, have been made using indirect calorimetry, and by prediction from heart rate. These results show that oxygen consumption under water of over 3 litres/minute is possible, and values over 2 litres are quite common. The diver's energy expenditure when inactive may be lower than found on land, presumably because the absence of gravitational effects reduces the energy required to maintain posture under water.

Typical gas consumption and energy expenditure levels are: for a slow swim (0.5 knot) the diver would have an air consumption of 20 l/min and an oxygen consumption of 0.8 l/min; a swim of 0.8 knot would cause an air consumption of 30 l/min and an oxygen consumption of 1.4 l/min; a fast swim (1.2 knots) would cause an oxygen consumption of about 3 l/min and an air consumption of 50 l/min (air consumption was measured at the depth the diver was swimming and oxygen consumption was measured at 1 ATA).

Increased gas density increases the work of breathing. Investigations show that, despite this, divers can perform useful work at depth. The limit to diving depth imposed by the respiratory effects of increased gas density is probably about 1500 metres (unless the divers are prepared to wear ventilators).

> *Gas density may prove to be the limiting factor for deep diving.*

It might be expected that the higher oxygen partial pressures in hyperbaric environments could improve physical performance. Chamber experiments, where the subjects exercised while breathing oxygen at 3 ATA, showed that the maximum aerobic work performance was not significantly increased.

Physically fit swimmers can swim for an hour at 65% of their maximum speed; runners can only maintain 55% of their maximum speed for 1 hour. This difference has been attributed to the ease of heat dissipation in water.

## Special senses

**Hearing** performance is changed by both high pressures and immersion. The changes in the ear in a gaseous medium are complex: in air the losses are greatest round 500 Hz and between 3 and 4 kHz. The loss tends to increase with pressure at all frequencies.

Immersion degrades the hearing by air conduction; water in the external ear canal dampens the vibration of the ear drum. Hearing by bone conduction is slightly improved because there is better transfer of energy from water to the skull than there is from air to the skull. Overall the result is that hearing is degraded by 30–70 dB. The loss is least at low frequencies. A wet suit hood or helmet causes further impairment.

The decrease in hearing threshold gives some protection against the noise generated by underwater tools, but it is not sufficient to prevent damage from using some tools. Sonars can cause distress at ranges over a kilometre.

**Balance disturbances** can be caused by pressure changes and thermal stimulation (see Chapters 10 and 28). **Visual** changes associated with the refractive properties of water causing an apparent change in size of objects when viewed under water have been discussed in Chapter 2. There is also a loss of acuity in association with both the low light intensity at depth or the presence of particles in the water. Scattering from these particles can complicate the problem if artificial light is used to increase illumination.

## Diver monitoring

There are several reasons for monitoring a diver: to improve safety, to study performance or physiology, and to monitor the equipment or the progress of the diving operation. Any monitoring system should be simple to use, to interpret and have a minimum of faults and false alarms. This is not to infer that it cannot be based on sophisticated technology.

Simple methods of monitoring dive depth, time, gas cylinder pressure etc. are available. The supervisor of a surface supply dive can use the movement in a line pressure gauge to monitor the divers' respiration.

The most desirable monitoring is that of communication. This may vary from the basic lifeline and signals to a complex helium speech unscrambler. Through water, ultrasonic equipment can communicate with a free diver. Simple speech monitoring will reveal stress, overexertion and anxiety – these often precede an accident. Television surveillance is also available, both within chambers and under water. It has frequently been of value as a safety monitor.

The **electrocardiogram** (ECG) is one of the easiest physiological parameters to measure and record. It has the disadvantage of interpretation problems if medical or paramedical staff are not present. Disposable stick-on electrodes are usable under dry suits if care is taken in their application. For divers using a wet suit, insulated electrodes are needed. The pulse rate, derived from the ECG recording, may be of value in demonstrating variations from normal and the degree of physical exertion. The ECG will also aid in diagnosis of cardiac abnormalities, which may include arrhythmias and/or cardiac ischaemia.

**Respiration** can be monitored by sound or temperature recordings near the mouth. The respiratory rate rises with physical exertion and psychological stress. It is a simple guide to the well-being, or at least the continued existence, of a live diver. Many experienced civilian dive instructors listen to the regulator noise transmitted through the water for signs of stress in their students. It is simple to multiplex ECG and respiration.

Monitoring of the diver's **temperature** may be performed either by rectal or tympanic membrane temperature sensors, or by a swallowed 'radio pill', with temperature being read by the FM radio waves that the pill transmits.

Monitoring of the diver and the atmosphere in compression chambers is simpler than monitoring a diver in open water. Not only may continuous measurements of temperature, carbon dioxide, oxygen and humidity be made on the chamber atmosphere, but there is also usually a pressure/time readout available. It should be possible to make hard wire recordings of electrocardiograph, electroencephalograph and electronystagmograph readings.

# Liquid breathing

In 1950, Stein and Sommerschein wrote that 'water with oxygen dissolved under pressure and properly adjusted for osmotic, ionic and density characteristics, etc. conceivably may sustain life when it surrounds the man and fills his lungs . . . there is no reason why, with water as a diluent for oxygen, man may not be able to work safely at any depth to which fish may go'.

In 1962, the first experimental evidence was presented, supporting these beliefs. Kylstra showed that mice were able to stay alive for hours while submerged in salt solutions equilibrated with oxygen at higher pressure. These animals inhaled and exhaled the salt solution, extracting oxygen from it in order to survive. Mice which were submerged in a hyperbaric oxygenated salt solution, to which a carbon dioxide buffer, THAM, had been added, lived markedly longer than in an identical but unbuffered salt solution. They even continued making respiratory movements for long periods when subjected to a depth equivalent of about 1 mile under the ocean (160 atmospheres).

Other experimental evidence also supports the theory. Anaesthetized dogs can breathe an oxygenated salt solution for 1 hour or an oxygenated liquid fluorocarbon for up to 8 hours, resume spontaneous breathing of warm air and survive afterwards. Pulmonary function testing on animals who have been ventilated with liquid fluorocarbon for 1 hour showed no abnormalities 72 hours later. These animals had serial pulmonary function tests for another year which were normal. Dogs, which have been ventilated with fluorocarbons, subsequently conceived and sired apparently normal offspring. One dog, pregnant at the time of the ventilation with hyperbarically oxygenated saline, subsequently delivered nine healthy pups.

Patients with alveolar proteinosis, cystic fibrosis of the pancreas, bronchiectasis, intractable asthma and accidental inhalation of radioactive dust, have been clinically treated in the past with unilateral lung lavage with isotonic saline, as a therapeutic measure. Apart from being beneficial, this showed no demonstrable lasting impairment of pulmonary function associated with it. A conscious man, whose trachea and larynx had been anaesthetized to allow intubation, but who otherwise received no medication, has tolerated the filling of one lung with saline as well as the flow of saline in and out of that lung.

Due to the fact that all the diluent liquid media are far more dense to breathe than air, it is inevitable that the flow rates through the respiratory passages will be impaired. The supply of oxygen and the removal of carbon dioxide from the lungs will be less with liquid breathing. It may be partly ameliorated by using the least dense liquid possible or by increasing the oxygen pressure. Oxygenated fluorocarbon liquid, at 1 ATA, will produce adequate arterial oxygen tensions (80 mmHg) in an anaesthetized normothermic dog for at least 8 hours. Oxygenation has also been adequate for 1 hour in hyperbarically oxygenated saline at 5 ATA. All mammals ventilated with liquid have developed arterial carbon dioxide tensions greater than 40 mmHg during the episode of liquid breathing. After resumption of gas breathing, it returned to normal within 15 minutes.

Small amounts of fluorocarbon can be detected in the blood within minutes of ventilating the lungs with this and it can be found in all major tissues for at least 1 year after breathing Caroxin F and D. To date there have been no adverse effects from this. Serum concentrations of $Na^+$, $Cl^-$, $Ca^{2+}$, $Mg^{2+}$ and $K^+$ are maintained at normal levels during and after ventilation with fluorocarbon liquids for up to 8 hours. No appreciable changes in serum electrolyte concentrations have been observed following therapeutic lung lavage with up to 40 litres of saline in humans.

There still remains a great deal to do in research into liquid breathing. Improved liquids need to be developed and tested. Both lungs need to be ventilated simultaneously with these liquids and they should supply normal oxygenation, normal carbon dioxide elimination, an absence of toxicity, high solubilities for oxygen and carbon dioxide, a low density and a low vapour pressure, as well as easy removal from the lungs and the body.

Other problems will arise, e.g. the production of an embolism from the liquids being breathed, the pressure equilibration of all other gas-containing cavities during the liquid breathing (sinuses, middle ear, mastoids etc.), as well as communication, speech and hearing implications, the effects on the integrity and turnover rate of lung surfactant during and following liquid breathing, together with the various methods of producing mechanically assisted ventilation.

## Diving mammals

Human beings, comparatively poor breath-hold divers, have often envied the remarkable performance of the diving mammals. In this section an interesting anatomical and physiological background is presented to illustrate the sophisticated mechanisms available to these animals. The most obvious adaptations to a marine environment is seen by the streamlined shape of the animal, and the placement of a blowhole in the dorsum of its body. The blowhole allows respiration with a minimum of the body out of the water; it is occluded during diving, and may be used for noise production on the surface.

The streamlined shape and the nature of the surface skin allows the dolphins to reach speeds of up to 20 knots with the expenditure of only 2 hp (1.5 kW). A naval architect would need to allow approximately 10 times the power to drive a similarly sized object at the same speed.

Diving animals face five potential problems: hypoxia, carbon dioxide accumulation, the effects of pressure changes (i.e. barotrauma), decompression sickness and cold or hypothermia. If they dive deep enough they could also be expected to experience high-pressure neurological syndrome.

Some of the adaptations are discussed below, but for a more complete discussion of them, the reader is referred to the recommended reading at the end of the chapter.

The early analysis of diving animals was based on results where the animal was forced to dive and had no control of when it could get its next breath. Recently, techniques have been developed which allow the study of unrestrained animals in the wild. From these studies we now know that seals, and probably other animals, have different physiological responses for short and long dives. For a long dive, mechanisms to conserve oxygen are activated. This selection is probably made to avoid unnecessary periods of anaerobic metabolism, which is less efficient than aerobic metabolism and lengthens the time required on the surface recovering between dives. By deciding on a shorter aerobic dive, the seal can maximize its fishing time. How it can voluntarily modify its physiological response depending on the expected length of dive is not known.

**Hypoxia** is avoided by a combination of physiological changes, the most striking of which are the circulatory adjustments. During a dive the heart rate of a seal, beaver or penguin may fall to less than a sixth of the surface value. During this intense bradycardia, central blood pressure is maintained at normal or even elevated values. An enlarged fibrous section of the ascending aorta is thought to expand during systole and contract during diastole, thus helping to maintain the pulse pressure wave. Circulation to the heart and brain is maintained at near normal rates. Flow to the viscera and the skeletal muscles falls to almost negligible amounts or becomes intermittent.

These circulatory adjustments keep the animal's vital organs functioning for a longer time on a limited oxygen supply. An interesting converse situation is that fish develop a bradycardia when removed from the water. Fish cannot absorb oxygen from the air, so it is a useful survival mechanism to conserve the remaining oxygen stores until the tide rises.

Other features which delay hypoxia are modifications that increase oxygen storage. Diving animals tend to have a higher haematocrit than non-diving animals. Blood volumes also tend to be higher and often much of this blood is stored in the spleen. During a dive the spleen contracts, feeding blood into the venous side of the circulation. These changes increase the quantity of oxygen carried in the blood.

In skeletal muscle, the myoglobin levels are increased, compared to terrestrial animals, and this also increases the oxygen storage. There can be a temporary reduction in the energy metabolism of many diving animals during the dive. The metabolic rate of a seal can fall to a quarter of its surface value. This may be the consequence of the changes that minimize oxygen usage, indicating the effectiveness of the oxygen conservation mechanisms.

**Carbon dioxide accumulation** during a dive is reduced by two mechanisms. The first is the bradycardia discussed above, resulting in the low blood flow to the skeletal muscles, with a corresponding fall in venous return. Thus the metabolites, carbon dioxide and lactic acid, can be held in the muscles until the end of the dive. There may then be a reactive hyperaemia and up to a three-fold increase in blood lactic acid concentration. Diving mammals, and also well-trained humans, tend to be less sensitive than normal to increased carbon dioxide tensions. The effect of this is to delay the breaking point further when the animal has to recommence breathing.

**Pressure changes** could cause barotrauma and are avoided by anatomical modifications. Unlike human beings, whales have relatively small residual lung volumes, using up to 90% of their lungs during quiet breathing. If they need to increase ventilation, they increase the frequency of respiration. With the low residual volume, it can be assumed that dives can be made to at least 90 metres before the lung volume decreases to the residual volume. Further reduction in volume does not cause pulmonary barotrauma in whales, their lungs being able to collapse without damage. This collapse allows the air to be restricted to the more rigid air spaces. On ascent the air expands and reinflates the lungs.

Some diving animals have vascular plexus in the middle ear and nasal sinuses. As the animal descends, the pressure in these cavities is relatively less than that of the ambient environment and the animal's body. These plexus distend in response to this relative negative pressure. The animal avoids ear and sinus barotrauma by allowing blood in the plexus to occupy the air spaces.

Another danger encountered by human beings during descent is the rupture of the round window of the inner ear. Some diving animals have developed very thick fibrous round windows, thereby preventing this problem.

**Decompression sickness** could occur in the deeper diving animals. Several of the modifications discussed above will reduce the animals' susceptibility to it. The slowing of the heart rate restricts the flow of blood, and therefore of nitrogen, to the tissues. There is some nitrogen uptake during the dive, but with the reactive hyperaemia following the dive, there is an increased gas elimination which tends to decrease the likelihood of decompression sickness. Contraction of the spleen supplies a nitrogen sink for the blood which has more nitrogen to mix with and this lowers the average blood nitrogen level.

The reduction in lung volume, associated with the collapse of the alveoli during the dive, stops nitrogen transfer from the lungs to the tissues once the animal has passed the depth where gas exchange ceases. The blood of some marine animals does not coagulate readily. This may contribute to avoiding decompression sickness by reducing the blood:bubble interaction which is thought to aggravate the effects of nitrogen bubbles.

The effectiveness of these mechanisms is illustrated by the activities of the sperm whale. This animal can make repeated dives to 1000 metres with no apparent ill effects. Because this is hard to understand from our knowledge of human physiology, various other mechanisms have been proposed, including the presence of 'bubble traps' within the circulatory system.

Measurements of the blood nitrogen levels of free-diving seals show that the arterial nitrogen peaked during descent at up to 2500 mmHg and fell during the dive to 1500 mmHg just before surfacing – these results suggest that the seal has no need for 'bubble traps'.

Reptiles have developed other evolutionary adaptations to avoid decompression sickness. In the turtle, this involves a right-to-left shunting of blood within the heart. The shunt opens during a dive so that blood bypasses the lungs and the excess nitrogen absorption is circumvented.

Sea snakes can exchange gas through the skin as well as the lungs. Any nitrogen absorbed from the lungs can be lost directly into the water. This is possible because of the relatively low nitrogen tension in sea water, normally remaining at approximately 0.8 ATA (in accordance with Henry's law).

One of the few natural sites, where water has a nitrogen tension in excess of 0.8 ATA, is in the turbulent frothy areas below dam spillways. In this zone, the air is caught in the waterfall and forced into solution at pressures greater than 0.8 ATA. The nitrogen at the increased pressure can dissolve into salmon which are migrating through these areas. They absorb the extra nitrogen below the dam and then develop decompression sickness as they ascend up it.

**Hypothermia** is avoided by a series of mechanisms and the body temperature of marine mammals is close to that of humans. Most marine mammals have a thick layer of insulating subcutaneous fat. The body shape is often more spherical than that of humans, reducing the surface area from which heat is lost. Those animals which do not have a thick subcutaneous fat layer, such as polar bears and some newborn seals, have a thick fur layer. They restrict their diving to shallow depths, otherwise the layer of trapped air becomes compressed and a less effective insulation.

A reduction of blood flow to the skin increases insulation of the fat layer and allows surface cooling which is not transmitted to the internal core. Well-developed countercurrent heat exchange systems also aid in conserving heat by cooling arterial blood and heating venous blood as it returns to the core. Examples can be found in the fins and flippers of whales and seals; here working muscles are close to the surface and have little fat insulation.

Some marine animals are poikilothermic and their metabolism is related to the water temperature, i.e. their activity rises in warmer water. Others, although classified as poikilothermic, have developed a functional warm-bloodedness. Pelagic tuna and the great white shark (Isuridae) have a countercurrent mechanism for conservation of heat from metabolism which allows them to function effectively in cold water.

# Recommended reading

ANTHONISEN, N.R. (1984). Physiology of diving. In: *The Physician's Guide to Diving Medicine*, edited by C.W. Shilling, C.B. Carlson and R.A. Mathias. New York: Plenum Press.

BOVE, A.A., PIERCE, A.L., BARRERA, F., AMSBAUGH, G.A. and LYNCH, P.R. (1973). Diving bradycardia as a factor in underwater blackout. *Aerospace Medicine* **44**, 245–248.

CASTELLINI, M.A. and KOOYMAN, G.L. (1989). Behaviour of free diving animals. *Undersea Biomedical Research* **16**, 335–363.

CLARK, J.M. (1982). Oxygen toxicity. In: *The Physiology and Medicine of Diving*, 3rd edn, edited by P.B. Bennett and D.H. Elliott. London: Baillière Tindall and Cassell.

DICK, A.P.K., VANN, R.D., MEBANE, G.Y. and FEEZOR, M.D. (1984). Decompression induced nitrogen elimination. *Undersea Biomedical Research* 11, 369–380.

EPSTEIN M. (1984). Water immersion and the kidney: implications for volume regulation. *Undersea Biomedical Research* **11**, 113–121.

FEDAK, M.A. (1985). Diving and exercise in seals: A benthic perspective. In: *Diving in Animals and Man*. The 1985 Kongsvoll Symposium. The Royal Norwegian Society of Sciences and Letters.

FLOOK, V. (1987). Physics and physiology in the hyperbaric environment. *Clinical Physics and Physiology* **8**, 197–230.

FOLK, G.E. (1966). *Environmental Physiology*. Philadelphia: Lea and Febiger.

KANG, B.S., HAN, D.S., PAIK, K.S., PARK, Y.S., KIM, J.S., KIM, C.S. et al. Calorigenic action of norepinephrine in the Korean women divers. *Journal of Applied Physiology* **29**, 6–9.

KYLSTRA, J.A. (1982). Liquid breathing and artificial gills. In: *The Physiology and Medicine of Diving*, 3rd edn, edited by P.B. Bennett and D.H. Elliott. London: Baillière Tindall and Cassell.

LANPHIER, E.H. (1969). *The Physiology and Medicine of Diving and Compressed Air Work*, edited by P.B. Bennett and D.H. Elliott. London: Ballière Tindall and Cassell.

LANPHIER, E.H. and CAMPORESI, E.M. (1982). Respiration and exercise. In: *The Physiology and Medicine of Diving*, 3rd edn, edited by P.B. Bennett and D.H. Elliott. London: Baillière Tindall and Cassell.

LANPHIER, E.H. and RAHN, H. (1963). Alveolar gas exchange during breathhold diving. *Journal of Applied Physiology* **18**, 471–477.

LE BOEUF, B.J., NAITO, Y., HUNTLEY, A.C. and ASAGA, T. (1989). Prolonged, continuous, deep diving by northern elephant seals. *Canadian Journal of Zoology* **67**, 2514–2519.

LUNDGREN, C.E.G. (1978). Monitoring signs in the diver. *16th Undersea Medical Society Workshop Proceedings*. Bethesda, Maryland: UMS.

NOVOTNY, J.A., MAYERS, D.L., PARSONS, Y.J., SURVANSHI, S.S., WEATHERSBY, P.K. and HOMER, L.D. (1990). Xenon kinetics in muscle are not explained by a model of parallel perfusion-limited compartments. *Journal of Applied Physiology* **68**, 876–890.

NUNN, J.F. (1989). *Applied Respiratory Physiology*, 3rd edn. London: Butterworths.

PAULEV, P. (1965). Decompression sickness following repeated breath-hold dives. *Journal of Applied Physiology* **20**, 1028–1031.

RAHN, H. (Ed.) (1965). *Physiology of Breathhold Diving*. Publication No.1341, National Academy of Sciences, Washington.

RIDGWAY, S.H. (1985). Diving by Cetaceans. In: *Diving in Animals and Man*. The 1985 Kongsvoll Symposium. The Royal Norwegian Society of Sciences and Letters.

RUBIN, R.T. (1969). Adrenal activity in anxiety. *Australia New Zealand Journal of Psychiatry* **3**, 207–212.

SCHAEFER, K.E., ALLISON, R.D., DOUGHERTY, J.H., CAREY, C.R., WALKER, R., YOST, F. and PARKER, D. (1968). Pulmonary and circulatory adjustments determining the limits of depths in breathhold diving. *Science* **162**, 1020–1023.

SCHOLANDER, P.F. (1964). Animals in aquatic environments: diving mammals and birds. In: *Handbook of Physiology Section 4: Adaptation to the Environment*. Washington: American Physiology Society.

STRAUSS, M.B. (1970). Physiological aspects of mammalian breath-hold diving. A review. *Aerospace Medicine* **41**, 1362–1381.

VAN LIEW, H.D. (1983). Mechanical and physical factors in lung function in dense environments. *Undersea Biomedical Research* **10**, 255–264.

WEATHERSBY, P.K., MEYER, P., FLYNN, E.T., HOMER, L.D. and SURVANSHI, S. (1986). Nitrogen gas exchange in the human knee. *Journal of Applied Physiology* **61**, 1534–1545.

# 4

# Diving equipment

## Introduction

The first part of this chapter deals with the equipment used by amateur divers. The more complex and unusual types of diving equipment which are used by commercial or military organizations are dealt with in the second half of the chapter. Attention is paid to the problems that the equipment can cause, particularly to the learner. This is of importance in understanding the medical problems that are related to the diving equipment. It may also help the reader to understand the stresses experienced by the novice diver.

# Equipment for amateur diving

## Breath-hold diving equipment

The simplest assembly of diving equipment is that used by many children, coral reef tourists and spearfishermen: a mask, snorkel and a pair of fins or flippers. In colder climates, a wet suit may be added for thermal insulation and a weight belt to compensate for the buoyancy of the suit.

### Mask

A mask is needed to give the diver adequate vision under water. The mask usually covers the eyes and nose, and it seals by pressing on the cheeks and forehead with a soft rubber edge to prevent entry of water. Goggles which do not cover the nose are not suitable for diving. The nose must be enclosed in the mask so that the diver can exhale into it to allow equalization of the pressure between the mask and the water environment. It should be possible to block the nostrils without disturbing the mask seal, to allow the wearer to perform a Valsalva manoeuvre. Full face masks that cover the mouth as well as the eyes and nose, or helmets that cover the entire head, are more commonly used by professional divers and are considered under 'Equipment for professional diving'.

A diver with visual problems may obtain a mask with the **optical corrections** ground in. Others mount ordinary spectacles (with arms removed) into their mask. Ocular damage can occur if hard corneal lenses are used for diving (see Chapter 30); also contact lenses may be lost if the mask floods. The lens part of the face mask should be hardened glass. People who are susceptible to allergies may prefer a mask with the rubber portion made from silicone rubber to reduce allergy problems.

All masks cause a restriction in vision. In most the diver can see about one-third of his normal visual field. The restriction is most marked when the diver tries to look down towards his feet and can be a danger if the diver becomes entangled. The more nervous beginner finds the visual restriction worrying, often fearing that there is a predator lurking just outside his vision. The visual field varies with the style of mask and experimentation is also needed to find which mask gives a good seal to minimize water entry. The diver needs to master a technique of expulsion of water from the mask. If it is not learned, a leaking mask can become a major problem.

### Snorkel

The typical snorkel is a tube, about 40 cm long and 2 cm in diameter, with a U bend near the mouth piece. A mouth piece is fitted to allow the diver to grip the tube with his teeth and lips. The tube is positioned to lead past the ear so that the diver can breathe through the tube while he floats on the surface looking down. Any water in the snorkel should be expelled before inhaling through it. Many attempts have been made to 'improve' the snorkel by lengthening it, adding valves etc. So far these attempts seem to have been unsuccessful. All snorkels impose a restriction on breathing, a typical snorkel restricting the maximum breathing capacity to about 70% of normal. The volume of the snorkel also increases the diver's anatomical dead space. As a consequence, increasing the diameter to reduce the resistance is not a viable option. These problems all add to the difficulties of a diver who may be struggling to cope with waves breaking over him (and into his snorkel) and a current that may force him to swim hard. There have also been anecdotal reports of divers inhaling foreign bodies that have previously lodged in the snorkel.*

### Fins

Fins, or flippers, are mechanical extensions of the feet. Fins allow the diver to swim faster and more efficiently, and free his arms for other tasks. The fins are normally secured to the feet

---

* The senior author's reported incident involving a cockroach has been discredited as a cockroach of the claimed size would not fit in a snorkel.

by straps or moulded shoes. Various attempts have been made to develop fins that give greater thrust with special shapes, valves, controlled flex and miracle rubber competing for the diver's money. Divers often get cramps, either in the foot or calf, with fins that are the wrong size, or if they are out of training. The loss of a fin may also cause problems for a diver if he has to swim against a current.

### Weight belt

Even without the buoyancy of a wet suit, some divers require extra weights to submerge easily. The weights are made from lead and are moulded to thread onto a belt. Usually the belt should be fitted with a quick release buckle, to allow a diver to drop the weights quickly and so aid his return to the surface. The situations where a quick release buckle should not be fitted are those where it would be dangerous to ascend, e.g. in caves where there is no air space above the water.

Unfortunately, divers often neglect to release the belt if they are in difficulties. The reason for this omission is not clear. It is possibly caused by defective training, because they almost never drop it during a drill. There have been cases of people in a panic touching the buckle, as is commonly done in a drill and leaving the belt on. The alternative drill of taking the belt off and holding it in one hand is recommended because the diver will drop it if he loses consciousness. If he needs two hands to correct his problem, he can replace the belt and remedy it. Another, less frequent difficulty with weight belts is that the weights can slip on the belt and jam the release mechanism.

> *In most fatal diving accidents the diver has not released his weight belt.*

This basic free-diving equipment is adequate to dive in shallow, warm water. Experience with this gear is excellent training for a potential scuba diver. The diver can gain the basic skills, without the extra complications caused by scuba gear. It will allow a more realistic self-assessment of the desire to scuba dive.

With the confidence gained in free diving, the diver is also less likely to become dependent on his breathing apparatus. In cold climates, a free diver needs a suit to keep him warm (suits are discussed below under 'Safety and protective equipment').

### Breathing apparatus

The simplest form of breathing apparatus consists of a gas source and a tap which the diver turns on to obtain each breath of air. This system works and was in use until the 1930s, but much of the diver's time and concentration may be taken up in operating the tap. In the most common breathing apparatus, the **Aqualung** or **scuba**, the tap is replaced by a one- or two-stage valve system. The flow of gas to the diver is triggered by the diver's inspiratory effect and closed by expiration or cessation of inspiration.

The operating principles of a simple demand valve system are shown in Figures 4.1 and 4.2. The air is stored in a cylinder at a maximum pressure which is determined by the design of the cylinder. For most cylinders this pressure, called the working pressure, is 150–200 ATA (2200–3000 lb/in$^2$ or 15.2–20.7 MPa).

The first stage of the valve system (Figure 4.1) reduces the pressure from cylinder pressure to about 10 atmospheres greater than the pressure surrounding the diver, and regulates its outlet pressure at this value. The valve is held open by the force of a spring until the pressure above the first-stage piston builds up and forces the valve seal down on the seat, shutting the gas off. The first-stage valve opens and closes as gas is drawn from the system by the diver. The water can enter the water chamber and helps the spring to hold the valve open. This adjustment of the supply pressure with water pressure is termed 'depth compensation'. It is designed to prevent the flow decreasing as the diver descends.

When the diver inhales he reduces the pressure in the mouth piece, or second-stage valve. As he does so the diaphragm curves in and depresses the lever (Figure 4.2a). The inlet valve opens and remains open until inhalation ceases. At this stage the diaphragm moves back into the position shown in Figure 4.2b.

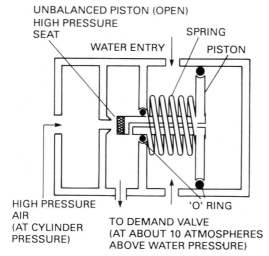

**Figure 4.1** First-stage reducer valve: the gas escapes from the cylinder until the pressure above the piston increases to a level where the force on the pressure can compress the spring, pushing the first-stage valve seat down and shutting the gas flow off. The valve opens again when the pressure above the piston (and in the hose to the second-stage valve) falls. This is normally because the diver has taken another breath

The second-stage valve is often called the demand valve.

Expired air passes out of the mouth piece through an expiratory valve. In the demand valve, air flow increases with respiratory effort because the valve opens more, allowing the diver to breathe normally. The purge button allows the diver to open the inlet valve to force any water out of the regulator. He may need to do this if he takes his regulator from his mouth while under water, which may be necessary if the diver has to share the air supply with another diver, a practice called 'buddy breathing'.

> *The scuba regulator provides the diver with a gas supply matched to his respiratory needs and depth.*

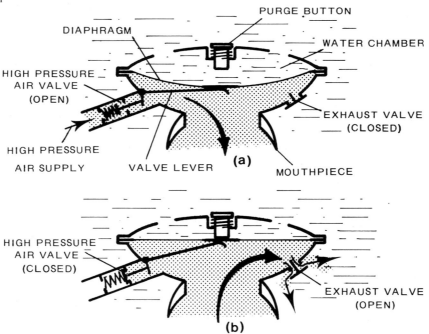

**Figure 4.2** Scuba demand valve during (a) inspiration, (b) exhalation. The arrows indicate air flow. During inspiration, the diver decreases the pressure in the mouth piece. This causes the diaphragm to curve in and tilt the air supply valve open. At the end of inspiration, air continues to flow until the pressure in the mouth piece equals the pressure in the water chamber; at this stage, the diaphragm will return to the position shown in (b), and the air supply valve shuts. During exhalation, the pressure difference forces the exhaust valve open and allows exhaled air to escape. The purge button is used to trigger a flow of gas from the supply without the need to inhale from the regulator

Most divers have little difficulty using scuba. When they first put it on, the weight and bulk will make them awkward, and may aggravate back problems. In the water, the buoyancy of the set balances its weight.

The lips should seal round the mouth piece and prevent the entry of water. Water can also enter through the diaphragm or the expiratory valve if either is faulty. A leak can generate an aerosol if the water reaches the inlet valve of the second-stage valve. The aerosol can cause distress to the diver and may cause a syndrome called salt water aspiration syndrome (see page 284).

Another problem associated with demand valves is that they may cause pain in the temporomandibular joint. This condition is considered in Chapter 30.

In very cold water the first stage of the regulator may freeze. This occurs due to the cooling of air as it passes through the first stage and the regulator can ice up with the piston frozen in the open position. The problem can be reduced by using a first-stage valve that is designed for operation in cold water.

Because the first stage regulates the pressure to the second stage, the inspiratory effort required to cause a flow does not vary until the cylinder is almost empty, when the pressure in the hose to the second stage falls and the flow decreases. The diver's first warning of the cylinder being almost empty would be an increased resistance on inhalation.

Most divers have a pressure gauge connected to the cylinder by a hose which gives them a measure of their remaining air supply. The contents of the cylinder are proportional to the pressure so the gauge is often called the 'contents gauge'. Divers tend to say they have 50 bars left rather than the volume this represents. A major problem is that a diver who is entranced by the scenery or concentrating on his task may run out of air because he forgets to check the gauge.

Another common system to prevent divers running out of air is a reserve valve. In operation, it resembles a boiler safety valve: the air escapes to the diver until the cylinder pressure falls to the level at which the reserve valve closes. The remainder of the air can be released by pulling a lever to open the reserve valve. The problem with this is that the valve lever may be bumped into the 'on' position, so the diver uses the reserve of gas without being aware of the opening of the valve.

A diver can also use a demand valve with air supplied by a hose from the surface. This equipment, surface supply breathing apparatus (**SSBA**), restricts the diver's range and depth to the length of his air supply hose. Its advantages are that the diver is freed from the cumbersome air tanks and his air supply can be as large as needed, instead of being restricted by his carrying capacity and need for mobility. The air for SSBA may be stored in large tanks or compressed as required. The use of a compressor, often called a '**Hookah**' system, is economically attractive because the air is compressed to a lower pressure than that required for storage tanks. The major disadvantage is that the diver gambles on the reliability of the compressor.

Two modified forms of SSBA have found support in some circles. In one, a small motor and air compressor is supported on a float on the surface. It supplies air to one or two divers. In the other, the diver(s) tow a float that supports an air cylinder. An advantage of these systems is that, if the hoses are short, the divers are unable to reach the depth needed to develop decompression sickness. A significant problem is that the user has no indication of when the gas supply will fail. Also the users may forget that they are still exposed to the other hazards of scuba diving. In some resort areas, people are renting these devices to novices who have had no training and who may be medically unfit to dive.

## Safety and protective equipment

The best safety measures available to a diver are proper training and commonsense. Almost all accidents are preventable and the authors do not ascribe the popularly held belief that these accidents are attributable to an 'Act of God'. They involve human, predictable, and thus correctable, mistakes. This point is developed in Chapter 8 where deaths and accidents are considered. Several items of equipment which reduce the hazards of diving, or assist with coping with them, are discussed below.

## Emergency air supplies

Emergency air supplies can take a variety of forms. In the early days it was common to rely on **buddy breathing**, a procedure where two divers share an air supply. Analysis of diving accident statistics showed that this often did not work in an emergency. The use of a second regulator attached to the scuba set, often called an **octopus rig**, has many supporters. Neither buddy breathing nor an octopus rig will be of use if the diver with gas is not available or is unwilling to cooperate. For this reason, a second source of air to each diver without assistance is now favoured. For cave divers this may be a second scuba set. For divers who can reach the surface more easily, a small cylinder of air with an attached regulator, such as the device sold under the name *Spare Air*, is becoming a popular option. Other people rely on the air contained in their buoyancy vest. In some vests, there is a separate air supply and a valve that allows the diver to inhale air from the vest.

## Thermal protection

Thermal protection is needed in cold water or on prolonged dives to minimize the risk of hypothermia. The protection is normally provided by insulated clothing which reduces heat loss. The most common protection is a **wet suit**, made from air-foamed neoprene rubber. The water which leaks into spaces between the suit and the diver soon warms to skin temperature. Foamed neoprene has similar insulation properties to wool felt. Its effectiveness is reduced by loss of heat with water movement, and increasing depth. Pressure decreases insulation by reducing the size of the air sacs in the foam; at 30 metres, the insulation of a wet suit is about a third of that on the surface. The compression of the gas in the foam also means that the diver's buoyancy decreases as he goes deeper. He can compensate for this if he is wearing a buoyancy vest. If he is not, he needs to consider reducing his weights, but this will mean he is too buoyant when he is closer to the surface. The buoyancy and insulation of a wet suit decrease with repeated use.

The other common form of thermal protection is the **dry suit**. This is watertight and has seals round the head and hand openings: openings with waterproof seals to allow the diver to get into the suit. The dry suit allows the diver to wear an insulating layer of warm clothes. A gas supply and exhaust valve are needed to allow the diver to compensate for the effect of pressure changes on the gas in the suit. The gas can come from the scuba cylinder or a separate supply.

The diver needs training in the operation of a dry suit or he may lose control of his buoyancy. This can lead to an uncontrolled ascent, when the excess of gas expands, speeding the ascent. If the diver tries to swim down, the excess gas may accumulate round his legs. Then it cannot be vented off through the exhaust valve; the excess gas can also expand the feet of the suit and cause the diver's fins to pop off, so he can find himself floating on the surface with the suit grossly overinflated – a most undignified posture.

Heat can also be supplied to a diver to help him keep warm. The most commonly used systems include hot water pumped down to him in hoses; various chemical and electrical heaters are also available. External heat supplies are more often used by commercial divers.

## Buoyancy compensators

This consists of an air-filled bag attached to the scuba, or an inflatable jacket, called an ABLJ (adjustable buoyancy life jacket) worn by the diver. It allows the diver to adjust his buoyancy or bring him to the surface and support him. The ability to change buoyancy allows the diver to hover in the water and adjust for any factor that causes his density to increase (e.g. picking up some object on the bottom). A buoyancy compensator with a reduced maximum lift is needed in cave and saturation diving because, in these situations, it may be dangerous to ascend.

The best buoyancy compensators can be inflated from the scuba or a small separate air bottle which can also be used as an emergency air supply. A vent valve is fitted so the diver can reduce buoyancy by venting gas from the compensator. Divers can lose control of their buoyancy while ascending – as the diver starts to ascend the gas in the vest expands, so the lift increases and the rate of ascent increases. This may lead to the diver imitating a leaping whale and an air embolism may result from the rapid ascent. The second problem is that the diver surfaces when he should have stopped for decompression.

## Depth gauge

Depth gauge, a watch and waterproof decompression tables are needed if an unsupervised diver is operating in a depth/time zone where decompression stops may be needed. Electronic, mechanical and capillary gauges are all used as depth gauges by divers. Capillary gauges measure pressure by the reduction in volume of a gas bubble in a graduated capillary tube. Some gauges record the maximum depth reached by the diver during the dive. This feature aids the diver in choosing the correct decompression table. The need to check the accuracy of some types of gauges is often overlooked and faulty gauges have lead to divers developing decompression sickness.

## Decompression meters

Decompression meters have been designed to replace tables and to shorten decompression from a dive where time is spent at several depths. Use of tables, where decompression is calculated on the basis of all the time being spent at the greatest depth, may require a long period of decompression. The choice of decompression meters in the 1990s is rapidly expanding, the meters available being electronic and combining data from the depths and durations of the dive (and any recent dives). The meter has a display which advises the diver when he should ascend to the surface and, if he needs to pause during the ascent, for excess gas to be eliminated from his tissues. It generates this information by comparing the dive conducted with a program and decompression data stored in its memory. The design of these meters is considered in greater detail in Chapter 11, when the reader will be given a better understanding of the decompression theory involved.

## Contents gauge

The role of this gauge has been discussed above. It indicates the pressure and, by extrapolation, the amount of gas remaining in the supply cylinder.

## Communication lines

As a consequence of the risks in diving, it is generally considered to be foolhardy to dive without some method of summoning assistance. Most commercial divers do this with an underwater telephone or signal line. Divers who do not want the encumbrance of a link to the surface can dive in pairs, commonly called buddy pairs. Each has the duty to aid the other if one of them gets into difficulty. The common problem in the use of the buddy system is to attract the attention of the buddy if he is looking elsewhere. The partner can be called to assist if the pair is linked with a buddy line. A light, 2–4 metre line, clipped to each diver, is all that is required. A tug, or the drag of a body, soon attracts attention. The line causes little inconvenience to a considerate, capable pair and is less of a distraction than looking to see if the buddy is alright every few seconds. Some divers oppose buddy lines, placing their faith in some other method of calling for assistance. When diving in caves, a continuous line to the surface is needed so that it can be followed if the team of divers becomes disoriented, or when visibility is lost due to torch failure or disturbed silt forming an opaque cloud; each diver should be clipped to the main line.

> *A buddy line is a simple reliable method of summoning assistance.*

## Float line

A floating line, dragging downstream or -tide from the boat, will aid recovery of divers when they surface downstream. Some call this the 'Jesus line' because it saves sinners, i.e. those divers who have erred and surfaced downcurrent from the dive boat. This is not needed if a lifeline or pick-up boat is being used, or if the current is insignificant.

### Shot line

A shot line or shot rope is a line that hangs down from the dive boat to the bottom, with a weight at the bottom end. It may be used to guide the diver to his work and back and it can also be the centre for a circular pattern search. It is often marked with depth markers, which can be used to show the decompression stop depths. The diver can hold onto the line at the depth mark. A **lazy shot** line is a weighted line that does not reach the bottom and is used for decompression stops.

### Lead line

A lead line is often used to assist the diver on the surface. It leads from the stern of the boat to the anchor chain. It allows the diver, who has entered the water at the stern of the boat, to reach the anchor when the current is too strong for him to swim to it.

### Dive boats

Boats used for diving range from canoes to large specialized vessels which support deep and saturation diving. The facilities required depend on the nature of the diving but there are minimum requirements. In some conditions a second safety boat may be needed because divers may need to be picked up after drifting away from the main vessel.

**Propellor guards**, or a safe propulsion system such as a water jet, are desirable if there is any chance of the engine being needed during diving operations.

A **diving platform** or ladder is needed on most boats to facilitate the diver's return from the water. Consideration should also be given to the recovery of an unconscious or incapacitated diver. This can be very difficult from a craft with enough freeboard to be used for diving in a seaway. Recovery into an inflatable craft is often a safer alternative; the body can be dragged, rather than lifted, into the boat. Also, the air-filled hull is less likely to injure a diver than a rigid hull.

**Diving flags**, lights or other signals, as required by the local maritime regulations, should be available. These offer legal, if not physical, protection from the antics of other craft. In most areas, boat 'attacks' cause more deaths than shark attacks.

The **first aid kit** and **emergency medical equipment** (see Chapter 33) should be chosen depending on local hazards and the distance from assistance.

## Equipment for professional diving

This section deals with the more specialized equipment used by professional and military divers. Most of their tasks involve comparatively shallow depths. The tasks could be conducted with scuba gear of the type described above. Equipment needs to be fitted with communications to allow the diver to confer with the surface support. Communications operate better in air, and so are commonly fitted into a helmet or full face mask. In these devices the air flow may either be continuous or on demand.

More specialized equipment is used for some military diving where an element of stealth is required. For these tasks an oxygen rebreathing system, which can be operated with no tell-tale bubbles, may be used. In dealing with mines, stealth is again required to avoid activating the noise or magnetically triggered circuits. If the mine is too deep for an oxygen set, a rebreathing system with an oxygen/nitrogen mixture can be used.

For even deeper tasks, where oxygen/helium mixtures are used, some method of reducing the gas loss provides cost and logistic savings. This can be achieved by the diver using a rebreathing system or returning the exhaled gas to the surface for reprocessing.

### Breathing systems

For most tasks, the professional diver is working in a small area for long periods. Consequently, he does not need the mobility of the scuba diver. His air normally comes from the surface in a hose, either supplied from storage cylinders or compressed as needed by a motor-driven compressor. The cable for the communication system and a hose connected to a depth measuring system are often bound to the air hose. Another hose with a flow of hot water may also be used to warm the diver. It is normal for the diver to have an alternative supply of air in a cylinder on his back and this supplies him with air if his main supply should fail.

**Free-flow systems** were used in the first commercial air diving apparatus. The diver was supplied with a continuous flow of air, which was pumped down a hose to him by assistants turning a hand-operated pump. The hand-operated pumps have gone but the same principle is still in use. In the most common system, called a **standard rig**, the diver's head is in a rigid helmet, joined onto a flexible suit that covers his body. The diver can control his buoyancy by controlling the amount of air in the suit. The main problem with the system is that the flow of fresh air must be sufficient to flush carbon dioxide from the helmet. The flow required to do this is about 50 l/min measured at the operating depth, well in excess of that needed with a demand system.

The other problem associated with free-flow systems and the high gas flow is the noise this generates. In the early days, the diver was also exposed to the risk of a particularly unpleasant form of barotrauma. If the pump or air supply hose broke the pressure of the water tended to squeeze the diver's soft tissues up into his helmet. Fitting a one-way valve, which stops flow back up the hose, stops this. For deep dives, where oxygen/helium mixtures are used, the cost of gas becomes excessive. Equipment for reducing the gas consumed may be fitted. For example, the US Navy Mark 12 rig can be fitted with a rebreathing circuit incorporating a canister of carbon dioxide absorbent to purify the gas. The gas flow round the circuit is generated by a Venturi system that does away with the need for valves to control gas flow. The rig is converted into a rebreathing system, which has a separate set of problems that are considered in a later section.

**Demand systems** have been developed to gain the reduction in gas consumption expected from a demand valve system. They also have the facility for the diver to talk under water. Several types of equipment are in common use. One type uses a full face mask, which seals round the forehead, cheeks and under the chin. The back of the diver's head may be exposed to the water, as in the *Aga* mask, or covered with a wet suit hood that is joined onto the face mask, as with the *Bandmask* and derivatives. Another type is fitted in a full helmet. An oronasal mask in the helmet reduces rebreathing of exhaled air. The helmets are often less comfortable than the face masks, but give better thermal and impact

protection. In each case, a demand valve reduces the gas consumption compared to a free-flow system.

These helmets may also be used at greater depths, where helium mixtures are used. A return hose may be used to allow collection of the exhaled gas at the surface for reprocessing.

All the systems mentioned above have the major advantage, compared to a demand valve held in the mouth, of reducing the chance of the diver drowning. This is important if he loses consciousness or has a convulsion while breathing oxygen. Some decompression schedules allow the diver to breathe oxygen to reduce decompression time. The increased safety and the advantages of a clear verbal communication system have lead to the adoption of helmets by most diving firms.

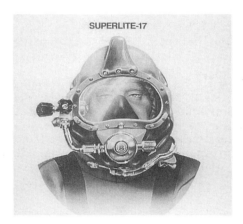

**Figure 4.3** The Superlite helmet made by Dive Systems International: the demand valve below the face plate releases gas into an oronasal mask to minimize the dead space. The knob on the demand valve allows the diver to adjust the valve to reduce inhalation effort. One of the valves on the diver's right is used to select the main or emergency gas supply. The second is used to release a flow of dry gas over the face plate to demist it

> *Sets that use helmets and full face mask reduce the risk of drowning and can allow the diver to converse with people on the surface.*

### Rebreathing systems

The major advantage of rebreathing systems is their economy of gas usage which is shown by the following example. In a demand system, a diver on the surface may have a respiratory volume of 20 l/min and an oxygen consumption of 1 l/min. He inhales 4 litres of oxygen per minute, and exhales 3 litres. This is lost into the water and is therefore wasted. A diver at 40 metres (5 ATA), consuming the same amount of oxygen, would have a minute volume of 20 litres at that depth which is equal to 100 litres at the surface. This contains 20 litres of oxygen and 19 of these are exhaled into the water and wasted. The oxygen wastage inherent in demand breathing apparatus is considerable even on the surface, and increases with depth. With closed circuit rebreathing equipment, the diver can extract all the oxygen in the supply. With semi-closed rebreathing systems, the wastage can be reduced to a fraction of that with a demand system.

The main disadvantage of rebreathing systems is that they are more complex than free-flow or demand systems and, in particular, they have a carbon dioxide absorbing agent which is prone to failure.

Due to the similarity between semi-closed and closed rebreathing sets, their common features will be discussed and then the points peculiar to each type will be discussed in separate sections.

The two common gas flow patterns found in rebreathing sets are shown in Figure 4.4. In the circuit set one-way valves are needed to control the direction of flow in the circuit.

Gas enters from a storage cylinder, through a flow-regulating device, into the breathing bag or counterlung and then to the diver. In most sets the flow regulator adds gas automatically. A manually controlled valve allows the diver to add extra gas; with this the diver can increase his buoyancy by adding the volume of gas in his breathing bag. He can also add fresh gas to dilute any contaminating gas in his set.

The breathing bag or counterlung is a gas storage bag which expands and contracts as the diver breathes. It normally incorporates a relief valve which releases surplus gas into the water and prevents excess pressure building up. Venting of excess gas is needed in closed rebreathing sets when the diver ascends and the gas in the counterlung expands. In semi-closed circuit sets there is a loss of excess gas through the relief valve.

The carbon dioxide absorbent is usually a mixture of calcium and sodium hydroxides. These chemicals react with carbon dioxide to form carbonates and water

$$M(OH)_2 + CO_2 \rightarrow MCO_3 + H_2O$$

**Closed circuit oxygen systems** are the simplest closed rebreathing sets. The breathing bag is filled with oxygen from the cylinder and, as oxygen is consumed, the volume of the bag

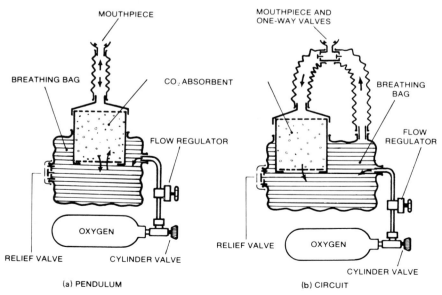

**Figure 4.4** Rebreathing oxygen sets

decreases. In some sets a trigger mechanism, which operates like a demand valve, releases more gas into the bag. In other sets there is a mechanism that releases a continuous flow of oxygen into the circuit. A manually operated method of adding oxygen to the breathing bag is also usually fitted. This will be needed when the diver puts the set on, when he goes deeper and the gas in the breathing bag is compressed, or when he needs to increase his buoyancy.

The set can be operated as a closed system because, unless something goes wrong, the gas in the breathing bag will contain a high concentration of oxygen, diluted with nitrogen that was in the lungs and body of the diver when he put the set on. It is standard practice to flush the set with oxygen at fixed intervals to prevent a build-up of diluting gases.

Possible problems with these sets include carbon dioxide toxicity if the absorbent fails, dilution hypoxia if the oxygen is impure or the diver neglects to flush nitrogen from his lungs and the counterlung, and oxygen toxicity if he descends too deep. To reduce the risk of oxygen toxicity, a depth limit of about 8 metres is often imposed on the use of these sets.

Closed oxygen rebreathing apparatus has the particular advantage that a small set may give long endurance. A set weighing less than 15 kg can allow dives of over 2 hours. The lack of bubbles and quietness of this set is also important in some specialized roles such as clandestine operations.

> *Rebreathing sets are quieter and have a greater endurance than compressed air sets. The extra hazards and costs involved restrict their use.*

**Closed circuit mixed gas systems** are comparatively new types of sets in which oxygen and a diluting gas are fed into the breathing loop at rates required to keep the oxygen partial pressure within safe limits, and to provide an adequate volume of the mixture. Figure 4.5 shows the fundamental features of this system. As with the oxygen set, the diver inhales gas from the storage bag and exhales through the carbon dioxide absorber back into the bag. As he uses oxygen, the partial pressure of oxygen in the bag will fall. This fall is detected by the oxygen sensor. At a certain level, a valve lets more oxygen into the circuit. If the volume of gas in the bag falls, a volume sensor triggers a second valve that adds diluting gas. Manual controls, and readouts indicating the oxygen concentration, may be fitted to allow the diver

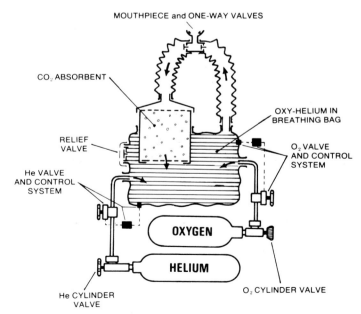

**Figure 4.5** Closed circuit, mixed gas, rebreathing set

to override the controls if the automatic valves fail. In some sets, he can also change from normal gas mixture to high oxygen mixtures to shorten his decompression time.

This system would appear to be the most efficient breathing system. It is more economical in terms of gas usage than any other equipment apart from the oxygen breathing apparatus. It enables a diver to go deeper for longer, and with less encumbrance than other equipment. As an example of the efficiency of this type of equipment, it has been stated that in a helium saturation dive programme involving a prolonged series of dives to 180 metres, the cost of helium for semi-closed diving apparatus was US$40 000. With a closed rebreathing apparatus, the cost would have been less than US$1000. These advantages must be balanced against the greater cost and complexity of the system; the latter can lead to fatal malfunctions.

**Semi-closed rebreathing systems** give some of the saving in gas obtained in the closed systems while avoiding the depth limits of the oxygen sets and the complexity of the closed mixed gas sets. The basic system as shown in Figure 4.4 can also be used for a semi-closed system, the main change being that a gas mixture is used instead of oxygen. The other component of the mixture, generally nitrogen or helium, dilutes the oxygen and increases the depth capability of the equipment.

In a typical semi-closed rebreathing system, the gas flow and composition are chosen for maximum efficiency for the proposed dive. First the composition of the gas is chosen, with as high an oxygen concentration as possible. A partial pressure of oxygen less than or equal to 2 ATA is generally used to prevent oxygen toxicity at the maximum depth. This level may be changed depending on the duration of exposure. The flow is then chosen so that the diver will receive sufficient oxygen while working on the surface.

These steps can be used in reconsidering the dive to 40 metres described above. A 40% oxygen mixture could be chosen (at 5 ATA the partial pressure of oxygen would be 2 ATA). If the maximum expected oxygen consumption on the surface was 3 l/min, then the flow would be set at about 12 l/min.

The oxygen concentration in the diver's inspired gas is an equilibrum between flow into the system, the diver's consumption and loss through the relief valve. It ranges from close to that in the supply bottle when the diver is resting, down to about 20% when the diver is working at the maximum expected rate. This ensures that the diver does not become hypoxic if he needs to surface rapidly.

A variety of methods has been devised to meter the fresh gas into the circuit. The example used above assumed a constant flow, and this may be obtained with a jet or valve if the flow through the metering device meets certain design conditions. In other sets, the flow is determined by the amount of gas the diver breathes, a small portion of each breath being lost into the water.

The semi-closed system with a flow of 12 l/min gives an eight-fold saving of gas compared with a demand system when the diver is consuming 1 litre of oxygen per minute. This saving would increase if the scuba diver was working harder and consuming more air. The high oxygen concentrations in these sets means that the diver may not absorb as much nitrogen as he would if he had been breathing air. This can give a decrease in the decompression needed.

Military divers are the main users of semi-closed sets. The reduced gas flow with these sets means that they can be designed to make little noise. If they are constructed from non-magnetic materials, they can be used for dives near mines.

The main problems with these sets have much in common with closed circuit equipment: carbon dioxide accumulation can occur if the absorbent fails; oxygen toxicity can occur if the diver exceeds his depth limit, or uses a mixture with too much oxygen in it; and hypoxia may result if the gas flow decreases, if the diver works harder than expected, or if a mix with too little oxygen is used.

## Chambers, habitats and underwater vehicles

Divers may use several special types of vehicles and living facilities. These include vehicles that are hoisted and lowered to transport divers to and from deep dive sites, propelled vehicles to increase the diver's range and endurance, and machines to carry underwater equipment. The accommodation to be considered includes underwater houses and pressurized houses at the surface.

**Submersible decompression chambers (SDC)**, often called personnel transfer capsules, are used to transport divers and any attendants from the surface to the work site, and may also be used as a relay station and store for gas and equipment. The most complex SDC may carry the diver at constant pressure from a deck decompression chamber to his work site, and back. The simplest SDC consists of a bell chamber that is open at the bottom and allows the diver to decompress in a dry environment, exposed to the same pressure as the surrounding water.

**Habitats** are underwater houses which accommodate divers in air- or gas-filled environments. They are used by divers to rest between excursions. Divers have lived in some of these habitats for weeks at a time.

**Deck decompression chambers (DDC)** can be small and used for surface decompression, a procedure that allows a diver to be decompressed in a dry chamber instead of in the water. Larger chambers can be used to treat divers with decompression sickness and other diseases that respond to compression; in this case the chamber may be called a **recompression chamber**. Deck decompression chambers are also used to house divers for prolonged periods under elevated pressure. In this case they are carried to their work by a submersible decompression chamber or a small submarine which keeps the diver in a pressurized environment; at the end of his job, possibly after several weeks, the pressure in the DDC is lowered slowly to return the diver to atmospheric pressure.

**Transport vehicles** can carry the divers at normal atmospheric pressure, at ambient pressure in a dry environment, or in a wet environment, including vehicles towed by a boat. A small motor and propellor which pulls the diver along gives increased speed with reduced effort. Some submarines have a lock system to allow divers to leave and enter under water.

**One atmosphere diving equipment** such as the **JIM** suit seals the diver in a pressure-resistant compartment. It has flexible arms with tools on the 'hands' for him to work under water. The early types of suit had legs that gave the diver the ability to walk on firm surfaces if there was little current. The diver had no control in mid-water and had to be lowered and hoisted from the surface. In other designs, such as the **WASP** system, the diver controls a set of propellers which make him a cross between a diver and a one-person submarine.

**Life support systems** are required to provide the occupants of all these vehicles, habitats and chambers with a respirable atmosphere. These work on the same principles as a diver's breathing apparatus, and in some vehicles he may even be wearing a breathing apparatus. The system must be self-contained for transport vehicles, but for habitats and submersible decompression chambers the gas is generally supplied for the surface.

Gas from the surface can be supplied in a free flow and escape out of the bottom or be recirculated through a purifying system. Simple gas purification systems can involve a hand-powered pump to force gas through a carbon dioxide absorption canister with a manually operated system for adding oxygen. The most complex systems are those found on large submersibles, nuclear submarines and chambers used for deep saturation dives. These have automatic closed systems with provision for removing trace contaminants and odours; they also regulate temperature, pressure and humidity.

**Gas reclaimers** are mainly used to recover helium for reuse. They help to lower costs by reducing the amount of gas used. One type cools the gas until the other gases are liquefied, leaving pure helium to be stored and used again. Other types use a chromatographic technique to separate the gases.

# Recommended reading

DAVIS, R.H. (1955). *Deep Diving and Submarine Operations.* London: St Catherine Press.

HAUX, G. (1982). *Subsea Manned Engineering.* London: Baillière Tindall.

PENZIAS, W. and GOODMAN, M.W. (1973). *Man Beneath the Sea.* New York: John Wiley & Sons.

*US Navy Diving Manual* (1988). NAVSEA 0944-LP-001-9010.

# 5

# The diver: stress responses, panic and fatigue

INTRODUCTION                    PANIC

PERSONALITY FACTORS             FATIGUE

STRESS RESPONSES                RECOMMENDED READING

## Introduction

Although compressed air diving has been possible for most of this century, it only became popular following development of the scuba equipment in the late 1940s.

At that time, only those who sought excitement and had a genuine love of the sea would embrace the sport of diving. Natural selection dictated that these would be aquatic people – with skills and personality suited to this and other water activities – the 'waterman' concept. Diving was merely an extension of this overall interest and ability.

In the 1960s, these 'natural' divers commercially exploited their talents and became instructors. They required of their trainees a level of water skills often in excess of that available to most people. Few trainees took up this challenge. Those who did were required to show personality characteristics that would be able to tolerate extremes of physical discomfort, environmental hazards and inadequate equipment.

During the 1970s, with increased availability of more user-friendly equipment, and the general change in attitude, away from the hunter/killer male chauvinist approach, there was a movement towards the ecologically aware and sensitive diver, equipped more often with a camera than a catch bag.

Thus the tough male stereotype of the pre-1960s was supplanted by the sensitive and sociable diver of the 1980s. The belief that diving should be available to all even resulted in a number of handicapped groups entering the scuba diving world. These included paraplegics, blind and deaf divers, as well as the introduction of 'friends of divers', i.e. children, members of the diver's family, other peer groups etc.

Some of the people now undertaking scuba diving are probably more accident prone – or at least less able to cope with accident situations – than those of the earlier years. New types of disorders are arising apart from the traditional diseases. The stress syndromes of diving are typical of these.

The ocean environment can be unforgiving, and may not make allowance for the personality of the new divers. Also, unfortunately, the user-friendly equipment may expedite diving training but promote new difficulties and dependency.

## Personality factors

The early divers were somewhat like the early aviators; they were adventure seekers, and often carried out their activities because of necessity. These included such groups as explorers, treasure hunters (salvage) and military divers.

With the increasing sophistication of equipment and the greater complexities of deep diving, the commercial divers of this decade are far more careful, obsessional and conscientious than their forebears.

The personality characteristics required for an amateur casual diver, who can choose the dive conditions and vary the duration, are quite different to those of the professional diver who may have to remain isolated in the underwater environment and be able to use underwater habitats for days or weeks at a time.

In this text, some of the observations that have been made on divers will be summarized.

### Traditional beliefs

A need for excitement, or environmental stimulus, is probably required for scuba diving.

Yarborough, in 1955, stated that the diver not only had to have an absence of physical defects, but should possess a stable psyche and a phlegmatic personality. The possession of a temperament free of alarmist characteristics was essential. This observation was later supported by the progressively increasing numbers of divers who died from 'panic'.

Dr Harry Alvis, in 1957, stated that divers were not the most normal of normal people. A special type of personality was required.

Sir Stanley Miles, in 1962, stated in the first sentence of his textbook on underwater medicine 'it is most important, right at the outset, to realize that the problems of man's adaptation to a watery environment are primarily those of temperament'.

Bowen and Miller, in 1967, stressed the hazardous nature of diving activities. Danger ('and drowning') was always one breath away. Cooperation was imperative for safety and yet the diver was necessarily a lonely person, dependent more on his own quick actions for his safety.

Caille (1969) stated that, of all divers, the greater physical and mental demands were made upon the military and naval personnel who fulfilled a combat role. There is only a small margin under water for deviations from normal health. No one could predict when and in what circumstances a candidate would be exposed to excessive stress (danger).

### Research observations

Many psychometric studies have been performed on divers, but as each group has different operational requirements, the results do not have widespread relevance. In general, full psychometric assessments probably do not have a predictive value that is commensurate with the time and cost of the investigations.

In most of the diving training during the 1950s and 1960s, there was a consistent 50% failure rate in **professional diving courses**. This meant that some sort of standard was being applied. In comparison, there is little or no failure rate in many of the recreational diving courses now being held – suggesting that few or no standards are really being applied, other than the ability to pay.

Ross, in 1950, conducted an investigation into Australian **Navy divers** and found that the characteristic required appeared to be sufficient self-control to face threatening situations, without disabling anxiety. He also noted the importance of an 'adventuresome approach, diligence in performing work, self-reliance, tolerance of discomfort and an indifference to minor injuries and illnesses'. Physical attributes such as stamina, athletic fitness and an affinity for strenuous effort were important.

In the training of the underwater demolition teams from the US Navy, **psychometric testing** revealed that mechanical and arithmetical comprehension were more highly correlated with success than other characteristics such as clerical ability.

Psychological tests on some groups of divers, such as **underwater demolition teams** (UDT), showed quite different traits to the tests performed on other diving groups. Nevertheless, there were some characteristics that continued to be present among most divers and these included objectivity, low neuroticism, aggression and self-sufficiency. Fear and anxiety were not acceptable characteristics.

Edmonds, in 1967, carried out a prospective assessment of 500 diving candidates, undergoing a diving course which had a 41% pass rate. A statistical analysis of the results showed that the diver was a psychologically stable, medically and physically fit individual who was not overtly worried by diving hazards, and had both the desire and ability to perform in the water environment. In comparison to the unsuccessful candidates, the diver was usually more mature, motivated by love of water sports (but not by adventure or comradeship), not fearful of the hazards likely to be encountered, physically fit, thick-set (high Cotton's Index of Build), a non-smoker and free of medical disorders, very capable of breath-holding and swimming, intelligent, self-sufficient, simple and practical.

Physical fitness, and especially aquatic fitness, were considered important characteristics for successful diving. A failure to complete a 200 metre swim in less than 5 minutes, without swimming aids, was an indicator of poor aquatic fitness.

After 3 years of detailed investigation, Edmonds had merely confirmed the anecdotal views of Yarborough and Ross, expressed many years previously.

Comparisons of divers to non-divers in the US Navy revealed that divers had less hospitalization for stress-related disorders, but higher for environmentally induced disorders. The interpretation that they did more but thought less is possibly an oversimplification.

**Different personality characteristics** are required for different types of professional diving. In saturation diving, the divers have to work together within a small enclosed area where an affinity and ability for teamwork and tolerance are needed. An abalone diver, who works in isolation for many hours each day, does not require such social skills (and often does not possess them). A navy diver who detonates or defuses underwater explosives needs good mechanical aptitude.

Divers performed quite differently on psychometric testing from their non-diving controls. Professional abalone divers, even in the 1980s, tended to be risk-taking types and this was shown up in the testing procedures carried out by Edmonds and his colleagues.

Similarly, the range of skills required for recreational divers varies with the type of diving. Nevertheless, self-reliance and a freedom from neuroticism (trait anxiety) seem common among all diving groups.

Morgan and his colleagues showed that **anxiety** (trait anxiety, neuroticism) was likely to predispose to panic response. **Introverted** people are more concerned with the exercise demands of diving, becoming more susceptible to exhaustion and fatigue, than extroverts.

## Stress responses

Stress responses assist in the survival of the species, but are of value to the individual only if not excessive. The stress response acts through the autonomic nervous system. This prepares the animal for 'fight or flight'. The respiratory and circulatory systems are stimulated, and there are biochemical and haematological changes to support this hyper-alert state. The animal is then ready for action in a state of high physiological excitation.

The stress responses can only be understood by having an appreciation of the complex interaction of human beings, technology and the environment in which it is used.

The reason that stress responses are ignored in most diving texts is that they are psychologically complex and ill-defined and do not lend themselves readily to academic study or pathological scrutiny. Nevertheless, they include three of the most common causes of accidents and deaths from scuba diving (see Chapter 8):

1. **Panic**: a psychological stress response related to anxiety:
2. **Fatigue**: a physiological stress response to exceptional exertion.
3. **Sudden death syndrome**: a pathological stress response of the heart (see Chapter 26 and page 85).

The induction of panic in the anxious diver, fatigue in the physically unfit and cardiac death in the medically unfit is more appreciated when one examines specific equipment problems (see Chapter 4) and environmental demands (see Chapter 7), and is cognisant of the diving and training techniques that influence these reactions.

## Panic

### Personality factors

Panic is a psychological response to stress and is probably the most common single cause of death while scuba diving. It is an extreme form of anxiety and is produced when an animal perceives or experiences a threat. The threat may be real (environmental or physiological) or imaginary (psychological). The latter can be as intense a stimulus in producing the stress response as the more obvious physical causes.

The psychological response of the diver to actual or perceived problems and hazards is based on his innate susceptibility (neuroticism). The diver must be aware of problems to be able to create an anxiety state of sufficient magnitude to be termed 'panic'. Under identical conditions, different divers will react in different ways, and those with a high anxiety tendency are more likely to react with panic.

Neuroticism is a measure of the individual's tendency to break down under stress. It is mainly inherited and can be assessed by various personality tests or by monitoring the physiological responses to stress. However, there are some divers who have specific anxieties to aquatic threats, e.g. drowning, claustrophobia, sharks etc., even with normal neuroticism levels.

Panic commences as a loss of confidence. The diver then experiences a loss of control over the situation, thereby producing a vicious circle in which further loss of confidence is experienced. Inappropriate behaviour very rapidly takes over, with the diver reaching a state in which self-preservation is threatened. Panic was implicated as a significant factor in more than 80% of scuba diving fatalities surveyed in Los Angeles County in 1970. It contributed to at least 39% of the deaths in the Australian survey of recreational diving fatalities.

**Anxiety** is often induced by certain diving tasks, especially those of buddy breathing, free ascent training, open ocean diving, diving alone etc., and it is known that the autonomic nervous system responses are exaggerated, before, during and after these experiences. As in all other diving techniques, repeated non-stressful diving experiences promote confidence and reduce the degree of generalized anxiety.

**Specific fears** or **phobias** associated with the diving and aquatic environments are also reduced by acquiring relevant experience. This is achieved by considerate and repetitive training under those environmental conditions. It is referred to by behavioural psychologists as 'conditioning' and it follows that a diver who is exposed to certain environmental conditions repeatedly, and with good tuition, in training and preparation for emergencies, is less likely to act irrationally or to panic when subsequently faced with those conditions.

Sensory deprivation can lead to the **blue orb syndrome** and is described in Chapter 29. Both this, and excessive sensory overload, will act by disrupting psychological equilibrium and predispose to panic. This can be made better or worse, depending on the thought processes of the victim. A beneficial influence will depend on such intangibles as volition, self-confidence, emotional stability, experience and aquatic skills.

---

*It takes as long to die from panic as it does to assess the situation rationally and initiate effective and corrective action.*

---

The sympathetic nervous system responses to fear will produce a terror-stricken facial appearance, pallor, dilated pupils, shallow rapid respirations, rapid jerky movements and irrational behaviour. The diver focuses excessive attention on either his equipment or the surface. All these can be observed by companion divers. The affected diver would add dyspnoea, palpitations and a sensation of panic to the symptom complex. Fear alone, without the addition of any other stress, can cause death.

There are many factors, any one of which can lead to a panic situation. Table 5.1 lists some of these which will be dealt with in more detail later. They basically all lead to a diver's inability to cope with his equipment or his environment. They tend to relate to each other. For example, if we look at the first cause in each column, it will be evident that a diver who is swimming against a tidal current will be

## CASE REPORT 5.1

### A composite report with many unwitting contributors

Nick was a recently qualified diver not using all of his own equipment, and diving in an area with which he was not familiar. He borrowed a wet suit, but it was a bit tight around the chest, restricting his breathing. He decided to overweight himself by two extra lead weights, because he felt that he may have some difficulty with descent under ocean conditions.

It was one of his first open ocean dives, and there had been some question regarding whether the conditions were suitable for diving. Even before entry into the water he was not entirely happy with himself.

Initially the dive was uneventful, other than Nick being a little apprehensive regarding his ability to outlast his companions. (*Note*: one of the more serious marine hazards is the diver who aims to dive deeper or longer, utilizing less air than his companions – thereby setting up a competitive situation and placing everyone in jeopardy, including himself.)

In this particular dive, Nick was convinced that he was using more air than his companions. This tended to aggravate his apprehension, and he spent considerable time wondering whether he was running out of gas. There was unfortunately no way to confirm this, as he was not wearing a contents gauge on the scuba regulator, and he felt that he was probably a long way from either the boat or the shore.

A mixture of inexperience and misplaced pride prevented him from surfacing to clarify his position, and at this time he noticed that he was becoming rather more anxious. His breathing rate increased and, as if to confirm his worst fears, he noticed a resistance to breathing through his regulator. He was then concentrating carefully on his breathing and noting that both it and his heart beat seemed to be fairly rapid. He considered the possibility of turning on his emergency reserve, and finally decided to do this, to see if it would have any effect on the respiratory difficulty.

A quick thought flashed through his mind that he was not enjoying this dive. He had spent a disproportionate amount of time either looking at his equipment, his buddy or the surface. He did not inform his companion that the reserve valve had been activated, hoping against hope that his companions would be equally short of gas. Another fear was that he was not making very much headway against the current, and he thought that he was probably still a long way from completing the dive, which would have brought him near a safe area to exit. He was now becoming far more apprehensive and there was greater resistance from the demand valve. He decided to leave his weight belt on for the moment, arguing that perhaps he could last out a little longer. He was becoming very anxious, with increased respiration and a greatly increased breathing resistance.

In fact, and putting it in its simplest terms, he was not getting enough air. The situation was serious. He decided to surface fast. During ascent, which was rapid but not rapid enough for Nick's peace of mind, he could see the surface, but despite previous assurances to the contrary he did not get a more adequate air supply as he ascended. He just reached the surface in time to wrench off his face mask and regulator, feeling about to 'blackout'. By expenditure of considerable effort he managed to keep his head above water for a few terrifyingly precious seconds before one of the small waves sloshed over him, with some getting into his mouth and causing him to cough. He struggled hard to maintain his head above water. Unfortunately, he was becoming very fatigued, exhausted, and wondered how long he could keep this up. Then strength and determination seemed to recede.

**Case report 5.1 (contd)**

His 'buddy' realized that Nick had disappeared, and after delayed reconnaissance of the area, he decided to ascend. By the time he reached the surface, Nick was no longer to be seen. His body was subsequently found within a few metres of where he had sunk (despite the tidal currents), with his weight belt still fastened, his buoyancy vest uninflated, ample air in his scuba cylinder – and at a distance so close to shore that he could well have swum under almost any conditions, using mask, snorkel and fins.

*Autopsy diagnosis*: drowning.
*True diagnosis*: death from panic.

Rereading the case history will reveal that anxiety and panic explains every facet; drowning explains only the final result.

more likely to become fatigued if he has reduced his efficiency by being overweighted. In some cases one factor will predominate, whereas in others a combination will produce the same eventual result. There are some circumstances in which any and all divers would panic. The art lies in avoiding these circumstances as much as possible and ensuring that your capabilities are not exceeded by the limitations of your equipment and the demands of the environment.

> 'A contented man is one who knows his limitations.'
>
> *An Old Man in a Pub*

Know your limitations and dive within them is a venerable admonition given to new divers. Every diver has certain limitations and apprehension is felt when he perceives these limitations are being exceeded. Then the first seeds of panic are sown.

## Fatigue

Fatigue is a common contributor to diving deaths (28%) and accidents, either due to personal, equipment or environmental problems which impose excessive demands on physical effort and result in exhaustion.

### Personal

Adequate physical fitness is essential in diving activities, which invariably, sooner or later, impose considerable physical demands. Fitness to undertake aquatic activities can be evaluated both by reference to past performance and present capabilities (swim speeds, breath-holding ability etc.). Age is associated with a reduction in physical fitness.

**Table 5.1 Contributors to panic**

| Personal factors | Equipment problems | Environmental hazards |
|---|---|---|
| Fatigue | Buoyancy | Tidal currents |
| Physical unfitness/disabled | Snorkel | Entry/exit techniques |
| Previous medical disorders | Face mask | Cold |
| Seasickness and/or vomiting | Weight belt | Surf |
| Alcohol or drugs | Wet suit | Kelp |
| Inexperience | Scuba cylinder | Caves, wrecks |
| Inadequate dive plan | Regulator | Ice and cold water |
| Techniques (buddy breathing) | Other equipment | Deep diving |
| Psychological characteristics | Reliance on equipment | Dangerous marine animals |
|    Neuroticism and anxiety | Loss of equipment | Poor visibility |
| Sensory deprivation | Misuse of equipment | Explosives |
| Vertigo and/or disorientation | Entrapment – lines | Boat accidents |
| Diving accidents | | |

In some situations, even unfit divers are not at risk. In others, even very vigorous, fit divers will be sorely tried.

Personality factors are also important. Given the same physical fitness and exercise load, the extrovert diver has more ability to ignore the environmental and physical demands, whereas an introvert is likely to be aware of the development of fatigue earlier. A neurotic diver, or one with high trait anxiety, will be more susceptible to fatigue at an earlier time than the more stoic diver.

Many other factors may influence the diver's fitness, such as the use of alcohol or drugs, the development of seasickness, medical disorders, diving accidents such as vertigo or disorientation, salt water aspiration etc.

## Equipment

The scuba cylinder, buoyancy compensator and other equipment cause excessive drag with normal swimming, regulators limit the respiration and protective suits limit movement. Greater swimming effort is needed to overcome negative buoyancy. Even experienced divers without assistance, supporting a 5 kg negative buoyancy (weights held above the water), can only remain on the surface for less than 10 minutes, before submerging.

## Environment

Most tidal currents in excess of 1 knot are beyond the capability of many divers for more than a few minutes. Cold exposure and hypothermia will aggravate fatigue (see Chapter 7).

*Note*: despite the plethora of reasons given for not diving – and the hazards described are only relatively few examples – it must have some positive aspects. Investigations into biochemical responses of experienced divers reveal that the 'buzz' hormones, plasma β-endorphins, are elevated during diving, but not with hyperbaric exposure per se. This response confirms our observations that diving is thrilling and hyperbaric work is boring.

## Recommended reading

BACHRACH, A.J. and EGSTROM, G.H. (1987). *Stress and Performance in Diving*. San Pedro, CA: Best Publications.

BACHRACH, A.J. and EGSTROM, G.H. (1990). *Diving Medicine*, edited by A.A. Bove and J.C. Davis, Chap. 12. Philadelphia: Saunders.

EDMONDS, C. (1972). *The Diver*. Project 2/72. Royal Australian Navy School of Underwater Medicine Report.

EDMONDS, C. (1987). *The Abalone Diver*. National Safety Council publication, Morwell, Victoria, Australia

EDMONDS, C. and WALKER, D. (1989). Scuba diving fatalities in Australia and New Zealand. Part 1. *SPUMS Journal* **19**(3), 94–104.

EGSTROM, G.H. (1990) In: *Diving Medicine*, edited by A.A. Bove and J.C. Davis. Philadelphia: Saunders.

MORGAN, W.P. and RAGLIN, J.S. (1989). Psychological considerations in the use of breathing apparatus. In *Proceedings of Undersea and Hyperbaric Medical Society workshop, Physiological and Human Engineering Aspects of Underwater Breathing Apparatus*, edited by C. Lundgren.

RESECK, JOHN JR. (1975). *SCUBA Safe and Simple*. New Jersey: Prentice Hall International.

# 6

# The female diver

## Introduction

Prior to the 1960s, diving was essentially a male-dominated sport. He was a tough adventurer, determined to prove his stamina and courage, while providing food for the little woman and the kids. He was able to demonstrate his ability as a hunter in the spearfishing massacres of the 1960s and 1970s.

During this period it was very common to see advertisements of a fully equipped male Adonis, standing majestically on a cliff top, spear gun held nonchalantly in one hand with a giant groper in the other. He was as much a victim of stereotypes as his bikini-clad mate, who gazed admiringly into his face, while resting her hand upon his forearm.

For those who were more attuned to slight deviations, there was also the occasional advert-ising poster showing an almost naked female glaring menacingly as she unsheathed her new diving knife or unbuckled her buoyancy compensator.

But the diving world was changing and the appearance of women divers was probably one of the significant factors in achieving this. Social activities have taken on a far more interesting aspect, and in the whole of the diving scene there is a greater warmth and brightness, gaiety and fun, and gentleness. There is now a diversity of interests in diving, and it no longer attracts the Neanderthal hunter who vandalized the marine environment. The reasons for diving now include an admiration of nature, photography, archaeology, exploration, marine biology etc.

There is no longer the need to argue the case for female divers. They did this very well for themselves and, during the 1960s and 1970s, there were a whole group of female adventurers who matched their male counterparts, fish for fish, depth for depth, thus undermining the supposed sexual dominance. During the 1970s and 1980s, a revolution of female instructors and scientists ensured the death of any belief in sexual bias in this sport.

Unfortunately, there are still some problems and, despite equality, the sexes are not identical. There must be some variations in the ability of males and females to adapt themselves to the diving environment.

## History of women in diving

Originally the shell divers of Asia were males. This changed hundreds of years ago – some say because of the better tolerance to cold exhibited by females, whereas others attribute it to the folklore that diving affects male virility. The Ama divers of Japan included some male divers, although they only dived during the summer months.

The Ama of Korea and Japan have been famous for their diving capability. They have dominated the breath-hold diving scene, and these women adapted well to their diving activities by increasing their basal metabolic rate, at least during the colder months, up to 30% above normal. This meant that they utilized more food to produce heat and energy which allowed them to endure the cold water. To conserve heat they developed increased body tissue insulation (about 10% above normal), a reduction in their blood flow to the skin (30% less than normal) and an ability to tolerate a lower water temperature before the shivering developed.

In Western society, there were both cultural and legal restrictions on the aquatic activities of females. In the early part of this century, it was customary to have the women swimmers bedecked in a full blouse plus skirt, long dark-coloured hose, rubber bathing slippers and a bathing hat. Presumably only a very competent swimmer would attempt to cope in the ocean with those restrictions!

In the 1940s, Simone Cousteau joined her illustrious husband, Jacques Cousteau, in using and becoming adept with the scuba apparatus called the Aqualung. Lottie Haas proved her expertise at diving and underwater photography, despite discouragement from her husband, the famous Hans Haas. She inspired others with her success in both roles in her autobiography *Girl on the Ocean Floor*.

In Australia, Valerie Taylor and Eva Cropp led a group of very enterprising and capable women who captured the admiration of the public with their skills and abilities at handling marine animals, immortalized in film and television productions. Dee Scarr demonstrated the same skills in the Caribbean.

Some female scientists excited the diving world. Eugenie Clark became known as the 'shark lady', because of her brilliant work in this field and Sylvia Earle, in 1969, led the first all-women team of aquanauts in the Tektite 2 habitat experiments. They stayed under water for 2 weeks in the Tektite habitat and were acclaimed for their diving and scientific professionalism. Sylvia showed rightful exasperation when she said, 'After Tektite, we were called aquanetts, aquabelles, aquachicks, aquababes, aquanaughties, and aquanuts. What would the reaction have been if newspapers had hailed the first lunar astronauts as "astronuts"?'.

Kati Garner was the first woman to graduate from the US Navy Diving School, which she did in 1973. Many others have successfully followed her.

Perhaps the most important contribution of women to diving has been in the instructional area. Many male instructors used the training period as an ego trip for themselves, denigrating the trainees' apprehensions, and issuing stories to demonstrate the instructor's prowess. With the advent of women instructors, there has been a removal of the old 'bravado' image of the instructor. Instead of a glib and deprecating response to questions, the diving trainee is now far more likely to be listened to, have his or her question considered and answered in a non-point-scoring way.

About one in three of the current trainees is a woman. The ratio of females in the diving death statistics is one in ten. Women divers are less likely to die than male divers, but to make the figures more meaningful the diving frequency of the sexes is needed.

# Scuba training

Experienced female divers are similar in personality profile to other highly trained athletes, and to other established divers. The average female, however, is not the adventurer described above, but a normal young woman who wishes to develop skills in a sport that had traditionally been considered to be a male activity. The society stereotype would suggest that she is more dependent and less self-reliant than her male counterpart, and also less mechanically minded and perhaps less physically strong. Although these observations may be correct, it need not be so.

As regards physical strength, experience and training are far more important than sexual differentiation. In the 1924 Olympics, the men's record for the 400 metre free-style swim was 16% better than the women's. In the 1972 games the difference was only 7% and the women in the 1970s were swimming faster than the men in the 1950s. This demonstrates the dominating effect of training over gender.

The technical/mechanical/mathematical training of girls is not as adequate as that of boys. Thus they have less self-esteem in these areas.

The dependency role of the female is a very socially determined factor. In some societies (e.g. the Mundugamor of New Guinea) it is the opposite and it is not so in many areas of the USA, whilst still being very much the norm in other areas. Women who behave in a stereotyped and dependent manner, who avoid mechanical issues or who believe lifting heavy objects is a male prerogative are likely to perpetuate this problem.

Chauvinism still does exist in some diver training classes, and many of the older divers have unwittingly contributed to this. A woman who would only dive 'when someone could look after her' is an unfortunate result of this attitude. Annette Donner realized this, understood the cultural basis for its development and described it in her reports. The male diver, who assists the female trainee by assembling all her scuba equipment, carrying it down to the water and then making all the decisions before and during the dive, is denigrating her ability as well as denying himself the comfort of a competent dive buddy. Anyone who is treated in this way is unlikely to develop into a reliable diver.

Dale Cyphert, during the PADI seminar on 'Women in Diving' (1977), documented many of the problems in training female divers. Combining males and females as buddies during the classes is likely to encourage sex stereotyping which prevents adequate training for the female student. Many instructors realize the danger in pairing a woman with her partner.

There are three frequent problems that emerge from the male/female buddy system during training. First, the woman is likely to adopt a culturally determined role as the 'weaker buddy', and continue in this role. With the male being dominant, it is possible that the female diver would finish the course without ever having to carry tanks, gear up, correct equipment malfunctions or cope with many environmental demands without assistance. Following this, the woman is likely to be dependent on her buddy, rather than being a buddy.

The second problem is inadequate communication. A male, if faced with a problem, is likely to approach the instructor and discuss it with him. A female is more likely to turn to her equally ignorant male buddy to obtain assistance and instruction. In this situation the man acts in a knowledgeable way, failing to show the vulnerability that the woman feels. The result is that the male will often be given competent and full instruction, whereas the female may get inadequate or non-authoritative information. It is even possible that instructors direct their tuition towards males, in the belief that the male is more able to grasp the intricacies of problems and understand the mechanical solutions.

The third result of the male/female buddy combination is that the woman is less likely to have an image of herself as a competent novice diver. Instead, she sees herself as 'a person who is taking scuba lessons', or an 'apprehensive beginner diver' – a follower, rather than a diving equal. The decisions about whether it is safe to dive, the dive plan, variations in the plan, depth and direction changes etc. are more likely to be left to her male partner. The male, especially if he is a novice, may well delude himself that he is superior and therefore knowledgeable about both his and his female buddy's capabilities – thus endangering them both.

In this way, cultural pressures may work against the development of the competent female diver. It can be overcome with a pre-diving class, teaching water and snorkelling skills before scuba and instilling a 'can-do' attitude, ensuring that the female students pass the course entirely on their own merits.

Female instructors tend to be more conservative, considerate and perceptive than their male counterparts, more able to reassure the pupils and allay their fears. A large amount of the time is spent in direct physical contact between the instructor and pupil. This is seen with readjusting equipment, helping gear up, assisting balance when putting equipment on, the passage of equipment from one diver to another, buddy breathing, and especially when hand-in-hand buddy diving. The latter technique is very valuable to allay the anxieties of a pupil during the first few dives.

Physical contact is very reassuring to the anxious student diver. Women in our society tend to be less inhibited about person-to-person contact, and it is in this area that the male stereotype is at a great disadvantage. Male instructors may be more reticent, either because of their own inhibitions or because they are apprehensive that the contact may be misunderstood. Fortunately, like all other stereotypes, these are rapidly weakened by experience and the more experienced instructors, both male and female, will use a great deal of touch to ensure that the pupil does get the reassurance that he or she needs.

## Anatomical differences

There are definite differences between the sexes which affect their diving capability. Women have lower performance, with less cardiovascular, respiratory and skeletal capabilities. The average male differs from the average female in terms of strength, buoyancy, respiratory function, thermal protection etc. Nevertheless, in each one of these there is a great deal of cross-over with most men and women being equivalent.

If we consider **muscle strength**, on average the male is stronger than the female. The female is smaller, has less muscle mass and in many cases does not exercise as much. Until the age of 11–13, children have similar weights, often similar habits, and therefore the strength difference is not very noticeable. From that time, a hormonal factor comes into play, and a small but definite difference develops, both from this and from cultural teaching, i.e. males tend to play more active sports than females. However, the normal individual variation is such that it ceases to be relevant in the diving context.

The development of osteoporosis as women age may well contribute to the complications of dysbaric osteonecrosis in excessive divers – but this has not yet been verified.

Women, due to their smaller stature and smaller lung size, require less oxygen and produce less carbon dioxide. Their respiratory minute volume is less, and therefore they need to carry less compressed air, which means that they may not require as large a scuba cylinder.

As a consequence of different sizes and shapes, women do require slight changes in the male-oriented diving equipment. Using inappropriately sized equipment can produce greater problems, and this can be seen in difficulty with:

- Obtaining well-fitting good quality face masks.
- Having to use unnecessarily heavy and large scuba cylinders.
- Coping with a back pack that is so long that it anchors the weight belt to the waist.
- Having buoyancy compensators which are far too large, with excessive drag.
- Quality fins, which may need socks, wet suit bootees etc. to produce a tight fit.
- Ill-fitting wet suits.

The above limitations are now much less, because the manufacturers acknowledge the importance of the female market. The 1960s advice to 'just wear children's gear' is no longer acceptable.

## Thermal variations

Women are better insulated than men – they have a thicker adipose (fat) layer beneath the skin. Sedentary women in their late teens and early twenties have a body fat of about 25%, dropping to less than 15% in trained athletes. Comparative figures for males are 15% and less than 10%. However, these advantages are lost in lean females. Women also have a greater ability to constrict blood flow to the limbs.

Even though there is much debate, overall these factors result in a potentially slower heat loss and a natural buoyancy of women, enhancing swimming and survival abilities.

The ability to cope with cold water exposure is an adaptation, i.e. it can be acquired by practice. It is unfortunate that many women seem to be far more sensitive to cold water, probably because of the lack of previous exposures. The Korean Ama proved that females are able to adapt, but the likelihood in Western society is, however, that the females will expose themselves less to cold water, and therefore be more sensitive during the diving course. This can be corrected by appropriate training in the aquatic environment prior to the course.

The one area in which the female is definitely more susceptible is that of hyperthermia (being overheated, sun stroke etc.). Females have a smaller number of functional sweat glands, and tend to sweat later than males, making it more difficult for females to get rid of heat than males. This is easy to counteract in the marine environment, by just hopping into the water.

All of the above factors are relatively minor.

# Menstruation

Whether or not a woman dives during her menstrual period depends on how she feels. Over the 3–5 days, she is likely to lose between 50 and 150 ml blood and cellular debris. This is an insignificant amount physiologically, but there has been a great deal of fear that even this small amount may attract sharks. There is no support for this belief, and in fact female divers have a much lower incidence of shark attack than males. One hypothesis to explain this is that the haemolysed blood associated with the menses may act as a shark deterrent, and not the opposite.

For comfort's sake most women would not wear menstrual pads but tend to wear the intravaginal devices, such as tampons.

Although the menstrual cycle may have some psychological and physiological effects, reducing the fitness to dive in some cases, examination of the statistics in the Olympic Games during the 1970s showed no significant performance decrement at any specific stage of the menstrual cycle.

It has been conjectured that the fluid retention and oedema which develop before and during the menstrual period could increase the possibility of decompression sickness (DCS). Aviation DCS was shown to be more frequent during and soon after the menses, suggesting that extra decompression may be needed at that time. Susceptible females would be prudent to avoid or modify their diving if they have **psychological** or **physiological problems** during this time, such as anxiety, tension, depression, malaise and muscle cramps, nausea and vomiting, or a propensity to sea sickness etc.

Another disorder which sometimes has a marked increase in incidence during the menstrual cycle is that of **migraine**. If divers suffer from this, especially in the premenstrual period, it is worth while either avoiding diving or ensuring that they do not do anything that can aggravate or precipitate a migraine-type syndrome (see page 406).

At premenstrual and menstrual periods, there may be a **congestion of the mucosal membranes**, possibly associated with the oedema and fluid retention. When this happens it may be more difficult to equalize the middle ears (because of the eustachian tube congestion), and it may also predispose towards sinus barotrauma.

It must be reiterated that these are uncommon and usually mild associated features of menstruation. Many women notice that during their periods the flow and abdominal cramps are less while diving.

# Oral contraceptives

Oral contraceptives have a similar pharmacological effect, in many instances, to pregnancy. They may also have similar effects to the premenstrual period. As such, there is a series of possible or potential problems, analogous to those described above. It is commonly believed that the contraceptive pill will or could aggravate the intravascular problems associated with severe DCS. Because of this the Tektite 2 female team stopped taking these pills 3 months prior to their saturation dive.

# Decompression sickness

It was noted that nurses undergoing flight training at the US Air Force School of Aerospace Medicine had an increased incidence of **aviation DCS**. Both the original work of Bassett and his reassessment at a 10-year follow-up suggested that there was a four-fold greater incidence of DCS, which was statistically significant (at less than the 0.005 level) for altitude exposure. DCS also seemed to be more delayed in onset, and there were more instances similar to 'migraine' or with neurological features.

Nunneley questioned whether the male aviators would have had the same degree of stress in exposure to altitude as the female nurses. He also questioned whether the difference could be due to the different physical fitness of the two different groups.

Fife described some NASA experiments in which, with the same exposure, 18% of the women had circulating bubbles, but 9% had DCS, whereas 23% of the men had bubbles but only 6% had the bends. As there were only 14 men and 14 woman in the study, it was not statistically significant.

Susan Bangasser (1979b) carried out a survey of **women divers**, and the incidence of DCS was 3.3 times that of males exposed to the same dive profiles. The incidence of DCS among women divers was 0.033% per dive, compared to 0.007% for men, but these figures could not be controlled for the effects of physical fitness. There was no relationship found between DCS and either menstruation or taking the oral contraceptive pill. Comparisons of the cases of DCS, experienced at the US Navy diver training centre at Panama City, did not show any increase among females.

Hart et al. (1981) demonstrated a higher rate of nitrogen loading for females than for males, in both subcutaneous and muscular tissue.

With hindsight, the **decompression tables** were not designed for females and perhaps the increased adipose tissue of females may well enhance the absorption of nitrogen and thus increase the likelihood of DCS. It would therefore seem very reasonable to add conservative safety factors to the decompression tables when used by women.

A specific, but minor, problem can develop under special circumstances with **breast implants**. Obviously any implant that has gas spaces would enlarge or contract with ascent and descent, respectively. All current commercial implants do not have gas spaces, but the material does slowly absorb gas under pressure and may result in bubble formation during ascent. This may expand the breast implant by up to 4% in typical recreational diving – probably insignificant. Decompression from saturation caused a 7–47% increase in exposures tested and may have implications for professional diving.

# Pregnancy

The question as to whether a pregnant woman should dive has created a great deal of concern. Exercise, as such, is not contraindicated in pregnancy – except for high-risk cases. There is a fear that the hyperbaric and diving environment may cause problems for the pregnant female and to the developing fetus. Nevertheless, the problems are complex, and the final decision must be left with the diver.

Although only 25% of the current diving population are women, they are mostly in the child-bearing age, and many are such enthusiasts that a 9-month interruption is not appreciated. For those whose career involves diving, the 9-month interruption is sometimes very disruptive.

There may be a conflict between personal liberty and a safe conservative attitude. It is likely that those who insist upon the former will continue to dive no matter what advice is given. It is also likely that the latter will not dive, because it could never be proven to be 100% safe.

The reason for concern is based mainly on general problems, animal experiments and the extrapolation from our knowledge of other situations that may influence the health of the pregnant mother and/or the fetus.

### Potential problems of the pregnant diver
(after Lanphier, 1987)

### *Maternal factors*

- Morning sickness and motion sickness
- Reduced respiratory function
- Circulatory competition with placenta

- Altered sympathetic response
- Reduced fitness and endurance; unusual fatigue
- Size: fit of suit, harness etc.; clumsiness leading to injury
- Effects of lifting heavy weights
- Increased fat and fluid – increased susceptibility to DCS
- Mucous membrane swelling – difficulty in equalizing middle-ear and sinus spaces

### Fetal factors

*General*

- Hypoxia from various mishaps
- Hyperoxia – blindness?, closure of ductus?, haemoglobin breakdown?, consumptive coagulopathy?
- Exercise hyperglycaemia; post-exercise hypoglycaemia
- Exercise hyperthermia
- Physical injury
- Leaking membrane – infection
- Marine animal envenomation– direct or indirect damage
- Decompression – bubbles – altered placental flow

*Early*

- Malformation related to maternal DCS
- Teratogenic effects of pressure: ?oxygen, ?nitrogen, ?dive-related medications, ?bubble formation, ?other
- Recompression treatment – exceptional exposure to $O_2$ and $N_2$
- Decompression – bubbles – birth defects

*Late*

- Prematurity (Ama diving)
- Decompression – stillbirth

Maternal bubbles are likely to be filtered as the blood passes through the lungs. In the fetus, the blood bypasses the lungs and goes direct through the ductus arteriosus and the open foramen ovale. Therefore, any bubble that does form in the fetus is potentially a life-threatening embolus if it enters the brain or heart, or it may cause damage wherever it lodges.

> *ANY bubbles in the fetus are more ominous than MANY bubbles in the mother.*

### General

*Maternal effects*

During the first trimester, and especially between the sixth and twelfth weeks, there is a variable but definite increased incidence of nausea, vomiting, gastric reflux and a propensity to sea sickness. These contribute to diving accidents and deaths (see Chapter 8).

From the fourth month onwards, there tends to be fluid retention and mucosal swelling, thereby making the middle-ear and sinus equalization process more difficult, and predisposing to barotrauma.

During pregnancy there is a progressive interference of respiratory function. The tidal volume increases at the expense of the expiratory reserve volume. There is also a progressive difficulty with the oxygenation of the blood flow through the lungs, and an increase in the resistance to airway flow. The latter may increase up to 50%, and is probably due to the effect of progesterone aggravating bronchoconstriction. The results of this respiratory impairment may be to reduce the woman's ability to cope with strenuous activity, and perhaps to increase the likelihood of pulmonary barotrauma.

The possibility of DCS during pregnancy may be increased by the increased blood flow, increased fluid retention, increased total body fat and increased blood clotting mechanisms.

The change in shape of a pregnant woman may have unfortunate side effects. The wet suit must be altered, to ensure that there is not any increased abdominal tension which will push the diaphragm even further up into the thoracic cavity, and aggravate the respiratory difficulties. The weight gain and the change in posture results in the woman being more unbalanced. Weight belts are difficult to position and dive exits are more difficult.

During the last 3 months there are a number of pregnant women who 'leak' amniotic fluid through the membranes of the fetus into the vagina, without being aware of it. They presume this slight discharge is normal. Unfortunately, should sea water gain entry to the womb, it would carry the danger of infection and/or premature labour. This is verifiable by testing with litmus, because the normal vaginal secretion is slightly acid whereas the fetal amniotic fluid is slightly alkaline. The possibility of uterine infections after the birth of the child must also be considered.

A variety of uncertain hypotheses to explain an increased risk of DCS in pregnant females has been presented, which these authors find difficult to interpret. They include:

- An increased blood flow in pregnancy which might increase the rate of gas transferred to tissues.
- The pressure of the distended uterus on the iliac veins and inferior vena cava which might reduce blood flow from the lower extremities, and interfere with the elimination of gas.
- Supine hypotension, tight-fitting wet suit, weights, weight belts or buoyancy compensator (BC) which have been considered as potential vascular restrictions.

### Psychological effects

The pregnant woman has many hormonal and psychological changes occurring during her pregnancy and postpartum period. It is likely that it is more difficult to learn any task during these periods, and the pregnant woman and the postpartum woman are likely to be far more emotional and anxious than non-pregnant women. Many women will find that they are not comfortable learning to dive during pregnancy and even many experienced female divers find that they are very apprehensive when diving for some months after the birth of the child.

### Effects on the fetus

During the first 3 months of pregnancy, the blood supply to the developing ovum is similar to that of other tissue. Unfortunately, diving may cause a reduction in oxygen levels of the blood, and one of the major problems for the fetus is hypoxia. This is believed to increase the possibility of both miscarriage and birth abnormalities. Oxygen transfer to the fetus across the placenta must be rapid and continuous to ensure successful growth.

Heavy exercise, stress or any increase in catecholamine levels, at least temporarily, reduces the uterine blood flow.

Hypoxia will develop in the pregnant female, as it will occur in any other diver, through salt water aspiration (from buddy breathing, inhaling of salt water on the surface, being towed, faulty demand valves and regulators etc.), but also due to the changes that develop within the pregnant female lungs (with the amount of blood going through the lungs exceeding the ability of the lungs to oxygenate it).

Later in pregnancy, following the development of the placenta and the special haemoglobin states which characterize the developing fetus, the fetus is more protected against changes in oxygen levels of the mother's blood. It may not, however, be able to accommodate the very significant drop in oxygen following salt water aspiration. There is also a fear that an impaired oxygen supply may result in hyaline membrane disease of the newborn child.

Other gas concentrations may also be altered in divers, e.g. an increase in the carbon dioxide levels due to the resistance of breathing with scuba, and a rise in the nitrogen level, which happens with all air diving. The harmful effects on the fetus, experienced with nursing sisters who inhale small quantities of anaesthetic gases in operating rooms, may well be analogous to the effect of breathing nitrogen under higher than normal pressures (nitrogen narcosis).

The fetus is susceptible to damage by many extraneous influences. It is this disruption of development that has prompted many women to avoid other toxins during their pregnancy, such as smoking, alcohol, stimulants etc. Other drugs which are incriminated include decongestants and anti-seasickness tablets, which are often used during diving activities.

Perhaps the most significant worry has been the speculation that either bubble formation (DCS) or hyperoxia (oxygen poisoning) may severely affect the developing fetus causing either abnormalities or death. Bubbles from DCS are less likely to be tolerated in the fetus, who cannot get rid of them, than in the mother, who can filter them out in the lungs.

In the fetus, the blood is shunted around the lungs and liver by special blood vessels, which only close once the oxygen level of the fetal blood is increased. There are two problems with this. First, the DCS could be more severe and destructive in its effects and, secondly, if the fetus is given a higher oxygen level (by the mother diving under water, or being given hyperbaric therapy), then these vessels could close prematurely and this causes another series of developmental problems in the fetus. A further possible effect of high maternal oxygen levels is to produce blindness in the fetus from retrolental fibroplasia.

## Animal experiments

Attempts to derive guidelines from animal research have shown conflicting results. DCS affecting the fetus was first observed by Haldane.

In 1968, McIver compressed female dogs to 50 metres (165 feet) for 30–120 minutes. Although the adults had serious DCS, only 4 of the 193 fetuses were affected. In 1974, Chen conducted a study on rats and produced similar results.

Because of the doubt regarding the ability to detect small bubbles in these studies, and the great difference in placental characteristics between these species and humans, Fife et al. (1978) from Texas A & M University experimented on pregnant sheep. This placenta approximates the human placenta more closely. The results were disconcerting: operatively they inserted Doppler flowmeters around the umbilical vessels. In all dives greater than 30 metres (100 feet) which exceeded the limits set by the US Navy tables, the ewes developed no circulating bubbles, but the fetuses were affected. The 30-m dive for 25 minutes (i.e. within the US Navy tables) also produced bubbles in the fetus. Even the 18-m (60 feet) dive produced some bubbles in the sheep fetuses. Although they were classified as threshold bends, the bubbles were clearly present. Several of the sheep aborted or delivered within 12–24 hours after a dive in which the fetus developed the bends (which was treated). It is not known whether these were induced miscarriages or early deliveries.

When these experiments were repeated, by Stock et al. in 1980, and Nemiroff et al. in 1981, it appeared that the insertion of the flowmeter itself could precipitate the bubble formation in an exposed animal. Thus the Texas work was brought into question, until in March 1985, Powell and Smith produced essentially the same results as Fife, but by detecting the fetal bubbles non-invasively.

Hyperbaric oxygen induced developmental abnormalities, abortion, stillbirth or birth defects in some studies. Hyperbaric oxygen effects on the fetus of rats by Miller, and rabbits by Fukikura, showed cardiac abnormalities and retrolental hyperplasia. Experiments attempting to demonstrate the damage of normobaric oxygen and hyperbaric air at moderate depths have been less informative. Studies by Bolton on rats and sheep did not verify the increased birth defects in animals, but required much larger numbers of animals than she had to draw conclusions.

If the mother developed DCS, bubbling in the fetus would presumably be more likely. Lehner et al. showed that all lambs delivered soon after maternal DCS were stillborn. Willson et al. showed that, if DCS develops in the mother, the likelihood of producing death of a fetus increases with the increasing maturity of that fetus. Explosive decompression also caused abortion in pregnant sheep.

Gilman et al. exposed hamsters to repetitive air dives and deduced that both DCS and deep air diving had harmful effects on the fetus. During early pregnancy, DCS in the mother produced frequent and severe teratogenic effects among the fetuses. At least one fetus from each female exposed to these conditions had serious malformations. The fetuses in the females who did not develop DCS were significantly smaller than the non-diving controls.

Alternatively, exposure of pregnant hamsters to hyperbaric oxygen, to approximate the treatment required for DCS, was found to have no adverse effect on fetal development or survival. Fetuses from females who were treated for DCS did not differ from controls.

It can thus be seen that there are conflicting reports from animal experiments, and these have not really clarified the situation for the pregnant woman.

## Human data

Investigation of the Ama, the free-diving females of Korea, suggested that both hypoxia and bubble production under certain conditions were potential problems for the fetus. The breath-holding Ama divers who dive up until a few days before childbirth have a 44.6% incidence of prematurity with an infant of less than 2.5 kg (compared to 15.8% in the non-diving females from the same district).

Susan Bangasser, in 1977, followed up a group of women who were pregnant when they were diving. Approximately 72 women were thus questioned, and it was found that more than one-third stopped during the first trimester (when they found out they were pregnant), more than one-third stopped in the second trimester mainly due to the increased size, but 20% continued diving. Most were very seasoned and competent divers. The deepest dive was 54 metres (180 feet) and there were five decompression dives performed. All babies were normal; however, there were some complications – one premature birth, one septic abortion, two miscarriages and two caesarian sections.

Margaret Bolton (1980) from the University of Florida carried out a survey of the effects of diving while pregnant. Information was collected on 20 women who had dived during pregnancy. There was a raised incidence of: abortion, stillbirth, low birth weight, death of the newborn in the first 28 days of life and congenital abnormalities. Among the 24 women who had reported diving to 30 metres or more, 3 had congenital defects. Although congenital abnormalities are a fact of everyday life, the incidence is normally about 1 in 50 pregnancies; therefore there would only be an even chance of one birth defect arising. The actual figure was thus six times higher. It is very difficult to draw conclusions from such low numbers, and Miss Bolton herself was cautious of such extrapolation.

Nevertheless, some of the congenital abnormalities were rather uncommon and specific case reports were worrying. One of Bolton's cases had a hemivertebra, one an absent hand and these two were from divers who dived in excess of 30 metres. Four others had congenital malformations (two with congenital heart disease and two with minor abnormalities). There were no recorded malformations in the babies of the mothers who did not dive during the pregnancy (69 controls, 109 subjects). More than 6% of the babies in the diving group were small for their presumed age, compared with only 1.4% in the control group.

Compared to their own controls, and to the population of the fit young women having children, Bolton's series is a cause for great concern, although it is not absolute proof in itself.

A Scandinavian study by Bakkevig et al. (1989) was made on 100 pregnancies in divers, 34 in which diving was continued and 66 in which it was not. The diving exposures were associated with five birth defects and the non-diving with one. The incidence of infant anomalies was thus 15% in the diving group and 1.5% in the non-diving group. None of the divers had DCS and the incidence of other pregnancy-related problems was the same in each group.

Jillian Turner and Ian Unsworth from Sydney, Australia, reported the case of a mother who dived 20 times in 15 days, during the end of the first trimester. Most dives were 18 metres or less and three were to 30 metres; one was to 33 metres. There were no diving accidents although there was one incident of rapid ascent. The only medication used was pseudoephedrine (Sudafed) on two or three occasions. The fetus had unusual malformations and the embryopathic timetable would suggest that the damage occurred around day 40–45 – she dived between day 40 and 55. Abnormalities in the fetus were a unilateral ptosis (drooping eyelid), a small tongue, micrognathia (a small lower jaw) and a short neck; the penis was adherent to the scrotum; the fingers were in fixed flexion with webbing between them and the thumb was abnormal; the hip joints were dysplastic and had a reduced range of movement, one hip being dislocated; and there were flexion deformities of the knees and other abnormalities of the feet. Arthrogryposis was present and presumed to have resulted from either muscle disease or abnormalities of the cells forming the anterior root ganglion, so the same embryopathic timetable may be applicable.

The toxicity to hyperbaric oxygen in the fetus, when the maternal animal has been exposed to it, may have implications in the rather worrying possibility of having to treat a pregnant female diver in the hyperbaric chamber, with either hyperbaric oxygen or, alternatively, hyperbaric air at a greater depth. Assali demonstrated gross changes in oxygen tensions and fetal blood flow, tending to neonatal patterns, when the mother is exposed to hyperbaric oxygen.

Nevertheless, about 800 pregnant women

have been treated in recompression chambers in Russia, with and without hyperbaric oxygen; it is not known whether these had significant problems such as premature closure of the ductus arteriosus, decreased placenta perfusion, increased pulmonary arterial pressure, retrolental fibroplasia etc.

Although we must be aware that the case against diving during pregnancy is as yet unproved, no one really wants to be associated with similar case histories, or their treatments.

> *The physiological implications of diving while pregnant are an academic's dream. But the answer is NO.*

## Recommendations

A number of researchers have recommended that if scuba diving be performed during pregnancy it should be limited to shallow depths.

For those who do consider that it can probably be continued, most would recommend the maximum depth of 9 metres (30 feet) or less. They would also agree that there should be a strict buddy diving situation, it should only be carried out in sheltered and safe areas and should be limited to those who are already skilled in this sport – thereby decreasing the physical exertion required, the incidence of diving accidents and the likelihood of salt water aspiration.

The Undersea Medical Society in 1978 held a workshop on this subject and it was recommended that, until further studies were made, women who are or may be pregnant should be discouraged from diving. The conclusion, promulgated by Lanphier in 1983 and supported in the Societies' Symposium on Women in Diving in 1988, was as follows:

1. Diving can increase the incidence of birth defects.
2. Fetal resistance to bubble formation (DCS) is offset by the dire consequences of this.
3. Maternal DCS late in pregnancy entails a higher risk of stillbirth. The risk may be increased by recompression.

There are insufficient hard data to say, unequivocally, that diving will produce danger to the fetus. Unfortunately, there is enough evidence to suggest that this could well be so. A 9-month respite from diving seems a small price to pay for a healthy child. Alternatively, a birth defect, with the possibility that it was caused by diving, would be a heavy burden, outweighing any benefit that diving in pregnancy could possibly confer.

These authors respect and commend Lanphier's conclusions.

## Recommended reading and references

BANGASSAR, S. (1979). Physiological concerns of women SCUBA divers, *I.Q. Proceedings*.

BANGASSAR, S. (1979b). Incidence of decompression sickness amongst women SCUBA divers. *Undersea Medical Society Proceedings*, Miami, June.

BAKKEVIG, M.K., BOLSTAD, G., HOLMBERG, G. and ORNHAGEN, H. (1989). Diving during pregnancy. *Proceedings of the 15th Annual Meeting of the EUBS*, Eilat, Israel, pp. 137–142.

BOLTON, M.E. (1980). Scuba diving and fetal well-being. *Undersea Biomedical Research* **73**.

COLE, M. (1988). Women and diving. *South Pacific Underwater Medical Society Journal* **19**(2), 56–60.

FIFE, W. (Ed.) (1987). *Women in Diving Workshop*. Bethesda, MA: Undersea and Hyperbaric Medical Society.

FIFE, W.P., SIMMANG, C. and KITZMAN, J.V. (1978). Susceptibility of foetal sheep to acute decompression sickness. *Undersea Biomedical research* **5**(3), 287–293.

HARASHIMA, S. and IWASAKI, S. (1965). Occupational diseases of the Ama. In: *The Physiology of Breathhold Diving and the Ama of Japan*, edited by H. Rahn. Washington DC: National Academy of Science.

HART, G.B., STRAUSS, M.B. and WELLS, C.H. (1981). Nitrogen loading in the human at 2 ATA air. *Undersea Biomedical Research* (Suppl.) **8**(1).

HUNT, W. (1979). In: *Fathom Magazine*. US Navy publication.

LEMON, R.A. (1978). Train Women Divers. *Undercurrent* **3** (12), 10–12.

PADI (1977). *Proceedings of the PADI Women in Diving Seminar*. Santa Ana, CA: PADI.

RANKIN, J.H.G., LANPHIER, E.N., STOCK, M.K. and ANDERSON, D.F. (1980). SCUBA diving in pregnancy. *7th Symposium on Underwater Physiology*.

TAYLOR, M.B. (1990). In: *Diving Medicine*, edited by A.A. Bove and J.C. Davis. Chap. 13 Philadelphia: Saunders.

ZWINGELBERG, K.M., KNIGHT, M.A. and BILES, J.B. (1987). Decompression sickness in women divers. *Undersea Biomedical Research* **14**(4), 311–317.

# 7

# Undersea environments

## Introduction

For the diver who is adequately trained and physically fit, who is aware of the limitations of his equipment and who has given attention to the specific requirements of different environmental diving conditions, the sea is rarely dangerous. Nevertheless, it can be hazardous and unforgiving if attention is not paid to all of these factors.

The induction of fear in the inexperienced and physical stress in the more skilled diver is easily appreciated on examination of each specific environmental situation and on becoming cognisant of the specialized techniques that are recommended to cope with them. These techniques will be mentioned in this and other chapters. The reason for including them in a medical text is that, unless the physician has some comprehension of the problems and dangers, his diving medical examinations and understanding of diving accidents will be less than complete.

Some aspects of the environment have physiological and pathological sequelae, and therefore have specific chapters devoted to them, e.g. the effects of cold (see Chapter 22), altitude and fresh water diving (see Chapter 2), explosives (see Chapter 25), depth (see Chapters 2, 3, 15, 16), marine animal injuries (see Chapter 24) etc. These receive little mention here. Others, which are covered more fully in diving texts, are considered in this chapter.

# Water movement

Because of the force of water movement, a diver can become a hostage to the sea.

## White water

The foaming effect of air bubbles or white water dramatically interferes with both visibility and buoyancy, as well as implying strong currents or turbulent surface conditions. A diver in white water is a diver in trouble. Under these conditions, the recommendation is usually to dive deeper.

## Surge

The to-and-fro movement or surge of water produces disorientation and panic in inexperienced divers who often try to swim against it. Others use the surge by swimming strongly with it, then holding on to rocks or corals when the surge moves in the opposite direction.

## Pressure gradients

Occasionally there is a continuous water flow, because of a pressure gradient through a restricted opening, which can siphon and hold (or even extrude) the diver. It is encountered in some caves, blue holes or rock areas near surf (an underwater 'blow hole'), in artificial structures such as the water inlets in ships' hulls, and outlets in dams and water valves. The pressure gradient may slowly draw the diver into the opening and then seal him, like a bath plug. Protection is by avoiding the area or covering it with a large grating.

## Tidal currents

These are very important to the diver. If used wisely, they take him where he wants to go. Otherwise they are likely to take him where he does not want to go. The latter event can be both embarrassing and terrifying, and it can also be very demanding physically.

Divers commonly relate their successful swims against currents of 4–5 knots. In fact, the average fast swim approximates 1.2 knots; for brief periods, it may be possible to reach up to 1.5 knots. The average swimmer can make very slow progress or none at all against a 1-knot current. A 0.5-knot current is tolerable, but most divers experience this as a significant problem, and so it is. They tend to exaggerate its speed as the hours go by, and especially during the après-dive euphoria.

Tidal currents are usually much faster on the surface than they are on the seabed. A helpful observation is that the boat will usually face the current with its anchor upstream and the stern of the boat downstream. Any diver worth his salt knows that it is safer to swim against the current for the first half of his usable air, and allow the current to bring him back to the boat for the second half of the dive. The **'half-tank' rule** is worked out by taking the initial pressure, say 200 ATA (3000 lb/in$^2$ or 20.7 MPa), subtract the 'reserve' pressure, say 40 ATA (600 lb/in$^2$ or 4.1 MPa), i.e. 160 ATA (2400 lb/in$^2$ or 16.6 MPa) and divide this by 2, i.e. 80 ATA (1200 lb/in$^2$ or 8.3 MPa). Thus for this example 80 ATA or 1200 lb/in$^2$ or 8.3 MPa is used on the outward trip and then the return is made.

Untrained divers tend to make unplanned dives. They submerge and 'just have a look around'. While they are having their look around they are being transported by the current, away from the boat, at a rate of 30 m (100 feet) every minute in a 1-knot current. When they consider terminating the dive, after they have used most of their air, they have a very hard return swim against the current; they have to surface, because of their diminished air supply, well downstream from the boat. This is a very difficult situation, and far more hazardous than that of the experienced diver who used the 'half-tank' rule, who surfaced upstream from the boat and floated back to it – but who also had enough air to descend underwater and return with ease if he wished.

The **lines** attached to the boat are of extreme importance when there are currents. First, there is the anchor line, and this is the recommended way to reach the seabed upstream from the boat. The anchor chain should not be followed right down to the anchor because this may occasionally move, and can cause damage to surrounding divers. More than one diver has lost an eye from this 'freak accident'. How may the diver reach the anchor line? A line may be attached to the top of the anchor line, and the other end to the stern of the boat. It should have enough play in it to allow divers to sit on the side of the boat and to hold it with one hand – the hand nearest the bow of the boat – using the other hand to keep the face mask and demand valve intact. On entry, he ensures that he does not let go of the line. He then pulls himself forward along this lead line to the anchor line, and descends.

Perhaps the most important line is a float line, or 'Jesus line'. This drags 100 metres or more behind the boat, in the direction of the current, and has some floats on it to ensure that it is always visible to divers on the surface. It is often of value to have one diver on this line while the others are getting into the water. He virtually acts as a back stop to catch the odd stray diver who has not followed instructions and is now floating down current. The Jesus line is also of immense value at the end of the dive when divers have, incorrectly, exhausted their air supply or when they come to the surface for some other reason and find themselves behind the boat. This would not have happened had a dive plan been constructed and followed correctly. Occasionally, however, it does happen to the best divers and it is of great solace to realize that the Jesus line is there, and ready to save the sinner.

Even divers who surface only a short way behind the boat in a strong surface current may find that it is impossible to make headway without a Jesus line. Under these conditions, they can descend and use their compass to swim back to the anchor line or inflate the buoyancy compensator, attract the attention of the boat lookout and hope to be rescued.

Buddy breathing, while swimming against a strong current, is often impossible. Even the octopus rig causes problems at depth, or when two people are simultaneously demanding large volumes of air, typical of divers swimming against a current. An alternative air supply (pony bottle) is of value, if it has an adequate capacity.

In dive planning, there should be at least one accessible fixed water exit, easily identifiable, that serves as a safe haven. This may be an anchored boat, in areas with tidal currents. The safety boat is a second craft – not anchored – and this, like any boat that is used among divers, needs a guard on its propellor. A pressure-tested distress flare (smoke) may be needed to attract the safety boat. Another recently developed device to attract attention is an inflatable elongated 2 m (6 foot) bag, called the 'safety sausage'.

There are other problems with currents, and these are particularly related to general boat safety and ensuring that there is a stable anchorage.

When the current is too strong or the depth too great for an anchored boat, a float or **drift dive** may be planned. This requires extreme care in boat handling. Divers remain together and carry a float to inform the safety boat of their position. It allows the surface craft to maintain its position behind them as they drift.

The concept of 'hanging' an anchor, with all personnel drifting in the water near it and the boat being at the mercy of the elements, has little to commend it. The raising of the diver's flag under such conditions, although it may appease some local authorities, is often not recognized by the elements, reefs or other navigational hazards, including other boats which are moored.

Some currents are continuous, e.g. the Torres Strait, the standing currents of the Gulf of Mexico and the Gulf Stream off Florida but tidal currents are likely to give an hour or more of slack water. At these times, diving is usually safer and also more pleasant as there is less sediment to interfere with visibility. To ascertain the correct time for slack water, reference has to be made to the tidal charts for that area. The speed of the current can be predicted by the tidal height.

## Surf

Entry of a diver through the surf is loads of fun to an experienced surf diver. Otherwise, it can be a tumultuous, moving experience, and is a salutary reminder of the adage 'he who hesitates is lost'. The major problem is that people tend to delay their entry at about the line of the breaking surf. The diver, with all his equipment, is a far more vulnerable target for the wave's momentum than any swimmer.

The recommendation is that the diver should be fully equipped before entry into the surf, and not spend time pottering with face masks and fins until he is well through the surf line. The fins and face mask must also be firmly attached, as it is very easy to lose equipment under these conditions. The diver walks backwards into the surf, looking over his shoulder at the breakers and also towards his buddy. The face mask and snorkel have to be held on during the exposure to breaking waves. The regulator must be attached firmly to the jacket, with a clip, so that it is easily available to him at all times.

When a wave does break, the diver presents the smallest possible surface area to it, i.e. he braces against the wave sideways, with his feet well separated, and he crouches and leans, shoulder forward, into the wave as it breaks. As soon as possible he swims (in preference to walking) through the wave area, preferably going under the waves. If he has a float, then this is towed. It should never be pushed between the diver and the wave.

Exit should be based on the same principle as entry. However, the wave may be used to speed the exit by swimming or backing with it, after it has broken.

## Entrapment environs

Being held under water, with a limited air supply, will result in drowning. A variety of materials can trap the diver, including kelp, lines (even 'safety' lines), fishing nets and fishing lines. If there is no compromised air supply, a buddy, a calm state of mind and a diving knife will help cope with most circumstances. All three may be needed.

### Kelp

Giant members of this large brown algae or seaweed may grow in clear water to depths of 30 metres (100 feet). The growth is less in turbid or unclear water. It usually grows on hard surfaces, e.g. a rocky bottom, a reef or wreck. It is of interest commercially because it is harvested to produce alginates, which are useful as thickening, suspending and emulsify-

ing agents; it is also used in stabilizing the froth on the diver's glass of beer.

Kelp has caused many diving accidents, often with the diver totally bound up into a 'kelp ball' which becomes his coffin. The danger of entanglement is related to panic actions and/or the speed and activity of the diver while in the kelp bed. Divers who are accustomed to kelp diving usually take precautions to ensure that there is no equipment that will snag the strands of kelp, i.e. they tend to wear knives on the inside of the leg, tape the buckles on the fin straps, have snug quick-release buckles and do not use lines. They descend vertically feet first, to where the stems are thicker and there is less foliage to cause entanglement. The epitome of bad practice in kelp diving is to perform a head-first roll or back roll, as it tends to result in a 'kelp sandwich with a diver filling'.

The kelp is pushed away by divers as they descend and ascend, i.e. they tend to produce a clear area within the kelp, into which they then move. They ensure that they do not run out of air, as this situation will produce more rapid activity. If they do get snagged, they avoid unnecessary hand and fin movements. Kelp can be separated either by the use of a knife or by bending it to 180° when it will often snap (this is difficult to perform while wearing gloves). It is unwise to cut kelp from the regulator with a knife without first clearly identifying the regulator hose. Some divers have suggested biting the strands with one's teeth. This may be excellent as regards dietary supplementation, the kelp being high in both B vitamins and iodine, but it does seem a little over-dramatic.

Kelp can be useful in many ways to the diver. It allows a good estimate of clarity of the water by assessing the length of plant seen from the surface. The kelp blades tend to lie in the direction of the prevailing current. In kelp beds there is usually an abundance of marine life, and the kelp gives other benefits such as dampening wave action both in the area and on the adjacent beach. It can also be used as an anchor chain for people to use when they are equalizing their middle ears, as well as to attach other objects such as floats, diver's flags, surf mats, specimen bags etc.

Kelp does float, and it can often be traversed on the surface by a very slow form of dog paddling or crawl, i.e. actually crawling along the surface of the water, over the kelp. This can only be done if the body and legs are kept flat on the surface, thus using the buoyancy of both the body and the kelp, and by using the palms of the hands to push the kelp below and behind during forward movement. Any kicking that is performed must be very shallow and slow.

## Cave and wreck diving

These are perhaps the most dangerous situations encountered by recreational divers. Caves are often more complex than they first appear. Planning involves not the setting of goal-oriented objectives, but the delineation of maximum limits. Maximum safe depths for cave diving is 40 m (130 feet).

The diver descends, often through a small hole, passes down a shaft, goes around a few bends and is faced with multiple passages, in total darkness. Under these conditions, and to make this particular type of diving safe, it is necessary to be accompanied by a diver who has considerable cave experience – in that cave – and whose judgement is very trustworthy. It is equally important that the equipment is both suited to cave diving and can be totally replaced with spares during the dive. Apart from the obvious environmental difficulties inherent in diving through a labyrinth of caves, there are added specific problems.

Safety in cave diving is not usually achievable by immediate surfacing. Thus all necessary equipment must be duplicated.

Air pockets found in the top of caves are sometimes irrespirable, due to low oxygen and high carbon dioxide levels. Sometimes the roof is supported by the water and when this is replaced by air from the divers' tanks, it can collapse.

The minimum extra safety equipment includes a compass, two lights, a safety reel and line. It is a diving axiom that entry into a cave is based on the presumption that the return will have to be carried out in zero visibility.

For visibility, each diver takes two lights; however, other factors can interfere with their value. A great danger in cave diving is the silt which can be stirred up when the diver swims along the lower part of the cave. If there is little water movement, the clay silt can be very

fine and easily stirred up. It is for this reason that the fins should be small ones, and the diver should try to stay more than a metre away from the bottom of the cave. Visibility can be totally lost in a few seconds as the silt curtain ascends – and it may remain for weeks. Sometimes it is inevitable as the exhaled bubbles dislodge silt from the ceiling. Mixing of salt and fresh water also causes visual distortion and blurring.

The usual equipment includes double tanks manifolded together, making a common air supply, but offering two regulator outlets. With the failure of one regulator, the second one may be used for the air supply – or as an octopus rig. The second regulator must have a long hose because often the divers cannot swim next to each other. Due to space limitations, buddy breathing is often impractical under cave conditions. An extra air supply (pony bottle) is a bonus.

The ideal equipment for recreational divers to explore many caves is a reliable compressed air surface supply, with a tender and a complete scuba back-up rig.

All the instruments should be standardized, e.g. the watch goes on the left wrist, the depth gauge above it, the compass on the right wrist and the contents gauge attached to the harness under the left arm. The gauges and decompression must be modified for fresh water and altitude, if these are applicable. The knife is strapped to the inside of the left leg, to prevent entanglement on any safety lines. The buoyancy compensator is often bound at the top, to move the buoyancy centre more towards the centre of gravity (because cave divers do not need to be vertical with the head out of water). There is no requirement for excess buoyancy, because safety in cave diving is not usually equated with a direct ascent; therefore carbon dioxide cylinders should be removed and replaced with exhausted ones to prevent accidental inflation of vests. One principle of cave diving is that safety lies in retracing the entry path by the use of lines and not, as in the normal open ocean diving, by ascent.

The techniques of cave diving are also very stereotyped. Specialized training in cave diving, dive planning, the use of reels and lines, and lost diver protocols is essential.

Usually no more than three divers should go on a single dive and, on completion of the dive, each should have a minimum of one-third of his initial air supply. If there is water flow within the cave, and the penetration is with the flow, this rule is not conservative enough – because the air consumption is greater returning against the current.

Vertical penetrations need a heavy shot line moored or buoyed at the surface and weighted or fixed at the bottom. The reel is used for horizontal penetrations, not vertical, otherwise entanglement is likely with rapid ascents, especially if divers precede the lead diver. Thin, non-floating lines in particular cause entanglement if they are slack.

Most people who have difficulties with cave diving have not followed the recommended rules, and unfortunately cave diving problems tend to lead to multiple fatalities. The number one enemy of cave divers is panic.

Wreck diving has potentially similar problems to some cave and ice water diving. In addition, it has the hazards of instability of the structure and the dangers of unexploded ordinance, sharp objects, and toxic cargo and fuel.

Silt in wrecks is usually heavier than that in still water caves. Thus, the sudden loss of visibility which can occur when silt is stirred up may be less persistent. The diver should ascend as far as is safe, and wait until the silt cloud settles down.

## Cold water and under ice

In these situations the obvious problem is that of hypothermia. It is so obvious that most people will avoid it by the use of dry suits, or efficient wet suits. (See Chapter 22 for the effects of a cold environment on physiological performance.)

A major difficulty is the tendency of many single hose regulators to freeze, usually in the free-flow position, after about 20–30 minutes of exposure to very cold water (less than 5°C). This is aggravated if there is water vapour (potential ice crystals) in the compressed air and if there is a rapid expansion of air, which produces further cooling in both the first and second stages. The first stage or the second stage may then freeze internally.

Expansion of air as it passes from the high tank pressure to the lower demand valve, and then to environmental pressures (adiabatic expansion), results in a drop in temperature. It

is therefore not advisable to purge regulators if exposed to very cold temperatures. Freezing from increased air flow is also produced with hyperventilation or panic. Octopus rigs also become more dangerous to use under these conditions, or at great depth, because of the increased air flow. An emergency air source (pony bottle) has replaced buddy breathing and octopus rigs.

'External' ice is formed in and around the first (depth-compensated) stage of the regulator, blocking the orifice and interfering with the spring. Moisture from the diver's breath, or water in the exhalation chamber of the second stage, may also freeze the demand mechanism, causing free flow of gas and 'internal' freezing with no flow.

Modifications designed to reduce freezing of the water in the first stage include the use of very dry air and the replacement of first-stage water with silicone, oils or alcohols, which require lower temperatures to freeze, or with an air flow from the regulator. The newer, non-metallic second stages are less susceptible to freezing. Despite all this, regulator freezing is common in polar diving. Surface supply with an emergency scuba or twin tank/twin regulator diving, as with cave diving, is probably safer. It must be presumed, in under-ice diving, that the regulator will freeze.

Under ice there is little use for snorkels and so these should be removed to reduce the likelihood of snagging. Rubber suits can become sharp and brittle. Zippers are best avoided because they freeze and may also allow water and heat exchange. Buoyancy compensators should be small and with an independent air supply.

As a general rule, and if well-fitting dry suits are unavailable, the minimum thickness of the neoprene should increase with decreased water temperatures, e.g.

< 5°C – 9 mm thick wet suit
< 10°C – 7 mm
< 20°C – 5 mm
< 30°C – 3 mm

Hood, gloves and booties should be of a similar thickness.

Unheated wet suits do not give sufficient insulation at depth (beyond 18 m or 60 feet) when the neoprene becomes too compressed and loses much of its insulating ability. Then non-compressible wet suits, inflatable dry suits or heated suits are required.

Ice diving is in many ways similar to cave diving. It is essential that direct contact must always be maintained with the entry and exit area. This should be by a heavy duty line attached to the diver with a bowline knot. The line must also be securely fastened at the surface, as well as on the diver. The dive should be terminated as soon as there is any suggestion of either shivering, diminished manual dexterity, other effects of cold or a reduced gas supply.

The entry hole through the ice should be at least two divers' wide. Allowing room for only one diver to enter ignores two facts: first that it tends to close over by freezing and, secondly, that two divers may need to exit simultaneously. There should be a surface tender with at least one standby diver. If the penetration under the ice is in excess of a distance equated with a breath-hold swim, then a back-up scuba system is a requirement. A bright light, hanging below the surface at the entry hole, is also of value.

## Deep diving

'Divers do it deeper' represents a problem with ego trippers and a challenge to the adventure seekers. Unfortunately, the competitive element sometimes overrides logic, and divers become enraptured, literally, with the desire to dive deeper. They then move into a dark, eerie world where colours do not penetrate, where small difficulties expand, where safety is further away and where the leisure of recreational diving is replaced with an intense time urgency.

Beyond the 30 m (100 feet) limit, the effect of narcosis becomes obvious, at least to observers. The gas supply is more rapidly exhausted; buoyancy, due to wet suit compression, has become negative – with an inevitable reliance on fallible equipment, such as the buoyancy compensator. The reserve air supply lasts less time, and the buoyancy compensator inflation takes longer and uses more air. Emergency procedures, especially free and buoyant ascents, are more difficult. The decompression tables are less reliable and ascent rates become more critical.

Many of the older, independent instructors would only qualify recreational divers to 100 feet. Now, with instructor organizations seeking other ways of separating the diver and his money, speciality courses may be devised to entice the diver to 'go deep'.

## Night diving

Extra care is needed for night diving due to impaired visibility. Emergency procedures are not as easy to perform as during the day and there is a greater anxiety. For inexperienced divers, it is advisable to remain close to the surface, the bottom or some object (anchor, lines etc.). Free swimming mid-water, and without objects to focus on, causes apprehension to many divers.

Preferably the site should be familiar, at least in daylight, without excessive currents or water movements and with easy beach access, or between the boat and the shore. From a boat entry, the diver sometimes encounters surface debris that was not obvious.

Any navigational aid needs to be independently lighted. This includes the boat, the exit, buoys, buddies etc. A compass is usually required. A chemical Cyalume light should be attached firmly to the tank valve, and at least two reliable torches should be carried. The snorkel should have a fluorescent tip. A whistle and a Day/Night distress flare are sometimes of great value in summoning the boatman, who does not have the same capabilities of detecting divers at night.

Marine creatures are sometimes more difficult to see. Accidents are more likely from a partly buried stingray or needle-spined sea urchins.

Signals include a circular torch motion (I am OK, how about you?) or rapid up and down movements (something is wrong). The light should never be shone in a diver's face, because it blinds him momentarily. Traditional signals can be given, by shining the light onto the signalling hand.

## Altitude diving

The conventional idea of diving is that a diver descends from the sea level (1 ATA) and returns to 1 ATA when he has finished his dive. A diver might, however, have to dive in a mountain lake where the pressure on the surface is less than 1 ATA. The problems are related to the physics of altitude.

For the sake of simplicity, the following description is based on the useful, but questionable, traditional belief that the ratio between the pressure reached during the dive and the final pressure determines the decompression required. If this ratio is less than 2:1 then a diver can ascend safely without pausing during ascent. This means that a diver can dive from the sea surface (1 ATA) to 10 metres (2 ATA) and ascend safely. A diver operating in a high mountain lake, surface pressure 0.5 ATA, could only dive to 5 metres (1 ATA) before he had to worry about decompression. This statement ignores the minor correction required in a fresh water lake – fresh water is less dense than salt water.

Another pressure problem occurs when a diver, who dives from sea level, flies or ascends into the mountains after his dive. For example, a 5-metre dive (1.5 ATA) could be followed by an immediate ascent to a pressure of 0.75 ATA, with little risk. Deeper dives or higher ascents may require the diver to pause at sea level if he is to avoid decompression sickness. If the diver ascends, in a motor vehicle or aeroplane, the reduced pressure will expand 'silent' bubbles or increase the gas gradient so as to produce larger bubbles, aggravating the diseases of pulmonary barotrauma and decompression sickness.

Another problem of diving in a high altitude lake is the rate at which a diver may have to exhale during ascent. A diver who ascends from 10 metres (2 ATA) to the surface (1 ATA) would find that the volume of gas in his lungs has doubled. Most divers realize this and exhale at a controlled rate during ascent. They may not realize that a similar doubling in gas volume occurs in the last 5 metres of ascent to the surface, where the pressure is 0.5 ATA. The same effects are encountered with buoyancy control, which can more rapidly get out of control at altitude.

The diver's equipment can also be affected or damaged by high altitudes. Some pressure gauges only start to register when the pressure is greater than 1 ATA. These gauges (Bellows and Bourdon tube types) would try to indicate a negative depth, perhaps bending the needle,

until the diver exceeded 1 ATA. Thus the dive depth would have to reach over 5 m (17 feet) before it even started measuring.

The other common depth gauge, a capillary tube, indicates the depth by an air/water boundary. It automatically adjusts to the extent that it always reads zero depth on the surface. The volume of gas trapped in the capillary decreases with depth. For a diver starting from 0.5 ATA this gauge would start at zero, but would show the diver when he had reached 10 metres' depth when he was at 5 metres. Theoretically, the diver could plan his dive and decompression according to this 'gauge' depth, but only if he was very courageous.

Divers who fly from sea level to dive at altitude, as in high mountain lakes, may commence the dive with an already existing nitrogen load in excess of that of the local divers, who have equilibrated with the lower pressures. Thus the 'sea level' divers are in effect performing a repetitive dive.

Decompression tables which supply acceptable modifications for altitude exposure, include the Buhlmann tables and the Canadian DCIEM tables (see Appendix IV).

Some decompression meters are damaged by exposure to altitude (e.g. as in aircraft travel) and none is applicable to altitude diving or saturation excursions.

## Fresh water

The main problem with fresh water is that it is not the medium in which most divers were trained. Thus their buoyancy appreciation is distorted. Acceptable weights in sea water may be excessive in fresh water.

There are also many organisms that are killed by sea water, but which thrive in warm fresh water (see Chapter 23).

## Recommended reading

*Australian Antarctic (ANARE) Diving Manual* (1990).
*British Sub-Aqua Club Diving Manual*, current edition.
EXLEY, S. (1981). *Basic Cave Diving*. Jacksonville, Florida: National Speleological Society.
*NOAA Diving Manual*, current edition.
*US Navy Diving Manual*, current edition.

# 8

# Why divers die: the facts and figures

# Background

The causes of diving deaths depend on the populations being investigated, the equipment used and the environment. Thus, oxygen-rebreathing navy divers will have very different causes of death than air-breathing, surface-supplied shell divers or helium-breathing, deep oil rig divers.

The USA Underwater Diving Fatalities Statistics (McAniff, 1981, 1988) have until recently been compiled almost single-handedly by John J. McAniff, Director of National Underwater Accident Data Centre (NUADC), University of Rhode Island. These records, which go back to 1970, include more than 2600 fatalities, and are unsurpassed in their scope.

> Most accidents involve multiple factors that are mutually interacting.
> *Mark Bradley, on diving fatalities*

In an Australia and New Zealand (ANZ) series, the deaths are less numerous, but data are much more detailed and are comprehensively catalogued (Edmonds and Walker, 1989). All factors were recorded that were likely to have contributed materially to the sequence of events which led to death, or prevented action being taken which would have led to a successful rescue.

The Japanese statistics supplied by Mano and his colleagues (1990) are less detailed, but with almost 100 000 newly qualified divers per year they should soon be comparable with the Australian and US figures.

Thus the NUADC detailed the diving activity, whereas the ANZ series define the conditions that contributed to the deaths. The populations are very similar, probably because of similar socioeconomic conditions and affiliated diving instructor organizations. The figures are therefore complementary, and can be compared with general diving population surveys, as supplied by the Diver Alert Network (DAN) (Wachholz, 1988).

This chapter considers mainly recreational scuba divers and the statistics have been restricted to the 1980s, because the instruction and equipment of earlier years would distort the lessons for today.

# Diving data

These data give an overview of the diver, the type of diving, and the behaviour of the diver and the observers.

## Diver profile (Table 8.1)

In most cases the accident came as a great surprise to all associates of the deceased, but in 9% the victim had been specifically advised by a diving medical expert, and sometimes by a dive instructor, that they were unfit for scuba diving.

**Table 8.1 Diver profile**

|  | NUADC | ANZ |
|---|---|---|
| Average age (years) | 33.1 | 32.9 |
| First scuba dive (%) | 5.4 | 8 |
| Under training (%) | 9.0 | 5 |
| Multiple deaths (%) | 9.8 | 4 |
| Diving alone (%) | 17.5 | 21 |
| Male:female ratio | 9.1 | 9:1 |
| Age > 50 (%) | 9.7 | 8 |

## Activity

Two-thirds of these divers were either recreational diving or amateur fishing (mainly shellfish), 7% were photographers, 5% were cave diving, 3% were wreck diving, 2% were instructing, 2% were night diving, 1.5% were ice diving (NUADC). In 14% of cases the fatal dive was a repetitive one.

## Age

During the 1980s, there was an increase in NUADC fatalities of individuals over 50 years of age. The trend has continued, reaching 18% of the fatalities during 1986 and 1987. It is not possible to determine whether this reflects an increased risk with age and/or more aged divers.

The age range in the ANZ series was 13–65 with the majority between 21 and 35, and a small increase around 46–50. The latter was related to the 'cardiac deaths' which had their peak in this age group.

## Depths

The depths of the dive, the initiating problem and the unconsciousness (or death) are related. A small number in the ANZ survey never descended at all and over a quarter first encountered their trouble on the surface. Despite the wide range of diving depths, at least half either died or lost consciousness on the surface.

In the Japanese series, two-thirds of those who died were diving at less than 10 metres and one-quarter never left the surface.

## Duration

In 17%, the diver succumbed in the first 10 minutes of the dive; in 56% the problem developed following an exhaustion of the air supply (either on reserve, low-on-air (LOA), or out-of-air (OOA)); in 8% it was intermediate between these times.

It would seem reasonable to conclude that, in planning a dive, accidents could be anticipated to occur more often at the start or at the end.

## Experience

In the NUADC series:

- 5.4% died during their first ever dive with scuba.
- 3.9% died in their first open water dive.
- 21.4% died in an early open water dive.

Thus, it can be seen that almost one-third of the cases were early entrants into the sport:

- 8.7% were under instruction at the time of death.
- 33.3% (one-third) were considered to have 'some experience'.
- 36% were considered to be very experienced.

The Japanese statistics show that nearly half of their deaths occur in novice divers (less than 1 year's experience) and 30% happened during the first open water dive.

However, experience is relative; in the ANZ series

- 8% died in their first dive.
- 5% were under instruction.

- 49% had enough experience to undertake the dive that killed them.

## Responses

Once a problem has developed, even though the surface was sought in most cases, the weight belt was ditched by the **victim** in only 9% of cases and the buoyancy compensator (BC) was not inflated, either on the surface or at depth in 48%.

The **rescuer** assisted with the air supply (11%), ditched the victim's weights (12%), inflated the victim's BC (10%), and assisted in rescue and first aid (23%).

When the buddy remained with the victim, or eventually found him, there was usually an appropriate response. Only rarely (1%) did the rescuer become a victim.

The buddy breathing seemed to cause some problems, especially during ascent – it failed in 4% of cases. The NUADC had studied 24 cases of failed buddy breathing from a single regulator in 1945–1970. They stressed the following findings:

- Over half were attempted deeper than 20 metres.
- In no instance did the assisting buddy die and the victim survive (this should encourage would-be rescuers to share their air).
- In 29% of cases, the victim or buddy's face mask was displaced, considerably complicating an already difficult operation.
- In 12.5%, air embolism supervened. It is easy to imagine overinflation of the lungs occurring during the situation involving considerable victim anxiety, regulator sharing, purging and ascending.
- In 12.5% the victim refused to return the mouth piece and/or fought for it.

These figures support the argument for an alternative and independent source of air.

## Overview of contributing factors

The factors contributing to death were comprehensively investigated in the ANZ survey. The number of factors increased with the detail available of the dive. A 'sole cause', such as a shark attack or an inexplicable burst lung, was a rarity, except in the divers who dived alone, when the records were probably incomplete.

Each victim was recorded only once in each major category (medical disorders, equipment faults and environmental) (Table 8.2).

**Table 8.2 Major categories**

|  | NUADC* | ANZ series |
|---|---|---|
| Medical disorders (%) | 55.7 | 74 |
| Equipment faults (%) | 9.5 | 35 |
| Environmental (%) | 34.8 | 62 |

* The NUADC series, which had less information available on each death, did not 2t use identical classifications, and only recorded one contributing factor – and then in only 73% of cases. The ANZ series had much more detail and thus more identifiable contributing factors.

As well as these major categories, certain **diving techniques** or activities were likely to have contributed to the final event. These are

- Inadequate air supply (56%).
- Buoyancy problems (52%)
- Other equipment misuse (35%).

# Medical contributions

These include psychological (e.g. panic, fatigue), physiological (e.g. vomiting, extreme physical unfitness) and pathological conditions (e.g. pulmonary barotrauma, cardiac disease) leading to death.

Unless specified otherwise, all figures given for the ANZ series in the following analyses refer to a percentage of the total fatalities.

## Autopsy findings (Table 8.3)

Even though an understanding of the events cannot be obtained by autopsy findings alone, they are indicative of the final event. The results in the ANZ survey were derived more from the autopsy data, than from the formal coronal findings.

## Medical contributions: ANZ survey
(Table 8.4).

In assessing medical problems which contributed to the death, drowning was excluded as it represented only the inhospitable 'final act' after losing consciousness under water.

**Table 8.3 Autopsy findings: cause of death**

|  | ANZ 124 causes for 100 victims | NUADC |
|---|---|---|
| Drowning (%) | 86 | 74.2 |
| Pulmonary barotrauma (%) | 13 | 24.5 |
| Cardiac (%) | 12 | 9.1 |
| Aspiration of vomitus (%) | 6 | < 1 |
| Trauma (%) | 3 | 1.5 |
| Asthma (%) | 2 | – |
| Marine animal injury (%) | 1 | – |
| Coincidental (%) | 1 | – |

**Table 8.4 Medical contributions (excluding drowning)**

|  | Pre-existing | Fatal dive |
|---|---|---|
| Panic (%) | – | 39 |
| Fatigue (%) | – | 28 |
| Vomiting (%) | 1 | 10 |
| Nitrogen narcosis (%) | – | 9 |
| Drugs (%) | 8* | 7 |
| Very physically unfit (%) | 4 | 4 |
| Severe disability (%) | 3 | 3 |
| Severe visual loss (%) | 3 | 3 |
| Alcohol (%) | – | 2 |
| Motion sickness (%) | 2 | 2 |
| Gross obesity (%) | 8* | 2 |
| Carotid sinus reflex (%) | – | 1 |
| Salt water aspiration (%) | – | 37 |
| Pulmonary barotrauma (%) | – | 13 |
| Cardiac disease (%) | 3 | 12 |
| Asthma (%) | 9 | 8 |
| Respiratory disease (%) | 5 | 7 |
| Hypothermia (%) | – | 3 |
| Hypertension (%) | 8* | 2 |
| Ear problem (%) | 2 | 2 |
| Diabetes (%) | 1 | 1 |
| Others (%) | – | 1 |
| Epilepsy (%) | 1 | – |
| Decompression sickness (%) | – | nil |
| Contaminated air supply (%) | – | nil |

* Not necessarily considered as contributing factors, but included because other related disorders coexisted. Excluding these, in 25% of the cases there was a pre-existing medical disqualification for scuba diving. This compares to an overall 'failure rate' of almost 10%, during the 1980s, among applicants for scuba diving, who were examined by specialists in diving medicine.

In the final assessment only the past medical or physiological disorders which were thought to influence the death of the victim were included in the above table. The past medical history was available only rarely. For this reason, the 'pre-existing' figures must be considered as underestimates of the true situation.

In this geographical area, patients who had diabetes, epilepsy, cardiac surgery, or asthma were not considered suitable for diving activities – both in the obligatory medical examination and in the signed declarations required by diving instructor organizations.

Salt water aspiration, while the diver was still conscious, was in most cases overtaken and pathologically obscured by its logical extension, drowning.

### Stress responses, panic and fatigue

These subjective symptoms are 'soft' data that can only be presumed from a detailed description of the diving activitives. Nevertheless, they occur frequently throughout the fatality case reports. To dismiss them because of the inability to demonstrate morbid pathology would be to ignore two of the major purported contributory causes of diving deaths (Bachrach and Egstrom, 1987).

Shilling, in *The Physicians Guide to Diving Medicine*, reported that 'overexertion, fatigue, exhaustion, respiratory embarrassment, panic and resultant accident is the repeated sequence of events leading to a fatality'.

Webster believed that physical exhaustion was the cause of death in over half the diving fatalities of earlier years.

### Panic (39%)

Panic is a psychological stress reaction to anxiety. The threat of death is a reasonable cause of anxiety and, under selected circumstances, anyone will panic. Difficulty in obtaining air is a very frequent cause and the inhalation of water was associated with panic in 19% of the cases.

Panic occurred when unusual circumstances were present, such as greater than customary depth, compromised air supply, buoyancy problems, being left alone, poor visibility, strong water movement, unpleasant surface conditions (a long swim to the boat) or any equipment malfunction or perceived malfunction caused by overbreathing a snorkel or regulator.

The results include rapid ascents and inappropriate actions, such as abandoning regulator, snorkel or mask, and a failure to respond appropriately, such as ditching weights, inflating BCs etc.

The high incidence of novice divers' deaths from panic in the Japanese studies was due to trying to cope with surface conditions and

difficulty with middle-ear equalization during shallow dives.

### Fatigue (28%)

Fatigue is a physiological stress reaction to a muscular effort which was often underestimated by the victims. Under sufficient physical stress anyone can become fatigued. Salt water aspiration, panic and cardiac disease all occurred more frequently than would be expected in these cases.

Fatigue often developed when cold, trying to ascend when overweighted or during an attempt to swim against a current. The latter is especially noticed when the victim swims against the equipment drag, if overweighted and with an inflated BC. It is more likely to happen, but is certainly not restricted, to those who are physically unfit or disabled. Panic, water aspiration, cardiac disorder and asthma may be precipitated.

### Vomiting (10%)

After exclusion of those cases in which vomiting happened after removal of the victim from the water or as a terminal event, it either initiated or complicated the accident in 10% of the cases.

The more common causes included sea sickness and salt water aspiration. Both were associated with adverse sea conditions, and the latter with surface swimming, snorkelling and problems with the regulator 'leaking'.

### Nitrogen narcosis (9%)

Although this contributed to the death in 9% of cases, it was never the sole or major cause. It was always produced by depths greater than 30 m (100 feet) and aggravated by poor visibility, as in caves. It resulted in inappropriate behaviour such as rapid ascents or panic. It was also probably causal in interfering with buoyancy control, buddy breathing and rescue attempts.

### Drugs (7%)

Evidence of breathing gas contamination and narcotic intake was sought in most cases. They were rarely contributors to the death. Alcohol and cannabis were occasionally contributors, but presumably most divers are aware of the dangers of combining these with diving. The relationship between alcohol intake and drowning is described elsewhere (see Chapter 21).

Prescribed drugs included drugs for asthma (in 9% of deaths) and antihypertensives, such as beta-blockers (in 5%). These diseases and their therapies were much more frequently present than in the general diving population (about 1% in each case), and so their contribution to the fatalities must be a cause of concern. In only 7% was it considered likely that drugs contributed to the death.

The high incidence of deaths among these drug takers could either be due to the effects of the drug or the underlying disease.

### Salt water aspiration (37%)

While still conscious, evidence of this was present in 37% of cases; it was usually an interim factor, following some other event, such as using a snorkel in white water or an out-of-air (OOA) situation. Problems with the regulator unexpectedly caused this in 12%. Buddy breathing was also a cause.

The result of the inhalation of water is seen in the associations between this and other medical contributions to death, such as panic, fatigue, cardiac disease, asthma and hypothermia.

### Pulmonary barotrauma (13%)

This was evident in 13% of cases and was the major single, pathologically verifiable cause of death (excluding drowning). In some cases the extensive pulmonary damage was obvious, but in others it was complicated by the effects of subsequent drowning.

The suddenness of these cases made other observations more difficult; however, some associations were noted. They included narcosis, panic, asthma and other lung diseases. Other behaviour which caused this involved excessive depth exposure, vomiting under water, regulator failure and excessive buoyancy which resulted in rapid or emergency ascents.

### Cardiac disease (12%+)

In accepting this diagnosis, very gross pathology or an excellent clinical description was required. If all autopsy and clinical diagnoses of cardiac disease were accepted, the incidence would have risen to 21%.

Of the 12% of divers who definitely died of cardiac disease, the average age was 43.6 years (s.d. = 7.6), with the median (5%) in the 46–50 year age group and 3% between 51 and 55 years. They tended to die quietly in the water, usually soon after entry or at the end of an otherwise uneventful dive, except possibly for exertion and aspiration of water. Three had a history of heart disease and another four had hypertension requiring treatment.

With so many possible trigger factors (previous pathology, exertion, cold exposure, prescription drugs including beta-blockers, hypoxia from aspiration of sea water etc.), for both myocardial ischaemia and ventricular fibrillation, it would be hard to incriminate one specific aggravating factor.

### Asthma (8%) (Table 8.5)

Although only 1% of divers are asthmatic (probably less where medical examinations or questionnaires are required before diving), at least 9% of the deaths were in asthmatics and, in at least 8%, it was a contributory factor.

**Table 8.5 Asthma**

|  | *Percentage* |
|---|---|
| Autopsy cause of death | |
| Drowning | 7 |
| Pulmonary barotrauma | 2 |
| Medical contributions | |
| Salt water aspiration | 5 |
| Fatigue and/or panic | 5 |
| Technique problems | |
| Compromised air supply | 6 |

Most of the deaths are in clinically mild asthmatics who are otherwise physically fit young men.

The factors for asthma provocation in scuba diving are the following:

- Exertion (from overweighting, equipment drag, swimming against tides etc.).
- Inhalation of cold, dry air (adiabatic expansion of dehumidified compressed air).
- Hypertonic saline inhalation (bubbling or leaking regulators).
- Breathing against a resistance (increased gas density, regulator problems, low air supply).
- Hyperventilation and hypocapnia.

When these factors are considered, and it is realized that many of these stresses are used clinically to initiate asthma as diagnostic provocation tests (Reed, 1988), then the problems with this disorder are understandable. In a number of cases the diver was returning to obtain a bronchodilator spray; in others it had been used immediately before the dive.

Asthmatics, even more than others, had multiple contributions to death. The relative frequency of a compromised air supply, salt water aspiration, panic and fatigue, prior to drowning, was evident.

### Respiratory disease (7%)

Another 7% had respiratory disease other than asthma; they included acute and chronic respiratory infections, pleural adhesions, cystic disease and other intrapulmonary pathology.

## Diving techniques

Certain diving procedures or techniques that involve human judgements were perceived as having an influence on diving deaths. These include: out-of-air situations, buddy diving and buoyancy problems.

### Air supply

From the fact that 56% of the problems developed after the air supply had reached reserve levels (low-on-air and out-of-air), it was concluded that the divers found it more difficult to handle problems under those conditions. This tallied with the observations on the number of 'surface' deaths, and the problems of coping with surface swimming conditions.

Most problems develop from the time the victim became aware that the air supply was compromised. Snorkelling on the surface was employed by divers attempting to conserve an air supply and coincided with the development of problems in 8% of cases.

An LOA situation was produced by using either a smaller cylinder than normal or by diving with less than the customary air pressure (9%). In the case of small cylinders, not only is there less air supply than that available to the other divers, but when the LOA situation develops the actual amount of reserve air is much less than usual. In some of the cylinders, holding only 800 litres (28 cubic feet), there are only a few breaths of air once the LOA situation is reached at depth.

### Buddy diving

The buddy system, which has universal support among recreational diving groups and instructors, appeared to have more verbal than factual application. Many who claimed to be buddies were divers who merely shared the same boat.

In the ANZ series, 21% dived solo from the start, 13% voluntarily separated before any problem developed, 25% voluntarily separated after a problem commenced, 20% were separated by the problem and only 14% were not separated at all, i.e. correctly practised buddy diving.

By far the most common reason for voluntary separation was that one diver (the subsequent victim) was OOA or LOA, with the buddy deciding to continue the dive alone. Occasionally the buddy accompanied the victim to the surface and then left him to return alone.

The problem which sometimes separated the buddies were: uncontrolled ascents, underwater and surface currents – sometimes sudden and unexpected. Among the small numbers who were true buddy divers, there were some practices which seemed to detract from the buddy concept: in 15% there was not one buddy, but two or more. This led to considerable confusion as to who exactly was responsible for whom. In 6% the victim was following the 'buddy'. Under this situation, any observation by the lead diver would have been fortuitous. To attract the lead diver's attention required energy, air and time-consuming behaviour on the part of the victim, who could rarely afford it. The experienced diver was invariably the one who took the lead, and therefore had the luxury of a buddy observing him at all times.

In some cases there were groups of people being led on a dive. The procedure used was that the first diver to exhaust his air supply would inform the dive leader that he was now 'on or near reserve'. The dive leader would then take time to determine who else was in or close to an LOA situation. These two divers were then buddied to the surface and returned to base. Thus the dive leader managed to select the two heaviest air consumers, and usually the two least experienced divers, and buddied them together into a situation in which either one was likely to develop a complete OOA situation during ascent, while performing a safety stop, or on the surface. This illogicality seemed to be accepted practice in some 'resort' areas.

> *Over a third of the victims were either diving alone or separated voluntarily before the problem developed.*
> *One-quarter voluntarily separated afterwards!*

In the NUADC series the dive buddy's activity was less verifiable than in the ANZ survey, but still only 25% of the buddies claimed to stay with the victim. There were 48 double deaths, 4 triple deaths and 1 quadruple death, i.e. the total number of fatalities in which there was more than one death was 9.8% in the NUADC series. These were mainly cave divers.

## Buoyancy

Many of these problems came under the 'equipment faults' category, but an appreciable number were clearly errors of judgement and were therefore included as difficulties in diving technique. Buoyancy problems contributed in 52% of the deaths (47% with negative buoyancy and 8% with positive buoyancy).

The wet suits available for most of that decade required a weight compensation as follows: 1 kg weight for each 1 mm thickness, 1 kg extra for 'Long John' extensions and a hood, 1 kg for aluminium tanks and 1–2 kg for individual variation in buoyancy.

In excess of this, the diver is overweighted and requires extra effort, hyperventilation or reliance on the BC, to remain buoyant on the surface. Using this criterion, it was found that 40% of the divers who died were **overweighted** on the surface. At depth, the problem of overweighting was compounded by the loss of buoyancy from the wet suit.

Apparently, many divers have replaced the skills of buoyancy control with heavy reliance on the BC. They are purposely overweighting 'to get down', and the BC is inflated to return to the surface. In these cases, the BC is relied on, not to trim buoyancy with depth, but to return the diver to the surface. Such a procedure introduces the potential for accidents.

The BC problems included:

- Accidental inflation.
- Confusion with use – some victims repeatedly confused inflation with dump valves.
- Overinflation during ascent – Boyle's law and the 'Polaris missile' effect.
- Inadequate and very slow inflation at depth – especially if LOA.
- Effort required to overcome drag when swimming under water and on the surface.

The American Academy of Underwater Sciences, in a symposium in 1989, pointed out that, of the cases requiring recompression therapy, half were related to loss of buoyancy control.

## Weights

As in previous surveys, it was found that very few of the victims, only 9%, successfully ditched their own weight belts. In 40% this omission probably contributed to the victim's death. Failure to ditch the weights, when in difficulty, presumably reflects on training techniques.

## Equipment problems

The problems with air supply have been described above. The failure to ditch weight belts, and many of the problems with buoyancy that were clearly errors of judgement, have also been recorded above as technique or procedural faults.

**Table 8.6 Equipment contributions (faults 35%, misuse 35%)**

| Equipment | Percentage |
|---|---|
| Regulator | 15 |
| Fins | 13 |
| Buoyancy compensator | 12 |
| Scuba cylinder | 9 |
| Weight belt | 6 |
| Harness | 6 |
| Mask | 5 |
| Protective suit | 5 |
| Lines | 4 |
| Gauges | 2 |
| J valve | 2 |
| Snorkel | ? |

In the ANZ survey on diving deaths, equipment faults contributed to 35% of the deaths and equipment misuse to 35% (Table 8.6). There was an overlap between these. Equipment faults were defined as problems that could not have been reasonably attributed to any action of the diver during that dive; it is not considered an equipment fault if the diver has injudiciously chosen the wrong equipment. This would be included under the 'misuse' category.

### Regulator (15%)

In 14% there was a fault in the regulator and in 1% it was misused. The laboratory testing of the regulators after the incident showed many minor discrepancies. The ones which contributed to the death were verified by either the case history or the in-water test, in which the accident conditions were simulated.

The contributing faults were:

| | |
|---|---|
| Salt water inhalation | 8% |
| Increased breathing resistance | 4% |
| Catastrophic failure | 2% |

The subsequent production of panic, salt water aspiration and fatigue was often complicated by negative buoyancy (overweighting), and surface swimming with excessive equipment drag and tidal currents.

### Fins (13%)

Flipper or fin loss was surprisingly frequent and difficult to interpret. In 3% there was a definite misuse, in that the fins were either not worn or too loose. In another 10%, one or both fins were unaccountably lost. In all these cases, other difficulties were present. The loss of a fin interferes with propulsion, and is as likely to be a result of panic or excessive leg movement as it is a contributory factor to panic, fatigue or negative buoyancy.

### Buoyancy compensator (12%)

In 8% there was a malfunction of the buoyancy compensator (BC). In 6% there was a misuse of the BC.

The main faults included failure to achieve buoyancy because of inflation mechanism malfunction or failure to retain the air.

Misuse involved such actions as over-inflation, producing the 'Polaris missile' type ascent, or mistaking inflation mechanisms with dump valves. Sometimes the high pressure hoses were not correctly connected and, in other cases, there was difficulty with attempted ditching procedures.

### Scuba cylinder (9%)

In these cases there was rarely a fault in the equipment, but it was either inappropriately chosen or was misused in some other way. The causes were either: an initial low air fill in 3%; too small a cylinder in 3%; the cylinder valve not turned on in 2%; and loss of the cylinder in 1%.

### Weight belt (6%)

In 3% this was fouled, such as by being worn under other equipment and harness. In another 3%, it was unable to be released due to entanglement with lines, the weights slipping onto the quick release buckle, and the strap being too long and jamming the release on the belt.

### Harness (6%)

In 4% there was a fault in design or performance. With some, it was possible to ditch all the equipment and yet leave the weight belt on. This could be considered a fault in the design for open water diving. Sometimes it was difficult to undo the harness, even for the would-be rescuers. Occasionally the tank fell through the harness.

In 3% there was misuse in that the harness was placed over the weight belt.

### Mask (5%)

Broken straps, displacement and failure to achieve a watertight seal were the main problems.

### Protective suit (5%)

In 4%, the suit was considered to be so tight as to cause difficulties to the diver, including dyspnoea, panic, claustrophobia and fatigue. Tightness around the neck produced the carotid sinus syndrome (see page 401).

## Lines (4%)

These resulted in entanglements when misused.

## Gauges (2%)

Problems included not only incorrect information (air supply, depths), but explosive blow-offs and snagging.

## J valve (2%)

Both faulty design and misuse resulted in reduced air availability.

## Snorkel

It was impossible to determine the number of problems with snorkels. These were not well documented in scuba deaths, even though there is evidence that deceased divers were having trouble snorkelling on the surface. Some were in difficulty because they either did not have a snorkel or were not skilful in its use.

Others seemed to have difficulty with achieving sufficient air supply while swimming against a current or when overweighted on the surface.

## Absence of equipment

In many instances, not usually considered here as equipment misuse or failure, there were situations in which equipment should have been available and, had it become available, may have resulted in a less serious outcome.

## Environmental contributions (Table 8.7)

These include both the natural hazards (e.g. tidal currents, sharks) as well as non-scuba-related, artificial hazards (e.g. boats, dam outlets). Environmental problems contributed to 62% of the diving deaths.

If the diver attempted to dive under conditions for which he was clearly untrained and inexperienced, then this is seen as an error of judgement. In 47% there was either no experience of the type of diving environment being

encountered, or inadequate experience to cope with that environment. The training or experience was considered to be sufficient for the planned dive in less than 50% of cases.

## General

About 66% of all sport diving fatalities in the USA occur in salt water. As regards the fresh water diving, diving in caves appears to be the dominant cause, although diving in dams, sinkholes and at altitude also incur specific hazards (see Chapter 7). Most divers are trained to dive in the more dense sea water, and the problems with buoyancy are appreciably different in fresh water.

Such situations as fresh water diving, altitude exposure etc. are not described here, as they in themselves do not cause the death other than by influencing medical or equipment problems.

**Table 8.7 Environmental contributing factors (62%)**

| Environment | Percentage |
|---|---|
| Excessive water movement | 36 |
| Depth | 12 |
| Poor visibility | 6 |
| Cold | 5 |
| Marine animals | 5 |
| Caves | 5 |
| Exit/entry problems | 5 |
| Entanglement | 4 |
| Boats | 3 |
| Diving under a ledge or boat | 3 |
| Night diving | 2 |

## Excessive water movement (36%)

This is by far the major environmental problem contributing to diving deaths. In 15% the **tidal current** was too great for the diver to negotiate. In 15% there were rough surface conditions contributing, often involving 'white water' – surf and surging water around rocks. One effect of white water is to reduce the diver's buoyancy and make surface swimming more strenuous. It also indicates turbulence and fast water movements, which interfere with communication and visibility. In 3% there was an **unexpected and sudden underwater surge** which put the divers into difficulty. In 2% it was a normal **to-and-fro surge** which caused the problem.

Due to the involvement of surface swimming in many of these situations, the effects of an exhausted air supply, overweighting and excessive 'drag' of equipment led to panic and fatigue as well as to the sudden death syndrome. There was also an increased incidence of salt water aspiration and provocation of asthma.

In 2% death was caused by being trapped and drawn into a **pressure outlet** (a valve) in a fresh water dam. It was often not appreciated that the outlets in dams, although not very deep, nevertheless produced a considerable pressure difference and, in both cases, the body was drawn into an outlet pipe. Although the flow of water was not great in either case, the pressure gradients were, once the diver's body had been drawn onto and then obstructed the orifice.

Similar pressure effects can occur in caves and near rocks if there are springs or currents.

## Depth (12%)

Sometimes the depth itself was excessive for that person. In 4% it was considered a major cause, and in 8% a probable one. In most of these cases it was the greatest depth to which that diver had dived.

Excessive depth produced the problems of more rapid air consumption (thus an inadequate air supply, OOA or LOA, at depth or during ascent), nitrogen narcosis, negative buoyancy, slower BC inflation and more reliance on BC integrity, less visibility, more difficult free ascents, panic etc.

## Caves (6%)

These include caves in the ocean (especially along drop-offs and coral reefs) and in fresh water. Multiple fatalities are common in cave diving.

The specific problems included nitrogen narcosis, entanglement in lines, panic, loss of visibility due to the absence of light or to silt (making the torches ineffectual), sudden catastrophic water surges or equipment failure etc.

## Poor visibility (6%)

This was especially encountered in night, cave, white water and deep diving. It greatly increased the dangers of panic, disorientation and nitrogen narcosis.

## Marine animal injury (5–8%)

There is a tendency to belittle the importance of marine animals, and with many such injuries the pathologist may not observe the lesion (e.g. from a cone shell, sea snake or blue ringed octopus bite).

In some cases the divers initiated the problem, but in an appreciable number the animal instigated the proceedings. They included fatal and non-fatal shark bites, other bites (from eels, octopus, cuttle fish etc.), stings from fish, coelenterates, urchins etc. The injury sometimes initiated the fatal sequence of events.

## Entry and exit problems (5%)

These were encountered during rock platform and boat diving, surf and night diving, ice, wreck and cave diving. It was usually complicated by excessive water movement (see above).

## Cold environment (5%)

The cold environment was considered to be a contributing factor in 5%, because of inadequate protection or excessive exposure.

The effects included hypothermia, reduced dexterity and strength, fatigue and the sudden death syndrome. In other series, the influence on equipment malfunction and decompression sickness have been noted.

## Entanglement (4%)

Entanglement from environmental hazards occurred in only 4%. In 3% it involved lines used by divers, and in 1% it involved kelp. Not included in this figure is the entanglement in the harnesses or diving equipment.

The specific difficulties with line entanglement were aggravated by poor visibility, incorrect choice of lines and allowing lines to become slack.

Other causes of entanglement, in other surveys, included fishing line, nets, anchor cables, underwater wrecks and land falls in caves.

## Trapped under ledge or boat (3%)

This led to difficulty when the diver attempted to ascend to safety.

In an emergency, there may be inadequate time or composure to swim back down to avoid an obstacle between the diver and the surface.

## Boats (2–3%)

Problems with tidal currents, causing the diver difficulty with finding and reaching the boat, often complemented the deaths with fatigue, panic, cardiac disease, overweighting etc. These were not included in the 2–3% of cases in which the boat was instrumental in causing physical damage to the diver.

## Night diving (2%)

This figure may be an underestimate because, unless the night conditions very obviously contributed to the death, they were not recorded. The problems included vision loss, navigational difficulty, entanglement, panic etc.

# Summary, conclusions and recommendations

The purported low death rates among recreational divers in the early 1980s were shown to be based on overly optimistic figures and creative statistical interpretations (Monaghan, 1988a,b; PADI, 1988). So also was the alleged improvements in safety among scuba divers.

The death rates of 16–20 per 100 000 now being proposed, together with the death rate per dive increasing to 1 in 95 000, have compelled the diving industry to review and appreciably modify its claims of safety.

The NUADC has conscientiously recorded the number of diving deaths in North America over many years. DAN is now committed to continuing this valuable activity.

The ANZ series documented all the known contributing adverse factors. It differentiates medical disorders, diving techniques, equipment faults and misuse, and environmental factors. The ANZ cases demonstrate that, although diving may be safe under most circumstances, when a number of adverse factors combine, the diver is often unable to cope with the complexities of his equipment and environment.

## Medical contributions

The fact that 9% of the divers who died were specifically told by diving experts that they were unfit to dive suggests that sometimes good advice goes unheeded. At least 25% of the divers who died were medically unfit to undertake scuba diving, and should not have been diving.

A significant number of asthmatics and hypertensives undergoing treatment, as well as patients suffering from cardiac disease, diabetes and epilepsy, were represented in the ANZ series. Their presence was difficult to comprehend, considering that the candidates were required to pass specialized medical standards for diving, as well as to complete a health questionnaire issued by the diving instructor organizations, before they were accepted for training. The physicians and the instructors were not adequately applying these standards.

A report suggested (Marshall, 1985) that the failure of physicians to apply the medical standards is due to ignorance of these standards and a failure on the part of the physician to appreciate the problems of scuba equipment and the demands of the ocean environment. The reasons for the instructors not applying the standards is still conjecture, and may well be based on commercial, rather than ethical, standards. In either case, the current system has not adequately succeeded in selecting out the high-risk patients. Physicians and dive instructors are still confusing physical fitness (needed for many sports) and medical fitness (a freedom from medical diseases incompatible with safe diving). Both are required. Many of the deceased divers were said to have been very fit physically, despite having such medical diseases.

If drowning is excluded as only the final event in a sequence of adverse happenings, then the stress problems of panic and fatigue dominate the medical contributions. They are not fully appreciated in some series because these do not feature in autopsies. They are interwoven with faults in technique (or training), and with many equipment and environmental provocations (Walker, 1980–88).

The importance of these stress factors is contrasted with the great rarity of the 'high profile' diving diseases of decompression sickness and gas contamination, which were absent in the ANZ series and present in less than 1% of the NUADC series.

The importance of other major contributors which leave little or no evidence at autopsy, such as salt water aspiration, nitrogen narcosis, drug intake, vomiting and asthma, can only be comprehended by a detailed dive history. These do not show up as much in the NUADC series, because of the limitations of the data collection and the decision to only include one contributing factor in most cases.

Current diving medical examinations and diver training need to be modified to reflect the relative importance of these contributing factors.

The NUADC and ANZ series show reasonable agreement on the importance of pulmonary barotrauma and cardiac disease. The latter seems to be an increasing problem. The importance of astute medical selection and then adequate training of divers is dominant in the prevention of these.

The DAN survey (Wachholz, 1988) showed that established divers are a relatively healthy group. Of 2633 divers, with an average age of 40 years, 5.8% had hypertension, 1.2% had asthma (0.9% took bronchodilators) and 1.1% had diabetes.

## Diving techniques

These are more related to diver training than to diver selection. The inexperienced and overconfident male was overrepresented in both the NUADC and ANZ series. Diving well within the limitations of the diver, and the equipment, was not a well practised activity among these divers.

The majority who die do so after voluntarily inducing a compromised air situation (using up most or all of the air available). They are then forced to surface to breathe, or to conserve their emergency air supply. Returning with plenty of air was not common.

The traditional admonition that the surface is the danger area for divers was supported by the figures showing that at least half the cases lost consciousness and died there. Nevertheless, the surface was unavoidable. In 56% of cases, the diver was in a compromised situation as regards his air supply.

The surface problems were frequently aggravated by the decision not to ditch weights. This also contributed to many of the cases that developed at depth, where a failure to appreciate buoyancy factors resulted in excessive exertion being required.

The training technique of older experienced instructors, which requires trainees to practise removal and replacement of the weight belt on each dive, could well be reinstituted. This practice alone would at least have prevented the deaths in which the belt was eventually found to be unreleasable.

Instruction to unbuckle the weight belt and hold it at arm's length in all demanding situations was either not taught or not applied in any of these cases. Yet had this been done and the situation deteriorated, the belt would have been dropped successfully and the diver made positively buoyant – assisting slow ascent and permitting surface swimming without being overweighted. If the situation had not deteriorated, the diver could have replaced his belt without penalty.

The extreme effort in swimming on the surface with scuba gear, heavy weights and an inflated buoyancy compensator (Brookspan, 1988; Graves, 1988; Wong, 1988) did not seem to be appreciated widely among this diving population.

The technique of overweighting – 'to get down' – and the subsequent strong reliance on the inflation of the buoyancy compensator to ascend and remain on the surface presumably makes instruction far easier. The failure to learn the skills of buoyancy control, without an overinflation/overweight trade-off, is an expensive lesson not to learn. Dependency on equipment may well be related to the failure to ditch it in an emergency.

Buddy diving, as envisaged in the manuals, is in a minority in these cases. The majority of divers dived alone and died alone.

Even in the less detailed NUADC reports, less than half dived as a buddy pair, and only a quarter claimed to have stayed together. The ANZ series showed that:

- Over one-third of the victims were either diving alone or separated voluntarily before the problem developed.

- One-quarter voluntarily separated after a problem developed.
- One-fifth were separated by the problem.
- Only one-seventh genuinely remained as buddy divers.

It seems as if the buddy concept, if used at all, was mainly employed when it was not needed. More buddies voluntarily separated from the victim at the start of problems (usually when LOA) than actually stayed together.

Even when it is applied, the less experienced diver, or the one who will consume more air, is initially given the task of following the more experienced diver until he runs out of air – and he is then sent to the surface to swim back alone or is buddied with another LOA diver.

Traditionally, buddy diving was recommended and the need was self-evident because of the recognition that diving was a potentially hazardous activity. As diving is now promoted as being a safe sport, perhaps the need for buddy diving is appreciated less. For uneventful dives this attitude is adequate. For others it is not.

The observations in both the NUADC and ANZ fatality series for the 1980s should emphasize the need for buddy diving. This involves the divers genuinely taking responsibility for each other for the whole time, until they return to shore or safety. It needs to be taught, understood and practised.

The need for an adequate independent emergency air source is evident. Buddy breathing from a single regulator involves too many problems. Even octopus breathing was inadequate in many circumstances.

### Equipment problems

There is a popular misconception that the equipment nowadays is so technically advanced that it is reliable. This is not so. The regulators, which caused our scuba pioneers so much concern, were still common contributors to the deaths in the 1980s.

The new equipment, such as power-inflated buoyancy compensators, seemed to cause as many problems as they solved – although perhaps this is as much due to inadequate training and excessive dependence, as to faults in equipment design. (See Chapter 4 for discussion on the value and limitations of equipment.)

### Environmental hazards

Even with improved training and reliable equipment (not that the authors concede either factor), the environmental hazards are unlikely to change. Divers tend to overestimate their own abilities and to underestimate the power, unpredictability and capriciousness of the sea. The more aware diver has great respect for the ocean and its inhabitants. Training in one diving environment does not automatically transpose to others.

Some environmental hazards are dealt with in Chapter 7.

---

*High standards for scuba diving are as important for safe diving now as they ever were. They include: physical fitness, a freedom from many medical diseases, training in accident prevention and management, an appreciation of the limitations of equipment, a healthy respect for a potentially hazardous environment.*

---

## Professional diving

Professional diving fatality statistics (Bradley, 1981) vary with the type of diving. Oil rig divers of the Gulf of Mexico had a death rate of 2.49/1000 per year, whereas those of the deeper and more treacherous North Sea reached 4.82 for the same period. Despite the careful medical selection and rigorous training in these groups: 6–7% had a medical factor which contributed to the death; 19–28% died from decompression sickness (DCS) or cerebral artery gas embolism (CAGE); 15–17% showed poor judgement or panic; cold was a factor in up to 11%; heavy seas were a factor in up to 15%; equipment problems contributed in 33–41%.

Other full-time professional diving groups (abalone divers, commercial divers) have similar death rates − 3 to 6/1000 per year.

Some navies employ rebreathing equipment, and then the common causes of death are carbon dioxide or oxygen toxicity, or hypoxia.

The US Navy diving fatality investigations suggested that inexperience contributed in 25% and panic was an important factor in 30%.

# References and recommended reading

BACHRACH, A.J. and EGSTROM, G.H. (1989). *Stress and Performance in Diving*. San Pedro, CA: Best.

BRADLEY, M.E. (1981). An epidemiological study of fatal diving accidents in two commercial diving populations. *7th Symposium on Underwater Physiology*. Undersea Medical Society, Maryland.

BROOKSPAN, J. (1988). Technical issues. *NAUI News*, Sept./Oct., pp. 46–47.

EDMONDS, C. and WALKER, D. (1989). Scuba diving fatalities in Australia and New Zealand. *SPUMS Journal* **19**(3), 94–104.

EDMONDS, C. and WALKER, D. (1990). Scuba diving fatalities in Australia and New Zealand. *SPUMS Journal* **20**(1), 2–4.

EDMONDS, C. and WALKER, D. (1991). Scuba diving fatalities in Australia and New Zealand. *SPUMS Journal* **21**(1), 2–4.

GRAVER, D. (1988). Advanced buoyancy control. *8th Annual Symposium*, pp.49–54. American Academy of Underwater Sciences.

McANIFF, J.J. (1981). *United States Underwater Diving Fatality Statistics 1970–79*. US Department of Commerce, NOAA, Undersea Research Program, Washington DC.

McANIFF, J.J. (1988). *United States Underwater Diving Fatality Statistics/1986–87*. Report number URI-SSR-89-20, University of Rhode Island, National Underwater Accident Data Centre.

MANO, Y., SHIBAYAMA, M., MIZUNO, T and OHKUBO, J. (1990). Safety of sports diving. In *Man in the Sea*, vol. 2, edited by Ya-Chong Lin and K. K. Shida. San Pedro; CA: Best.

MARSHALL, W.F. (1985). *Underwater medicine. A study of the current level of knowledge of primary care physicans*. Project SM402. Department of Medicine, University of Queensland.

MONAGHAN, R. (1988a). The risks of sport diving. *SPUMS Journal* **18**(2), 53–60.

MONAGHAN, R. (1988b). *Australian diving death rates comparison with USA and Japan*.

PADI (1988). *Diving Accident Management in Australia*. North Ryde, Australia: PADI.

REED, C.E. (1988). Editorial. Changing views of asthma. *Sandoz Journal of Medical Science* **27**(3), 61–66.

WACHHOLZ, C. (1988). Analysis of DAN member survey. *DAN Report*.

WALKER, D. (1980–88). Reports on Australian and New Zealand diving fatalities. Serially presented in the *South Pacific Underwater Medicine Society Journal*.

WONG, T.M. (1988). Buoyancy and unnecessary diving deaths. *SPUMS Journal* **19**(1), 12–11.

# 9

# Pulmonary barotrauma

## General

Pulmonary barotrauma (PBT) of ascent is the most serious of the barotraumas, and causes concern in all types of diving operations. It is the clinical manifestation of Boyle's law as it affects the lungs and is the result of over-distension and rupture of the lungs by expanding gases during ascent. It is also called 'burst lung' or pulmonary overinflation. It happens in both compressed air divers and submariners, especially when exposed to free ascent or buoyant ascent training. Free ascent refers to an ascent without equipment; buoyant ascent refers to an ascent using specialized buoyancy equipment.

Lanphier (cited in Shilling et al., 1976) believed PBT to be second only to drowning as a cause of death among recreational scuba divers. Support for its importance comes from the fatality statistics of both North America and Australia (see Chapter 8).

In navy submarine escape practice, with extremely high standards of diver selection, training supervision and with immediate medical and recompression facilities available, the incidence of PBT is approximately 1 in 3000 free ascents and the incidence of death from this disorder is 1 in 50 000 free ascents. Under recreational scuba diving conditions, these figures are likely to be underestimates.

## Aetiology

PBT may involve much of the lung, such as when the expanding lung gases are not exhaled during ascent. Alternatively, it may involve only localized areas of pathology following obstructed air flow or altered compliance in associated airways.

Normally, intrapulmonary and environmental pressures are equalized by exhalation during ascent. The pressure change necessary to cause PBT is approximately 70 mmHg near the surface, i.e. a force which could cause an increase in lung volume of about 10%. Hence, generalized PBT may result when the ambient water pressure falls by 70 mmHg or more below the intrapulmonary pressure, i.e. with an ascent from a depth of about 1 metre to the surface. Greater transpulmonary pressure gradients may be resisted, without tearing the lungs, and especially with the support of abdominal or thoracic binders (and possibly wet suits). It is more likely to occur after full inspiration prior to ascent. A diver whose total lung volume is 6 litres at 10 metres depth (2 ATA)

will need to exhale 6 litres of gas surface equivalent in order to maintain his normal 6-litre lung volume at the surface (1 ATA). If he commenced his ascent with the lungs only half-full, at only 3 litres, he could have surfaced in safety. Once the total lung capacity is reached, the lung tends to stretch against an increasing resistance until the elastic limit of the pulmonary tissues is exceeded, and tearing results.

Predisposing pathology includes previous spontaneous pneumothorax, asthma, sarcoidosis, cysts, tumours, pleural adhesions, intrapulmonary fibrosis, infection and inflammation etc. These disorders may result in local compliance changes or airway obstructions.

Precipitating factors include inadequate exhalation caused by panic, faulty apparatus or water inhalation.

Although many cases of PBT may be due to voluntary breath-holding during ascent, or to

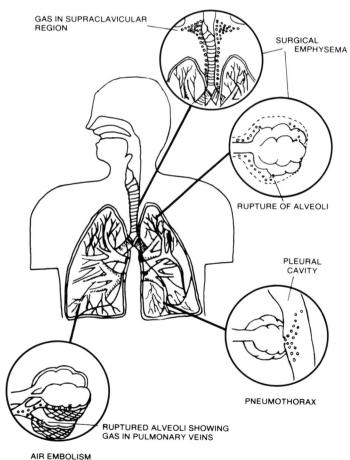

GAS IN SUPRACLAVICULAR REGION

SURGICAL EMPHYSEMA

RUPTURE OF ALVEOLI

PLEURAL CAVITY

PNEUMOTHORAX

RUPTURED ALVEOLI SHOWING GAS IN PULMONARY VEINS

AIR EMBOLISM

**Figure 9.1** Pulmonary barotrauma of ascent

the pathological lesions mentioned above, attitudes towards these aetiologies are changing. About half the ascent trainees who develop PBT have been observed to carry out correct exhalation techniques. Many of these divers were also passed as medically fit before the dive and showed none of the causative pathology afterwards. A frequent finding with some of these subjects is a reduction of compliance at maximum inspiratory pressures, i.e. the lungs are less distensible (more stiff), and are exposed to more stress than normal divers' lungs, when distended.

There are four manifestations of PBT of ascent which may occur singly or in combination:

1. Pulmonary tissue damage.
2. Mediastinal emphysema.
3. Pneumothorax.
4. Air embolism.

In a Royal Navy series of 109 PBT submarine escape training accidents, the pathology in the majority of the cases was cerebral arterial gas emboli (CAGE); however, 15 with arterial gas emboli also had mediastinal emphysema, 7 with arterial gas embolism also had pneumothorax (3 bilateral, 4 unilateral), 4 had only mediastinal and cervical emphysema and 1 had only unilateral pneumothorax.

---

*Expansion of intrapulmonary gas during ascent may cause pulmonary barotrauma with:*
- *Pulmonary tissue damage*
- *Mediastinal emphysema*
- *Pneumothorax*
- *Air embolism*

---

## Clinical features

### Pulmonary tissue damage

After the diver surfaces, an explosive exhalation of expanded gases may be accompanied by a characteristic sudden high-pitched cry. Dyspnoea, cough and haemoptysis are symptoms of lung damage, and widespread alveolar rupture may cause death from respiratory damage.

Abnormal investigations include arterial gas measurements, haematological assessment and chest X-ray examinations etc. Perfusion imaging of the lungs has also been employed. These tests are usually not possible during the all-important few minutes after ascent.

### Mediastinal emphysema

Mediastinal emphysema is more likely to present in scuba divers who have a history of breathing against the high regulator resistance from a low-on-air tank, and who are not exposed to the depths and extremely rapid ascent rates of the free ascent trainees in the submarine escape training tank.

It also tends to be delayed in onset, perhaps due to:

- The gradual tracking of the gas.
- Increase in pulmonary pressures during coughing or exertion.
- The nitrogen movement from tissue to bubble – due to a nitrogen load from the diving exposure.

In some cases there may be hours between the dive and the patient presenting with symptoms.

After alveolar rupture, gas escapes into the interstitial pulmonary tissues. This gas may track along the loose tissue planes surrounding the airways and blood vessels, into the hilar regions, and thence into the mediastinum and neck (subcutaneous emphysema). It may also extend into the abdomen as a pneumoperitoneum. When the pleura is stripped off the heart and mediastinum, a pneumoprecordium may be misdiagnosed as a pneumopericardium (Figure 9.2).

**Symptoms** may appear rapidly in severe cases, or may be delayed several hours in lesser cases. They may include a voice change into a hoarseness or a brassy monotone, a feeling of fullness in the throat, dyspnoea, dysphagia, retrosternal discomfort, syncope, shock or unconsciousness.

The voice changes are described as 'tinny' and have been attributed to 'submucosal emphysema' of the upper airways and/or recurrent laryngeal nerve damage.

**Clinical signs** include subcutaneous emphysema of neck and upper chest wall, i.e. crepitus under the skin (described as the sensation of egg-shell crackling, by divers), decreased areas of cardiac dullness to percussion, faint heart sounds, left recurrent laryngeal nerve paresis, and cardiovascular effects of cyanosis, tachycardia and hypotension.

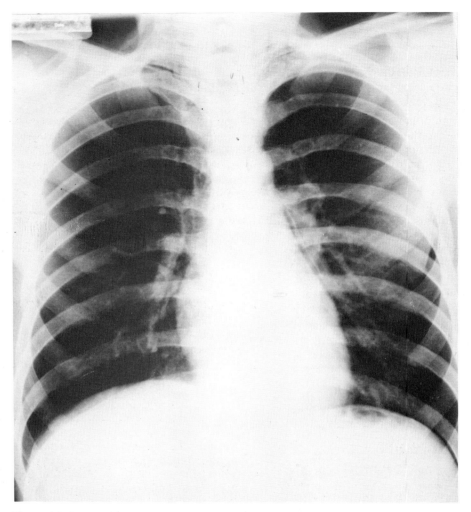

**Figure 9.2** Pulmonary barotrauma of ascent: chest X-ray showing mediastinal emphysema causing the 'tram track' sign, from air stripping the pleura from the edge of the cardiac shadow

Precordial emphysema may be palpable and give the pneumoprecordium or Hamman's sign – crepitus related to heart sounds. Sometimes it can be heard at a distance from the patient; other times it can only be diagnosed on auscultation. An extension of the mediastinal gas into the tissues between the pleura and the pericardium, rather than gas in the pericardial sac, has produced cardiac tamponade with its clinical signs.

There may be radiological evidence of an enlarged mediastinum with air tracking along the cardiac border or in the neck.

*Note*: pneumoprecordium is often mistakenly diagnosed because of the Mach phenomenon, where there is an apparent translucency surrounding dense structures such as the cardiac shadow.

> *Surgical emphysema may also be called mediastinal emphysema or subcutaneous cervical emphysema, depending on where the extra-alveolar gas has tracked.*

## CASE REPORT 9.1

RJN, a 19 year old, was having his second dive in scuba equipment at a depth of 5 metres when he noted a slight pain in his chest. He then noted a restriction in his air supply and thought he had exhausted his gas. He opened his reserve valve and ascended to the surface. He was asymptomatic after the dive but later, during physical training, he noted that he was breathing heavily and felt weak. A few minutes later he noted slight retrosternal chest pain. During lunch, he noted a fullness in his neck (a 'tightness') and dysphagia.

An hour and a half after the dive, he decided to see the doctor because he was not feeling well. It was then noted that his voice was altered in quality and that he had subcutaneous emphysema in both supraclavicular fossae, bilateral generalized crepitus over the chest and a positive Hamman's sign. Chest X-ray showed gas in the upper mediastinum and neck. An electrocardiogram showed ischaemic changes in leads II, III and aVF.

He was treated with 100% oxygen and improved rapidly.

Chest X-ray and electrocardiogram were normal 6 days later. Subsequent lung function studies showed that pulmonary compliance was reduced below predicted values.

*Diagnosis:* PBT with mediastinal emphysema and coronary artery embolism.

## CASE REPORT 9.2

MJC was an experienced diver, aged 25 years, who had suffered from a slight cold during the week preceding the dive. On surfacing from a dive to 10 metres for 50 minutes he noted some bleeding from the nose. He was otherwise well.

Four hours later he complained of an aching sensation in his chest and noted that his voice had a 'tinny' quality. On examination, pulse, blood pressure and heart sounds were normal. Evidence of mild bronchospasm was noted in the left upper anterior chest. Subcutaneous supraclavicular emphysema was also noted and mediastinal emphysema seen on a chest X-ray. Radiography of the accessory nasal sinuses showed mucosal thickening in both antra.

He was treated with 100% oxygen by mask and reservoir bag and was asymptomatic the next day. Haemoglobin, white cell count, serum electrolytes, blood gases and simple lung function studies were normal. Subsequent lung tomograms were also normal and showed no evidence of bullae or cysts.

*Diagnosis:* PBT presenting with mediastinal emphysema. This followed a generalized infection of the respiratory mucosa probaby blocking the smaller respiratory airways and resulting in air trapping in certain sections of the lung during ascent.

## Pneumothorax

If the visceral pleura ruptures, air enters the pleural cavity and expands during further ascent. It may be accompanied by haemorrhage, forming a haemopneumothorax. The pneumothorax may be unilateral or bilateral, the latter being more common from the dramatic emergency ascents (Figure 9.3).

> *Pneumothorax from diving has the same clinical features and management as pneumothorax from other causes.*

Symptoms usually have a rapid onset and include sudden retrosternal or unilateral, sometimes pleuritic, pain, with dyspnoea and an increased respiratory rate.

Clinical signs may be absent, or may include diminished chest wall movements, diminished breath sounds and hyper-resonance on the affected side; movement of trachea and apex beat to the unaffected side with a tension pneumothorax; signs of shock; X-ray evidence of pneumothorax; and arterial gas and lung volume changes.

If necessary, chest X-rays can be performed through the windows of most recompression chambers, giving results satisfactory enough to confirm the diagnosis. It is prudent to conduct a few trials before being confronted with a genuine case, and this will indicate suitable adjustment of exposures, which vary for different distances and penetration materials.

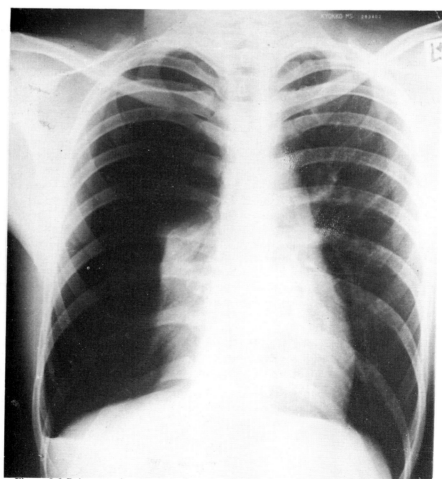

**Figure 9.3** Pulmonary barotrauma of ascent, causing a large, right-sided pneumothorax with a slight haemothorax

A pneumothorax under pressure becomes a tension pneumothorax during ascent. Tension pneumothorax may also develop from coughing or exposure to altitude or aviation pressures. Rarely a pneumoperitoneum may accompany the pneumothorax.

## Air (gas) embolism

This is a dangerous condition and is the result of gas passing from the ruptured lung into the pulmonary veins and thence into the systemic circulation, where it can cause vascular obstruction, hypoxia and infarction. Air embolism is more commonly associated with mediastinal emphysema than with pneumothorax.

In one large series of cerebral arterial gas embolism (CAGE), 8.6% occurred during ascent, 83.6% occurred in less than 5 minutes after ascent, and in 7.8% they occurred between 5 and 10 minutes after ascent. There were no cases occurring in excess of 10 minutes.

During overdistension of the lung, the capillaries and small vessels are stretched and these may tear, along with other lung tissue. Since these vessels are small and often compressed by distended air sacs, air embolism does not usually result until overdistension is relieved by exhalation. Only a small volume in the systemic arterial system is necessary to produce severe disturbances. Serious effects may result from blockage of cerebral or coronary vessels by bubbles in the order of 25 µm to 2 mm in diameter, or by otherwise interrupting blood flow (perfusion injury). Death may follow coronary or cerebrovascular embolism. Other tissues affected may include spleen, liver, kidneys or limbs.

Most of the clinical series refer to CAGE as the dominant site of pathology. Due to the buoyancy of circulating bubbles, CAGE is more likely to occur with the subject in the vertical position (common, under the diving situation, with ascent). Air emboli are more likely to enter the coronary system when the subject is in a horizontal position.

> *Air embolism may result in death when cerebral or coronary blood flow is occluded.*

Serious symptoms which develop immediately after ascent must be regarded as air embolism and treated accordingly, until a definitive diagnosis has been made.

The manifestations are usually acute and may include:

- Loss of consciousness; other neurological abnormalities such as confusion, aphasia, visual disturbances, paraesthesiae or sensory abnormalities, vertigo, convulsions, varying degrees of paresis; gas bubbles in retinal vessels; abnormal electroencephalograms (generalized slowing or flattening of waves) and brain scans etc.
- Cardiac-type chest pain and/or abnormal electrocardiograms (ischaemic myocardium, dysrhythmias or cardiac failure).
- Skin marbling; a sharply defined area of pallor on the tongue (Liebermeister's sign).

In one series of 88 cases of CAGE, mainly from free ascent practices, 34% had collapsed unconscious within seconds of surfacing, 23% had become confused, disoriented or uncoordinated after emerging from the water, 17% had presented with a paresis (six cases with an upper monoparesis and six with a hemiparesis).

In another series, presented by Pearson, 15% had complete remission within 4 hours, 53% had some spontaneous improvement pretherapy; 77% with coma improved to some degree before treatment. These spontaneous improvements were not always sustained and 15% died. Four per cent had a previous incident of CAGE.

Of divers who experience symptoms of CAGE, many will show a partial, or even a complete, recovery within minutes or a few hours of the incident. This recovery presumably reflects a movement of the embolus through the cerebral vasculature. Even those who become comatose may improve to a variable degree after the initial episode.

Unfortunately, the recovery is unreliable. It may not occur or it may not be sustained. Recurrence of symptoms has an ominous prognostic significance.

Interest has centred on the pathological implications of the air emboli, and a differentiation has been attempted between those who die immediately, and those who initially improve with recompression therapy, then relapse.

Recurrence of symptoms or deterioration of the clinical state may be due to:

- New embolization (coughing, straining, Valsalva manoeuvre).
- Recycling of gas emboli which pass through both arterial and venous systems.
- Redistribution of gases trapped elsewhere (heart, pulmonary vessels etc.).
- Positioning effect or buoyancy determining bubble movement.
- Local vascular damage, perfusion and reperfusion injury.
- Local cerebral damage, blood–brain barrier disruption, oedema.

### Differential diagnosis

The differential diagnosis for a patient who rapidly ascends from 30 metres (100 feet) or more and becomes unconscious or develops neurological signs within some minutes of ascent, but with no respiratory manifestations, can cause problems. Some would label the case as air embolism, whereas others would claim it to be a manifestation of fast-tissue decompression sickness, with intravascular bubbles. The same treatment may be very effective in both cases, irrespective of the aetiology. Tables listing the differences between these two disorders tend to oversimplify the question of diagnosis.

Unfortunately, the interrelationship of decompression sickness and PBT is sometimes not only of academic interest. If the diver has been exposed to depth and durations that significantly increase the tissue inert gas loading, this will influence the therapy if the diver develops PBT. This situation is not uncommon because both disorders – decompression sickness and PBT – are likely to develop in the diver who has overstayed his duration at any-depth, and then been forced to make a rapid ascent when he runs out of air. Under these circumstances, it is wise initially to treat for the PBT problem, but to avoid recompression tables with rapid ascent rates. These may be acceptable for treatment of air embolism, but not for decompression sickness (e.g. 6A of the US Navy Diving Manual).

It is possible that gas emboli may trigger off a decompression sickness incident if these emboli are seeded into a supersaturated solution, e.g. in venous blood taking nitrogen from the tissues to the heart and lungs. The presence of 'combined CAGE and decompression sickness' is well recognized, but fortunately not very common.

## Pathophysiology

### General

A great deal of controversy surrounds PBT, its cause, pathophysiology, differential diagnosis and treatment.

There is evidence to believe that there may be many subclinical cases of PBT. Of chest X-rays performed on 170 consecutive free ascent trainees in New London, two had mediastinal emphysema which was asymptomatic. Swedish workers demonstrated electroencephalography disturbances compatible with cerebral air embolism in 4 of 112 subjects who had performed a free ascent. Imaging

---

**CASE REPORT 9.3**

AI was a relatively inexperienced diver, aged 19 years and in good health. He was performing a free ascent from 10 metres. On reaching the surface, he gave a gasp, his eyes rolled upward and then he floated motionless. While being rescued from the water it was noted that blood and mucus were coming from his mouth and that he was unconscious. Resuscitation was commenced immediately, using oxygen. He was noted to be groaning at this time but soon after appeared dead. Resuscitation was continued while he was rushed to the nearest recompression chamber. Thirty minutes after the dive he was compressed to 50 metres but with no response. Autopsy verified the presence of PBT.

*Diagnosis:* air embolism resulting from PBT of ascent.

**Table 9.1 Presenting signs and symptoms in 114 Royal Navy submarine escape training accidents and 74 diving accidents involving arterial gas embolism***

| Sign and symptoms | Percentage incidence | |
| --- | --- | --- |
| | Submarine escape training | Scuba diving |
| Coma with convulsions | 7 | 18 |
| Coma without convulsions | 29 | 22 |
| Stupor and confusion | 14 | 24 |
| Collapse | 8 | 4 |
| Vertigo | 14 | 8 |
| Visual disturbance | 6 | 9 |
| Headache | 2 | 1 |
| Unilateral motor changes | 17 | 14 |
| Unilateral sensory changes | 10 | 8 |
| Unilateral motor and sensory changes | 6 | 1 |
| Bilateral motor changes | 1 | 8 |
| Bilateral sensory changes | 1 | 1 |

*Data compiled from case histories and records of initial post-accident examinations. In the case of submarine escape training accidents, the examinations were always carried out within 5 minutes of onset of symptoms.

techniques are now used to identify cerebral pathology (see page 109).

Occasionally PBT develops in free diving (without equipment). In such cases the presentation is with mediastinal emphysema and/or pneumothorax. Divers with reduced compliance could conceivably produce mediastinal emphysema or pneumothorax by their own normobaric respiratory efforts, as they can develop great transpulmonary pressures. This may account for the few reported cases of PBT in free diving.

Scuba divers with reduced compliance are also likely to suffer PBT with short ascents, when performed after inhalation. Any diver who, like the asthmatic, tends to breathe with higher than average lung volumes, is also more likely to burst his lung with minimal ascent provocation.

Pressure gradients formed between peribronchiolar and perialveolar tissues during expansion of gas, may lead to tearing of these structures. If elastic tissue is less in one area, or if fibrosis is greater, then this tearing effect will be more likely. Distension of fresh cadaver lungs resulted in tearing at the site of fibrotic adhesions.

Autopsy findings suggest that pneumothorax is more associated with adhesions, pleural damage and bullae, which indicate a physical weakness in the lung tissue but which may not be discernible clinically or radiologically. Parenchymal damage with interstitial emphysema is not so clearly related to such pathology. In some cases, the cause of death is obvious, as from gross parenchymal damage to the lungs. In other cases, it is less clear.

A theoretical hypothesis is that forced exhalation itself produces airway closure leading to air trapping, which then expands with ascent (but presumably does not open the airways) and causes the lung to burst. This hypothesis awaits clinical and experimental support.

There are two types of alveoli: partitional and marginal. The marginal ones are those that rest on blood vessels and are the source of interstitial gas in PBT. The gas escapes into perivascular sheaths over the pulmonary blood vessels. When the pressure gradient is created, the gas takes the line of least resistance, tracking along the sheaths to the hilum of the lung, giving rise to mediastinum emphysema or pneumomediastinum.

## Arterial gas emboli (AGE)

The **cardiovascular** symptoms following arterial air embolism could result from five or

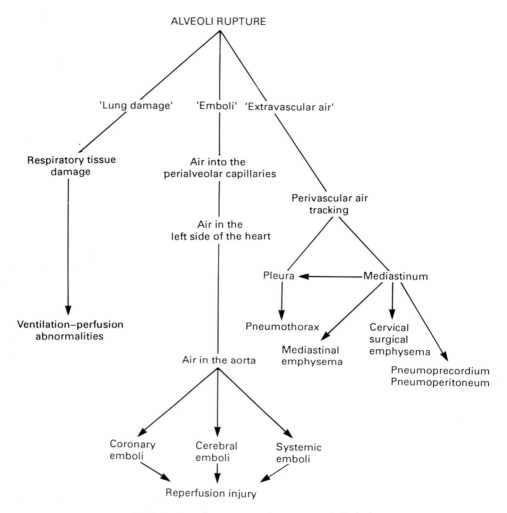

**Figure 9.4** Pulmonary barotrauma of ascent – pathological sequence

more mechanisms acting alone or in combination:

1. Air enters the coronary arteries leading to myocardial infarction with resulting dysrhythmia and ischaemic damage
2. A bolus of air in the ventricle produces an air lock which interfers with cardiac pumping action.
3. Air enters the cerebral circulation initiating hyperactivity of the automatic nervous system, resulting in changes in blood pressure, cardiac dysrhythmias, and even ventricular fibrillation and death.

4. Cerebral air embolism produces apnoea and other respiratory problems which could aggravate the cardiovascular changes.
5. Air bubbles in the vascular system cause ischaemia, haemorrhages, coagulopathies, endothelial damage in vessels, solid materials coating the air emboli, perfusion and reperfusion injury affecting cerebral or cardiac function.

Some of these mechanisms would theoretically be overcome by adequate cardiopulmonary resuscitation, which has often been administered to the fatal cases. Recompression is the mainstay of therapy, and could affect all the above mechanisms, except for the last.

### Cerebral arterial gas emboli (CAGE)

As well as having severe autonomic disturbances aggravating the cardiac disorder, there is also the likelihood of multiple cerebral lesions with vascular damage, perfusion and reperfusion injury, oedema, haemorrhage and necrosis. The pattern is not usually similar to that of a single vessel involvement, as in the more conventional cerebrovascular accidents of general medicine, but to that of multiple vessel involvement. The neuropathology will be influenced not only by the original lesion, but also by the effects of treatment and the duration of survival.

In animal experiments which demonstrate the influence of bubbles on the cerebral circulation, it is evident that the bubbles will coalesce in arterioles, 25–100 μm diameter and, if they span three branches or generations of vessels, obstruction is possible. Even small bubbles may affect the vascular endothelium, without necessarily causing obstruction. The vessel wall may be damaged and cause perfusion abnormalities, haemorrhages, collection of coagulation products, platelets and leucocytes, and disruption of the blood–brain barrier.

Small bubbles which temporarily obstruct the arterioles are sausage shaped, with the arterial pulsation on the proximal end of the bubble pushing it through the vessel, which may dilate and assist passage.

Fortunately, most emboli redistribute spontaneously from the arterial to the venous circulation. This redistribution occurs within the first 10 minutes following emboli production, and coincides with the reflex rise in arterial pressure. There is also a rise in intracranial pressure and a rise in cerebral blood flow which has considerable regional variations, with coexisting hyperaemia and ischaemia, causing impaired cerebral function. Convulsive seizures aggravate neuronal damage, as does the accumulation of metabolic acids, increased by glucose administration.

The coalescence of intravascular bubbles, together with a deposition of leucocytes, platelets, fibrin and lipid material at the gas–blood boundary, tends to stabilize gas bubbles and may be demonstrable within 5 minutes. An early effect, which may escalate even after the embolus passes, is the endothelial damage to the blood vessels. Thus cerebral blood flow may initially decrease, despite vasodilatation distal to the damage and, when the bubble passes on and the blood flow returns, cerebral damage may still be demonstrable by somatosensory evoked cortical potentials showing a diminution of the P2 wave.

### Therapy experiments

When there is a possibility of further embolization, it is advantageous to convert air or nitrogen bubbles into oxygen. In animal experiments, oxygen gas emboli are more rapidly removed as oxygen is metabolized by surrounding tissues. This has an application in therapy.

Positioning of embolized animals determines, to some degree, the distribution of the emboli. Although early experiments demonstrated the effect of buoyancy, with bubbles travelling to the brain in the upright animal, the extrapolation of this observation to first aid therapy led to some questionable practices – such as the use of the head-down, supine 'modified Trendelenburg' position. More recent work has thrown doubt on the value of even a 30° head-down position as regards bubble distribution in dogs, and has demonstrated a positively damaging effect in the presence of existing cerebral pathology. The current advice is to maintain a horizontal position until the embolism is dealt with.

There is a growing tendency to prefer the conventional oxygen tables to the 50-metre air dip, followed by the oxygen tables. This avoids the problems of the extra nitrogen load, but may not achieve the compression value of reducing the bubble to a size and frictional resistance which will allow the arterial pressure to force it through the arteriole into the capillary and venous system.

Compression seems very effective in the redistribution of emboli. Most workers would agree that, if initial pressure to 18 metres is unsuccessful, further pressurization is of questionable benefit. Some experimenters have found no improvement in bubble redistribution by increasing depth, so that 10 metres on oxygen is as effective as 18 metres, or 30–50 metres, with air.

Laboratory-produced CAGE in animals subjected to different therapeutic recompression regimes, and using somatosensory evoked cortical responses, supports the belief that 18 metres' pressure on oxygen is as effective, or more effective, than 50 metres on air.

Many experimental drug regimes have been tried in animals exposed to gas emboli and DCS, and it has been claimed that they have potential for extrapolation to humans. Most of these claims have not been substantiated. Anticoagulants, antilipaemics, anti-inflammatory agents, surfactants, plasma expanders etc. have all been the source of copious research grants.

Recent animal experiments in CAGE treatment, have suggested that: fluid replacement is needed to maximize cerebral blood flow; there is increased brain damage if the animal is placed in a head-down position; the hypertensive spike causes injury only in the arteries that have been cleared of air emboli; steroids are only of value if given hours before the embolism; and steroids increase glucose levels, worsen cerebral neuronal damage and extend infarction areas.

Lignocaine, given to animals after the hypertensive phase of the CAGE and in the same dosages as used for cardiac dysrhythmias, may have a beneficial effect by causing cerebral vasodilatation and leucocyte suppression. It has also been shown to blunt the rise of intracranial and blood pressures and improve somatosensory evoked cortical potentials, following experimental CAGE.

Currently, fashionable agents include antipolymorphonuclear leucocyte drugs and perfluorocarbon emulsion infusions (to increase gas solubilities and reduce blood viscosity, platelet accumulation and coagulation).

# Treatment

## Aggravation of PBT

Once PBT has resulted in the distribution of gas within body tissues, it may be aggravated by other factors. Further ascent in a chamber or under water, or ascent to altitude during air transport, will expand the enclosed gas and cause deterioration in the clinical state of the patient.

Physical exertion, increased respiratory activity, breathing against a resistance, coughing, Valsalva manoeuvre etc. may also result in further pulmonary damage, or in more extraneous gas passing through the lung tissues or into the pulmonary vessels.

If the diver has exposed himself to depths and times resulting in tissue loading by inert gas, this gas will have a pressure gradient between the tissue and the bubbles, resulting in transport by diffusion into the latter. A situation develops which has facets of both PBT and decompression sickness and may require more energetic recompression therapy.

Another way in which the entrapped gas from PBT may be temporarily increased in volume is by breathing a lighter, more rapidly diffusible gas, e.g. helium, in the otherwise correct belief that this may improve ventilation. The anaesthetic, nitrous oxide, rapidly diffuses into tissues, causing expansion of bubbles.

## Pulmonary tissue damage

Treatment involves the maintenance of adequate respiration with 100% oxygen to ensure acceptable arterial gas levels. The treatment is similar to that of near-drowning or the acute respiratory distress syndrome. Positive pressure respiration could increase the extent of lung damage and should be used only if absolutely necessary. Support for the cardiovascular system may be required, and attention should be paid to the electrolyte and fluid balance (see Chapter 13).

## Mediastinal emphysema

The need for therapy may not be urgent in mediastinal emphysema. However, for those cases which occur, exclusion of air embolism or pneumothorax is necessary and, if in doubt, treatment for these should take precedence. Management of mediastinal emphysema varies according to the clinical severity. If the patient is asymptomatic, only observation and rest may be necessary. With mild symptoms, 100% oxygen administered by mask without positive pressure will increase the gradient for removal of nitrogen from the emphysematous areas. This may take 4–6 hours.

If symptoms are severe, therapeutic recompression using oxygen is necessary. Tables 5 or 6 of the *US Navy Diving Manual* are often employed. A shallow oxygen table, such as Comex 12m without air breaks (to prevent further nitrogen entry), is more logical and should be used if the diver is comfortable at the lesser depth. It also avoids the complications of oxygen toxicity, which can be confused with lung or cerebral damage from PBT.

Cannulation to remove a localized pocket of retrosternal air has been proposed but this is rarely, if ever, indicated.

## Pneumothorax

Treatment depends on the clinical severity and the depth at which it is diagnosed. The possibility of associated air embolism must be excluded. Mild cases require only surface administration of 100% oxygen, without positive pressure. This will often appreciably reduce the size of the pneumothorax within a few hours. The patient may also need bed rest and analgesics. Physiotherapy may be required later.

A pneumothorax may also respond rapidly to high oxygen pressures at depth – as when it occurs in a compression chamber or when a patient is recompressed for other reasons, such as CAGE. This works because of the higher inherent unsaturation both at depth and with the use of oxygen. It has been estimated that extrapleural air would decrease as much as 30 times faster for a patient breathing oxygen at 18 metres sea water depth, as it would with breathing air at sea level (see Chapter 11, page 148).

Serious cases, often with more than 20% lung collapse, may need to have the gas removed rapidly by needle aspiration and/or intercostal cannulation and underwater drainage or Heimlich valve, with or without low pressure suction. This may be needed while the patient is undergoing recompression therapy. Therapeutic recompression performed for other manifestations of PBT gives rapid initial relief from the pneumothorax. Because the pneumothorax is likely to be re-expanded during ascent, thoracocentesis and/or the use of 100% oxygen (or as high an oxygen pressure as is safe) is indicated. Pneumothorax may be aggravated or reproduced by coughing, which

is sometimes produced in chambers, especially due to condensation while decompressing.

If an underwater drain has been inserted, it should be clamped close to the chest wall prior to compression, or air and water may flood the thoracic cavity.

With a pneumothorax, air treatment tables are preferably avoided. It may be converted into a tension pneumothorax, thus requiring emergency thoracocentesis and removal of intrapleural air. Ascent must be halted until this is completed, and then recommenced with great care. Repetitive needle aspiration is an alternative.

Offshore chambers may be very infective – especially with *Pseudomonas* sp. and *Staphylococcus aureus*. Such problems need to be considered in making the decision to rely on surgical intervention or the use of oxygen with inherent unsaturation.

## Air embolism

Treatment of air embolism is urgent, must be instituted immediately, and usually takes precedence over other manifestations of PBT. The effect of delay on treatment outcome is to increase mortality and morbidity. The likelihood of achieving a cure was reduced to 50% when delay of recompression exceeded 4 hours.

### *Positioning*

The 'modified Trendelenburg' position or the head-down left lateral position was recommended in the past. Some authorities even recommended a 45° angle, which is virtually impossible to maintain even in a conscious cooperative patient, let alone a seriously ill victim requiring resuscitation.

To prevent further brain damage, and possibly to reduce the likelihood of a further CAGE, the patient should be nursed horizontally, on his back or lying on his side in the 'coma' position (preventing the tongue from causing airway obstruction, or if there is a possibility of aspiration of stomach contents or sea water). The legs should not be elevated, as this may increase cerebral venous pressures as well as central venous pressure possibly causing paradoxical embolism.

A similar position should be maintained in transit to the chamber, while the chamber is being compressed and for an uncertain period of time (possibly some hours) while breathing oxygen. The patient is initially allowed to sit or stand only while breathing 100% oxygen, so that gas emboli which may still exist are likely to be predominantly oxygen, not nitrogen.

A sudden deterioration in the clinical state, with an apparent redevelopment of the embolism, may follow the resumption of an erect (sitting or standing) position. Whether this is due to a redistribution of gas in the circulatory system, or a perfusion failure from other causes (e.g. orthostatic hypotension effect on a precarious circulation) is unknown.

### Oxygen

Oxygen (100%), via a close-fitting mask, should be administered in transit to the chamber:

- To improve oxygenation of hypoxic tissues
- To dissolve the mobile emboli
- To ensure that any subsequent ones are composed of oxygen, instead of nitrogen
- To dissipate the blocked emboli more rapidly

Oxygen may also be used intermittently following recompression therapy, for similar reasons and to reduce the growth of existing bubbles (see Chapter 13).

### Recompression

Immediate recompression is necessary, and a recompression chamber should always be available near surfacing positions for all free ascent or submarine escape training. The choice of therapy is limited by the facilities available.

The patient is kept horizontal for at least the first 30 minutes of 100% oxygen breathing in the recompression chamber before being allowed to move and possibly redistribute emboli.

There is insufficient practical experience available to most physicians in the treatment of CAGE. Most 'clinical series' are retrospective reports of other physicians' patients, and it would be rare for any one doctor to be available at the time in more than a handful of cases of acute and serious 'pure' air embolism from PBT. There are no genuinely controlled therapeutic trials available or possible. Thus there are various approaches to recompression therapy.

Many groups use the conventional 18 metre oxygen tables. By reducing bubble size, this may assist the bubbles to pass through the arterial circulation into the capillary and venous systems, where they may become trapped in the lungs or redistribute to other areas. The denitrogenated state of the blood then assists in rapid bubble resolution. Oxygenation of damaged tissues and a reduction of cerebral oedema are bonuses.

A variation in this technique is to expose the patient to an initial 50 metre short exposure on air, to enhance the redistribution of blocked arterial emboli by decreasing their length to less than 20%, and proportionately reducing the resistance to forward flow, prior to the oxygen tables. More traditional clinicians extend the duration at depth and may even employ long air and saturation exposures, foregoing the value of hyperbaric oxygen.

The 30 metre 50% oxygen/nitrogen Comex tables may be an acceptable compromise between these opposing concepts.

More radical approaches have been employed. On theoretical grounds and based on animal work, it could be argued that the 50 metre 'dip' may be indicated only for 5 minutes or so, and that it is only warranted in serious and recent cases. If the emboli have not moved into the venous system after 5 minutes at 50 metres, there is no evidence that they will disperse other than by dissolving the nitrogen gas from them. For this to occur there needs to be an increase in the nitrogen gradient, and this can be done best with oxygen breathing – and is delayed by nitrogen (air) breathing.

To avoid compounding the problem by adding more nitrogen, the use of gas mixtures has been proposed, such as high oxygen/low nitrogen mixtures at the 50 metres' depth and during ascent to 18 metres, and Heliox to replace the air breaks during the 18 metre oxygen tables. These authors support such modifications.

Repetitive hyperbaric oxygen treatment may be of value in those neurologically impaired patients who have not recovered fully. These are continued until improvement has stopped.

### Symptomatic therapy

A possible cause of death from air embolism is from a cardiac lesion, and so cardiopulmonary resuscitation before and during recompression may be necessary. Despite the common hazards of hyperoxia and highly conductive wet environments, some chambers are equipped for using defibrillation techniques. With appropriate precautions these are claimed to be safe.

Circulatory and respiratory support may be necessary while the recompression facilities are being obtained. Prevention and/or treatment of secondary complications such as myocardial infarction, dysrhythmias, renal failure, cerebral oedema or haemorrhages, respiratory insufficiency etc. should be carried out. The treatment of these disorders are based on conventional medical principles.

Rehydration may be both important and needed. Intravenous fluids (saline, electrolytes) should correct haemoconcentration, and may contain glucose only if long-term infusion is needed. Dextrose or glucose is not usually indicated, because hyperglycaemia may decrease neuronal survival by increasing lactic acid and provoke glycosuria and more haemoconcentration.

Neuropsychological testing may demonstrate transitory or permanent cerebral damage after CAGE, and many have abnormal EEGs during and after treatment. The abnormality is excessive or disorganized slow wave activity – localized or generalized. It tends to improve over some weeks, at least in cases effectively treated.

Brain scans, such as computed tomography, MRI and SPECT, may assist in the diagnosis and management of decompression sickness and CAGE. Blood flow imaging techniques, such as xenon-enhanced CT scans, or damaged tissue detected by positron emission tomography (PET), may determine the site and degree of pathology. Radioactive technetium in HMPAO, injected prior to recompression therapy, can cross the blood–brain barrier and be detected at leisure by SPECT days, weeks or months later; this is now being employed in sophisticated treatment centres and is more helpful in postrecompression diagnosis and evaluation of treatment. It may show areas of infarction and oedema. Such studies would take second place to recompression therapy in the acute phases.

Drugs are not very valuable in most cases of CAGE, despite many attempts to affect the complications of blood–bubble interactions. Heparin and aspirin are not indicated.

The administration of steroids is often used to reduce vasogenic cerebral oedema. Dexamethasone is used by the Royal Navy in a loading dose of 16 mg. Following this, 6–8 mg are given every 6 hours via the intramuscular route, for up to 72 hours. It has been considered that this may reduce the incidence of relapse.

The value of steroids is dubious, unverified in most studies and some claim it is detrimental. They take many hours to have effect, whereas the blood–brain barrier disruption from CAGE is immediate and extravasation of fluid usually takes less time. Steroids are only likely to be of value if given hours before the event.

Other regimes to reduce cerebral oedema include diuretics such as mannitol, frusemide and hypertonic solutions orally, e.g. 50% glycerol in water. Their value is unproven and they have not received much clinical support. The complications are often not appreciated.

The use of controlled hyperventilation has not been shown to be of value in CAGE and the reduction in blood flow in ischaemic areas may be detrimental.

Other drugs have been proposed to produce vasodilatation (although many vessels are already dilated) and vasoconstriction elsewhere (to produce an 'inverse steal' syndrome); naloxone, calcium channel blockers, agents that reduce blood viscosity and reactivity or that affect cerebral metabolism have been proposed, but are still experimental.

Intravenous procaine has been used in the past, and lignocaine (lidocaine) in more recent times, to reduce cardiac dysrhythmias. It also reduces the rise in intracranial pressure and catecholamine effects. It is claimed to increase the rate of neural recovery, but it is also epileptogenic. Adequate clinical trials are needed.

For other adjuvant treatment, see 'Cerebral decompression sickness' (see Chapter 13).

### Underwater recompression

Extreme measures such as reimmersion to 30 metres in water should be avoided in all but the most exceptional circumstances, and then only if:

1. Sea conditions are suitable.
2. Adequate air supply is available.
3. Several experienced support divers are present.
4. The patient is fully conscious, or equipment is suitable for sustaining the unconscious patient.

An alternative or complementary regime to the water recompression on air at 30 metres is the water recompression on oxygen at 9 metres and this is discussed in Chapter 13 and Appendix VIII.

### Relapses

In a Royal Navy series of CAGE patients, some degree of relapse was seen in 32% of cases.

The relapse may be profound and delayed as much as 6–8 hours. It may be due to:

- Regrowth of emboli during decompression.
- Re-embolization from the initial causative lung lesion.
- Redistribution of existing emboli (possibly when repositioning the patient).
- Vasogenic oedema secondary to the blood–brain barrier damage.
- Reperfusion abnormalities.

Endothelial damage is an initiating factor in a complex chain of events leading to progressive failure of perfusion, despite an initial restoration of blood flow after the initial embolic blockage.

### Diving after PBT

In general, an incident of PBT is a contraindication for further scuba diving. The reasons are two-fold: first, the diver has demonstrated a pulmonary abnormality and, secondly, pulmonary damage has been sustained and will produce local scarring on healing and predispose to further problems by alterations of compliance.

Recurrences of PBT tend to be worse than the first incident, with an increased risk to life. Being neurologically incapacitated in the water is a serious situation. The incidence of such incapacity rose from 25% to 75% on recurrences.

## Prevention

Attempts to prevent pulmonary barotrauma, or reduce its incidence, have centred around increased standards of fitness for divers, modification of training and diving techniques, and the development of safer equipment.

### Dive training

Dangerous diving practices to be avoided include delayed or skip breathing, buddy breathing at depth and during ascent, ditch and recovery training and emergency free ascent training when there are no experienced medical staff and full recompression facilities on site.

Deep diving increases the danger by exhausting the air supply more rapidly, causing narcosis and less attention to the air contents gauge, and results in a deeper and longer free ascent.

The faster the ascent, the greater the danger of PBT. Certain diving equipment will reduce the likelihood of out-of-air situations and subsequent uncontrolled ascents, e.g. the use of tank pressure (contents) gauges, octopus rigs, and carrying an alternative and independent air supply ('pony bottle').

### Medical selection

Predisposing pathology includes previous spontaneous pneumothorax, asthma, sarcoidosis, cysts, tumours, pleural adhesions, intrapulmonary fibrosis, infection and inflammation etc. These disorders may result in local compliance changes or airway obstructions.

Cases of penetrating chest wounds may increase the risk of CAGE or pneumothorax. Pleurodesis ensures a protection from pneumothorax, at the expense of an increasing risk of CAGE and mediastinal emphysema.

Basal plural thickening may indicate adhesions, which have been shown to be a cause of pulmonary tearing during the overinflation of the lungs of fresh cadavers.

The medical standards are dealt with in Chapter 35 and involve: the exclusion of candidates with any degree of significant pulmonary pathology as described above, the imposition of respiratory function tests demonstrating efficient capability of exhalation and often a pre-diving chest X-ray. In most cases, a single full plate chest X-ray is acceptable. However, some groups insist upon both maximum inspiratory and maximum expiratory X-rays, hopefully to demonstrate the air trapping in the latter view. If this is a serious consideration, more sophisticated lung function tests are indicated. High resolution CT scans of the lungs, without contrast, are excellent for demonstrating emphysematous cysts, pleural thickening etc.

There was no identifiable predisposing factor in 43% of the cases of PBT. In the remainder, the causes were largely avoidable with adequate training and dive planning.

## Syncope of ascent

The so-called syncope of ascent is a cause of a transitory state of confusion, often described as either disorientation or lightheadedness, and associated with a sensation of imminent loss of consciousness. It is caused by inadequate exhalation of the expanding lung gases during ascent, with resultant distension of the lungs and an increase in intrathoracic pressure causing an impairment of venous return. It is analogous to cough syncope.

Syncope of ascent most commonly occurs during rapid ascents, when the pressure gradients are magnified, and also when the diver attempts to retain the air in his lungs, instead of exhaling it. In the past, free ascent training from 18 to 30 metres was carried out by divers and submariners, and was a typical situation in which this disorder occurred – it caused considerable problems with differential diagnosis.

As there is no actual lung pathology, it is technically incorrect to describe this as pulmonary barotrauma, but it could sometimes be a step in the progression to this disease.

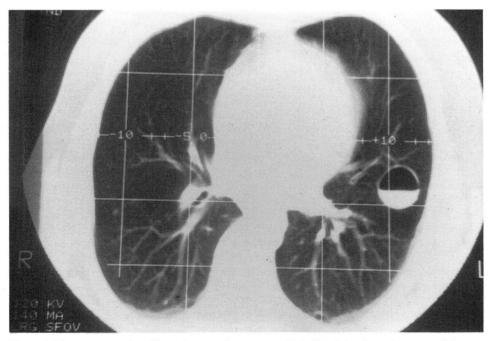

**Figure 9.5** Lung cyst produced by pulmonary barotrauma. This CT of the chest shows an axial scan through the lower zones. In the left lower zone, there is a 3-cm diameter cyst which contains a fluid level. It resolved within a month

### CASE REPORT 9.4
(described by a diver/doctor, in his incident report)

On Day 1 a bounce dive was carried out to 492 feet by the diver using a helium/oxygen system. The dive job was carried out successfully and was completed without incident in 13 minutes. During decompression upon reaching 90 feet, the diver reported a tightness in his chest, some shortness of breath and discomfort while breathing.

The diver was recompressed to 100 feet where he had complete relief and felt normal. The chamber atmosphere was at this point changed over to a saturation atmosphere and the diver was decompressed at a saturation decompression rate. The Diving Superintendent at this point informed Mr A. on shore that a treatment procedure was being carried out.

When the diver reached 85 feet the symptoms redeveloped and other treatment procedures were instituted. The diver was recompressed to 185 feet and brought out on a treatment schedule.

Decompression was uneventful with the diver feeling fine until Day 2 at 02:53 hours, where, at 105 feet, the diver had the first recurrence of symptoms. The diver was recompressed according to the treatment schedules and then decompressed. He experienced a second recurrence of the symptoms at 85 feet during decompression and he was once more recompressed to 185 feet for therapeutic decompression at 14:33 hours. At this point a special treatment was instituted at Mr A.'s instructions. He had now diagnosed the case as a burst lung problem and discounted any kind of bend.

On Day 3 at 13:00 hours, upon reaching 75 feet during his decompression, the diver complained of restriction to his breathing whereupon he was recompressed to 125 feet where he obtained complete relief. It was decided to attempt decompression once more to see if the diver could be decompressed all the way or if there would be a further recurrence of symptoms. At 23:25 hours while reaching 83 feet in the decompression the diver again complained of breathing difficulties. Recompression to 135 feet relieved all symptoms.

At this point it was decided by Mr A. that the problem could not be an ordinary decompression problem and was reasonably certain that the symptoms were the result of a pneumothorax. A doctor was called and arrangements were made to go to the rig in the morning of Day 4. The doctor was informed of the treatment to date and of the diagnosis and was asked to bring the necessary needles with him to vent a pneumothorax.

On Day 4 at 10:49 hours Mr A. and the doctor arrived at the rig. At 13:49 hours while the diver was at 80 feet the doctor made a cursory examination of the diver without taking his temperature and diagnosed the diver's condition as 'full blown pneumonia and pleurisy of the left lung' and ruled out the possibility of a pneumothorax. The doctor was challenged on the fact that the diver obtained relief by recompression; however, he stated that this would be the case with pneumonia and that he had previously treated a very similar case.

At this point the doctor took over the treatment and instructed the diver to be decompressed at the rate of 3 feet per hour and emphasized the fact that the diver would experience severe chest pains during decompression due to the pneumonia. By the afternoon of Day 4 the diver was treated with penicillin injections and, due to severe pain, an injection of pain killer was administered by the rig medic at 22:45 hours of Day 4.

The doctor left the rig by evening of Day 4 stating that it was a routine case and that he would be available ashore for consultation. By the morning of Day 5, the diver had

**Case report 9.4 (contd)**

been decompressed to a depth of 60 feet and his condition had steadily deteriorated. Mr A. at this point requested the opinion of a second doctor regarding the diver's treatment and condition. Attempts were made by Mr B. to obtain another doctor to go to the rig but he was unsuccessful.

The attending doctor was notified of these attempts and of the worsening of the diver's condition. During Day 5 the diver received injections of penicillin and pain killer with little apparent effect. During the early hours of Day 6, further drugs were administered and the diver's condition was worsening. The doctor had been summoned and examined the patient at 03:40 hours while the diver was at 39 feet.

The doctor stated that the diver's condition had improved, that the pneumonia was disappearing and that the decompression rate was to be increased so that the diver could be transferred to a hospital as soon as possible.

At 09:00 hours the diver's pulse had stopped and by 09:15 he was pronounced dead by the doctor.

*Cause of death*
1. Death resulted from a pneumothorax of the left lung (postmortem finding).
2. Cause of pneumothorax unknown; however, it was learned that the diver had a slight chest cough on the day before the incident and complained to the rig medic of some pain on the left side of his chest, and over the central area.

## Pulmonary barotrauma of descent

This is known by the divers as 'lung squeeze'.

Descent barotrauma is not common in breath-hold diving, and very rare with open circuit diving apparatus. The actual depth limit for breath-hold diving is probably determined by two factors:

1. Residual lung volume: the total lung volume decreases with increasing depth, in accordance with Boyle's law. Once the actual volume approximates the residual volume, lung compressibility is limited, and subsequent descent results in pressure gradients which are equalized by pulmonary congestion, oedema and haemorrhage. Further descent may also result in collapse of the chest wall.

2. Individual variations in the dilatory response of the pulmonary vascular bed to an increased pulmonary vascular-to-alveolar pressure gradient. It has been found that, in deep breath-hold dives, the pulmonary venous bed dilates and blood displaces air in the thorax, decreasing the effective residual volume. This extends the depth which can be reached in safety.

*Pulmonary barotrauma of descent is rare.*

An average full lung contains 6 litres of air at the surface, but this is compressed to 1.5 litres at 30 metres. This approximates the normal residual volume, and further descent may be hazardous. The individual pulmonary vascular response determines the final volume limitation. Breath-hold dives to a depth of 100 metres have been achieved because of a combination of increased dilatation of the pulmonary venous bed, a large vital capacity and a small residual volume. The minimal residual volume, which if further reduced will result in pulmonary damage, has not been determined.

In diving with open circuit apparatus, inhaled gases are at the same pressure as the surrounding environment and the diver, thus preventing pulmonary barotrauma of descent.

Pulmonary barotrauma of descent is possible in the following situations:

- Breath-hold diving.
- Loss of surface pressure supply with failure or absence of a non-return valve. This may occur with surface supply and standard diving.
- Failure of the gas supply to compensate for the rate of descent. This is more common with standard diving in which there is no automatic relationship between the gas supply and the ambient pressures, and in which the diver is overweighted and has negative buoyancy.

Clinical features are poorly documented but include chest pain, haemoptysis with haemorrhagic pulmonary oedema and death. Treatment is based on general principles. Intermittent positive pressure respiration may be needed. Initially, 100% oxygen should be used with replacement of fluids, treatment of shock etc. The use of positive end-expiratory pressure would seem hazardous and predispose to subsequent gas embolism, but may be necessary (see Chapter 21).

## Recommended reading

ADOLFSON, J.A. and LINDEMERK, C. (1973). Pulmonary and neurological complications in free escape. *Forsvarsmedicin* **9**(3), 244–246.

BUTLER, B.D., KATZ, J., LEIMAN, B.C. et al. (1987). Cerebral decompression sickness: Bubble distribution in dogs in the Trendelenberg position. *UHMS Annual Meeting.*

CALDER, I.M. (1985). Autopsy and experimental observations on factors leading to barotrauma in man. *Undersea Biomedical Research* **12**(1), 165–182.

COLEBACH, H.J.H., SMITH, M.M. and NG, C.K.Y. (1976). Increased elastic recoil as a determinant of pulmonary barotrauma in divers. *Respiratory Physiology* **26**, 55–64.

DAUGHERTY, C.G. (1990). Inherent unsaturation in the treatment of pneumothorax at depth. *Undersea Biomedical Research* **17**(2), 171–177.

DUTKA, A.J. (1985). A review of the pathophysiology and potential application of experimental therapies for cerebral ischaemia to the treatment of cerebral arterial gas embolism. *Undersea Biomedical Research* **12**(4), 403–421.

DUTKA, A.J. (1990). Therapy for dysbaric central nervous system ischaemia. Adjuncts to recompression. In: *UHMS/NOAA/DAN Workshop in Diver Accident Management*, edited by P.B. Bennett and R. Moon. Duke University.

ELLIOTT, D.H., HARRISON, J.A.B. and BARNARD, E.P.P. (1975). Clinical and radiological features of 88 cases of decompression barotrauma. *Proceedings of Sixth Underwater Physiology Symposium.*

GORMAN, D.F. (1987). The redistribution of cerebral arterial gas emboli. *PhD Thesis in Medicine,* University of Sydney.

GORMAN, D.F. and BROWNING, D.M. (1986). Cerebral Vasoreactivity and Arterial Gas Embolism. *Undersea Biomedical Research* **13**(3), 317–335.

HOFF, E.C. (1948). *A Bibliographical Source Book of Compressed Air, Diving and Submarine Medicine*, Vol. 1. Bu Medical Department of Navy, Washington, DC.

LEITCH, D.R. and GREEN, R.D. (1986). Pulmonary barotrauma in divers and the treatment of cerebral arterial gas embolism. *Aviation Space and Environmental Medicine* **57**, 931–938.

MACKLIN, M.T. and MACKLIN, C.C. (1944). Malignant interstitial emphysema of the lungs and mediastinum. *Medicine* **23**, 281–358.

PEARSON, R.R. (1984). *The Physicians Guide to Diving Medicine*, edited by C.W. Shilling, C.B. Carlston and R.A. Mathias, New York: Plenum Press.

POLAK, I.B. and ADAMS, H. (1932). Traumatic air embolism in submarine escape training. *US Navy Medical Bulletin* **30**, 165.

SCHAEFFER, K.E., McNULTY, S.P., CAREY, C.R. and LIEBOW, A.A. (1958). Mechanism in development of interstitial emphysema and air embolism on decompression from depth. *Journal of Applied Physiology* **13**, 15–29.

SCHAEFER, K.E., ALLISON, R.D., DOUGHERTY J.H. and PARKER, D. (1968). Pulmonary and circulatory adjustments determining the limits of depths in breathhold diving. *Science* **162**, 1040.

SCHAEFER, K.E., McNULTY, S.P., CAREY, C.R. and LIEBOM, A.A. (1958). Mechanism in development of interstitial emphysema and air embolism on decompression from depth. *Journal of Applied Physiology* **13**, 15–29.

SCHILLING, C.W., WERTS, M.F. and SCHANDELMEIER, N.R. (Eds) (1976). *The Underwater Handbook*. New York: Plenum Press.

STRAUSS, M.B. and WRIGHT, P.W. (1971). Thoracic squeeze diving casualty. *Aerospace Medicine* **42**, 673–675.

UMS Workshop No 13. (1977). *Arterial air embolism and acute stroke*. Bethesda, Maryland: UMS publication.

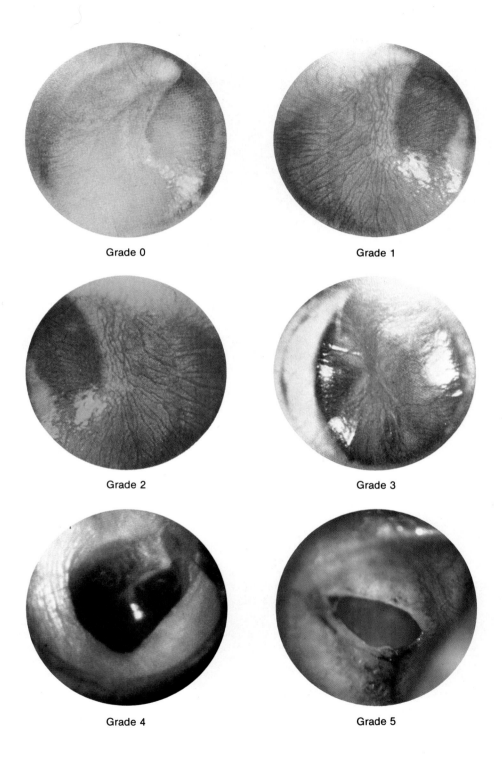

**Plate 1** Middle-ear barotrauma of descent: grades 0–5, graded by otoscopy

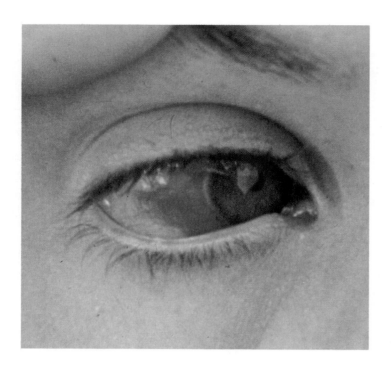

**Plate 2** Facial barotrauma of descent (mask squeeze), causing subconjunctival haemorrhages and facial oedema when this diver did not equalize the pressures within the mask during descent to 15 metres

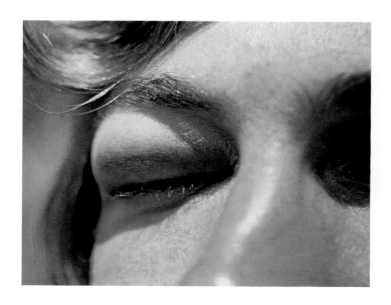

**Plate 3** Orbital surgical emphysema: following a recent vehicle accident, this diver performed a Valsalva manoeuvre at a depth of 9 metres. The otherwise asymptomatic fracture to the lamina papyracea allowed gas to pass from the nasal cavity to the orbit, causing surgical emphysema which expanded on ascent, occluded the palpebral fissure and produced subcutaneous haemorrhage

# 10

# Ear, sinus and other barotrauma

## Introduction

Barotrauma is defined as the tissue damage resulting from the expansion or contraction of enclosed gas spaces, and is a direct effect of gas volume changes causing tissue distortion. It is probably the most common occupational disease of divers, experienced to some degree by almost all.

Middle-ear barotrauma is the most common form of barotrauma; however, pulmonary barotrauma of ascent (see Chapter 9) is the most important. Ear barotrauma is a contributor to panic and diving deaths in novice divers, and to permanent hearing loss in experienced divers.

In the earlier literature on caisson workers' and divers' disorders, the common barotrauma symptoms were hopelessly confused with decompression sickness symptoms (especially those affecting the cranial nerves, and specifically the eighth nerve). This confusion has extended to animal experiments and the interpretation of many clinical reports.

There are two types of barotrauma – descent and ascent. Both are caused by the effects of Boyle's law (see Chapter 2). The volume

> Barotrauma refers to damage to tissues resulting from changes in volume of gas spaces which, in turn, is due to the changes in ambient pressure with descent and ascent.

change is proportionally greatest near the surface, and so it is in this zone that barotrauma is most noticeable.

Barotrauma of descent is that damage which occurs during compression in a chamber or descent in water, i.e. as a result of increasing pressures of the surrounding environment. Pressure imbalance is due to an inability to equalize pressures within the body cavities as the depth increases. The volume of contained gas decreases in accordance with Boyle's law. Because some cavities are surrounded by bone, no collapse can occur, and the space may be taken up by engorgement of the mucous membrane, oedema and haemorrhage. This, together with the compressed gas, assists in equalizing the pressure balance. It is commonly called a 'squeeze'.

Barotrauma of ascent is the result of the distension of tissues around the expanding gas. This occurs when environmental pressures are reduced, i.e. on decompression in a chamber or ascent in water. Divers use the misnomer 'reverse squeeze' to describe it.

> *Middle-ear barotrauma of descent is the most common disorder encountered by divers.*

## Ear barotrauma

This constitutes the major cause of morbidity among divers. There are two main types depending upon whether the injury is due to descent or ascent and the barotrauma is subdivided accordingly to the anatomical sites. The two types may occur separately or in combination in the external ear, the middle ear or the inner ear. General information on the ear in diving, including references to barotrauma, is also included in Chapter 27.

### External-ear barotrauma of descent
(external-ear squeeze, reversed ear)

Due to the fact that the external auditory canal communicates with the environment, water enters and replaces the air in the canal during descent. If, however, the external meatus is blocked, this water entry is prevented. Then the contraction of the contained gas cannot be compensated for by tissue collapse, but may be achieved by outward bulging of the tympanic membrane, followed by congestion and haemorrhage. These results are observed when the pressure gradient from water to air within the blocked external auditory canal is 150 mmHg or more, i.e. in as little as 2 metres of water.

The common causes of blockage of the external auditory canal include: cerumen, exostoses, foreign bodies such as mechanical ear plugs, tight fitting hoods and mask straps.

Clinical symptoms are usually mild. Occasionally, a slight difficulty in performing the Valsalva manoeuvre is experienced. Following ascent there may be an ache in the affected ear and/or a bloody discharge.

Examination of the external auditory canal may reveal petechial haemorrhages and blood-filled cutaneous blebs which may extend onto the tympanic membrane.

Treatment for this condition includes maintaining a dry canal, careful cleansing of the canal with 1.5% hydrogen peroxide solution, warmed to body temperature, removal of any occlusion and prohibition of diving until epithelial surfaces appear normal. Secondary infection may result in a recurrence of the pain, and require antibiotics.

This condition is easily prevented by ensuring patency of external auditory canals and avoidance of ear plugs or hoods which do not have apertures over the ear to permit water entry.

External-ear barotrauma of ascent is theoretically possible if there was a small opening of the external ear and a rapid ascent. It could also occur as a sequel to descent barotrauma when the material in the external ear prevented gas expansion. It has never been seen by these authors.

### Middle-ear barotrauma of descent
(middle-ear squeeze)

This is by far the most common medical disorder experienced by divers, and it follows the failure to equalize middle-ear and environmental pressures via the eustachian tubes. An abnormal pressure difference (gradient) is established and is responsible for the tissue damage.

Diving marine animals avoid this disorder by having an arteriovenous plexus in the middle ear. This fills up during descent and empties on ascent, accommodating the volume changes.

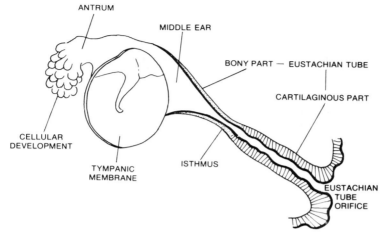

ANTRUM

MIDDLE EAR

BONY PART — EUSTACHIAN TUBE

CARTILAGINOUS PART

CELLULAR
DEVELOPMENT

TYMPANIC
MEMBRANE

ISTHMUS

EUSTACHIAN
TUBE
ORIFICE

**Figure 10.1** Middle-ear cleft

---

> *Any condition which tends to block the eustachian tube predisposes to middle-ear barotrauma.*

## Pathophysiology

The eustachian tubes usually open when the pressure gradient between the pharynx and middle-ear cavity reaches 10–30 mmHg. These figures equate to an underwater depth of 27 cm (1 foot). Equalization of pressures occurs when the eustachian tubes open. This can be achieved by yawning, moving the jaw or swallowing, or by inflating the middle-ear cavity using the Valsalva manoeuvre. It is termed 'clearing the ears' by divers.

If the eustachian tubes are blocked during descent, a subjective sensation of pressure will develop when the environmental pressure external to the tympanic membrane exceeds that in the middle-ear cavity by 20 mmHg, or 25 cmH$_2$O depth. Discomfort or pain may be noted with a descent from the surface to 2 metres, a 150 mmHg pressure change and a volume reduction of less than 20% in the middle-ear cavity. If the middle-ear pressure is then equalized, for another 20% middle-ear volume reduction and its associated ear pain to occur, the diver must descend to 4.4 metres, then to 7.3 metres, then to 10.8 metres etc. Thus, the deeper he goes, the fewer autoinflation manoeuvres are required per unit depth. If autoinflation is delayed beyond a certain point, a locking effect may develop and prevent successful autoinflation. It is due to the eustachian mucosa being drawn into the middle ear and obstructing the tube.

If this diver continues his descent without equalizing, mucosal congestion, oedema and haemorrhage within the middle-ear cavity are associated with inward bulging of the tympanic membrane. This tends to compensate for the contraction of air within the otherwise rigid cavity. The tympanic membrane will become haemorrhagic (the 'traumatic tympanum' of older texts). Eventually it may rupture, although this is not common.

There is a time factor in the development of middle-ear pathology, with greater damage resulting from longer exposure to unequalized middle-ear pressures.

Blockage of the eustachian tubes may be due to mucosal congestion as a manifestation of upper respiratory tract infections, allergies, otitis media, mechanical obstructions, such as mucosal polyps, or individual variations in size, shape and patency.

---

> *Factors leading to blockage of the eustachian tube include:*
>
> - *Upper respiratory infections and allergies.*
> - *Alcohol ingestion*
> - *Premenstrual mucosal congestion*
> - *Mucosal polyps*
> - *Descent to the point of 'locking'*
> - *Deviation from upright position*
> - *Cigarette smoking*

Opening of the eustachian tubes is more difficult in the inverted position, as when the diver swims downwards. It is easier if the diver descends feet first.

Divers should be advised of the dangers of delaying middle-ear autoinflation and of using excessive force in achieving it.

### Symptoms

These consist initially of discomfort followed by increasing pain in the ear if descent continues. This may be sufficiently severe to prevent further descent. Occasionally a diver may have little or no symptomatology despite causing significant barotrauma. This occurs in some divers who seem particularly insensitive to the barotrauma effects, and also when a small pressure gradient is allowed to act over a prolonged time, e.g. when using scuba in a swimming pool or when not autoinflating the ears on the bottom, following the final metre or so of descent.

Occasionally there is a sensation of vertigo during the descent, but vertigo is not as common as in middle-ear barotrauma of ascent or inner-ear barotrauma (see later), both of which can follow or be due to middle-ear barotrauma of descent. A patulous eustachian tube (page 379) can also follow either descent barotrauma or the forceful attempts at Valsalva techniques to overcome it.

Most difficulties are encountered within the first 10 metres due to the greater volume/pressure changes occuring down to this depth. Eventually, rupture of the drum may occur, usually after a descent of 1.5–10 metres (100–760 mmHg pressure) from the surface. This causes instant equalization of pressures by allowing water entry into the middle-ear cavity. If this occurs, pain is automatically relieved; however, nausea and vertigo may follow the caloric stimulation by the cold water. It is seldom dangerous and quickly settles as the water temperature within the middle-ear cavity approaches that of the body.

Following a dive which has resulted in descent barotrauma, there may be a mild residual pain in the affected ear. Blood or blood-stained fluid may be expelled from the middle ear during ascent, and present in the nasopharynx or the nostril on the affected side. Blood will rarely be seen in the external ear, from the haemorrhagic tympanic membrane.

A full or blocked sensation may be experienced in the ear. This is sometimes associated with a mild conductive deafness involving low frequencies, and is due to some dampening effect on the ossicles. It is usually only temporary. Fluid may be felt within the middle ear for a week or so, before full resolution.

Middle-ear barotrauma is classified into six grades based on the otoscopic appearance of the tympanic membrane. The grades are shown in the box on page 119.

Damage involves the whole of the middle-ear space and not the tympanic membrane alone.

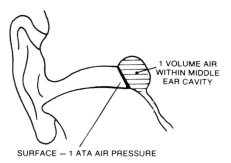

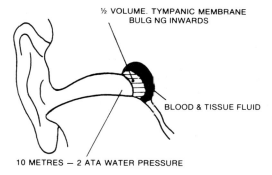

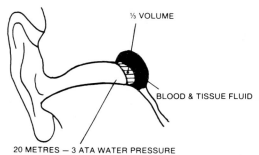

**Figure 10.2** Middle-ear barotrauma of descent

**Middle-ear barotrauma of descent – grading**

*Grade 0* – Symptoms without signs
*Grade I* – Injection of the tympanic membrane, especially along the handle of the malleus
*Grade II* – Injection plus slight haemorrhage within the substance of the tympanic membrane
*Grade III* – Gross haemorrhage within the substance of the tympanic membrane
*Grade IV* – Free blood in the middle ear as evidenced by blueness and bulging
*Grade V* – Performation of the tympanic membrane

The **clinical management** consists of:

- The prohibition of all pressure changes such as diving and autoinflation techniques until resolution.
- Occasionally (very rarely) systemic or local decongestants.
- Antibiotics only where there is evidence of a pre-existing or developing otitis media, gross haemorrhage or perforation (see Case 23.2).

In treating many thousands of middle-ear barotrauma cases, these authors have not often used antibiotics or decongestants.

Serial audiometric examination should be undertaken to exclude any hearing loss, and to assist in further action if such loss is present. Impedance audiometry may be used to follow the middle-ear pathological changes, if there is no perforation.

*Serial audiograms should be performed on all but the most minor cases of middle-ear barotrauma.*

Diving can be resumed when resolution is complete, and autoinflation of the middle-ear cleft has been demonstrated. If there is no perforation (grades 0–4), recovery may take up to 2 weeks. With perforation (grade 5) it may take 1–2 months, if uncomplicated and managed conservatively. Although the tympanic membrane may appear normal much earlier, recurrent perforation frequently results from a premature return to diving. There does not appear to be any indication for such active procedures as tympanoplasty, unless healing is incomplete, or if the lesion recurs with minimal provocation.

It is important to identify clearly the contributing factors to the disease in each case, or whether it is likely to recur.

### Prevention

Prevention of this disorder consists of ensuring patency of the eustachian tubes prior to diving, and good training in autoinflation. This is best checked by otoscopic examination of the tympanic membrane during a Valsalva manoeuvre, when the tympanic membrane will be seen to move outwards slightly. The degree of force needed to autoinflate, and the degree of movement of the drum, will provide an estimate of the probable ease of pressure equalization for subsequent dives. If one or other tympanic membrane appears to move sluggishly, or if much force is necessary, then decongestant nasal drops or sprays may help to improve the patency of the eustachian tubes. This can also be improved by training and attention to technique (see later).

The use of **decongestants** to improve eustachian tube patency prior to diving is to be discouraged. They reduce descent barotrauma problems but increase ascent barotraumas. From the safety aspect, it is preferable to be prevented from descending than to be prevented from ascending.

The rebound congestion of the mucosa is cited by otologists as a reason for avoidance of decongestants, but the diving clinician is more concerned with the systemic problems of sympathomimetics and the increased incidence of middle-ear barotrauma of ascent seen with these medications. The reason for the latter may be that decongestants are more effective in improving nasal air flow and thereby affecting the pharyngeal cushions of the eustachian tube, than in influencing the tubal mucosa or middle-ear orifice, which may be affected by the same pathology. Decongestants, both local and general, will only be effective in the marginally obstructed tube, thereby allowing slow descent and permitting some degree of descent barotrauma and resultant congestion of the middle-ear orifices of the tube, which block on ascent and cause middle-ear distension and barotrauma (see later).

In most cases, and especially in the novice diver, practice, instruction in middle-ear autoinflation and use of correct diving techniques, are much more effective than drugs in improving eustachian tube patency.

---

*Avoid diving with disorders which block the eustachian tube and sinus ostia, including:*

- *Upper respiratory infections.*
- *Upper respiratory allergies.*
- *Alcohol ingestion.*
- *Premenstrual mucosal congestion.*
- *Cigarette smoking.*

*Gross nasopathology such as septal deviations, polyps etc. may require repair.*

---

Instruments are available to measure the force or pressure necessary to open the eustachian tubes. A much improved estimation of eustachian tube patency and middle-ear pressure changes is possible when impedance audiometers are employed clinically. (See Chapter 27 for more information.)

When dealing with patients who have not adequately autoinflated their middle ears during descent – despite the ability to perform this in the clinic – the following errors are commonly observed.

1. Not autoinflating early enough, e.g. waiting until the sensation of pressure is felt. This results in the 'locking' of the eustachian tube referred to above. Commonly the novice diver, instead of performing a Valsalva manoeuvre before descent, will concentrate on his struggle to descend and will often be 2–3 metres underwater before he 'remembers his ears'.
2. Attempting to autoinflate while in the horizontal or, worse, the head-down position. Eustachian tube patency is reduced as the subject deviates from the upright posture. This may be related to the greater ease of pushing gas upwards in a virtually fluid or incompressible environment (the eustachian mucosa and tissue) or impedance of gas flow by eustachian mucosal congestion with increasing venous pressures.
3. If only one ear is difficult, it is advisable to cock that ear toward the surface while attempting autoinflation. This stretches the pharyngeal muscles and puts the offending tube in a vertical position, capitalizing on the pressure gradient of the water.

---

## CASE REPORT 10.1

JQ performed three scuba dives, to a depth of 5 metres. He was not able to equalize the pressure in his middle ear during descent, but in the first dive he did manage to achieve this after he had reached 5 metres. Following this first dive, his ears felt 'full' or 'blocked'. He then went down to 3 metres 'to see if I could clear them' for his second dive with the same result. On the third dive, he felt pressure in his ear during descent, and again could only equalize them once he had reached the bottom; considerable pressure was required for autoinflation. After ascent he again noted that his ears felt blocked and he again attempted to equalize them, this time using considerable pressure. Suddenly pain developed in the right ear, and it gave way with a 'hissing out'. On otoscopic examination of the left ear there was a grade III aural barotrauma with a very dark tympanic membrane, haemorrhage over the handle of the malleus and the membrana flaccida, and a small haemorrhage anterior to the handle of the malleus. The right ear had similar features with a large perforation posterior to the tip of the handle of the malleus. Daily audiograms revealed a 15 dB loss in this ear throughout the 250–4000 Hz range. This hearing loss disappeared after 2 weeks when the perforation had almost healed.

*Diagnosis:* middle-ear barotrauma of descent.

4. Ignoring the intercurrent mucosal congestion from such factors as infections, irritants
such as cigarette smoke, drug snorting or
allergies.

5. Previous overt or subclinical middle-ear
barotrauma of descent may also cause congestion of the middle-ear spaces and eustachian tube blocking – after successful
descents. Equalizing becomes harder as diving continues, with delayed or omitted
middle-ear autoinflation, until the middle
ear is almost totally full of fluid. Then there
is little problem with diving, but at the
expense of middle- or inner-ear damage.
This problem can be avoided by early and
successful autoinflation.

### Middle-ear autoinflation techniques

Passive opening of the eustachian tubes is the
ideal way to equalize pressure between the
middle ear and the nasopharynx, although it is
not always possible. Most amateur divers use
an active technique which will inflate the middle ears to prevent the pain and discomfort
during descent, and perhaps even permanent
damage that can occasionally result from
middle-ear barotrauma. During ascent, passive
equalization of ear pressures is more common,
and active techniques are rarely needed.

It is part of the routine diving medical examination to ensure that the diving candidate can
equalize his middle ear actively, and this is
achieved by using a positive pressure technique
described to the patient, while the examiner is
observing the tympanic membrane and its
movement. The latter is seen either by focusing
on the otoscopic light reflex or on another part
of the tympanic membrane. As the candidate
autoinflates the middle ear, the tympanic
membrane moves outwards.

The following techniques are recommended.
Different candidates perform them with different degrees of ease. In each case practice of
the technique is recommended on land, before
subjecting the novice to hyperbaric and aquatic
conditions which interfere with the application
of this new skill.

The *Valsalva* manoeuvre is probably the
most easily understood. It involves occluding

the nostrils, closing the mouth and exhaling so
that the pressure in the nasopharynx is increased. This separates the cushions of the
eustachian tube and forces air up this tube into
the middle ear. The pressure required to achieve this varies from 20 to 100 cmH$_2$O.

The force necessary for the successful
autoinflation will vary with the diver's *body
position*. Using the Valsalva technique, novice
divers average 40 cmH$_2$O in the head-up,
vertical position, and in the horizontal, ear-up
position. In the horizontal, ear-down position
they need 50 cmH$_2$O. In the vertical,
swimming-down position they average about
60 cmH$_2$O.

The *Frenzel* manoeuvre involves closing the
mouth and nose, both externally and internally
(this is achieved by closing of the glottis) and
then contracting the muscles of the mouth and
pharynx upwards. Thus, the nose, mouth and
glottis are closed and the elevated tongue can
be used as a piston to compress the air trapped
in the nasopharynx and force it up the eustachian tube. Pressure of less than 10 cmH$_2$O
may achieve this manoeuvre.

As divers become more experienced, they
tend to utilize such techniques as jaw movements, starting a yawn, swallowing, lifting the
soft palate etc. which allow for autoinflation of
the middle ear without pressurizing the nasopharynx.

The voluntary opening of the eustachian
tubes (beance tubaire voluntaire, BTV) refers
to the opening of the eustachian cushions and
allowing the pressure difference between the
middle ear and nasopharynx to move air. This
tends to be performed by experienced divers
who, over the years, have developed the muscular skill. The same principles are used in the
physiological replenishment of the middle-ear
air contents and is achieved by thrusting the
lower jaw downward and forward while keeping the mouth closed (or around the mouth
piece).

The *Toynbee* manoeuvre involves swallowing with the mouth and nose closed, and is of
special value in relieving the over-pressure in
the middle ear during ascent. It is also of value
during descent when movement of the eustachian cushions produce a nasopharyngeal
opening of the eustachian tube, with an equalization of pressures between the nasopharynx

and the middle ear. Thus the final pressure in the middle ear with the Toynbee manoeuvre may be negative (less than environmental).

A combination of the techniques has also been proposed. A very successful one is the combination of the Toynbee and Valsalva, often referred to as the *Lowry* technique. This involves the closing of the nostrils, then a swallowing movement which is made continuously with a Valsalva manoeuvre. The diver is thus advised to 'hold your nose, blow and swallow at the same time'. Despite the rather confusing instruction, the technique is extremely valuable in resistant cases. It is easily learnt with practice, on land.

The *Edmonds* technique is rather similar, and involves the opening of the eustachian cushions by rocking the lower jaw forward and downward (similar to the start of a yawn), so that the lower teeth project well in advance of the upper teeth, and performing a Valsalva manoeuvre at the same time.

When examining potential divers, attempts to demonstrate either the Frenzel or the BTV are not usually successful. In the authors' practice, the Valsalva manoeuvre is tried first, followed by the Toynbee, the Lowry and then the Edmonds technique. If there is any difficulty remaining with equalization, then the candidate is advised to repeat the most effective procedure a few times a day, and achieve success before commencing his diving course.

Academic arguments abound as to which is the best technique. Whichever one works is the best. The major problem is not the danger of middle-ear autoinflation, but the danger of not doing it.

Some techniques (Valsalva, Lowry, Edmonds) have the disadvantage of a transitory pressure that may extend into the thorax – but have the advantage of distending the middle ear and thus allow further descent without the problems of a negative middle-ear pressure developing and producing middle-ear congestion and eustachian tube locking. These are therefore better for divers who have trouble with middle-ear autoinflation.

Other techniques (Toynbee, BTV) are ideal if there is easy and frequent middle-ear autoinflation. They either equalize the pressures passively or produce negative middle-ear pressures. Wave action or descent can some-times cause a negative middle-ear pressure with congestion and eustachian tube locking, and these techniques may aggravate this.

Experienced divers, who have mobile tympanic membranes like small spinnakers, can often descend to great depths before they need to equalize their middle-ear pressures. They also autoinflate their ears using less pressure.

Most patients referred to us with inability to autoinflate their middle ears have suffered more from inadequate instruction than eustachian tube obstruction. To ascertain the extent of this problem, 200 consecutive otoscopic examinations were recorded on potential diving candidates. Autoinflation was successful using either the Valsalva, Toynbee, Lowry or Edmonds techniques in 96% of subjects, with 4% being unsuccessful in one or both ears.

Middle-ear autoinflation, together with sinus autoinflation, seems easier and less barotrauma has been noted with helium/oxygen breathing than with air breathing.

During ascent, the middle ear opens passively, with a pressure gradient of around 50 cmH$_2$O (70 in the head-down position).

## Middle-ear barotrauma of ascent

This refers to the damage from distension by enclosed gases within the middle ear, expanding with ascent. Due to the fact that this damage may prevent ascent, it is usually considered more serious than middle-ear barotrauma of descent – which allows unhindered return to safety.

Gas which has entered the middle ear by autoinflation at depth is at the surrounding environmental pressure, and on ascent it obeys Boyle's law. If the eustachian tube restricts its release, the expansion of gas within the middle-ear cavity can cause symptoms. These may include sensations of pressure or pain in the affected ear, vertigo due to increased middle-ear pressure difference, i.e. alternobaric vertigo (see page 386) or tinnitus.

The vertigo is most pronounced when the diver assumes the vertical position, and least in the horizontal. The spinning is towards the ear with the higher pressure. It tends to develop when the middle-ear pressures differ by 60 cmH$_2$O. Relief of the over-pressure in the affected middle ear may be heard, with air felt hissing out of the eustachian tube.

Hearing loss in the affected ear, if present, may be either conductive or sensorineural and may follow damage to the tympanic membrane or the middle-ear structures. Inner-ear barotrauma, as described previously, is a possible complication. Seventh nerve palsy is also a complication (see page 137).

Middle-ear barotrauma of ascent usually follows recent, but sometimes mild, middle-ear barotrauma of descent or the use of nasal decongestants. In each case, the common factor is probably a congestion and therefore blockage of the eustachian tube – laterally with the ascent and medially with the descent. It is often a complication of decongestant use (see above).

Otoscopic examination often reveals evidence of tympanic membrane injection or haemorrhage. Congestion of blood vessels is

common, but is less than with descent barotrauma. It is more pronounced around the circumference of the tympanic membrane than along the handle of the malleus. The tympanic membrane may appear to be bulging.

During the dive, these divers endure the discomfort as they ascend. Occasionally the Valsalva technique, jaw movements or performing a Toynbee manoeuvre (swallowing with the nostrils occluded) will relieve the discomfort, as may pressure applied to the external ear (by pushing the water column in the external ear, with the tragus or middle lobe). Equalization is usually easier if the affected ear is facing the sea bed, thereby utilizing the pressure gradient along the now vertical eustachian tube.

Fortunately, most effects are short-lived, and treatment should consist of prohibition of diving until clinical resolution has occurred and normal hearing and vestibular function are demonstrated. Vestibular function may often be tested while undergoing pressure changes in a recompression chamber, to replicate the sequence of events and verify the aetiology. Antibiotics are indicated if there is evidence of infection or gross haemorrhage, and decongestants are sometimes used to improve the eustachian tube patency.

Decongestants, especially topical ones, are rarely of use in preventing this disorder unless they help prevent a causal middle-ear barotrauma of descent. Usually they have the opposite effect (see above). Systemic decongestants are more effective, being more likely to influence the mucosa of the middle ear, but they have other disadvantages.

Prevention is usually best achieved by avoiding these nasal decongestants and by training of the diver in correct middle-ear equalization techniques (see above). Unless the descent barotrauma is prevented (this causes the initial eustachian tube congestion), the ascent barotrauma is likely to recur.

Once middle-ear barotrauma of ascent has been experienced, particular care should be taken that, if it does recur, the diver will have adequate air to allow for descent and gradual ascent. A low-on-air situation could cause extreme discomfort or danger, if the diver's ascent is restricted.

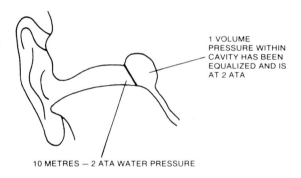

1 VOLUME
PRESSURE WITHIN CAVITY HAS BEEN EQUALIZED AND IS AT 2 ATA

10 METRES – 2 ATA WATER PRESSURE

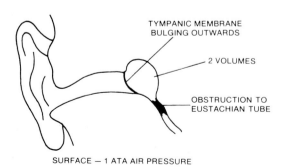

TYMPANIC MEMBRANE BULGING OUTWARDS

2 VOLUMES

OBSTRUCTION TO EUSTACHIAN TUBE

SURFACE – 1 ATA AIR PRESSURE

**Figure 10.3** Middle-ear barotrauma of ascent

## Inner-ear barotrauma

There is always the possibility of a sensorineural hearing loss in divers who have experienced ear barotrauma of any type, who have had difficulty in equalizing middle-ear pressures by autoinflation or who subsequently apply force to achieve this. In these cases, the hearing loss may immediately follow the incident, or may develop over the next few days.

Tinnitus is a very common association. Some patients, but certainly not all, may complain of vertigo, nausea and vomiting etc. The hearing loss is of the sensorineural type, either partial, predominantly involving high frequencies, or total, involving the whole range of frequencies. There may be no otoscopic signs.

Combined cochlear/vestibular injury is experienced in 50%: only cochlear injury in 40% and only vestibular in 10%.

---

> *In the event of otological barotrauma, a sensorineural or combined hearing loss, or demonstrable vestibular damage, implies inner-ear barotrauma.*

---

### Pathophysiology

An inner-ear (labyrinthine) window fistula is one pathological manifestation of inner-ear disease. It is usually also a complication of middle-ear barotrauma of descent or of a forceful Valsalva manoeuvre. There are two postulated mechanisms for this disorder: in one, the tympanic membrane moves inward because of the pressure gradient, resulting in the foot plate of the stapes being pushed inwards. This causes a displacement of perilymph through the helicotrema, so that the round window membrane bulges outwards. If, at this stage, a forceful Valsalva manoeuvre is performed, there is an increase in the pressure within the middle-ear cleft leading to the tympanic membrane being very rapidly returned to its normal position, the stapes moving outwards and the round window being pushed inwards. The reversed flow of perilymph may not be sufficiently rapid to avoid damage to the inner-ear structures, e.g. rupture of the round window membrane with loss of perilymph. The other explanation for this pathology involves a pressure wave transmitted from the cerebrospinal fluid through a patent cochlear aqueduct during the Valsalva manoeuvre, and 'blowing out' the round window into the middle ear. This has been demonstrated in animal experiments, with a rise in cerebrospinal fluid pressure of 120 mmHg. It is also thought to be one of the mechanisms for the occurrence of round window fistulae in weight lifters. The aqueduct constricts with age and may explain why children are more susceptible.

Other forms of inner-ear damage have been postulated but require further investigation. It is probable that cochlear and vestibular haemorrhages and internal inner-ear membrane ruptures are as common a pathology as round window fistulae – but less amenable to treatment. Stretching of the round window, with the entry of air into the cochlea, has also been described. Animal experiments suggest that the pathologies are likely to be multiple. End-artery spasm, thrombosis, gas or lipid embolism etc. are aetiological proposals that have little experimental or clinical support.

Inner-ear barotrauma may be due to external-ear barotrauma and middle-ear barotrauma of ascent. It has occurred in unconscious patients (including drowning) and guinea-pigs, suggesting that a forceful Valsalva manoeuvre is not a prerequisite. It has been reported from dives as shallow as 7 feet (2 metres) and has been observed in a surfer who merely dived under a wave. Animal experiments reproduce the pathology with equivalent depths of 1–6 metres.

It has been suggested that the pathology may be implied by the clinical syndrome. Inner-ear haemorrhage is often associated with signs of middle-ear barotrauma (diagnosed on otoscopy or with conductive deafness). A tear of Reissner's membrane results in an isolated loss in one or two frequencies (tested on 100-Hz increments between 400 and 1300 Hz). Progressive deterioration of sensorineural hearing, or persistence of vestibular symptoms, may indicate inner-ear window fistulae.

Oval window fistula, probably due to damage from the stapes footplate, has been observed, often with a severe vestibular lesion which may persist until surgical repair.

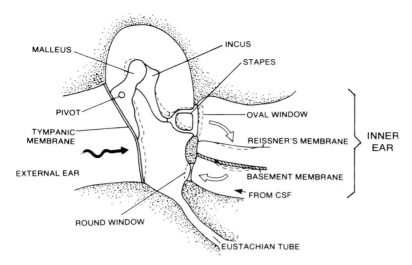

**Figure 10.4** Pressure wave (e.g. sound) passing from external, through middle, to inner ear

## Symptoms

Symptoms associated with inner-ear baro-trauma may include:

- A sensation of blockage in the affected ear.
- Tinnitus of variable duration.
- High frequency hearing loss.
- Vestibular disturbances such as nausea, vomiting, vertigo, disorientation and ataxia.
- Clinical features of an associated middle-ear barotrauma.

Deafness may be instantaneous or delayed and is of the sensorineural type, either a total (all frequencies) or selective high frequency loss (4000–8000 Hz). It also may be variable and altered by changing head positions – possibly due to the buoyancy of air in the perilymph. Impairment of speech discrimination may precede the delayed and progressive hearing loss.

There is often an associated conductive hearing loss which resolves over the subsequent 1–3 weeks. Bone-conduction audiograms are indicated.

Vestibular symptoms vary from almost unnoticeable to incapacitating.

A progressive sensorineural loss or vertigo which develops hours or days after the baro-trauma incident is likely to be due to a **fistula of the round window** with leakage of the peri-lymph into the middle ear, or air into the perilymph. The latter may only develop during or after ascent. Expansion of gas during ascent, or a rise in pressure in the middle ear by forceful middle-ear equalizing, may force air across the round window into the perilymph. Many of these cases develop the first symptoms after the completion of the dive, while performing energetic tasks, e.g. pulling up the anchor. This may be due to damage to the middle ear (including the round window) by the earlier barotrauma, and the eventual window rupture follows a rise of pressure in the cerebrospinal fluid, the cochlea aqueduct and the perilymph. If left uncorrected, the sensorineural hearing loss may become total and permanent.

Sensorineural hearing loss, which involves the high frequencies (4000–8000 Hz) only and which is unchanged and continuous from the time of the barotrauma, is likely to be due to **haemorrhage and/or trauma** of the cochlea. Tinnitus is usual and sometimes very troublesome. Vestibular symptoms are also possible. These cases are more frequent than the round window fistulae described above. Middle-ear surgical exploration is *not* indicated, because this is not a harmless procedure and, in rare cases, it can induce further or complete hearing loss.

Unfortunately, the clinical differential diagnosis between cochlear/vestibular trauma and fistula of the round window, based on the above criteria, is by no means certain. Once this disorder has happened to a diver, he seems predisposed to similar incidents, which further aggravate both the tinnitus and the hearing loss.

---

*Inner-ear barotrauma is suspected in the presence of hearing loss, tinnitus, vertigo or ataxia.*

---

In order to demonstrate inner-ear barotrauma, serial investigations may be necessary. Any combination of middle-ear barotrauma symptoms, vertigo, tinnitus and hearing loss should be immediately and fully investigated by serial measurements of clinical function, daily audiometry up to 8000 Hz and positional electronystagmography. Caloric testing is indicated only if the tympanic membrane is intact or if the technique guards against pressure or fluid transmission into the middle ear (see page 373).

A test proposed to support the diagnosis of round or oval window fistula, as opposed to other causes of inner-ear damage, is that of positional audiometry. The patient lies horizontal with the affected ear uppermost, for 30 minutes, and the hearing improves more than 10 decibels in at least two frequencies. The theoretical explanation for this improvement is that air is displaced from the perilymph-leaking windows. The test requires validation.

Investigations which may be of value include temporal bone polytomography, CT scans and other imaging techniques. Until now, they have not been particularly helpful in diagnosis or treatment, but this should change with more experience.

Cochlear injury is permanent in over half the cases, whereas vestibular injury is usually temporary.

## Treatment

Once damage has been confirmed, treatment should be initiated promptly. This includes:

1. Measures should be taken to avoid any increase in cerebrospinal fluid pressure, such as performing Valsalva manoeuvres, sneezing, nose blowing, straining with defaecation, sexual activity, coughing, lifting weights or physical exertion. Divers very commonly perform middle-ear auto-inflation almost as a matter of habit. It will therefore be necessary to advise the patient that under no circumstances should he attempt autoinflation or associated activities. If these activities are performed, the already damaged round windows may not withstand the pressure wave.

2. Immediate bed rest with the head elevated and careful monitoring of otological changes; this is given irrespective of which of the other treatment procedures are followed.

3. Bed rest should continue until all improvement has ceased and for up to a week thereafter, to allow the inner-ear membranes to heal and the haemorrhages to settle. Loud noises should be avoided.

4. If there is no improvement within 24–48 hours in cases of severe hearing loss, or if there is further deterioration in hearing, operative intervention must then be considered.

5. Reconstructive microaural surgery is indicated when there is deterioration or no improvement with bed rest, and severe hearing loss or incapacitating vertigo. With developing hearing loss, repair to the round or oval window will prevent the further leakage of perilymph and has proved curative in some cases, sometimes restoring hearing acuity. It cures vertigo and reduces tinnitus, both of which may be grossly disabling. If a fistula is not visualized during middle-ear exploration, a graft should still be applied to both windows, as sometimes the fistula is intermittent. A fistula may be demonstrated with intravenous fluorescein or abdominal pressure.

6. Prohibition of diving and flying – this is absolute for the first few weeks following a labyrinthine window fistula. If medical eva-

cuation by air is required, an aircraft with the cabin pressurized to ground level is necessary. For most cases, but especially those precipitated by minimal provocation and who have poor eustachian tube function or nasal pathology, it is prudent to advise against any further hyperbaric (diving) exposure. The same applies if permanent hearing loss, tinnitus or vestibular asymmetry persists. The authors would also advise against piloting aircraft because of the danger of alternobaric vertigo, which has followed some cases of unilateral inner-ear damage.

7. Treatment for vertigo – this is based on routine medical principles. It is usually suppressed by cerebral inhibition within a few weeks, but may be precipitated by sudden movement or other vestibular stimulation (caloric or alternobaric). It may persist if the fistula remains patent.

8. Other regimes – vasodilators (nicotinic acid) have been recommended by some, but little evidence exists to show any favourable effect. Aspirin is to be avoided because of its anticoagulant effects.

9. The significance of air entry into the perilymph, as a cause of the pathology, has yet to be determined. As an experimental procedure, we sometimes add 100% oxygen breathing to the above regime for 4–6 hours a day for 3 days.

Hyperbaric oxygen therapy has been used in some cases, but requires further confirmation before it can be generally recommended. These authors have tried it, but subsequently had to proceed to surgery. It has the potential for aggravating the fistula and increasing the perilymph flow into the middle ear during descent – both from the relatively negative middle-ear pressures and the need for Valsalva manoeuvres. It has given an apparent 'cure' in cases of middle-ear barotrauma with conductive generalized hearing loss, mistaken for the less common window fistula. In these cases, if the middle ear is autoinflated with descent, the gas expansion removed the middle-ear fluid on ascent.

---

**CASE REPORT 10.2**

This diver, who had been exposed to gunfire in the past, experienced considerable pain and difficulty in equalizing both middle ears during a dive to 10 metres. He continued to dive despite the pain and performed forceful autoinflations. He noted tinnitus, and also experienced ear pain and vertigo during ascent. Otoscopic examination of the tympanic membrane revealed the effects of barotrauma. The diver became progressively more deaf, with a sensorineural pattern in both ears, over the next few days. Transient episodes suggestive of vertigo were also noted. As both ears were affected, it was considered essential that exploratory surgery be performed, and this was carried out. A fistula of the round window was observed, together with a frequent drip of perilymph fluid into the middle ear. The round window was packed and subsequent audiograms over the following month revealed a considerable improvement in hearing. A similar procedure was performed 5 days later in the other ear, with the same result.

In retrospect, this diver gave a clear history of increasing difficulty in autoinflation over the previous 2 years, and admitted that he had not been concerned about this. Examination revealed a gross septal deformity with associated chronic rhinitis. ENG with caloric testing a month postoperatively revealed a spontaneous, right, beating nystagmus, but with a caloric response from both sides and directional preponderance to the right.

*Diagnosis:* inner-ear barotrauma (with fistula of the round window), due to middle-ear barotrauma of descent and forceful autoinflation, resulting in sensorineural hearing loss.

# Sinus barotrauma

### Sinus barotrauma of descent (sinus squeeze)

If a sinus ostium is blocked during descent, mucosal congestion and haemorrhage compensate for the contraction of the air within the sinus cavity. During ascent, expansion of the enclosed air expels blood and mucus from the sinus ostium. Ostia blockage may be the result of sinusitis with mucosal hypertrophy and congestion, rhinitis, redundant mucosal folds in the nose, nasal polyps etc. (see Figure 10.6).

## *Symptoms*

Symptoms include pain over the sinus during descent. It may be preceded by a sensation of tightness or pressure. The pain usually subsides with ascent but may continue as a persistent dull ache for several hours. On ascent, blood or mucus may appear in the nose or pharynx.

The pain is usually over the frontal sinus, less frequently it is retro-orbital, and maxillary pain is not common but may be referred to a number of upper teeth. Although the teeth may feel hypersensitive, abnormal or loose, they are not painful on movement. Coughing, sneezing or holding the head down may ag-

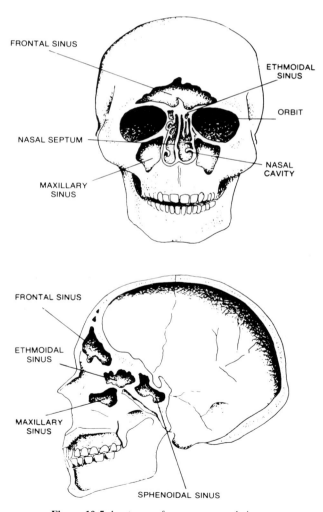

**Figure 10.5** Anatomy of accessory nasal sinuses

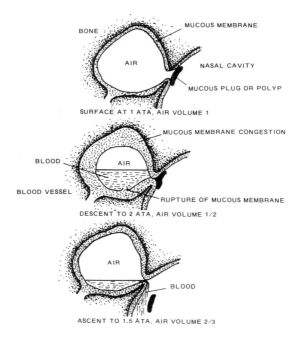

BONE

MUCOUS MEMBRANE

AIR

NASAL CAVITY

MUCOUS PLUG OR POLYP

SURFACE AT 1 ATA, AIR VOLUME 1

MUCOUS MEMBRANE CONGESTION

BLOOD

AIR

BLOOD VESSEL

RUPTURE OF MUCOUS MEMBRANE

DESCENT TO 2 ATA, AIR VOLUME 1/2

AIR

BLOOD

ASCENT TO 1.5 ATA, AIR VOLUME 2/3

**Figure 10.6** Diagrammatic changes of sinus barotrauma of descent followed by ascent

## CASE REPORT 10.3

DN, a 22-year-old sports diver, occasionally noticed a trace of blood from his face mask following ascent. He had often complained of nasal blockage and had various treatments for this, including cautery. His first dive to 12 metres for 10 minutes was uneventful. After a brief surface interval he again descended, but was unable to proceed beyond 6 metres due to a severe tearing headache in the frontal region. He equalized his face mask and this provided some relief. He then continued the descent feet first but still had some slight pain. On reaching the bottom, the severe sharp pain recurred. During ascent, it lessened in severity but, on reaching the surface, he noted mucus and blood in his face mask. A dull frontal headache persisted for 3 hours after the dive. Examination revealed a deviated nasal septum to both right and left, with hyperaemic nasal mucosa. X-rays showed gross mucosal thickening in both maxillary sinuses, the right being completely opaque. There was also some slight shadowing on the right frontal sinus. The radiological signs cleared over the next 2 weeks. As the airways were patent on both sides of the nasal septum, operative intervention was not indicated. The patient's nasal mucosa returned to normal after he abstained from cigarette smoking.

*Diagnosis:* sinus barotrauma of descent.

gravate the pain and make it throb. Numbness over the maxillary division of the fifth nerve is possible (see page 138).

The superficial ethmoidal sinus near the root of the nose occasionally ruptures and causes a small haematoma or discolouration of the skin between the eyes.

Discomfort persisting after the dive may be due to fluid within the sinus (remaining from the dive), infection (usually starts a few hours post-dive) or the development of chronic sinusitis or mucoceles.

Sinus X-ray examination, CT or MRI scan may disclose thickened mucosa, opacity or fluid levels. The opacities produced by the barotrauma may be serous or mucous cysts. The maxillary and frontal sinuses are commonly involved. The ethmoid and spenoidal sinuses may also be affected. The new imaging techniques can clearly demonstrate these.

### Prevention

This is achieved by refraining from diving with upper respiratory tract infections, sinusitis or rhinitis. Cessation of smoking will reduce the likelihood of mucosal irritation and sinus barotrauma. Correction of nasal abnormalities may be needed. Slow descents and ascents will reduce the sinus damage where there is marginal patency of the sinus ostia.

Positive pressure techniques during descent, such as the Valsalva manoeuvre, assist in aeration of the sinuses as well as the middle ears, as opposed to the passive equalization methods.

### Treatment

This consists of temporary cessation of all diving and flying, with correction of any predisposing factors. Patients with a sinus or upper respiratory tract infection may require antibiotics and decongestants. Surgical drainage is rarely indicated.

Even the mucoceles and chronic sinus pathology usually resolve without intervention, if diving is suspended.

### Sinus barotrauma of ascent

This may follow the occlusion of sinus openings by mucosal folds or sinus polyps, preventing escape of expanding gases. The ostium or its mucosa will then blow out into the nasal cavity, with or without pain, and haemorrhage commonly follows. This disease is aggravated by rapid ascent, as in free ascent training, emergency ascents, submarine escape etc.

If the expanding air cannot escape through the sinuses, it may fracture the walls and track along the soft tissues (see page 134). Rupture of air cells may cause localized and sudden pain of a severe degree, often affecting the ethmoidal or mastoid sinuses on ascent. Occasionally the air may rupture into the cranial cavity and cause a pneumocephalus (see page 136). (see also pages 130–132.)

### Clinical series

(Fagan, McKenzie and Edmonds, 1976)

A series of 50 consecutive cases of sinus barotrauma revealed the following findings.

In 68% the symptoms developed during or immediately upon descent – signifying sinus barotrauma of descent. They developed during or immediately upon ascent in 32% – signifying sinus barotrauma of ascent. Pain was the predominant symptom present in all cases of descent and in three-quarters of ascent barotrauma. It was present in the frontal area in 68%, in the ethmoidal area in 16% and in the maxillary area in 6%. In one case, it was referred to the upper dental area, but was verified to be of sinus aetiology by the radiological abnormality in the adjoining maxillary sinus, and the absence of any relevant dental pathology.

Epistaxis was the second most common symptom, occurring in 58% of cases. It was rarely more than an incidental observation and not very severe. It was the sole symptom in one-quarter of the barotrauma of ascent cases.

In 22% there was a history of previous sinus barotrauma. Fifty per cent had a history of recent upper respiratory tract inflammation, e.g. nasal congestion, discharge or sneezing. Fifty per cent gave a history of intermittent or long-term symptoms referable to the upper respiratory tract, e.g. nasal and sinus disorders, recurrent infections, hay fever etc.

In 48% of cases, the ears also showed some effect of barotrauma on examination of the tympanic membrane. There were nasal abnor-

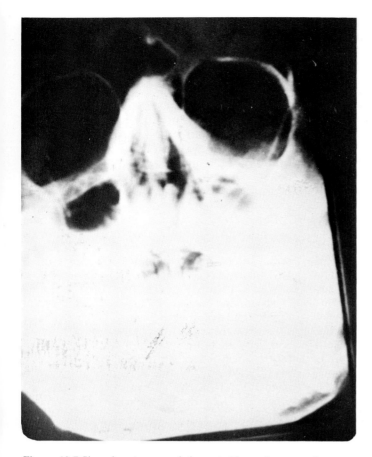

**Figure 10.7** Sinus barotrauma of descent: X-ray demonstrating gross opacity in right maxillary sinus

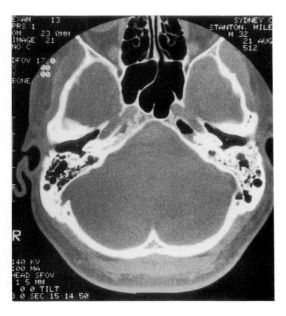

**Figure 10.8** Sinus barotrauma affecting the sphenoid and mastoid regions. CT scans have replaced traditional radiology in identification of problematic cases. The CT scan of the brain on bone setting through the skull base shows a fluid level within the antromedial air cell of the left petrous temporal bone line. In addition, there is loss of pneumatization of the left mastoid air cells

malities such as septal deflection, mucosal changes or the presence of polyps or abnormal secretions in 24%. In 34% of cases, there was tenderness of the sinus on palpation or percussion.

Radiological examination of the sinuses was performed within 24 hours. The maxillary sinus was affected with either mucosal thickening or fluid level, in 74% of cases, the frontal in 24% and the ethmoidal in 15%. A fluid level was present in the maxillary sinus in 12% of cases.

Most cases required no treatment. Those few that did responded rapidly to short-term use of nasal decongestants. Indications for antibiotics included a pre-existing or subsequent sinusitis or upper respiratory tract infection. Neither sinus lavage nor surgery was required in any case. For the routine clinical management of sinus barotrauma, radiographs and scans are not indicated as they do not substantially influence the course of treatment. It was noted that, although symptoms were predominantly from the frontal sinuses, the radiological changes were most often present in the maxillary sinuses. The explanation is conjecture, but perhaps the long and tortuous duct leading to the frontal sinuses enhances the possibility of blockage and therefore descent pain, whereas its position, passing vertically downwards, may promote drainage. The maxillary sinus, having a small ostium and placed well above the floor of the sinus, would be more prone to tearing and therefore haemorrhage, and would be likely to retain the fluid within the sinus.

## Dental barotrauma

This has been called aerodontalgia when applied to altitude exposure. Gas spaces may exist in the roots of infected teeth or associated with fillings which have undergone secondary erosion. During descent, the space is filled with the soft tissue of the gum or with blood. Pain may prevent further descent. If symptoms are not noticed on descent, then gas expansion on ascent may be restricted by the blood in these spaces, resulting in pain.

Another form of dental barotrauma occurs in cases involving a carious tooth with a cavity

and very thin cementum. As pressure differences across the cementum develop, the tooth may cave in (implode) on descent or explode on ascent, causing considerable pain. Fast rates of ascent or descent will tend to precipitate this disorder.

Pressure applied to individual teeth may cause pain and identify the affected tooth.

A third form of dental barotrauma involves the tracking of gas into tissues, through interruptions of the mucosa, e.g. after oral surgery, dental extractions or manipulations. Scuba regulators produce positive oral pressures, forcing gas into tissues.

Preventive measures include: biannual dental checks (including X-ray examinations), avoidance of all diving after dental extractions and surgery until complete tissue resolution has occurred (i.e. intact mucosal surface), slow descent and ascent.

Treatment consists of analgesia and dental repair. The differential diagnosis of sporadic or constant pain in the upper bicuspids or the first and second molars, but not localized in one tooth, must include referred pain from the maxillary sinus or the maxillary nerve (see page 138). This may also present as a burning sensation along the mucobuccal fold.

## Mask, suit and helmet barotrauma

### Facial barotrauma of descent (mask squeeze)

A face mask creates an additional gas space external to, but in contact with, the face. Unless pressure is equalized by exhaling gas through the nose, facial tissues will be drawn into this space during descent.

Clinical features include puffy, oedematous facial tissues especially under the eyelids, purpuric haemorrhages, conjunctival haemorrhages and, later, generalized bruising of the skin underlying the mask (Figure 10.10).

This condition is rarely serious and prevention involves exhaling into the face mask during descent. Treatment involves avoidance of diving until all tissue damage is healed.

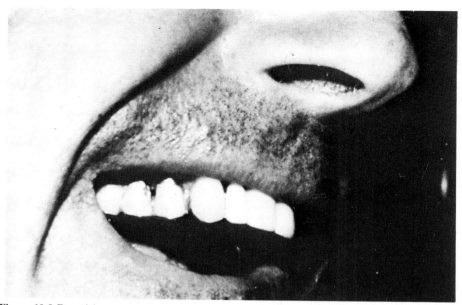

**Figure 10.9** Dental barotrauma showing collapse of the first right bicuspid during a dive to 20 metres. Previous dental treatment converted an open cavity into one covered by a silver amalgam filling

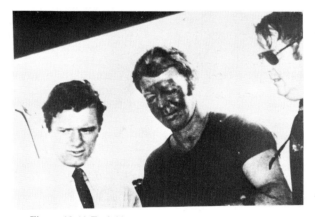

**Figure 10.10** Facial barotrauma of descent (central figure). This severe 'mask squeeze' developed with failure of the surface supply of compressed air to a full face mask (which did not have a non-return valve). Facial haemorrhage and swelling delineate the mask area

## Skin barotrauma of descent (suit squeeze)

This condition is encountered mainly with dry suits or poorly fitting wet suits. During descent, the air spaces are reduced in volume and trapped in folds in the skin. The skin tends to be sucked into these folds, leaving linear weal marks or bruises. The condition is usually painless and clears within a few days.

## Head and body barotrauma of descent
(diver's squeeze)

A rigid helmet, as used in standard diving, may cause this trauma. If extra gas is not added during descent to compensate for the effects of Boyle's law, the suit and occupant may be forced into the helmet, causing fractured clavicles, bizarre injuries or death. The sequence of events may present dramatically if the heavily weighted diver falls off his stage. There is a similar result when the diver loses his compressed air pressure, e.g. due to a compressor or supply line failure. To prevent this, a non-return valve is now required in supply line connections.

The clinical features include dyspnoea and a heavy sensation in the chest, bulging sensation in the head and eyes, swelling in the areas associated with rigid walls, e.g. the helmet, and then oedema and haemorrhages within the skin of the face, conjunctiva, neck and shoulders, bleeding from the lungs, gastrointestinal tract and nose, and in the ears and sinuses. These pathological changes are due to the effects of barotrauma on the enclosed gas spaces, and to a pressure gradient forcing blood from the abdomen and lower extremities into the thorax, head and neck, due to the negative pressure differential in the helmet. Similarly induced haemorrhages occur in the brain, heart, respiratory mucosa and other soft tissues.

### Suit barotrauma of ascent ('blow up')

During ascent in a standard diving ('hard hat') suit, the expanding gas must be able to escape. If it does not, then the whole suit will expand like a balloon and cause a rapid and uncontrolled ascent to the surface. This may result in barotrauma of ascent, decompression sickness, imprisonment of the diver and physical trauma. With the decreasing use of standard diving this emergency is now not encountered very often – but a less impressive manifestation is possible with divers who use an inflatable object, such as a buoyancy vest, dry suit, counterlung etc., and inflate this accidentally.

A clinically dissimilar and relatively minor symptom is noted by divers in an upright position using equipment which has a counterlung, or breathing bag, positioned below the head and neck. The pressure gradient from the bag to the diver's head results in a sensation of head and neck distension and bulging of the eyes.

## Gastrointestinal barotrauma

Gas expansion occurs within the intestines on ascent, and may result in eructation, vomiting, flatus, abdominal discomfort and colicky pains. It is rarely severe, but has been known to cause syncopal and shock-like states.

Inexperienced divers are more prone to aerophagia, predisposing to this condition. Swallowing to equalize middle-ear pressures is one cause of aerophagia. Performing Valsalva manoeuvres while in the head-down position may also result in air going into the stomach. Carbonated beverages and heavy meals are best avoided before and during exposure to hyperbaric conditions.

Treatment involves either slowing the rate of ascent, stopping ascent or even recompression. The simple procedure of releasing tight-fitting restrictions such as belts, girdles etc. may give considerable symptomatic relief.

Although not common, notable examples of gastrointestinal barotrauma are recorded. Two Norwegian divers were badly affected during 400-foot diving using helium/oxygen, on *HMS Reclaim* in 1961. An Australian lad, responding very well to hyperbaric oxygen therapy for gas gangrene, drank 'flat' lemonade at 2.5 ATA and deteriorated into a shock state with abdominal distension and pains before ascent was terminated. A group of officials celebrating the successful construction of a caisson in the UK experienced a similar embarrassing fate, from imbibing flat champagne. One case of burst stomach, following a rapid and uncontrolled diving ascent, has been recorded – requiring surgical exploration and repair.

## Miscellaneous barotrauma

### Localized surgical emphysema

This may result from the entry of gas into any area where the integument, skin or mucosa is broken and in contact with a gas space. Although the classic site involves the supraclavicular areas in association with tracking mediastinal emphysema from pulmonary barotrauma, other sites are possible. **Orbital surgical emphysema**, severe enough to occlude the palpebral fissure completely, may result from diving with facial skin, intranasal or sinus injuries. The most common cause is a fracture of the nasoethmoid bones. The lamina papyracea, which separates the nasal cavity and the orbit, is of egg shell thickness. When these bones are fractured, any increase in pressure in the nasal cavity or ethmoidal sinus from ascent or Valsalva manoeuvre, may force air into the orbit (Plate 3).

Surgical emphysema over the mandibular area is common with buccal and dental lesions. The surgical emphysema, with its associated physical sign of crepitus and its radiological verification, tends to occur in loose subcutaneous tissue.

Treatment is by administration of 100% oxygen by a non-pressurized technique, and complete resolution will occur within hours. Otherwise, resolution may take a week or more. Recompression is rarely indicated, but diving should be avoided until this resolution is complete and the damaged integument has completely healed.

## Pneumoperitoneum

This has been observed following emergency ascent, with movement of air from a ruptured pulmonary bulla, dissecting along the mediastinum to the retroperitoneal area, and then released into the peritoneum to track under the diaphragm. It is also possible that previous injury to the lung or diaphragm, producing adhesions, could permit the direct passage of air from the lung to the subdiaphragmatic area.

Another possible cause of pneumoperitoneum is, as described above, from a rupture of a gastrointestinal viscus – from barotrauma of ascent. The condition may be detected by chest X-ray or positional abdominal X-ray (gas under the diaphragm).

Treatment is by administration of 100% oxygen by a non-pressurized technique. Usually complete resolution will occur within hours. Management of the cause (pulmonary or gastrointestinal) is required and surgical management of a ruptured gastrointestinal viscus may be needed.

## Pneumocephalus

Occasionally, the cranial gas spaces (mastoid, paranasal sinuses) are affected by an ascent barotrauma, when the expanding gas ruptures into the cranial cavity. This may follow descent barotrauma, when haemorrhage occupies the gas space and its orifice is blocked.

The clinical presentation may have all the features of a catastrophic intracerebral event, such as a subarachnoid haemorrhage. Excruciating headache immediately on ascent is probable, although the effects of a space-occupying lesion may supervene. Neurological signs may follow brain injury or cranial nerve lesions.

It is likely that the condition could be aggravated by excessive Valsalva manoeuvres ('equalizing the ears') or ascent to altitude (air travel). Diagnosis can be verified by positional skull X-ray or CT scan (Figure 10.11).

The treatment includes: bed rest, sitting upright; avoidance of Valsalva, sneezing, nose blowing or other manoeuvres that increase nasopharyngeal pressures; 100% oxygen inhalation for many hours; and follow-up X-rays to show a reduction of the air volume. If untreated, the disorder may last a week or so and subsequent infection is possible. On theoretical grounds, recompression or craniotomy could be considered in dire circumstances.

The sudden bursting of gas into the cranial cavity could presumably cause significant brain damage.

## Bone cyst barotrauma

Occasionally, pain may develop from an intraosseous bone cyst, probably with haemorrhage into the area, during descent or ascent, and may last for hours after the dive. The pelvic bones are most often involved in the ilium and near the sacroiliac joints. An X-ray or CT scan may demonstrate the lesions (Figure 10.12).

## Cranial nerve palsies

Cases occasionally present with cranial nerve lesions attributed to neurapraxia. This can be due to implosive tissue-damaging effects during descent, the distension in enclosed gas

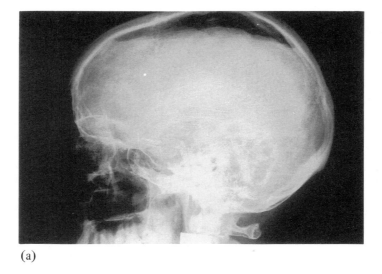

(a)

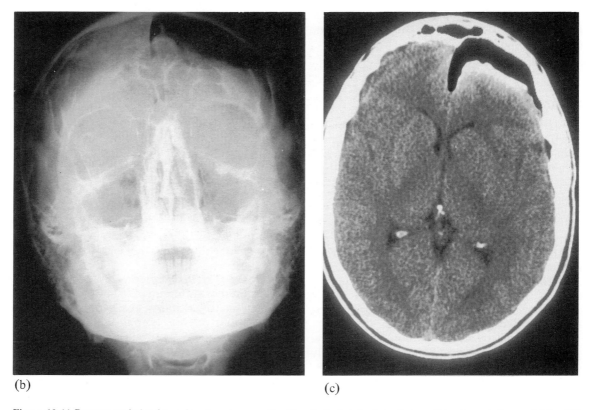

(b)                                           (c)

**Figure 10.11** Pneumocephalus from sinus barotrauma: the films include (a) a lateral view, (b) a frontal view and (c) a CT scan. (c) There is a pneumocephalus which is loculated on the left and has some 'mass effect' causing depression of the underlying brain, on the CT scan. (Courtesy of Dr R.W. Goldman)

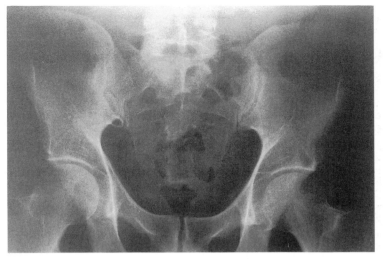

(a)

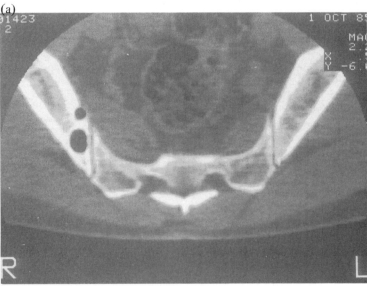

(b)

**Figure 10.12** Bone lysis: causing bone pain during descent and/or ascent. (a) X-ray of pelvis: a rounded translucency is seen in the right ilium adjacent to the lower part of the right sacroiliac joint. (b) CT scan: two rounded air bubbles are seen in the right ilium. One lies anteriorly in the cortex and the other lies within the medulla. (Courtesy of Dr B.L. Hart)

spaces during ascent or both. It is possible that air could be forced into the nerve canals as the gas expands with ascent. The nerve damage varies greatly, often being transitory but occasionally long-lasting. These presentations are usually associated with barotrauma symptoms and signs, as described earlier.

With the cases produced due to ascent, there may be a delay of many minutes after the dive and the diver may be aware of the feeling of distension of the gas space. The relief as gas escapes may coincide with improvement in the neurapraxia. This infers that the cause may be ischaemic, with a middle-ear or sinus pressure in excess of the mean capillary perfusion pressure.

The **seventh or facial cranial nerve** may be affected, causing 'facial baroparesis', because of its passage through the middle-ear space. Recorded in both aviators and divers, it is more frequent following ascent, presents as a unilateral facial weakness similar to Bell's palsy, and tends to recur in the same patient. Paralysis of the facial nerve makes frowning impossible, prevents the eye from closing on that side and causes drooping of the lower lid (which may result in tears running down the face because they do not drain into the nasolacrimal duct). The cheek is smooth and the mouth pulled to the good side. Whistling becomes impossible and food collects between the cheek and gum.

A metallic taste may be noticed at the start of the illness, as may impaired taste in the anterior part of the tongue on the same side, due to chorda tympani involvement. Hyperacusis may be due to paralysis of the stapedius muscle.

A possible reason for an individual's susceptibility to this disorder is perhaps found in the anatomy of the facial canal. This opens into the middle ear in some people and shares its pathology. A history of typical middle-ear barotrauma is usually present, with all the provoking factors (see above). If there is an ascent barotrauma with a distension of the middle ear, this can be relieved by performing a Toynbee manoeuvre, pressure via the external ear, oxygen inhalation, decongestants or, if needed, recompression (see Middle-ear barotrauma, page 116).

The **fifth or trigeminal nerve** may likewise be influenced by gas pressure changes in the maxillary antrum and sinus barotrauma (see above). The most common presentation is with involvement of the maxillary division, especially the infraorbital nerve, which traverses the sinus. Hypoaesthesia can be demonstrated for a variable time after the sinus barotrauma incident. It may involve the cheek, side of nose, lower eyelid, upper lip, maxillary teeth and gums. It may also be a cause of pain from sinus barotrauma referred to the upper teeth on the same side (see Sinus barotrauma, page 128).

## Others

Other gas spaces have been observed in the body, such as in the kidneys, the intervertebral disc and nucleus pulposus, but these have not yet been identified as having dysbaric manifestations.

## Recommended reading

AXELSSON, A. MILLER, J. and SILVERMAN, M. (1979). Anatomical effects of sudden middle ear pressure changes. *Annals of Otology* **88**, 368–376.

CAMPBELL, P.A. (1944). Aerosinusitis – its cause, course and treatment. *Annals of Otology* **53**, 291–301.

EDMONDS, C (1991). Peripheral neurological abnormalities in dysbaric disease. In: *Neurological Dysbarism workshop*, edited by T.J.R. Francis and D.J. Smith, in press.

EDMONDS, C. and THOMAS, R. (1972). Medical aspects of diving. *Medical Journal of Australia* **2**, 1300.

EDMONDS, C., FREEMAN, P., THOMAS, R., TONKIN, J. and BLACKWOOD, F. (1973). *Otological Aspects of Diving*. Sydney: Australasian Medical Publishing Co.

EIDSVIK, S., and MOLVAER, O.I. (1985). Facial baroparesis. *Undersea Biomedical Research* **12**, 495–463.

FAGAN, P., McKENZIE, B. and EDMONDS, C. (1976). Sinus barotrauma in divers. *Annals of Otology Rhinology and Laryngology* **85**, 64–65.

FARMER, J., KENNEDY, R.S., McCORMICK, R.G. and MONEY, K. (1976). *Audio-vestibular Derangements, National Plan for the Safety and Health of Divers*. U.M.S.

FARMER J.C. (1989). Ear and sinus problems in diving. In: *Diving Medicine*, edited by A.A Bove and J.C. Davis. New York: Grune & Stratton.

FORTES-REGO, J. (1974). Etiologia de paralisia facial periferica. *Arquivos de Neuro-Psiquiatria (Sao Paulo)* **32**, 131–139.

GARGES, L.M. (1985). Maxillary sinus barotrauma. *Aviation Space and Environmental Medicine* **56**, 796–802.

GOLDMANN, R.W. (1986). Pneumocephalus as a consequence of barotrauma. *JAMA* **255**, 3154–3156.

GRUNDFAST, K.M. and BLUESTONE, C.D. (1978). Sudden or fluctuating hearing loss and vertigo in children due to perilymph fistula. *Annals of Otology* **87**, 761–771.

HART, B.L., BRANTLY, P.N., LUBBERS, P.R., ZELL, B.K. and FLYNN, E.T. (1986). Compression pain in a diver with intraosseous pneumatocysts. *Undersea Biomedical Research* **13**, 465–468.

HILL, L. (1912). *Caisson Sickness*. London: Edward Arnold.

HOFF, E.C. (1948). *A Bibliographical Sourcebook of Compressed Air, Diving and Submarine Medicine*. Vol. 1. Bu Medical Department of Navy, Washington DC.

HOFF, E.C. and GREENBAUM, L.J. JR (1954). *A Bibliographical Sourcebook of Compressed Air, Diving and Submarine Medicine*, Vol 2. ONR and Bu Medical Department of Navy, Washington DC.

MOLVAER, O.I. and EIDSVIK, S. (1989). Inner ear barotrauma. *Proceedings of 15th Annual Meeting EUBS* 89, Israel, pp. 321–326.

NEWMAN, T., SETTLE, H., BEAVER, G., and LINAWEAVER, P.G. (1974). Maxillary sinus barotrauma with cranial nerve involvement. *Aviation Space and Environmental Medicine* **46**, 314–315.

ORNHAGEN, H. Pressure equilibration in the middle ear. In: *Hyperbaric Medicine and Underwater Physiology*, edited by Shiraki and Matsouka. Kitakyushu, Japan: UOEH.

PARELL. G.J. and BECKED. G.D. (1985). Conservative management of inner ear barotrauma resulting from scuba diving. *Otolaryngology Head and Neck Surgery* **93**, 393–397.

ROSE. D. M. and JARCZYK. P. A. (1978). Spontaneous pneumoperitoneum after scuba diving. *JAMA* **239** (3), 223.

# 11

# Historical and physiological concepts of decompression

## Historical

Bubbles may develop in the body of the diver, aviator or caisson worker, whenever he ascends and is exposed to a reduction in environmental pressure (decompression), causing symptoms of decompression sickness (DCS). They may cause limb 'bends' if located in the joints or periarticular tissues. In the peripheral nerve myelin sheath, they may cause a wide variety of symptoms, whereas other local bubbles can form in the spinal column and the brain. In the skin a range of pathologies depends on the histological site of the bubble, whereas in the lymphatic drainage they can cause localized patches of lymphoedema (Plate 4). Deafness and/or vertigo may result if the inner ear is involved, and osteonecrosis if gas develops within the bone marrow.

An appreciation of the history and the physiology of decompression is needed to understand this disease.

**Von Guericke** developed the first effective air pump in 1650. Robert Boyle exposed experimental animals to the effects of increased and decreased pressures and, in 1670, reported these experiments. This included the first description of decompression sickness (DCS) – a bubble moving to and fro in the waterish humour of the eye of a viper. The snake was 'tortured furiously' by the formation of bubbles in the 'blood, juices and soft parts of the body'.

Cases of DCS in humans were noted by **Triger** in 1841. He designed and constructed a caisson, intending to sink pylons in wet soil for the construction of a bridge across the Loire River near Chalonnes, France. Two labourers experienced severe pains after emerging from a 7-hour exposure to pressure. Relief was obtained by rubbing the affected area with alcohol – a treatment that with some variations in the route of administration has become a tradition among divers. Pol and Watelle, in 1854, published a report indicating the nature of the disease, together with case histories to demonstrate the relationship between pressure, duration of exposure, rapidity of decompression and the development of DCS.

**Hoppe-Seyler** repeated the Boyle experiments and, in 1857, he described the obstruction of pulmonary vessels by bubbles and the inability of the heart to function adequately under those conditions. He suggested that some of the cases of sudden death in compressed air workers were due to this intravascular liberation of gas. He also recommended recompression to remedy this.

**Le Roy de Mericourt**, in 1869, and **Gal**, in 1872, described an occupational illness of sponge divers, attributed to the breathing of compressed air, and equated this with the caisson workers' disease. A host of imaginative theories were proposed during the nineteenth century to explain the aetiology of this disorder.

In 1872, **Freidburg** reviewed the development of compressed air work and collected descriptions of symptoms of workers given insufficient decompression after exposure to high pressure. He compared the clinical course of severe and fatal cases of DCS to that of the venous air embolism occasionally seen in obstetrics and surgery. He felt that rapid decompression would be responsible for a rapid release of the gas that had been taken up by the tissues under increased pressure. He suggested that the blood was filled with gas bubbles which interfered with circulation in the heart and lungs.

'Caisson disease' or 'compressed air illness' was described in 1873 by **Smith** as a disease depending upon increased atmospheric pressure, but always developing after reduction of the pressure. It was characterized, he noted, by moderate or severe pain in one or more of the extremities and sometimes in the trunk as well. There may or may not be epigastric pain and vomiting. In some cases, there may be elements of paralysis which, when they appear, are most frequently confined to the lower half of the body. Cerebral symptoms, such as headache, vertigo, convulsions and loss of consciousness may be present.

**Paul Bert**, in 1878, demonstrated in a most conclusive manner that DCS is primarily the result of inert gas bubbles (nitrogen in the case of compressed air divers and caisson workers)

which had been dissolved according to Dalton's and Henry's laws, and then released into the gas phase in tissues and blood during or following decompression. He used various oxygen concentrations to hasten decompression, demonstrated the value of oxygen inhalation once the animal developed DCS, and proposed the concept of oxygen recompression therapy.

**Andrew Smith**, a surgeon from the Manhattan Eye and Ear Hospital, noted in 1894 the origin of the term 'bends'. Since pain in the hips and lower extremities was generally aggravated by an erect position, the victims often assumed a stooping posture. Such sufferers among the workers on the Brooklyn Bridge caissons in New York were the objects of good-natured ridicule by their comrades, who likened their angular postures to a fashionable stoop in walking, termed the 'Grecian bend', which was practised by sophisticated metropolitan women at the time. He was aware of the value of recompression, but this was unacceptable to some of his patients. Instead he used hot poultices, ice packs, hot baths, ergot, atropine, whiskey and ginger – or morphine if the others failed. He constructed the first specialized treatment chamber.

The factors which control bubble size and bubble resorption were discussed by **Zuntz** 1897.

The nitrogen bubbles circulating in a blood grow in size as a result of nitrogen diffusion from tissue fluids. Once formed, a gas bubble will diminish in size only gradually because the tension of nitrogen in the bubble is only slightly higher than alveolar nitrogen tensions. As circulation stops, the resorption of bubbles can only be effected by very slow diffusion through bloodless tissue layers to the nearest free blood vessels. It is no wonder that under such circumstances, Paul Bert as late as the fourth day after decompression still found bubbles in the blood vessels of the spinal cord centres.

**Moir**, in 1896, working on the Hudson river caisson tunnel, reduced the DCS death rate from 25% of the work force to under 2% by the use of recompression therapy.

**Snell**, in 1897, was one of the first investigators to observe that the risk of DCS was increased when, due to faulty ventilation in caissons, the concentration of carbon dioxide in the atmosphere was increased.

The two-volume monograph by **von Schrotter** and his colleagues in 1990 is one of the most comprehensive and detailed reports published on the histopathology of DCS.

During the early part of the twentieth century there was considerable controversy regarding the speed and manner in which divers and caisson workers should be decompressed. An English physiologist, **John Scott Haldane,** proposed his critical supersaturation ratio hypothesis – and most of the current decompression tables have their basis in his work. For this reason, a more detailed look at this development is indicated. Boycott, Damant and Haldane (1908) submitted a *Report to the Admiralty of the Deep-Water Diving Committee* and set down the knowledge and hypotheses on which their decompression table calculations were based.

Haldane exposed goats to 45 feet of seawater pressure (2.36 ATA) for up to 2 hours before rapidly decompressing them to the surface (1 ATA). With this pressure drop (1.36 ATA), a few of the animals just started to develop bends. The same pressure drop from 165 feet (6 ATA) did not produce bends. In fact the animals did not develop bends despite a drop of 3 ATA! Thus the bends was not thought to be due to the constant pressure drop.

## Tissue gases and bubbles*

To prevent this disease forming, a number of theories were developed which aimed to permit safe decompression.

### Haldane hypotheses

Haldane's discoveries, on which most of the current decompression tables are based, are explained as follows. During exposure to increased pressure, nitrogen is absorbed by the body. Blood, in accordance with Henry's law,

---

*It is important for any aspiring researcher in this field, if he wishes to make new discoveries, NOT to read the reports of Behnke or the reviews of Hoff and Greenbaum, of work done more than half a century ago.

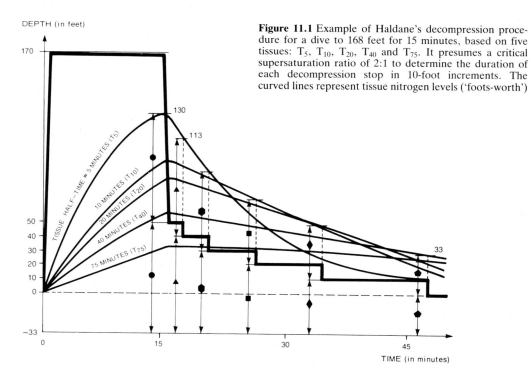

**Figure 11.1** Example of Haldane's decompression procedure for a dive to 168 feet for 15 minutes, based on five tissues: $T_5$, $T_{10}$, $T_{20}$, $T_{40}$ and $T_{75}$. It presumes a critical supersaturation ratio of 2:1 to determine the duration of each decompression stop in 10-foot increments. The curved lines represent tissue nitrogen levels ('foots-worth')

becomes saturated with nitrogen in the lungs, at ambient (environmental) pressure. It is then carried through the arterial system to the capillaries and diffuses into the tissues, eventually producing the same nitrogen pressure there as in the lungs. However, the blood supply and the solubility of nitrogen varies with different tissues and so the time taken for different parts of the body to become saturated will be different. It was decided to simulate the body by considering it to be represented by five distinct tissue types. **Haldane's first hypothesis** was that the uptake and elimination of nitrogen followed an exponential curve, and he postulated that the body could be represented by the five separate tissues having theoretical half-times of 5, 10, 20, 40 and 75 minutes.

The exponential uptake and elimination of a gas in solution is analogous to the radioactive 'half-life' concept with which most physicians are familiar. Tissue half-times are explained thus: if a subject is exposed to a gas, then half its absorption in any specific tissue will occur in a specific time, e.g. in 5 minutes the $T_5$ tissue will absorb half the total volume of gas that it is able to absorb in unlimited time. Over the next time interval of 5 minutes, the $T_5$ tissue will again absorb half of the remaining gas potential that it needs to become saturated. In 10 minutes, the $T_{10}$ will absorb half the total volume of gas that it is able to absorb etc. Thus in 20 minutes the $T_5$ tissue will have received one-half plus one-quarter plus one-eighth plus one-sixteenth, i.e. it will become 15/16 saturated with nitrogen. The $T_{20}$ tissue will only be half-saturated in the same 20-minute period. It was presumed that the elimination of gas during decompression could be expressed by a similar but opposite exponential function.

Numerically, if a piece of tissue, called $T_x$ (T = tissue, $x$ = half-time, in minutes), can absorb a total of, say, 16 ml gas, then it will absorb:

8 ml during the first $x$ min
4 ml during the second $x$ min
2 ml during the third $x$ min
1 ml during the fourth $x$ min etc.

**Haldane's second hypothesis** followed the observation that divers could tolerate a rapid decompression producing a supersaturation of gas within tissues, yet still not produce DCS (i.e. the tissue has more than enough gas in

solution to saturate it). It was believed that the environmental pressure could be halved, with the gas tensions in tissues being as much as twice the environmental pressure, producing a supersaturation and yet not resulting in bubbles or DCS. Haldane believed that decompression could be performed from 2 atmospheres to 1 atmosphere, 4 atmospheres to 2 atmospheres and 6 atmospheres to 3 atmospheres, i.e. a 2:1 ratio of maximum depth to the first decompression stop, in safety. Haldane then devised methods of ascent whereby the nitrogen pressures in each of the five hypothetical tissues never exceeded the environmental pressure by more than a 2:1 ratio – now known as a 'critical ratio' supersaturation hypothesis.

Haldane devised two commonly used tables: Table 1 involved decompressions of less than 30 minutes, and therefore for shorter dives – was later found to be far too conservative, compared to what was able to be achieved in practice; Table 2 involved longer decompressions, but an unacceptable number of bends.

## Neo-haldanian developments

The Haldane method was adopted and the Admiralty extended this to the 64 metre (210 feet) depth, although Haldane recommended its use only to 50 metres (6 ATA or 165 feet), as the limit of diving operations. The Haldane concept was carried to other countries, including France, Russia and the United States of America, where variations were made to the tables to make them safer.

Although haldanian 'tissues' were mathematical concepts, not representative of anatomical tissues, these organs do have different half-times. Thus, although they are made up of many 'tissues':

- Blood has the shortest half-time, but the spinal cord half-time is only 12.5 min.
- Skin and muscles have a half-time of 14–30 min for helium, 37–79 for nitrogen.
- Joints and bones have a half-time of 115–240 min for helium, 304–635 for nitrogen
- Inner ear has a half-time of 55–90 min for helium, 146–238 min for nitrogen.

The **US Navy experience** was that the 2:1 critical ratio hypothesis of Haldane was too conservative for dives where the fast tissue limits decompression (short dives), and not conservative enough for dives limited by the slow tissues (long duration dives). With the changes that were then made to the allowable critical ratio, divers could come up from short dives at considerable depths to a much more shallow first stop, thus increasing the nitrogen gradient which thereby increased elimination of the nitrogen from body tissues.

Yarbrough found that the critical supersaturation ratio seemed to vary not only with each hypothetical tissue, but also with the duration of exposure, and changed the tables used by the US Navy. Des Granges, Dwyer and Workman showed that the ratios also changed with depth – so that a simple 2:1 ratio developed into a series of tables of '**M values**', produced by **Workman**, showing the maximal allowable supersaturation for each hypothetical tissue at each depth. The result was a valiant and valuable attempt by the neo-haldanian workers to fit the physiology of diving to the Haldane model. Incorporating the work of VanDerAue and including a 120-minute tissue resulted in the US Navy tables of 1956, which are used today.

Slower tissues, such as muscles, tendons or joints, sometimes act paradoxically according to these beliefs. Even if bubbles do not develop, uptake of nitrogen may continue in these tissues even after the diver has surfaced – the nitrogen coming from the faster tissues which had taken up more nitrogen (see Figure 2.4). This may happen at any depth after an ascent, with uptake of gas continuing into 'slower' surrounding tissues from the 'faster' ones. Radioactive xenon studies suggest that gas takes much longer to leave tissues than predicted by the perfusion-limited models described above – and on which the conventional decompression tables are based.

Other observations also did not fit the classic haldanian theories.

To overcome some of the problems that arose with the decompression tables, it was found necessary to increase the number of hypothetical tissues from the original five, some workers using three times this number. It was also necessary to consider tissues even slower than $T_{75}$, some having a half-time of up to 1000 minutes for extreme exposures.

## Other hypotheses

**Leonard Hill**, in 1912, produced both experimental and theoretical evidence questioning the value of stage decompression over continuous uniform decompression. In the arguments between Haldane and Hill, the practical value of the Haldane tables in reducing decompression time made these more acceptable. The time at depth was less and Hill could not adequately explain why Haldane's technique avoided DCS. Hill's technique is now applied to decompression for saturation exposures. Sir Leonard Hill's concept was that, to prevent bubble growth, decompression would depend on a maximum safe gradient between the tissue gas tension and the environmental or ambient pressure, $\Delta P$, rather than the ratio between these two. This is therefore a **critical pressure hypothesis**.

$$\Delta P = p - P$$

where $p$ equals tissue gas pressure, $P$ equals ambient or environmental pressure and $\Delta P$ equals the gradient moving gas from tissues to the environment.

The $\Delta P$ hypothesis suggests a linear, and not a staged, decompression. This concept is now used in long exposure dives and is also included in other theories of decompression. Albano of Italy suggested a minimum allowable pressure gradient across a bubble surface before it would enlarge, thereby applying this principle to bubbles as well as to gas in solution.

Three related concepts were proposed, which appear to have considerable importance in both decompression theory and DCS therapy. These were the **oxygen window** (Behnke), the **partial pressure vacancy** (Momsen) and the **inherent unsaturation hypothesis** (Le Messurier and Hills). It is described by Behnke thus: 'During the course of blood transport through the capillaries, the oxygen is unloaded in different quantities to the various tissues. This results in available space for transfer of inert gas from tissues to lungs.' A similar but even greater oxygen utilization takes place in these tissues. It is this, the difference between the environmental pressure and the tissue gas tension, which allows divers to ascend a safe distance without the tissue gas tension exceeding that of the environment, i.e. without super-saturation and therefore without the likelihood of bubble formation.

During the early 1960s, two Australian workers, **Hugh Le Messurier** and **Brian Hills**, observed the type of diving performed by Okinawans who reached depths of up to 90 metres (300 feet) on air for as long as an hour, twice a day, 6 days a week. During the peak of the pearl diving industry, there were as many as 900 divers working out of the small coastal township of Broome, in Western Australia. These people had accumulated great experience, without preconceived scientific knowledge, and empirically produced a decompression regime which cost thousands of lives during its development, but finally resulted in relatively safe decompression tables which were very economical of time.

These decompression schedules were significant in that they required about two-thirds the time needed by the US Navy decompression tables. Also, when the US Navy tables caused DCS, the remedy used was to extend the shallow decompression. Brian Hills suggested that the problem developed during the initial ascent, and therefore the added stops should be at greater depths. Hills used deeper decompression stops than customary, but then surfaced directly from 7.5 to 9 metres (25–30 feet). Even the relatively minor variation of transferring the conventional 3-metre (10-feet) stop to 6 metres (20 feet) reduced the DCS incidence by 40% in a UK trial.

Hills, in 1966, developed his 'thermodynamic' model of DCS from these observations, and introduced a most important concept of 'unsaturation' in the understanding of bubble prevention and resolution. Hills believed that the gas bubbles developed during decompression with the US Navy tables and that these merely controlled the size of the bubbles – similar to the view expounded by Behnke in 1951.

The concepts of unsaturation can be illustrated by considering representative values for the partial pressures of respiratory gases for a person on the surface. This is depicted in Figure 11.3a and Table 11.1.

It will be noted that the total gas tension in tissues and venous blood is less than the barometric pressure; thus the tissues are unsaturated. Other workers suggest that tissue unsaturation is greater than the 60 mmHg (760 − 700) (or 8 kPa) indicated here. The importance of this tissue unsaturation in diving is that an instantaneous reduction of the total pressure caused by ascent equivalent to at least 60 mmHg must take place before the tissues become saturated with gas. After this ascent, the alveolar nitrogen partial pressure is less than the tissue nitrogen partial pressure so that a nitrogen pressure gradient is established. Elimination of nitrogen and the re-establishment of tissue unsaturation results. The clinical importance of the different tissue uptake speed is seen in two examples.

In astronaut exposures to 0.2 ATA, DCS can be prevented by denitrogenation of the body through the prior breathing of 100% oxygen for 3 hours. If, however, the astronaut breathes air for 5 minutes after the denitrogenation, DCS will develop at altitude. The fast tissues are the only ones that could be involved in this sequence. Similarly, the occasional DCS from a brief exposure to 5 ATA by divers, with a sudden ascent to the surface, should not cause surprise.

Once the diver has reached the surface from a non-saturation dive, 'slow' tissues such as

**Table 11.1 Partial pressures of respiratory gases at 1 ATA**

| *Sample* | *Gas partial pressure* | | | | |
|---|---|---|---|---|---|
| | $O_2$ (mmHg) | $CO_2$ (mmHg) | $N_2$ (mmHg) | $H_2O$ (mmHg) | *Total* (mmHg) |
| Inspired air | 158 | 0.3 | 596 | 5.7 | 760 |
| Expired air | 116 | 32 | 565 | 47 | 760 |
| Alveolar air | 100 | 40 | 573 | 47 | 760 |
| Arterial blood | 100 | 40 | 573 | 47 | 760 |
| Venous blood | 40 | 46 | 573 | 47 | 706 |
| Tissues | $\leqslant 30$ | $\geqslant 50$ | 573 | 47 | 700 |

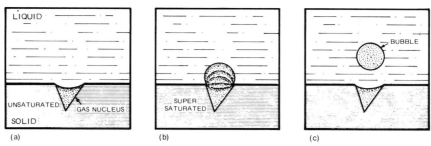

**Figure 11.2** Nucleation of gas emboli with decompression

joint structures can continue to absorb nitrogen from the faster ones, until they equilibrate.

In 1951, Harvey postulated the importance of **bubble nuclei** in the formation and development of bubbles in DCS. Hawaiian workers, including Kunkle and Yount, integrated this with the unsaturation hypothesis and extended the concept of bubble formation and growth. An oversimplified explanation is as follows: the pressure in a bubble ($P_b$) is due to the gas molecules it contains. If $P_b$ is greater than the surrounding pressures, the bubble will grow. If $P_b$ is less, it will be reduced in volume. The surrounding pressures are the environmental or ambient pressure ($P_a$), the tensions due to the tissue displacement ($P_t$) and the surface tension of the bubble ($P_y$). All these tend to constrict the bubble.

If $P_b > P_a + P_t + P_y$, the bubble will grow.

Bubble growth can follow decompression, when the pressure of the gases (especially nitrogen) in the bubble reflects the pressure at greater depth, and the $P_a$ has been reduced by decompression, decreasing the right side of the equation and producing bubble growth.

Localized falls in tissue pressure may be caused in areas of turbulence and during tissue movements.

The effect of surface tension will vary with the size of the bubble:

$$P_y = 2_y/r$$

where $P_y$ = pressure due to the surface tension, $y$ = surface tension and $r$ = radius of bubble.

For larger bubbles, $P_y$ is reduced and may become negligible. For smaller bubbles, $P_y$ is increased and may become so great as to force the bubble back into solution. It is difficult to understand how extremely small bubbles can persist, except in protected areas. Thus tissue bubbles of less than 1 μm will probably disappear, whereas those greater than 1 mm may cause symptoms.

It is believed that for bubbles to form during or after decompression, 'nuclei' of gas need to be present for the other gas molecules to pass into and enlarge. Supersaturation as such will not produce bubbles in pure water (without nuclei) until this supersaturation is about 1000 atmospheres! The 'nuclei' or gas pockets occur in the natural state, and may be illustrated by the bubbles of carbonated beverages developing more frequently on the rough surface of the glass.

In Figure 11.2, the gas is trapped in a small crevice producing a gas nucleus. The walls of this are hydrophobic (non-wettable), thereby preventing water from running in and eliminating the gas cavity. The gas/liquid interface tends to flatten due to surface tension (which, in the case of a free bubble, would tend to collapse it). As the gas pressure in the bubble is in equilibrium with tissue gas tensions, it is probably slightly less than the hydrostatic pressure in the liquid and therefore the gas interface will be concave.

When supersaturation of gas develops and gas molecules diffuse into the gas nucleus, it expands with its interface bulging into the fluid. Surface tension will tend to oppose the growth, but if a critical gas volume is reached a bubble will bud off the nucleus and be carried away in the liquid (e.g. in the blood). In the tissues, the gas bubble may remain stationary, but in either case the nucleus is left to generate more bubbles while the state of supersaturation exists.

Other ways of attracting gas molecules out of solution are by producing local areas of very

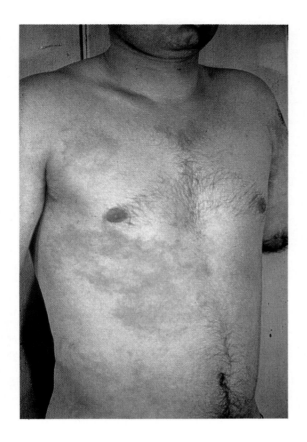

**Plate 4** Skin lesions of decompression sickness. This diver, who had had an upper limb amputation, developed 'bends' pain in the phantom limb, and skin bends over the body. Both responded rapidly to recompression therapy. (Photograph by courtesy of Dr Ramsay Pearson)

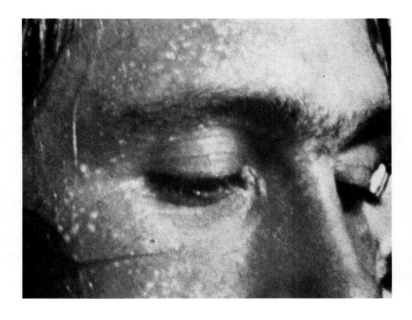

**Plate 5** Decompression sickness: skin lesions of isobaric counterdiffusion. The subject breathed a neon/oxygen mixture at 1200 feet (360 metres), while exposed to a chamber of helium/oxygen. Gross itching accompanied the intradermal bubbles. (Photograph by courtesy of Professor C. J. Lambertsen)

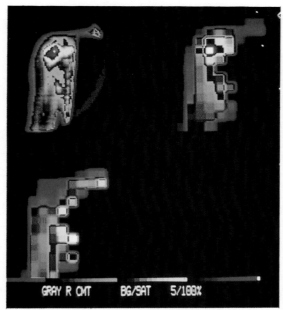

GRAY R CNT    BG/SAT    5/100%

**Plate 6** This is a further MDP scan taken after Figure 14.9a, using a technique called 'parametric scanning' or 'functional imaging'. The images are colour-coded on a scale which uses blue for 'cold' and white for 'hot'. The image at the top left is merely a way of quantifying the sort of qualitative image shown in Figure 14.9a and is the appearance 2–3 hours after the injection of MDP, when there is less background 'glare' from MDP which has not been taken up by bone, and which has been washed out of other tissues and excreted. The picture at the top right is a scan 30 minutes after giving the MDP and is not a measure of osteoblastic activity. In this case, there is a larger 'hot' area compared to the first image. The third image in the bottom left corner is an expression of the accretion rate constant for technetium measured on a minute-by-minute basis over the first 30 minutes. The accretion rate constant is directly proportional to perfusion and it is clear that an area in the shoulder joint in this image is 'cold' and therefore not well perfused. This, in turn, means an area of infarction which, in time, can be expected to become X-ray positive. This particular lesion was X-rayed again 3 weeks after the scan and the tomogram in particular showed an affected joint. Pain and restriction of movement were noted at this stage. (Courtesy of Dr Ramsay Pearson)

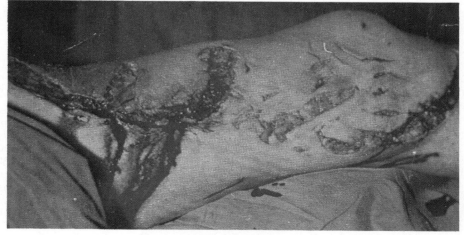

**Plate 7** Curved and concentric lacerations of shark bite – often with teeth left in the wound (see Chapter 24). (Photograph courtesy of Dr G. D. Campbell)

low pressure. Such may be seen with 'tribo-nucleation' – the shearing of joint surfaces over each other, in tendons and in the turbulent and vortical motions in the circulation.

High pressures may reduce the size of gas nuclei to such an extent that water enters the crevice and the nucleus disappears. When the walls of the crevice become wet, the gas forms a bubble and the bubble's surface tension is great enough to compress it further and force it back into solution.

Exposure to pressure, insufficient to produce DCS, may be adequate to remove some nuclei. This may account for the reduced incidence of DCS in divers and caisson workers after they have been exposed to repeated and regular diving. This is called acclimatization, and may be lost after a week of non-exposure. It may also explain the necessity to gradually 'build up' to deep diving exposures.

**Studies with gelatin**, initiated by Le Messurier in Australia and further developed by Strauss and Yount in Hawaii and Vann at Duke University, have clarified the behaviour of bubble nuclei when exposed to pressure changes. There is some agreement that the differences in pressure between the gas in the tissue and gas in the environment needs to be kept small to prevent bubble production. This therefore supports the critical pressure $\Delta P$ hypothesis. The bubble-free profiles would then have a small first 'pull', to take up the unsaturation, and then be linear to ensure that the meniscus of the bubble nucleus never bulges sufficiently to cause a separated bubble.

**Van Liew** and others later demonstrated these concepts by experiments utilizing gas analyses in induced gas pockets. Figure 11.3 illustrates some of these changes and is the basis of much of our recompression procedures. It demonstrates the gas gradients used to dissolve bubbles.

Nitrogen is lost much faster from solution in tissues, than from bubbles. Thus, if an air-breathing diver has been saturated at 2 ATA and then rapidly ascends to the surface (1 ATA), and if a bubble has not developed in tissue A, but has in tissue B, then the gradient from the tissue to the arterial blood is as shown in box.

Ignoring the other factors, such as distortion effects from the bubble, it is seen that the gradient to remove nitrogen from solution in

| | | |
|---|---|---|
| Tissue A: | $N_2$ pressure | = 1179 mmHg |
| Blood: | $N_2$ pressure | = 573 Hg |
| Gradient: | | = 606 mmHg |
| Tissue B: | bubble $N_2$ pressure | = 633 mmHg |
| Blood: | $N_2$ pressure | = 573 mmHg |
| Gradient: | | = 60 mmHg |

the tissues is 10 times that from a tissue bubble, and therefore it will take much longer to get rid of the nitrogen in bubble form.

Even with identical pressure exposures, various tissues will have different factors determining bubble development, including vascularity of the tissue, solubility of the gas and its diffusion coefficient.

Recent work by Danish researchers on bubbles in adipose tissue showed that the breathing of Heliox after air dives resulted in rapid resolution of nitrogen bubbles. The inflow of helium, because of its lower (1:4) solubility in adipose tissues, was less than the outflow of nitrogen. The bubbles, which grew while the animals were breathing air, were eliminated at the same rate with either oxygen or Heliox breathing. They also cast doubt on the concept of gas nuclei persisting after the bubbles had shrunk to submicroscopic levels (10–20 $\mu$m), because they were unable to re-expand such bubbles with nitrous oxide breathing. This gas has a solubility of 30 and 45 times that of nitrogen and helium respectively, and should rapidly expand such bubbles.

Behnke had already realized the value of the unsaturation of **oxygen window concepts** by using oxygen inhalation to hasten decompression. He treated DCS with oxygen at 9 metres (30 feet) and then proposed use of oxygen/nitrogen mixtures at greater depths. The value of oxygen was perhaps brought into question by a description of 'oxygen bends' by Donald. This was something of a red herring as subsequent analysis by Brian Hills revealed that the animals so afflicted had large quantities of inert gas and that the contribution of oxygen to the disease was minimal.

The next important development in comprehending the physiology of decompression was the appreciation of the importance of bubble production during apparently normal uneventful dives. Note was made in Haldane's original thesis that the body could withstand various pressure reductions which would produce a specific volume of gas. However, his decompression schemes relied on the belief that gas

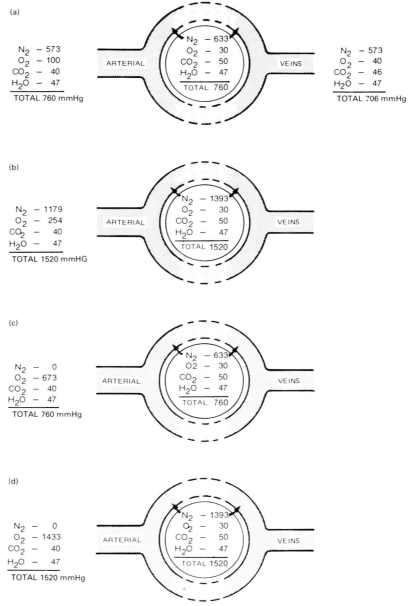

**Figure 11.3** Theoretical gas pressures in bubbles and blood, when the diver breathes air or oxygen at 1 ATA and 2 ATA. (a) $N_2$ gradient of 60 mmHg, breathing air at 1 ATA; (b) $N_2$ gradient of 214 mmHg, breathing air at 2 ATA; (c) $N_2$ gradient of 633 mmHg, breathing $O_2$ at 1 ATA; (d) $N_2$ gradient of 1393 mmHg, breathing $O_2$ at 2 ATA

phase separation (bubbles) did not occur with his staging techniques.

One of the main tenets of Haldane's concept was that gas elimination followed the same exponential manner as gas uptake. Behnke

first proposed the presence of 'silent' bubbles, while discussing DCS due to altitude exposure in 1942. Silent bubbles were so called because they had no clinically obvious effects, and were not specifically associated with DCS. If verified, the presence of these bubbles would not be consistent with the exponential gas elimination curve, because bubbles interfere with the movement of gas along pressure gradients in solution.

In 1960, **Hannes Keller** introduced his own approach to decompression theory, which he demonstrated by carrying out a dive to 210 metres (700 feet) in the lake at Zürich. A dive to 300 metres (1000 feet) in the open ocean was not as successful, resulting in the death of his companion. Keller's dives were followed by his Swiss colleague, Buhlmann, exploring these new avenues.

In 1961, **Goodman** suggested that future developments in decompression should include the use of different gases during decompression staging, with each one being breathed in turn, until the zero decompression limit is reached for that pressure–time relationship. He also suggested exploration of the use of nitrogen/oxygen mixtures for the treatment of DCS – an idea that was independently exploited by both the French and Australian workers during the following decade.

**Buhlmann** pioneered the use of mixed gas diving using various helium, nitrogen and oxygen mixtures in the belief that the gases would be taken up and released independently from solution. He developed curves relating the allowable safe supersaturation ratios for different half-time tissues at depth. The curves were interrelated in accordance with Graham's law (the diffusion coefficient is inversely proportional to the square root of the molecular weight of the gas). Buhlmann used fast compression rates for his deep dives. He progressively changed from helium to nitrogen as the inert gas during a continuous ascent, but as he approached the surface he would then switch to the maximum tolerable oxygen pressure. He also supported the belief that, if work was performed at depth, decompression times had to be extended.

**Inert gas counterdiffusion** was first described by Idicula and Lambertsen in 1973 in subjects who breathed one inert gas mixture while being surrounded by another. It was also termed 'isobaric counterdiffusion', deriving its name from the Greek prefix 'iso' meaning the same and 'baric' referring to pressure. Isobaric counterdiffusion therefore means the diffusion of gases in different directions, while at a fixed environmental pressure, i.e. without decompression. The production of bubble formation occurring without decompression introduced a new facet to DCS and its management. There are various forms of isobaric counterdiffusion.

### Superficial isobaric counterdiffusion

This develops whenever the inert gas breathed diffuses more slowly than the inert gas surrounding the body. This could occur when the diver breathes air while surrounded by a helium/oxygen mixture. The nitrogen moves from the skin capillary blood through the skin tissue into the environment at a slower rate than the fast diffusing helium passes from the environment into the skin capillary blood. This inequality of diffusion leads to a supersaturation at certain sites within the superficial tissues and presumably in the capillary blood as well. It was first noted at a stable depth of 1200 feet in a chamber filled with normoxic helium and the diver breathing a neon–oxygen mixture. It has also been observed in a helium environment, when the subjects changed the inert gas being breathed from helium to hydrogen.

The lesions produced by the developing bubble produce an intense itching of the skin (Plate 5).

The vestibular system is prone to decompression disease at great depths. This is thought to be due to counterdiffusion between the middle-ear space and the fluids of the inner ear through the round window, although others have suggested that the continuous gas embolism which accompanies superficial counterdiffusion may be the cause of the vestibular disease.

### Deep tissue isobaric counterdiffusion

With the entire body exposed to the same gas as that being breathed, superficial counterdiffusion cannot occur. Different rates of tissue uptake and elimination of the various gas mixtures breathed in sequence may possibly lead to tissue supersaturation or subsaturation in the isobaric state. After prolonged exposure to a nitrogen/oxygen mixture, breathing helium/oxygen results in more rapid entry of helium than loss of nitrogen from a particular tissue site. The sum of inert gas partial pressures therefore increases to above ambient and supersaturation will exist.

### Gas switching

DCS may be precipitated or worsened when a helium/oxygen breathing diver converts to air breathing. This is difficult to explain by counter-diffusion principles. It may be that air breathing interferes with pulmonary dynamics, because of the increased density, and that this may potentiate the DCS by reducing helium elimination. Some workers have found that in tissue, and specifically the central nervous system, oxygenation is less with the breathing of nitrogen/oxygen mixtures than with helium/oxygen mixtures at the same oxygen partial pressure.

## Intravascular bubbles

Doubts were raised regarding the haldanian hypotheses by Behnke in 1951, when he conjectured 'it may well be that what appears to be a ratio of saturation tolerance is in reality an index of the degree of embolisation that the body can tolerate'.

Large quantities of air can sometimes be tolerated in the venous system, if infused slowly. Up to 1 litre has been suggested, without causing death. However, less than 1 ml can cause death if it enters certain areas of the arterial system, such as the coronary or cerebral arteries. The difference in volumes is explained by the very capable pulmonary filtration of the bubbles preventing them from entering the arterial circulation, unless right-to-left shunts are present.

Because the obstruction of vessels by bubbles is dependent on the relative sizes of the bubbles and the vessels and also on the blood pressure forcing the bubbles through, obstruction is much more likely in the pulmonary artery than in the systemic arterial systems.

### Venous gas emboli (VGE)

Behnke's 'silent' bubbles became very audible following the development and application of sophisticated ultraonic techniques. Using these in 1963, Mackay detected bubbles in rats during decompression. Spencer and Campbell, in 1968, demonstrated gas emboli in decompressed sheep by the use of the Doppler ultrasonic bubble detection system. They also demonstrated bubbles in humans exposed to certain US Navy decompression tables. Evans and Walder, working in the UK, and Powell and Kent Smith working independently in the USA, verified and then extended these concepts. The following is a resumé of Doppler developments, and their relationship to DCS, over the last two decades.

Bubbles can be detected once they reach a size of 40–50 μm (sometimes as small as 20 μm, especially if there are a lot of them); even single bubbles of 150 μm can be detected. The characteristic sound of a bubble signal is a chirp or whistle, which can be confused with other sounds such as blood components, lipid and platelet emboli, superimposed on a background noise. The latter can be particularly troublesome, especially when the diver is active, shivering or cold. To obtain a good recording, an experienced observer is required. It is not a perfect instrument for use in the field and it is important to remember that it demonstrates bubbles, which are not synonymous with DCS.

Nevertheless, the Doppler technique is a very valuable research technique and has increased our understanding of decompression and its sequelae. The use of bidirectional ultrasonic localization for the demonstration of extravascular bubbles complements the Doppler technique for the detection of intravascular bubbles, and gives a more complete picture of how the body handles bubble development and movement during and after decompression.

Although bubbles may appear in the arterial or capillary systems, most of the current measurements relate to their movement within the venous system. They are released freely into the veins, either due to their own growth or because of disruption by movement of the tissue or limb. The bubbles then pass through the right side of the heart and in many cases become lodged in the pulmonary arterioles and capillaries. Up to 6% of the absorbed gas may be eliminated by having the bubbles trapped in this pulmonary filtration system. Most of the eliminated gas still passes in solution from the tissues to the pulmonary blood and then diffuses into the alveolar air.

For short deep air dives of 30–60 metres (100–200 feet), VGE can be detected within a couple of minutes of surfacing or while performing decompression stops. The number of bubbles heard reaches a peak within the first hour and then gradually diminishes over the next few hours. The specific time intervals will vary with different dive profiles, diver activity etc.

If there is an excess number of bubbles in veins, the pulmonary filtration system may become overloaded. Pulmonary hypertension then develops and, if this exceeds a rise of 120%, then the bubbles will tend to pass through the pulmonary system into the systemic system. Another effect of pulmonary hypertension is to open potential shunts in the atrial or ventricular septa, which may also allow paradoxical emboli into the arterial system. Clinically, when large quantities of gas emboli pass into the pulmonary filtering system and overload it, the syndrome of 'chokes' with right ventricular failure and circulatory collapse may develop. This is more likely when the pulmonary hypertension exceeds a rise of 150%. Spinal cord involvement is also associated with greater pulmonary gas loads. A large volume of gas in the right side of the heart may interfere with cardiac contraction and form an air lock.

Venous bubbles may influence specific organs in different manners (Figure 11.4). Spinal cord paraplegia may result from venous stasis produced by a gross accumulation of venous bubbles in the spinal venous plexus. Bubbles in the systemic arterial system may produce local brain damage, although there is some degree of tolerance to gas emboli within the cerebral system. Cardiac action may also allow some bubbles to pass through the coronary arteries, without consequence. It may be that the high flow rate and the squeezing action of the heart acting on its own blood vessels may protect the heart from the effects of some of these emboli.

Gas emboli have been demonstrated under many practical diving conditions. They were initially noted following the US Navy Tables of Exceptional Exposure. They have also been observed among sport divers performing no-decompression dives from the US Navy Standard Air Decompression Tables. Bubbles developed in slow decompressions from saturation dives, although they tended to be feeble

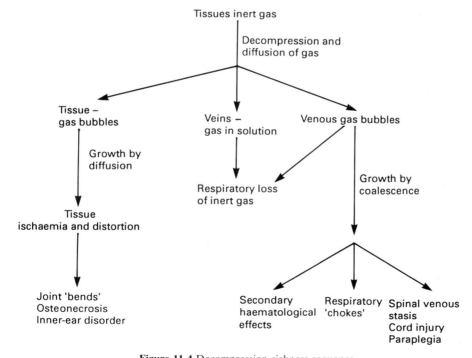

**Figure 11.4** Decompression sickness sequence

and fairly constant – unlike those described during the dives that are more likely to produce serious decompression cases. They were also noted in breath-hold dives performed by the Japanese Ama divers after 30 successive open ocean dives to 15 metres, with a total duration of each dive averaging just over 65 seconds.

Bubbles have been observed, as has DCS, from saturation dives to 9 metres (30 feet) and 7.5 metres (25 feet). The current depth for unlimited exposure is about 7 metres (22 feet), and most experienced diving physicians are aware of cases of DCS after diving at such depths – usually with aggravating factors such as very long exposure, extreme exertion etc.

Provocation of bubble formation and movement has been demonstrated by Doppler techniques in certain other environmental situations. This was observed under isobaric conditions (without any change of pressure) when animals were switched from air to helium/oxygen breathing at a depth of 40 metres (132 feet). Numbers of emboli may be increased enormously by limb manipulation, promoting the dislodging of gas bubbles held in the peripheral veins of that limb.

When a dive pattern is interrupted by a brief ascent to the surface and then a return to the bottom, the overall volume of nitrogen absorbed by the diver should be less than if he had remained at depth throughout. Despite this, there are a great number of gas emboli with the interrupted dive profile. The second decompression will produce more bubbles than would otherwise have been expected to occur had there been no intervening period at normal pressures!

In this bimodal profile, bubbles may be produced during either or both decompressions, and the bubbles produced by the first ascent, and trapped in the pulmonary circuit, may be compressed and therefore pass through the pulmonary bed into the systemic arterial system during the second compression. They may then expand in the tissue vessels during the second ascent – producing rapidly developing DCS.

There is a considerable individual variation in the likelihood of producing both gas emboli and DCS, but these two results are generally quantitatively related. Occasionally, bends or DCS will develop without VGE being present,

especially with saturation exposure or 'slow tissue' DCS.

Under good conditions, it is possible to use the presence of venous emboli as a practical guide to prevent DCS, avoid provocative conditions and indicate the need for specific preventive and therapeutic measures, which include the use of oxygen and recompression. Gas emboli, without DCS, were removed by breathing 100% oxygen at 1 ATA after some dives (Spencer et al.). Recompression to 9 metres (30 feet) on 100% oxygen cleared both gas emboli and DCS produced from deep exposures. Others showed the value of in-water oxygen decompression to reduce both VGE and DCS.

There is a much higher incidence of VGE than there is of DCS. The statistical relationship between the two is nevertheless very strong. A dive schedule which produces bubbles in 20% of divers may have a 5% DCS incidence.

**Spencer's grading** of bubbles heard precordially over the right ventricular outflow is as follows:

Grade 0    No bubbles signals on Doppler
Grade 1    An occasional bubble but with the great majority of cardiac periods free
Grade 2    With many, but less than half, of the cardiac periods containing Doppler signals
Grade 3    Most of the cardiac periods contain showers or single bubble signals, but not dominating or overriding the cardiac motion signals
Grade 4    The maximal detectable bubble signals sounding continuously throughout the heart cycle and overriding the amplitude of the normal cardiac signal

Grade 0 infers that there is little or no chance of DCS. Grades 1 and 2 are infrequently associated with DCS, whereas the higher grades of 3 and 4 are associated with a high incidence of DCS. The syndrome of 'chokes', together with the passage of bubbles into the arterial system through the pulmonary filter, is especially likely with grade 4 bubble detection.

Methods of decompression, and even of treating DCS, have been proposed on the basis of the quantification of bubbles by Doppler techniques. Although of value in research applications, clinically a patient is not a bubble. Bubbles and DCS may develop in tissues, and even in the less accessible vascular tissues, without being detected by Doppler.

### Arterial gas emboli (AGE)

Gas emboli may enter the arterial blood from:

1 Decompression of the blood.
2 Pulmonary tissue disruption, such as pulmonary barotrauma.
3. From venous (paradoxical) gas emboli, by:
  (a) patent foramen ovale or other cardiac septal defect;
  (b) failure of the pulmonary filter due to:
    (i) massive embolization,
    (ii) excessive pulmonary artery pressure,
    (iii) Valsalva technique,
    (iv) arteriovenous anastomoses;
  (c) bronchopulmonary anastomoses bypassing the pulmonary filter.
  (d) re-embolization after already passing through the arterial system.

Factors reducing the likelihood of in situ development of AGE include the higher arterial blood pressure and the relatively short circulatory time.

Even if bubbles do enter the arterial system, a calamity is not inevitable. The distribution will depend on the buoyancy of the bubbles, and many sites are either not critical, or may have alternative circulation. Possibly bubbles below 25 µm diameter may pass through cerebral and cardiac circulation, without effect. Many current surgical procedures produce small quantities of arterial bubbles without causing obvious damage.

## Bubble interaction with tissues or blood

Bubbles may impede circulation and cause congestion and oedema from the back pressure (venous emboli) or ischaemia (arterial emboli).

Other effects of gas emboli include:

- Damage to epithelium of vessels, with reduction in blood flow.

- An inflammatory reaction (neutrophils, platelets, fibrin) between the bubble and tissue/blood.
- Release of chemicals which have influence on blood flow and tissue viability.
- Destruction of surfactant.
- Coagulation and complement system activation.
- Increased local pressure, when there is a limit to tissue compliance without damage, e.g. in cells, osteoclast spaces, myelin sheaths, inner ear, spinal column, brain.

From these pathological changes, there may be more persistent damage from DCS than that expected of a treatable gas bubble.

## Decompression tables, techniques and computers

Every compressed air dive will require decompression – unless the diver remains under water forever. Nitrogen will be absorbed in excess of the norm, and it must be off-loaded. Decompression may occur at either shallower depths (staging) from the maximum, in which case the specific depths and durations are critical, or during ascent, in which case the rate of ascent is critical.

During the last two decades, there has been a plethora of **computer-designed decompression schedules**. Initially, they were based on the haldanian models, with variations in tissue numbers and half-times, in an attempt to explain anomalies of decompression. Subsequently, as with the University of Hawaii decompression tables, allowance has been made to include cavitation concepts in saturated solutions, a degree of inherent unsaturation from oxygen utilization, and the production of bubble-free decompressions using the gelatin models. Variations of breathing gas mixtures can be considered in the program, and attempts are made to produce bubble-free schedules which avoid both DCS and dysbaric osteonecrosis. As anticipated, the computer calculations propose dives with deeper first stops, but with a duration not dissimilar to the conventional tables for deep diving.

Significant changes have also taken place since the Haldane experiments, clarifying the safe **rate of ascent** for compressed air scuba diving. Haldane used 7–8 metres (25 feet) per minute ascent rate, slow enough to avoid bubble development in the fastest tissues and logistically to permit ascent in standard gear (hard hat). With the freedom of ascent with scuba, these rates were increased. With experience, they have now been decreased.

| 1956 – US Navy | 18 m/min | 60 feet/min |
|---|---|---|
| 1957 – Workman | 18 m/min | 60 feet/min |
| 1968 – RNPL | 15 m/min | 50 feet/min |
| (Hempleman) | (3 m/min between stops) | |
| 1966–76 – Hills | 12 m/min | 40 feet/min |
| 1975 – Buhlmann | 10 m/min | 33 feet/min |

Apart from the greater opportunity to off-load nitrogen during the ascent, other advantages of slow ascents probably include: reduced rate of VGE production; less pulmonary filter obstruction; and less chance of pulmonary damage (barotrauma or seeding of bubbles).

Not only is the total volume of gas very relevant, but so is the time over which it is released. Bolus doses of gas, such as produced during rapid ascents from short deep dives, are more likely to overload the pulmonary filtration system and thus cause early development of cerebral DCS than the same volume of gas from a shallow long dive, which may be in the slower deep tissues and cause a late joint bend.

The shallow safety stop, usually 5–10 minutes between 3 and 9 metres (10–30 feet), is of value not only in increasing the total decompression time, but also reduces by up to 50% the bolus volume of gas that the pulmonary filter has to cope with during that period. It reduces the nitrogen gradients between different tissues.

Oxygen can be used, both on the surface and under water, to increase inert gas elimination. Paul Bert, last century, observed the protective and therapeutic use of oxygen, breathed on the surface after diving. The duration of the oxygen inhalation needs to increase with the increased load in slower tissues, i.e. with longer dives. When this is used as an added safety factor, the duration of decompression is not lessened. At other times, it is used as a means of reducing decompression time, when the advantages and disadvantages need to be more carefully assessed.

There has been a move towards using VGE detection by Doppler as a device to demonstrate safety in diving table development. It is reasonable to denigrate a decompression table on the basis of its production of excessive VGE, because this is roughly correlated with DCS incidence in short duration dives. The ideal table will produce no bubbling, but this cannot be presumed from the absence of VGE, as these are probably late manifestations of bubble formation in tissues. DCS may occur without VGE being detected, especially in long duration and repetitive dives.

All currently used tables rely more on experience than knowledge, and are more effective in reducing slow tissue 'joint bends' than fast tissue neurological DCS.

Problems in developing a reliable mathematical model to predict DCS in humans were reiterated by Brian Hills, who was instrumental in proposing many such models during the perfusion vs diffusion arguments of the 1960s. Tissue perfusion observations reveal that arterioles and the associated capillary system will frequently and periodically shut down, whilst adjacent systems may perfuse normally. Thus, in the one tissue there may be both inert gas retention and inert gas washout! As he stated, one bubble was enlarging while a similar bubble in the same tissue was contracting. This observation would be difficult to incorporate into relatively rigid mathematical models.

## RNPL/BSAC decompression table

**Hempleman**, working at the Royal Naval Physiological Laboratory, introduced his single tissue model of decompression in 1952. There were several assumptions on which these tables were based. They are almost diametrically opposed to Haldane's concepts, the principles on which the US Navy tables are based. They are as follows:

1. Only one tissue type is involved in the production of type 1 (joint) bends.
2. The rate of uptake of gas in that tissue is limited by perfusion (blood supply).
3. The rate of uptake is greater than the rate of elimination because silent bubbles form in that tissue and interfere with maximal gas elimination, even in trouble-free dives.
4. A certain critical volume of gas can be tolerated without symptoms (compare the critical ratio hypothesis of Haldane).

5. Gas diffusion is analogous to the situation where the affected tissue adjoins arterial blood.

A 'limiting line' was proposed to demonstrate the dangers with deeper dives and longer decompressions. Although the allowable descent rate was 30 m/min, the ascent rate was reduced to 15 m/min.

Hempleman's tables result in longer decompressions and deeper first stops. They compared favourably with the US Navy tables in safety, at least for recreational diving depths (30 metres, 100 feet).

Unfortunately, because there are different mechanisms involved with various categories of DCS, the exclusion of one tissue DCS (limb bends) does not ensure protection of others, such as neurological DCS, and these are more likely if the RNPL/BSAC tables are used at greater depths.

New schedules were devised in 1968 and were known as the '1968 Air Diving Tables', incorporating a variable ratio of tissue nitrogen tension to environmental pressure. These tables were considered too conservative and the Royal Navy modified them, metricated them and presented them as the RNPL 1972 Tables.

For the RNPL/BSAC tables, the initial no-stop limits are sometimes considered too long. This is especially so with the deeper dives. Also, some surface intervals were too short.

In 1988, Hennessy modified the BSAC procedure for calculating repetitive dives and deleted the concept of the 'limiting line', by not permitting such exposures. The **BSAC-88 tables** are based on more conservative no-stop limits and a safe no-decompression depth of 6 metres, compared to 9, and makes allowance for the ambient pressure effects on bubbles during repetitive dives, as a source of extra inert gas. The rate of 'off-gassing' is presumed to decrease with each repetitive dive; thus each repetitive dive requires a more conservative decompression than the last. They consist of a set of seven tables, with Table A being used for the initial dive and other tables being determined by the presumed nitrogen retention and the surface interval.

These tables are comparable with the current Buhlmann and DCIEM tables for no-decompression diving. For dives requiring decompression stops they are often, but not always, more conservative than the US Navy tables, but usually less conservative than the Buhlmann or DCIEM tables.

## Bassett tables

The US Air Force commissioned Dr Bruce Bassett to validate schedules for flying after diving. This led him into believing that the US Navy tables had too high an incidence of DCS if they were 'pushed to the limit'. The DCS incidence was about 6% and Doppler bubbles were detected in approximately 30%. These findings were similar to those of Dr Merrill Spencer in Seattle.

With this information Dr Bassett reduced the no-decompression limits from the US Navy tables by reducing the allowable supersaturation in the various half-time tissues.

For the shorter no-decompression dives, Bassett recommended an ascent rate of 10 m/min, with a 3–5 minute safety stop at 3–5 metres for all dives greater than 9 metres, and a total time under water, rather than the bottom time, being used to calculate the repetitive group after a dive.

Knight and Lippmann modified the Bassett tables for repetitive dive use.

## DCIEM tables

The Defence and Civil Institute and Environmental Medicine (DCIEM) of Canada uses a different model for decompression, based on tissue compartments arranged in a series, rather than in parallel as with the US Navy (originally Haldane) model.

It is very well-researched table and, although it is based on the theoretical model, it has been modified greatly by extensive human testing with Doppler monitoring. The testing was performed in both cold water and under hard working conditions.

The single no-decompression times, and most repetitive dives, are more conservative than the US Navy tables.

## Buhlmann tables

The Swiss decompression expert, Professor Buhlmann, has conducted many theoretical and practical investigations on the Swiss model which includes 16 theoretical tissue compartments with half-times of 4–635 minutes. The testing of the tables at altitude has been more careful than for most other tables.

The permitted duration at deep stops often exceeds the US Navy tables, but the ascent rate is reduced to 10 metres. All no-decompression dives require a stop of 1 minute at 3 metres' depth.

It is believed that shorter initial dives will minimize bubble formation on the first dive and so improve the nitrogen off-loading during ascent. This allows longer times for the repetitive dives

### PADI tables

The initial PADI tables were, like the Bassett tables, more conservative than the US Navy tables.

The PADI Recreational Dive Planner is different and embraces a repetitive system based on the $T_{40}$ or $T_{60}$ tissue compartments rather than on the $T_{120}$, as in the US Navy tables. The result is that it allows longer repetitive dives after shorter surface intervals.

A small amount of somewhat selective and restricted practical testing of the tables was performed, using Doppler monitoring.

The repetitive dive planner comes in two forms: there is a table version, similar in design to the original tables; the other version is the 'wheel', and can be used for multilevel diving. The 'wheel' requires much more rigorous testing before it can be recommended.

### 'New' tables

The development of tables involves such a heavy cost, in terms of time and money, that it is most unlikely that any new tables could be tested comprehensively enough to be acceptable in the diving community, without many years of effort and huge financial backing.

This has not deterred many people from devising their own tables, because 'it seemed a good idea at the time', and attempting to inflict them on recreational divers on the basis of questionable mathematical concepts.

There are always rumours of new US Navy tables about to be released, as if this could be done without great time and effort. Even with the vast facilities available to them, the US

Navy would find it very difficult to produce new, well-tested tables under the current conditions.

Unfortunately, the perceptions usually exceed the facts. For table development, there not only needs to be a model on which the tables are based (to allow extrapolation to other situations), but also a testing of the tables against both a decompression database (such as is available in the USA and Canada) and also practical testing of the tables under conditions more likely to produce DCS. When such tables are tested, they will need to have a predictable decompression incidence allocated for each dive profile.

There are also new French tables, allegedly very well tested, currently being supplied to the recreational diver market (see Appendix III).

### Multilevel diving

This is being promoted, again without adequate research or testing, and there are a number of different techniques that can be used to allow for diving at multiple levels.

In all 'multilevel diving' it is necessary that the deepest part of the dive be carried out first and that, within 10–20 feet (3–6 metres), the dive should progressively become shallower. Multilevel diving in the other direction, i.e. going from shallow to deep, is particularly hazardous because any bubble formed will expand rapidly when the diver returns to the surface, as a result of the higher pressure gradient between the tissues and the bubble.

From current statistics it appears that, in a single dive, a square wave pattern is probably more likely to cause DCS than a multilevel dive, if the latter is carried out from deep to shallow.

Repetitive diving, when combined with multilevel diving, becomes a mathematical nightmare, and dive computers only supply answers to theoretical tissue models – not divers.

*Any decompression table or dive computer which permits less time for decompression will cause a greater need for recompression chambers.*

## Decompression meters (computers)

These instruments have been in widespread use since the late 1960s. None has yet received approval by conservative and safety conscious organizations, and many have been withdrawn despite extensive publicity and transient acceptance by the general diving population. The large number of models suggests that none is fully reliable. The constant replacement of recent models by the manufacturers leads to the same conclusion. Despite modern technology, the computers have a high mechanical and electronic (and expensive) failure rate.

Three concepts have been used:

1. **Mechanical models** of gas uptake and release, such as the movement of gas through restricted orifices. The SOS and Farallon meters were of this type. These models were gross oversimplifications of the dynamics of decompression and were inappropriate for the possible range of diving exposures – nevertheless the later SOS meters were moderately safe for single, shallow, no-decompression dives of less than 24 metres (80 feet).
2. Electronic models of the established **decompression tables**, such as the Suunto USN meter. As these offered no duration advantage over the tables, and no ability to 'cheat' the tables, they were not generally accepted by the diving community.
3. Electronic models using the **decompression theories** on which different tables were originally based (usually quoting the US Navy or Buhlmann tables), and integrating this with a theory of **multilevel diving**. Because these meters excluded the many safety factors of 'rounding up' the depths, durations and surface intervals used in the established tables, they allowed much greater underwater exposure with less decompression. In an attempt to reduce the inevitable increased danger of DCS, shorter no-decompression limits were often included and slower ascent rates were advised. Nevertheless, the dives permitted by these devices were shown to be dangerous, and this was supported by the clinical observations.

Subsequently, diving computer manufacturers have included more and more safety factors in an attempt to counter the many defects inherent in the meters. One of the major manufacturers, in 1989, released a more conservative booklet for their users, stressing the additional need for:

- training in diving computer use;
- acceptance of a DCS incidence;
- not diving in excess of 39 metres (130 feet), without specialized training and professional supervision;
- no repetitive dives deeper than 24 metres (80 feet) with surface intervals of less than 1 hour;
- in repetitive diving, successive dives should be shallower;
- in multilevel diving, use an ascending profile;
- always add safety margins;
- on all dives, stop at 10 feet for at least 5 minutes;
- do not begin using a meter, if diving has been undertaken within the previous 24 hours;
- extra care in altitude diving and flying after diving;
- back-up equipment and preparation for equipment failure.

The warnings are timely and address some of the problems with the meters. One major problem common to all models, and having both safety and financial implications, is the very high incidence of faults developing during underwater exposure.

## Recompression therapy tables

The history of this subject is dealt with elsewhere. Suffice it to say that the reverence with which some of these tables are held is a triumph of faith over knowledge.

In 1873, A.H. Smith first reported the treatment of DCS by recompression during the construction of the Brooklyn Bridge. Moir, during the construction of the Hudson River tunnel, reduced a 25% death rate in the workforce to less than 2% by recompression therapy.

The 50% recurrence rates observed following treatments in the first half of this century were reduced by the introduction of three principles:

1. Depth of treatment being the depth of relief plus 1 ATA, with a 6 ATA maximum.
2. A 12 hour 'soak' at 9 metres (30 feet).
3. The later addition of oxygen at shallow depths.

The US Navy air Tables 1–4 were promulgated in 1945 – before they were tried on patients. All tests were performed on asymptomatic, recently dived, healthy subjects. The high incidence of DCS production resulted in modifications, with Table 1 becoming 1A, Table 2 becoming 2A etc.

As the US Navy became more involved in treatment of civilian divers, with their less-controlled diving and often a delay in recompression, the failure rate moved from 6% to 43% in 1963.

Previously Behnke, in 1939, obtained excellent results by treating DCS with oxygen at 2 ATA. This was not acceptable to the navy at that time, probably for the same reason that the experience of Edgar End, who treated 250 cases with oxygen at 45 feet, was rejected. The regime was 'not sailor proof'. As an alternative to the oxygen treatment, Behnke also used Heliox (70% helium, 30% oxygen) at approximately 100 feet for treatment of caisson workers with air-induced DCS, in 1942. Half a century later, this is considered very avant garde.

Goodman and Workman reduced the failure rate to 3.6% by using oxygen at 18 metres (60 feet) for 90 minutes – a success rate that many today would envy. Later this was arbitrarily extended to 2 and 4 hours and, later again, air breaks were added in the belief that this would reduce the possibility of oxygen toxicity. A risk–benefit analysis of these modifications has still to be carried out.

Many would question whether the duration of oxygen breathing is not of more importance than the depth.

Now see Chapters 12 and 13.

# Recommended reading and references

BEHNKE, A.R. (1947). A review of the physiological and clinical data pertaining to decompression sickness. *USNMRI Project X-443 Report No 4.*

BECKMAN, E.L. (1976). *Recommendations for Improved air Decompression Schedules.* Sea Grant Technical Report, University of Hawaii.

BENNETT, P.B. and ELLIOTT, D.H. (1975–1982). *The Physiology and Medicine of Diving and Compressed Air Work.* London: Ballière Tindall.

BUHLMANN, A.A. (1983). *Decompression – Decompression Sickness.* Berlin: Springer-Verlag.

EDMONDS, C. (1989). Dive computers – the Australian experience. *Proceedings of the Dive Computer Workshop,* American Academy of Underwater Sciences.

FRYER, D.I. (1969). *Subatmospheric Decompression Sickness in Man.* Agardograph 125. Slough: Technivision Services.

GERSH, I. and CATCHPOLE, H.R. (1951). *Decompression Sickness,* edited by J. F. Fulton, pp. 165–181. London: Saunders.

GOODMAN, M.W. (1961). *The Syndrome of Decompression Sickness in Historical Perspective.* US Navy MRL, Report 368.

GRIFFITHS, P.D. (1960). Compressed air disease. *MD thesis,* University of Cambridge.

HAYMAKER, W. (1955). Decompression sickness. *Handbuch der Spexiellen Pathogrischen Anatomie und Pathologie,* Vol 14. München: Springer.

HYLDERGAARD, O. and MADSEN, J. (1985). Influence of heliox, oxygen and $N_2O–O_2$ breathing on $N_2$ bubbles in adipose tissue. *Undersea Biomedical Research* **16**(3), 185–193.

HILL, L. (1912). *Caisson Sickness.* London: Edward Arnold.

HILLS, B.A. (1977). *Decompression Sickness.* Chicago: John Wiley & Sons.

HOFF, E.C. (1948). *A Bibliographical Sourcebook of Compressed Air Diving and Submarine Medicine.* Navy Department, Washington DC.

KINDWALL, E.P. (1990). Historical review. In: *UHMS/DAN/NOAA Workshop on Diving Accident Management,* edited by R. Moon and P.B. Bennett, in press. Bethesda, MD: UHMS.

LAMBERTSEN, C.J. (ed.) (1978). *Decompression Sickness and its Therapy.* Allentown, PA: Air Products and Chemical Inc.

LIPPMAN, J. (1989). *The Essentials of Deep Diving.* Tuart Hill, West Australia: FAUI.

*Proceedings of Symposium on Blood Interaction in Decompression Sickness* (1973). Defence and Civil Institute of Environmental Medicine, Toronto, Canada.

STRAUSS, R.H. (1976). *Diving Medicine.* New York: Grune & Stratton.

UMS Workshop No. 12 (1977). *Early Diagnosis of Decompression Sickness.* UMS Annual Scientific Meeting, Toronto, Canada. 12 May 1977, UHMS, Bethesda, MD.

UHMS Workshop No. 38. (1989). *The Physiological Basis of Decompression,* edited by R. D. Vann. Bethesda, MD: UHMS.

# 12

# Decompression sickness: clinical manifestations

## Aetiology

Decompression sickness (DCS) is now known to be a dysbaric disease due to the liberation of gas bubbles from solution, into tissue or blood. Its sequelae range from generalized haematological changes to single organ involvement.

The development of a bubble in an enclosed space may damage tissue directly, or cause ischaemia by blocking vessels directly or increasing tissue pressure sufficiently to impair perfusion. The latter mechanism has been postulated for: neurological DCS, with distension of the dural membrane of the brain and spinal cord; inner-ear DCS, with osteoclast cells expanding in the bony vestibule of the inner ear; limb DCS, with pressure increase as gas is formed within tendons and muscle sheaths; and dysbaric osteonecrosis, with the increased intramedullary pressure in bone.

Asymptomatic bubbles, which do not produce clinical features, are termed 'silent' and may precede the overt manifestations in many cases. They may also be the foundation on which DCS develops during subsequent dives.

Although omitting decompression will predispose to DCS, the majority (86%) of USA recreational divers who develop DCS have apparently complied with the decompression tables. The British Sub-Aqua Club would suggest a figure of 40%. Those who omitted decompression are likely to have more severe DCS and a less satisfactory outcome to treatment.

## Predisposing factors

Some physiological and environmental factors are thought to increase the likelihood or severity of DCS. Most of these influence the blood supply to tissues and therefore the speed of gas uptake or release. These include exercise, environmental temperature, gender, age, obesity, injury and alcohol ingestion.

**Exercise** has various effects, which are sometimes contradictory. Exercise performed while at depth is likely to increase the blood supply to the muscular tissues, and increase the rate of inert gas absorption at that site, which is then the site of the DCS. It can increase decompression requirements by a factor of 3.

Thus some muscle, which has a blood perfusion of 3 ml/min per 100 g at rest, has a half-time of 23 min and will become 26% saturated with nitrogen during a 10-minute dive. With half-maximum exercise the perfusion rises to 30 ml/min per 100 g and the half-time to 2.3 min, and it becomes 95% saturated in a 10-minute dive. This exercise level increases the nitrogen absorbed in muscle by 69% in a 10-minute dive, or 16% in a 60-minute dive.

During or after decompression, severe exercise results in an increase in the speed of bubble development and in the number of bubbles – perhaps due to increased cavitation from tribonucleation of tissues, or the turbulence similar to shaking a bottle of champagne.

Mild exercise during recompression is of value in increasing the rate of gas elimination, perhaps by increasing tissue perfusion, if supersaturation and bubble growth have not been incurred.

---

**Factors influencing DCS**

*Exertion*
*Physical fitness*
*Temperature – cold water, hot shower*
*Sex – females*
*Age*
*Obesity*
*Dehydration*
*Increased carbon dioxide pressures*
*Alcohol intake*
*Physical injury*
*Adaptation*
*Dive profile*
*Rapid and multiple ascents*
*Repetitive and multi-day diving*
*Altitude exposure*

---

Resting after decompression may give the body a longer time to liberate the inert gas it has absorbed during the dive, although occasional movements are warranted to ensure that paralysis or incoordination has not developed without the diver being aware of it. Thus, the routine practice of periodically walking the length of the compression chamber during decompression and therapy is to be commended.

**Physical fitness**, perhaps due to its relationship to more efficient muscular use and blood flow, seems to be of some protective value to divers.

**Temperature** may influence DCS in a complex manner, by its influence on perfusion (increased temperature producing increased blood flow) and solubility (lowered temperature producing increased gas solubility). Divers who are exposed to cold at maximum depth may have less tissue perfusion and DCS in no-decompression dives than divers in warm water and with hot water suits.*

If the diver becomes mildly hypothermic, which is not uncommon in longer dives, the ability to eliminate the nitrogen is decreased, and DCS is more likely. In some studies the perfusion rate in muscle was halved, thus doubling the required duration of decompression.

---

* Although this seems unfair to the fashion-conscious diver, the same problems develop during the après-dive, with the hot water jacuzzi.

Divers who become cold during decompression have a lowered perfusion of tissues during ascent, less gas uptake from the tissues and more DCS. The opposite occurs in warmer conditions. During decompression it is better to be warm, because the nitrogen elimination is increased (as are xenon and krypton, in experimental conditions).

After the dive, exposure to sudden and excessive heat, such as with a hot shower, produces increased superficial blood flow and lowered solubility of gas, resulting in a bolus of nitrogen being mobilized, with gas phase separation and delivery to the lungs. Both skin and generalized DCS manifestations could develop.

**Females** may have a higher incidence of DCS than males. In altitude exposures, this is thought to be a four-fold increase, and in divers more than three-fold. The explanation may be a physiological difference between the sexes, or the effect of social conditioning (physical fitness, cold exposure etc.). Studies have shown higher blood perfusion in females, both in subcutaneous tissues and in muscle (see Chapter 6).

There is no support for the hypotheses that the contraceptive pill increases the incidence, but menstruation may.

**Age**: increasing age increases DCS incidence, possibly due to impaired perfusion or to already damaged vessels being more susceptible to other flow interferences. Abnormalities and degenerations within joint surfaces also increase the likelihood of tribonucleation in the aged. A 28 year old has twice the likelihood of an 18 year old in aviation DCS statistics.

**Obesity** increases the tissue mass available to absorb more inert gas. The fattest 25% of the diving population, as judged by skinfold thickness, have a ten-fold incidence of DCS. Not all surveys demonstrate an association between fat content and DCS among normals (excluding the obese). Overweight and obesity can be measured by body mass index (see page 456) or skinfold thickness.

Nitrogen is 4.5 times more soluble in fat than in water and non-fatty tissues. In active adult populations, women have 20–30% body fat compared to 10–20% for men.

**Dehydration**, caused by the environment, exercise, water loss from respiration and immersion, and the impracticability of fluid replacement while diving, will reduce perfusion of tissues and thus the elimination of inert gas.

**Increased carbon dioxide** pressures, from the effects of pressure, exercise or breathing resistances with equipment, may cause increased perfusion during the dive, with increased nitrogen loading. It is also a factor with inadequate ventilation in caissons, chambers and helmets.

**Alcohol** over-indulgence may influence judgement at the time, but more commonly the dehydration, vasodilatation and heat loss which develops in the hours afterwards will aggravate DCS.

**Physical injury**, such as a sprained joint or a previous episode of DCS, predisposes to DCS due to scarring and the alterations in local tissue perfusion. Thus, some clinicians are concerned that spinal operations, such as a laminectomy, may be associated with spinal DCS risk.

**Dive profiles** may influence the likelihood of DCS. The deeper the dive and the more decompression required, the greater the incidence of decompression sickness. Surface decompression (returning to the surface before being recompressed) is also more dangerous.

For a single depth/duration exposure, DCS is more likely with a direct ascent to the surface than a gradual ascent interrupted by reasonable and shallower stops, i.e. with a safety stop or multilevel diving. The opposite will occur if there is increased depths at successive levels.

The no-decompression dive durations allowed by the US Navy tables, if followed without any added safety factors, have a 1–5% incidence of DCS. Many of the dives permitted by the tables, such as the 150-foot (45 m) dive for 60 minutes, are notorious for producing DCS and are usually avoided by experienced divers. (See pages 153–156 for a discussion on different tables.)

**Multiple ascents** during the dive may, by initiating venous gas emboli which are trapped in the pulmonary filter but escape to the arterial system during subsequent compressions, increase the likelihood of DCS. A dive exposure which will probably produce joint DCS is more likely to induce neurological DCS if excursions are made to the surface during the profile. Surface decompression procedures, repetitive dives with short surface intervals (<2 hours) and arterial gas emboli from pulmonary barotrauma may have similar effects.

**Repetitive dives**: if a diver exposes himself to increased pressures within 24 hours of a previous dive, the residual nitrogen remaining within his tissues will increase the likelihood of DCS. Mild or insignificant cases may be made much worse. Advice is often given to recreational divers to take a day off after every 3 days of repetitive diving.

If asymptomatic bubbles have been produced by diving, then subsequent diving even longer than 24 hours afterwards will probably precipitate an episode of DCS.

Travelling to **altitude** to dive, or exposure to altitude after diving, may provoke DCS by producing or expanding existing bubbles. Air travel may also predispose to DCS because of the dehydration effect in the cabin altitude, if not rectified by a compensatory fluid intake. More often, aviation exposure can induce DCS days after a dive, especially from repetitive, long or saturation dives. Flying is not advisable for at least 24 hours after normal, non-decompression, recreational diving. In an Australian DCS series, 8.6% were induced by altitude exposure.

Breathing different **gas mixtures**, such as nitrous oxide after air diving, decompressing on air after diving on Heliox, or breathing a slow diffusing gas while in a fast diffusing gas environment, may produce local or general pressure gradients which cause bubbles to develop. Existing bubbles may also expand if faster gases are breathed, e.g. breathing Heliox after producing air bubbles (see Chapter 11).

Decompression staging in a horizontal **position** results in an increased rate of gas elimination, as compared with the vertical or seated positions. In water, decompression has similar advantages over dry decompression, although this is not mirrored in practical situations because of the many adverse factors during diving compared to dry compression.

One factor reducing the likelihood of developing DCS is **adaptation** or **acclimatization** – the repetitive and recent exposure to increased pressures. DCS is more probable during the first week of diving operations, and following lay-off periods of more than a week. Although the more susceptible divers would be select-

ively eliminated at an early stage, this is not the whole explanation. It appears as if, with regular diving, a slight degree of resistance to DCS can develop for that diving depth. The incidence of DCS in caisson workers is halved in the second week and again in the third week.

The currently fashionable explanation for adaptation is the removal of naturally occurring gas nuclei, which are thought to be the nidus on which the bubble develops. This is also the reason why divers and caisson workers are advised to work up to their maximum exposures gradually.

Many other possible aggravating factors have been proposed, both endogenous (serum complement, lipids, smooth muscle activating factors etc.) and exogenous (smoking, migraine, oral contraceptives etc.). They require more confirmation.

## Classification

In highlighting the problems with this disease, Behnke reviewed a series of 55 cases, and concluded that on no single point did all cases agree.

Despite this diversity, both in symptom complexity and severity, attempts were made to classify the disease, to facilitate diagnosis and treatment by non-medical personnel.

A classification into **type I** (mild) and **type II** (serious) DCS was introduced as an attempt to differentiate cases, so that identification, prognosis and therapy could be more standardized. Unfortunately, this clinical classification was not well defined or applied appropriately.

Type I was described as (musculoskeletal) pain-only bends. Skin manifestations were also allocated to this subdivision. Recently, the US Navy Diving Manual pragmatically defined type 1 DCS as having the following characteristics: (1) extremity pain only, skin rash or lymphatic disease, with (2) a normal neurological examination before treatment and (3) symptoms resolved within 10 minutes at 2.8 ATA, on oxygen.

Type II includes those presenting with symptoms other than pain or skin involvement, or with abnormal physical signs.

**Table 12.1 Decompression sickness grading**

| *Type I* ('pain only') | *Type II* ('serious') |
|---|---|
| Limb or joint pain – dysfunction | Central nervous system disorder |
| Itch | Inner ear |
| Skin rash | Lungs |
| Localized swelling | Cardiac |
| | Type I symptoms developing under pressure |
| | Other manifestations |

Although the use of type I is reasonably clear when it is applied to acute DCS affecting the musculoskeletal system ('joint bends'), recent investigations reveal many subclinical neurological manifestations – depending on the sophistication of the investigation. Also, some skin manifestations are of ominous significance.

Potentially serious type II cases involve the central neurological, cardiovascular, respiratory and gastrointestinal systems. Nevertheless, in most DCS series, peripheral nerve symptoms are allocated to the same group as spinal and cerebral manifestations. A differentiation has not been made between vestibular and cerebellar presentations, despite the excellent prognosis of the former compared to the latter.

The classification is so commonly modified, even by its own proponents, that it appears to have lost any merit that it originally had. The qualifying designation of the organs affected appears to be the only logical approach, e.g. DCS affecting the inner ear and musculoskeletal systems. Introducing new nomenclature, such as 'dysbaric illness' or 'decompression injury', does not clarify the situation.

**Type III** DCS has been postulated as another, more serious, manifestation when the intravascular bubbles (AGE and then VGE) from pulmonary barotrauma seed the circulation and tissues, which are loaded with inert gas from previous dive exposures. The pressure gradient from the supersaturated tissues causes inert gas to diffuse into the bubbles which are at environmental pressure. The result is that a rapidly developing DCS (often spinal) evolves from an existing or resolving CAGE case.

> *DCS is best classified according to the organ or tissue affected.*

## Onset

DCS develops after the subject has commenced decompression or ascent. Most cases present within 6 hours of the dive (Table 12.2).

> *Over 50% of cases of DCS develop symptoms within 1 hour of the dive and 90% within 6 hours.*

DCS is more likely to develop rapidly under the following conditions:

- Deep dives, in which fast tissues are loaded and release gas rapidly.
- Rapid ascents, increasing the inert gas gradient.
- With pre-existing bubbles from other dives.
- Gross decompression omission.
- With the predisposing factors referred to above (see pages 160–162).

Slower onset of symptoms is observed with:

- More shallow dives.
- Marginal decompression omission.
- Slower ascents.

**Table 12.2 Onset of symptoms**

| Population characteristics | Time of onset from surfacing (percentage incidence) | | | | | | | | |
|---|---|---|---|---|---|---|---|---|---|
| | 0–30 min | 30 min to 1 hour | Second hour | Third hour | 4–6 hours | 7–12 hours | 13–24 hours | Over 24 | Unknown |
| Royal Navy divers (n = 137) | 57 | 10 | 13 | 14 | | 6 | 1 | | |
| Canadian Navy divers (n = 127) | 62 | 12 | 9 | 6 | 9 | 3 | 1 | | |
| US Navy divers (I) (n = 935) | 54.7 | | 12.1 | | 19.5 | 6.6 | 2.3 | 0.3 | 4.5 |
| US Navy divers (II) (n = 113) | 34.5 | | 14 | 33.6 | | 10.6 | 4.4 | | |
| Hawaiian civilians (I) (n = 100) | 66 | 6 | 4 | 3 | 2 | 5 | | 4 | |
| Hawaiian civilians (II) (n = 122) | 66 | 6 | 9 | | 7 | | 5 | | 2 |

The following figures must only be interpreted with an appreciation of the diving populations and profiles.

A series of 115 cases of DCS in recreational and semi-professional divers in Australia and Singapore reflected the influence of uncontrolled deep air diving with rapid ascents: 10.4% developed the initial symptom during the dive, while staging; 57% developed their first symptoms within 10 minutes of surfacing.

The Australian/Singapore series was similar both in onset and in symptomatology to the Hawaiian series. The US Navy series were heavily weighted for saturation exposures.

A well-regulated diver who develops DCS from a conservative diving profile is more likely to develop a milder DCS well after the dive. A diver who dives repetitively, deeper, with omitted decompression and less controlled ascents, develops a more serious DCS, more rapidly.

# Generalized

Perhaps the most common presentations of DCS are generalized symptoms described as weakness, apathy, weariness, tiredness or malaise. Other less tangible presentations include deviations from normal personality and/or behaviour.

# Musculoskeletal

## Pathology

Although the musculoskeletal symptoms are common presentations of DCS in humans, the pathology is not well understood. Radiological evidence of gas in joint spaces, periarticular areas, fascial planes and tendon sheaths is occasionally seen, but this is not necessarily the causative lesion. Gas in a joint space is not usually painful.

Extravascular bubbles in the subperiosteal area, tendons, ligaments, joint capsule, fascia and muscles and thought to cause the pain of 'bends'. These tissues are tight, and the development of a bubble is likely to distort and stretch tissue or its nerve supply. Application of local pressure will reduce this effect and produce relief in 60% of cases. Crepitus can sometimes be felt and this, with the associated pain, can be massaged away.

Bubbles in the articular vascular supply have been proposed, but are unlikely as recurrences tend to be in the same site. Myelin sheaths of peripheral nerves and referred neurological pain have also been incriminated, and verified in some cases.

## Clinical

This is also termed 'joint bends', 'type I', 'pain-only bends', 'decompression arthralgia' etc. First, there is an ill-defined discomfort or numbness poorly localized to a joint, periarticular or muscular area. The subject may protect or guard the affected area, although in the early stages he may get some relief by moving the limb. Over the next hour or so the discomfort develops into a deep dull ache, then a pain with fluctuations in intensity, sometimes throbbing and occasionally with sharp exacerbations. Limitation of movement is due to pain, and the limb is placed in a position which affords the most relief. The duration of pain is often related to the severity of symptoms.

The shoulder is the more common joint affected in recreational divers, in approximately one-third of cases. In caisson workers, aviators and deep saturation divers, the knee 'bend' is more common. Other joints, about equally affected, are the elbows, wrists, hands, hips, knees and ankles. Often, when two joints are involved, they are adjoining ones, and frequently the localization is between joints, over the scapula, on tendon insertions etc. The involvement is rarely symmetrical.

The application of local pressure, by means of a sphygmomanometer cuff, may result in considerable relief and thus be of diagnostic value. The site of pain can sometimes be transferred by massage of the area. Occasionally a recent or old injury might predispose to DCS.

> *Localized pain in or around a joint may sometimes be relieved by application of local pressure, e.g. from an inflated sphygmomanometer cuff.*

In the mild cases, fleeting symptoms are referred to as 'niggles', and may only last a few hours. The pain of the more severe cases usually increases over 12–24 hours and, if untreated, abates over the next 3–7 days to a dull ache. Local skin reactions may occur over the affected joint (see Plate 4).

An uncommon presentation of DCS in which the gas in the joint capsule, is seen with shallow long-duration air dives, such as those performed by professional shell fishermen. They dive for many hours on consecutive days to depths of less than 15 metres, usually without decompression. The DCS is painless and develops many hours after the ascent. The only symptom is the loud crunching noise with joint movement. It is referred to as the 'squelching shoulder' by abalone divers. It usually clears by the next morning and can be detected by X-ray or CT scan of the joint. A similar condition has been described in aviators.

---

## CASE REPORT 12.1

PR, a 37-year-old sports diver, performed dives to 30 metres and 15 metres on Saturday. There were several hours between the dives but the duration of each was unknown. The same dives were repeated on Sunday. His decompression meter did not prescribe decompression stops and all dives were incident free. After the last dive he drove home 200 km, feeling tired and happy. On getting out of bed the next morning, he developed a sudden severe sharp pain in the right ankle. The pain steadily increased in intensity and prevented weight bearing. There was no history of injury to the joint, no history of arthritis and no other symptoms or signs. Recompression to 2.8 ATA breathing 100% oxygen provided improvement within 15 minutes. After 30 minutes there was no pain at rest but it was still present on forced extension. Ascent was commenced at 12 min/m and was uneventful. After reaching the surface he was completely asymptomatic, able to walk and bear weight with no pain.

*Diagnosis:* DCS arthralgia ('type I' bends).

## CASE REPORT 12.2

LS, aged 34 years, dived on compressed air to 50 metres for 10–12 minutes. He surfaced without decompression and, after having lunch, dived again to 50 metres for 6 minutes. The surface interval was approximately 105 minutes. His decompression meter prescribed a 10-minute stop at 3 metres on the second dive. He was well after surfacing, but 3 hours later felt a few twinges in his right elbow and right shoulder with some tingling in the right hand. Ten hours later he was awakened from sleep with severe pain in the right elbow and shoulder joints. He also noted some loss of power in the right arm. Examination revealed diminished sensation to pin prick and light touch over the right arm from the deltoid region. There was some loss of motor power in the flexors and extensors of the elbow and wrist. Administration of 100% oxygen resulted in slight diminution of pain in half an hour, but no improvement in power or sensation. Recompression in water to 9 metres breathing 100% oxygen resulted in considerable improvement. After 30 minutes his symptoms were completely alleviated but there was some slight tenderness around the shoulder joint. He was asymptomatic after decompression at 12 minutes per metre and the only residual sign following therapy was slight muscle tenderness and stiffness over the posterior deltoid. The next day he was completely symptom free.

*Diagnosis:* DCS arthralgia (type I bends), with peripheral nerve involvement.

## Neurological

These presentations have produced a great deal of interest and controversy. It has been cynically, but perhaps accurately, stated that the way to reduce the incidence of cerebral manifestations of DCS is to omit a full neurological examination.

Newer brain imaging techniques suggest that multifocal, small vessel, cerebral involvement, especially in the frontal and parietal lobes, is demonstrable with most neurological DCS cases and with CAGE.

### Onset

Civilian divers, who perform deep air dives (especially with fast ascent rates), tend to develop cerebral symptoms which reflect fast tissue DCS. Divers who do repetitive air dives for moderate durations produce more spinal problems, often with cerebral manifestations. Cerebral DCS often presents earlier than spinal DCS.

The shorter the time between surfacing and developing DCS, the greater the severity and the worse the prognosis. Of over 1000 cases the clinical distribution was: cerebral 22.7%, spinal cord 66.4% and combined 10.9%:

- 56% developed within 10 minutes of surfacing;
- 40% developed within 5 minutes of surfacing;
- only 15% were delayed more than an hour.

Cerebral DCS is fastest in onset, reflecting fast tissue bubble development and haemodynamic effects; 50% of cerebral DCS developed within 3 minutes. Peripheral nerve tends to be slowest, reflecting myelin release of inert gas. Spinal DCS is intermediate, reflecting both pathologies; 50% of spinal DCS developed within 9 minutes.

Myelin sheaths, being lipid structures, are capable of absorbing nitrogen more than helium. Cerebral, spinal and peripheral nerve DCS are more common with air diving.

With the very deep helium diving, and especially with excursions from deep saturation depths or from the initial pull during decompression from great depths, inner-ear disorders are more frequent.

The clinical subdivisions of neurological presentations are: cerebral, cerebellar, spinal, inner ear and peripheral nerve.

## Cerebral

In the neurological systems, the pathology includes perivascular haemorrhages, oedema and demyelination in the cortex and subcortex, cerebellum and brain stem.

## *Pathophysiology*

Gas bubbles form in the circulating blood following a short latent period after decompression. Most bubbles are filtered out by the lungs. Some bubbles, however, pass through the lungs, either by small arteriovenous anastomoses or the capillary lakes of Sjöstrand. These bubbles are small, about 25 μm in diameter. They then pass through the heart and reach the central nervous system and may damage or occlude multiple arterioles after coalescing into larger bubbles.

The intravascular bubbles which block cerebral arterioles are especially likely to enlarge if the diver has exposed himself to a nitrogen load in this 'fast' cerebral tissue – by breathing air (fat-soluble nitrogen) at greater depths and performing a fast ascent.

Other methods of 'arterialization' of the venous gas emboli include the passage of emboli through a patent ductus arteriosus (present in 30% of the population) or septal defects, especially when the pulmonary artery pressures increase with emboli blockage of the pulmonary circuit, producing a right-to-left intracardiac shunt (paradoxical emboli). Similar effects could be induced by straining, sneezing, coughing, Valsalva manoeuvre etc.

The greater the number of pulmonary emboli, the greater the pulmonary artery pressure and the greater the likelihood of paradoxical gas embolism and AGE.

The importance of a right-to-left shunt in the heart, through a patent foramen ovale, allowing VGE to become AGE, has been previously observed in autopsies. Moon and his colleagues (1989) elegantly demonstrated a higher than expected incidence of this disorder among severe DCS cases subjected to investigation. They examined 30 patients with a history of DCS for the presence of a patent foramen ovale by bubble contrast, two-dimensional echocardiography and colour flow Doppler imaging. The former technique was found to be more sensitive. Of the 18 patients with serious sign and symptoms of DCS, 61% had shunting, compared to a 5% prevalence with healthy volunteers as controls (this increased to 8.5% during the Valsalva manoeuvre).

An increase in right atrial pressure may cause cardiac dilatation and open a potentially patent foramen ovale, allowing paradoxical emboli. This could follow VGE blocking pulmonary arterioles, the Valsalva manoeuvre, straining or immersion in water (claimed to increase in right atrial pressures up to 12 mmHg).

Emboli can do damage by:

- Obstructing blood flow.
- Initiating solid envelopes of leucocytes, platelets, lipid and fibrin layers from the coagulation system.
- Damaging endothelium of the arterioles and disrupting the blood–brain barrier.

Re-perfusion injury, which develops after the emboli have passed and blood supply is returned to the ischaemic tissue, may explain some of the recurrences of symptoms – especially if they do not respond to recompression, which would be expected to reduce the effects of bubbles.

Other pathological possibilities for cerebral DCS include myelin sheath damage and other autochthonous bubbles, other emboli (lipid, platelet etc.), aggravated damage from raised intracranial pressure, coagulopathies etc.

## *Clinical*

The clinical manifestations depend on the site of vascular obstruction and collateral arterial supply, and are largely a matter of chance. They tend to affect multiple sites in the frontal and parietal lobes and represent impaired perfusion in the anterior and middle cerebral artery distributions.

Any cerebral tissue may be damaged by gas bubbles, and causes a great variety of manifestations, analogous to those of the diffuse cerebrovascular disease of general medicine. Especially noted are the homonymous scotomata, unilateral or bilateral, single or multiple. Others include hemiplegia, monoplegia, focal or generalized convulsions, aphasia, alexia, agnosia, hemisensory or monosensory disturbances, migraine and confusional states.

Raised intracranial pressure has been observed, and may be associated with severe headache. Sludging of blood in the venous sinuses, oedema or other cerebral pathology may also produce this effect.

Serial, non-cultural, psychometric assessments of cognitive function may be of value if given before, during and after treatment. They provide measurements of mental impairment and response to treatment. Permanent mental impairment has been claimed as sequelae of cerebral DCS. Brain-stem involvement may also result in cranial nerve and pupillary abnormalities.

Although it is usually impractical to investigate cases of cerebral DCS prior to the initiation of recompression therapy, this may be of great value during or after the first RCC treatment. In cases of homonymous hemianopsia, electroencephalographic slow waves have been reported over the affected occipital cortex. Serial electroencephalograms are usually indicated during convalescence.

Computed tomography (CT) or magnetic resonance imaging (MRI) may differentiate between areas of localized cerebral oedema or infarction and may show that the clinical manifestations, even if clinically rather nebulous, have a cerebral more than a psychological or spinal cord basis. Other, perhaps more sensitive, investigations, such as cerebral perfusion studies with technetium and single photon emission computed tomography (SPECT), may demonstrate the multiple and diffuse lesions – but should not be relied upon or take precedence over therapy.

Even after treatment of DCS, there is frequently evidence of neuropsychological dysfunction – as well as abnormal psychometric, electroencephalographic and brain imaging studies. This may last many weeks or months, and is similar to the post-concussion syndrome, with or without a symptomatic depression.

## Cerebellar

These lesions produce ataxia, incoordination with typical neurological signs of hypotonia, diminished or pendular tension reflexes, asynergia with dysmetria, tremor, dysdiadochokinesis, rebound phenomenon, scanning speech and nystagmus. The 'staggers', which is variously described as vestibular, posterior column, spinal cord and cerebral DCS, is probably more often due to cerebellar lesions, without nystagmus.

## Spinal

### Pathology

There are four common explanations for predominant spinal involvement in many DCS cases.

Spinal cord and anterior horn damage may occasionally be due to spinal artery obstruction from an embolus.

The rise in intrathoracic pressure when VGEs block the pulmonary arterioles causes interference with venous drainage of the spinal cord and subsequent damage to the cord. Pulmonary hypertension interferes with venous drainage through the anastomoses of the spino-vertebral–azygos system, with subsequent engorgement and thrombosis in the vertebral venous system. This causes oedema and infarction in the comparatively poorly vascularized area of the spinal cord – the mid-thoracic segment. This theory explains why spinal DCS is more common than cerebral DCS, despite the much greater blood supply (and thus emboli) to the brain.

The same situation will cause an impairment in the ability to remove gas from the cord tissue, and therefore result in 'autochthonous' or tissue bubbles – gas bubbles evolved from the nitrogen dissolved in white matter of the cord. These arise because the white matter has a high lipid content and this absorbs more nitrogen than the grey matter – which is relatively spared.

The spinal cord is a 'soft' tissue, but with a limited compliance, because of its confinement by the vertebrae and dura. If the volume of the canal is increased by 10% or more, the slack is taken up and the pressure within the cord escalates rapidly (waterfall effect). This can develop by either the engorgement of blood, production of gas or experimental injection of saline. Once the slack has been taken up, the escalating pressure could compress the venous system. This mechanism explains how spinal DCS cases can respond to recompression (reducing bubble size and cord pressure), but deteriorate with ascent (expanding bubble size and cord pressure).

## CASE REPORT 12.3

KG, a 21-year-old Torres Strait Islander, was learning to dive in the helmet and corselet equipment used by the local pearl divers. He was collecting shells at a depth of 17 metres and had made several brief ascents to the surface. At 9.00 a.m., after 2 hours in the water, he noticed the water level rising in his helmet and assumed that his air supply had ceased. Shedding his equipment he made a hasty return to the surface. He was not aware of the need to exhale. He surfaced conscious, but rapidly became dyspnoeic, confused and shocked. Soon after, he lost consciousness and his pulse could not be felt. External cardiac massage and mouth-to-mouth resuscitation were instituted and continued for several hours. On reaching the nearest island, intranasal oxygen, steroids and adrenaline were given. A doctor reached the island at 5.00 p.m. and found KG conscious but with episodes of confusion and irrational behaviour. He complained of pain in the right knee and the left loin. Marked weakness was noted in the lower limbs.

He remained stable until 10.00 p.m. when he became markedly confused, agitated and tachypnoeic. A chest X-ray revealed bilateral pneumothorax, small on the right, large on the left. Surgical emphysema of the neck was also noted. One hundred per cent oxygen by mask produced little improvement but a repeat chest X-ray showed the right pneumothorax had almost resolved while the left was growing. A left intercostal catheter and underwater drain produced considerable improvement.

Intravenous fluids were also commenced because of low urine output. Several small haematemeses were noted through the night and intravenous diazepam was required to prevent him thrashing about. At this stage, he would not tolerate an oxygen mask and his level of consciousness fluctuated from delirium to stupor.

A pressurized aircraft was arranged to transfer KG 3000 km, to the nearest adequate treatment centre. He arrived at 8.00 p.m. the next day (34 hours after the dive). He was noted to be conscious but not answering questions. During several lapses of consciousness, he became totally unresponsive to pain and developed a divergent squint. Other findings included epigastric tenderness, supraclavicular surgical emphysema and reduced lower limb reflexes. An electrocardiogram was normal and chest X-ray showed mediastinal emphysema and pneumothorax occupying one-third of the left chest. The intercostal catheter was replaced to ensure it was working properly and a mask giving 100% oxygen was tolerated.

Due to the lack of improvement in his condition, it was decided to recompress him as a therapeutic trial.

At 2.00 a.m. KG was compressed to 18 metres. He was markedly agitated during descent due to pain of aural barotrauma. After 20 minutes at 18 metres breathing 100% oxygen, his level of consciousness improved markedly and he was able to comply with simple requests. Decompression at 3 min/m to 10 metres then 12 min/m to the surface was uneventful. Later that day, KG was fully conscious, oriented and able to describe his dive. Two days later he was walking unaided and had no symptoms apart from mild abdominal discomfort.

*Diagnosis:* pulmonary barotrauma of ascent, probably with air embolism aggravated by DCS. (See Case report 12.4.)

> *Spinal DCS often follows pulmonary involvement.*

### Clinical

The spinal cord changes are predominantly in the white matter, and are most often observed in the mid-thoracic, upper lumbar and lower cervical areas, with the lateral, posterior and anterior columns suffering in that order. Often there is sparing of some long sensory tracts.

Local spinal or girdle pains may precede other symptoms, developing into serious spinal cord disease. It is more common in patients who also have respiratory symptoms ('chokes'). The symptoms and signs are those of paraplegia or paraparesis, and include urinary retention with overflow incontinence.

The lower abdominal pain due to a distended bladder from spinal DCS is frequently misdiagnosed.

Somatosensory evoked cortical responses may be of value in demonstrating the extent of the spinal lesions and may also be carried out during therapy, to show the effects of this. This investigation is not as sensitive as the clinical manifestations, in many cases, and thus the absence of positive responses should not be used in an attempt to exclude spinal disease. Imaging techniques will hopefully be available in the near future to demonstrate the pathology.

### Inner ear

### Pathology

Several non-exclusive explanations have been proposed for inner-ear DCS:

1. Rupture of bone lining the otic spaces by bubbles developing within the enclosed osteoclasts. This current theory proposes that osteoclast cells lie in bone cavities that do not permit expansion if bubble nucleation and growth develops during decompression. This causes elevated pressures which rupture the bone lining into the otic fluid spaces. Haemorrhages and blood-protein exudates are seen in the vestibular and/or cochlear systems. Petrous bone fractures attest to the considerable local pressures generated.

Later there is a growth of ectopic bone and fibrous tissue into the semicular canals, and this has been demonstrated at autopsy in both experimental animals and humans.

2. Supersaturation and helium bubble formation: the inner ear can receive helium not only from its own blood supply, but also from gas which passes across the round and oval windows bordering the middle-ear space. The perilymph can thus become saturated with this gas and can reach a steady state of gas content quite rapidly. The bubbling that develops during decompression may then disrupt the delicate inner-ear structures. Pressure fluctuations in the middle ear reflect eustachian tube functioning as well as ambient pressures, and this may aggravate release of dissolved helium into gas phase.

3. Supersaturation by counterdiffusion across membranes, such as the round or oval window, results in bubbles at the interface between the middle and inner ear. The inner ear is unique in having the only localized extracellular fluid space which may not be dependent on the circulation for inert gas transport. Helium still occupies the diver's middle-ear space, even after he changes from Heliox to air breathing, and the situation across the otic fluids is not dissimilar to the classic counterdiffusion situation – breathing a slow heavy gas which saturates the blood and fast tissues, while a fast gas diffuses inwards from the environment (middle-ear space). This hypothesis explains the additive effects of the inert gas switching and decompression. Although decompression is not required to fulfil these conditions, it would be expected to aggravate the situation by causing the bubbles to expand.

4. Vascular emboli, either gaseous, lipid or thrombotic, in the end-arteries of the inner ear (without the anastomoses of other cerebral arteries) cause ischaemia. The rarity of inner-ear disease with generalized intravascular emboli makes this hypothesis questionable.

5. Impaired perfusion from the severe haematological effects of DCS.

6. Gas-induced osmosis: transfer of fluid between endolymph (perfused with blood) and perilymph (saturated with gas in the middle ear) could result in vestibular membrane damage.
7. Inner-ear membrane ruptures associated with tissue damage or hydrostatic forces consequent on bubble formation in an enclosed space. This would explain the confusion between the two pathologies, permitting both to exist and, in the future, the possibility of inner-ear reconstructive surgery must be considered.
8. Inner-ear haemorrhages develop rapidly, within hours of the insult, and are likely to convert a potentially correctable lesion to a permanent one.

### Clinical

The clinical manifestations are more definite, and the precipitating conditions are derived from practical observations by many clinicians. In deep helium or hydrogen dives, the most common serious problem is DCS affecting the inner ear. It usually occurs suddenly, and may respond to rapid recompression and enriched oxygen breathing.

The consequences of vertigo, such as near-drowning, vomiting, dehydration, electrolyte disturbances and distress, are more important in a patient who is already seriously ill with DCS, but are dramatic enough in their own right to endanger a diving operation.

If incorrectly diagnosed during decompression (e.g. if the symptoms are incorrectly attributed to seasickness), then further decompression may result in more damage to the vestibular apparatus.

Clinically, it may be characterized by cochlear damage (tinnitus, sensorineural hearing loss) and/or vestibular disorder (prostrating vertigo, nausea, vomiting, syncope).

It is especially noted with deep helium diving, in excess of 100 metres (350 feet), excursions from saturation diving or of switching inert gas mixtures during a dive. It is sometimes precipitated by a helium-breathing diver changing rapidly to air breathing.

A delay of onset of symptoms is not uncommon in cases of inner-ear barotrauma and in DCS. The development of symptoms during an action which increases intracranial and otic pressure, such as coughing, lifting anchors etc., makes inner-ear barotrauma more likely.

In cases of generalized neurological DCS, vestibular symptoms are misdiagnosed and often confused with cerebellar disease. Investigations, including electronystagmography, clarify the peripheral (vestibular) or central (cerebellar) nature of the disease. In these cases, the auditory involvement is only a minor part of the disease, and other manifestations dominate the clinical presentation and treatment.

Recompression therapy, if instituted within an hour, should result in cure. Objective tests of vestibular function can and should be performed under hyperbaric conditions, especially when doubt exists regarding clinical management. These investigations include electronystagmography and iced-water caloric tests, and are valuable in differential diagnosis, prognosis and response to treatment.

There are possible long-term sequelae. With permanent cochlear and vestibular damage the diver may not be able to continue with his occupation, and he may be restricted from other occupations such as flying or driving vehicles.

### Diagnosis

In deep **helium diving**, the diagnosis is relatively easy. It is often an isolated DCS symptom, presenting deeper than most symptoms, but others may supervene at more shallow depths. Ear barotraumas are less common with helium diving, probably due to the rapid diffusibility of the gas.

In shallow **scuba air diving**, isolated inner-ear DCS is less well documented and probably rare. To make the diagnosis, there must be reasonable conviction that the patient has exposed himself to a dive that could produce DCS. This can only be ascertained by reference to decompression tables and to the patient's own dive profile. Isolated inner-ear disease with shallow air diving is much more likely to be due to inner-ear barotrauma (see page 124).

Although vertigo and hearing loss have often been reported among scuba air divers and caisson workers with DCS, there is considerable doubt about the validity of the diagnosis.

In many of the cases reported, there were no manifestations of the disease except for otological disorder. It is likely that many of the permanent otologically damaged cases originally reported as DCS were really due to inner-ear barotrauma.

A differential diagnosis of inner-ear disease is given in Table 12.3.

### Vision

Bubbles have been observed in the ocular fluids and in the lens. The latter are longer lasting, but both may cause blurring of vision in one or both eyes. Bubbles under corneal lenses may also cause corneal damage and have this effect (see page 408).

Retinal lesions with intravascular bubbles and haemorrhages have been described. Vision is more commonly affected by interference with the neural pathways, with appropriate visual field defects, either directly from bubble development or indirectly by the cardiovascular effects of DCS.

Long-term retinal lesions, with low retinal capillary density at the fovea, microaneurysms and small areas of capillary non-perfusion, are said to be related to DCS incidence.

### Peripheral nerve

Bubble formation in the myelin of peripheral nerves will result in a patchy sensory damage or motor impairment, predominantly involving the limbs. In severe cases, there may be a glove-and-stocking distribution, but the usual presentation is with paraesthesia, numbness and weakness. Pain may be related to a major plexus, and may be long lasting.

The differentiation between peripheral nerve and an incomplete spinal lesion is important, because the prognosis is less worrisome if the clinical symptoms are due only to peripheral nerve involvement.

## Cutaneous

Skin manifestations range from being local and innocuous, to generalized and ominous, with a complete spectrum in between. If they develop with water exposure, they are more likely to be serious than with chamber exposures, in which the inert gas can be absorbed through the skin.

They have been variously described as follows.

### *Pruritis*

This is a common complication of diving in compression chambers and dry suits, more than in water environments and wet suits. It may be partly or wholly due to gas passing into the skin from the hyperbaric gas environment. This is especially likely when the environmental temperature is elevated. The increased temperature produces vasodilatation and accelerates the cutaneous uptake of nitrogen during compression. The elimination of gas is restricted by the vasoconstriction that accompanies the drop in environment temperatures during decompression.

It is often a transient effect, presenting very soon after decompression, and is not considered a systemic or serious manifestation of DCS. It is noticed mostly after short deep exposures, often with only one or two decompression stops. The areas affected are the forearms, wrists and hands, the nose and ears, and the thighs. The symptoms are transient and there is usually no objective sign available. In other cases, a slight folliculitis may be observed as red punctuate areas, when this presentation merges with the next. The symptoms are attributed to small gas bubbles in the superficial layers of the dermis, and especially near its entry via the epidermis and the sebaceous glands.

**Table 12.3 Differential diagnosis of inner-ear disease due to diving**

|  | Inner-ear barotrauma | DCS |
|---|---|---|
| Dive exposure | Any | Near or exceeding decompression limits |
| Onset | Descent, ascent or post-dive | At depth, ascent or post-dive |
| Associations | Ear barotrauma, exterior | Other DCS symptoms; deep or saturation dive |
| Gas breathed | Mainly air | Mainly helium or hydrogen |
| Treatment | Conservative/surgery | Recompression/oxygen |

### Scarlatiniform rash

This is a progression of the above. A pilo-erector stimulation, and perhaps a tissue histamine release, produces a red punctate rash. The distribution is predominantly over the chest, shoulders, back, upper abdomen and thighs, in that order. The rash may last for several hours.

### Erysipeloid rash

This is a further exension of the above and occurs over the same distribution, but with the involvement of endogenous gas interfering with venous drainage, it is a definite sign of systemic DCS. Some of the skin appearance is thought to be a reflex vascular reaction. The lesions are collections of papules which may merge to form large plaques with flat and firm borders. Coughing or performing the Valsalva manoeuvre will accentuate the venous markings (Mellinghoff's sign) (see Plate 4).

### Cutis marmorata marbling

This commences as a small pale area with cyanotic mottling. It may spread peripherally becoming erythematous with extension of cyanotic mottling. The area is warmer than the surrounding skin and swelling and oedema result in a mottled appearance. Recompression gives dramatic relief. The area may become tender to palpation in a few hours, but the other signs may have diminished or disappeared by then. Marbling of the skin is a cutaneous manifestation of what is occurring elsewhere in the body, and this is a serious sign of DCS. Gas bubbles are present in both tissues and blood vessels.

### Subcutaneous emphysema

This has the typical crepitus sensation on palpation, either in localized areas or along the tendon sheaths. It can be verified radiologically and should not be confused with the supraclavicular subcutaneous emphysema extending from the mediastinum, due to pulmonary barotrauma.

### Lymphatic obstruction

This presents as a localized swelling which may be associated with an underlying DCS manifestation. If it involves hair follicles, a peau d'orange or pigskin appearance with brawny oedema is characteristic. It is common over the trunk, but it is also seen over the head and neck.

### Counterdiffusion of gases

There have been occasional reports of skin and mucosal swellings due to counterdiffusion of gases. This results in bubbles forming in tissues from gases diffusing at different rates, but with the total gas pressure at the interface exceeding the environmental pressure. This is only likely when the subject's body is exposed to a readily diffusible gas, while he breathes a slower diffusing gas (see page 149 and Plate 5).

### Others

Formication may be the presentation in any of the skin manifestations described above, or due to involvement of the peripheral nervous system of the spinal cord. The neural involvement may also result in numbness, hypoaesthesia, paraesthesia or hyperaesthesia of the skin. Signs of inflammation may also occur over affected joints. Bruising is sometimes described over the chest and abdomen in serious cases, but this is not due to genuine tissue haemorrhages, because it blanches on local pressure.

# Gastrointestinal

Mildly affected patients may present only with anorexia, nausea, vomiting or retching, abdominal cramps and diarrhoea. When the condition is severe, local ischaemia and infarction of bowel, with secondary haemorrhages, may result. In such cases the use of drugs that encourage haemorrhage, such as aspirin or heparin, could be detrimental. In some of the DCS fatalities, gastrointestinal haemorrhage was the final cause of death.

## CASE REPORT 12.4

JH, a 28 year old, had been sport diving for many years. He was renowned for his ability to conserve gas by shallow breathing. On December 26 he was spear fishing using a single 72 cubic foot tank at a depth of 28 metres. He started to surface after 60 minutes in the water, but during ascent noted a tendency to swivel to one side. He was quite distressed by this on reaching 4 metres, so he descended again to 28 metres and the symptom cleared. He felt worried by the dive so surfaced without stoppages.

On reaching shore he felt 'queer', unsteady on his feet. After resting a few minutes, he drove home but complained of feeling unwell and extremely weary. He then retired to bed. Three hours later he was found collapsed over the toilet seat. He appeared confused but was complaining of nausea, headache, abdominal pain and a full feeling in the neck. He was noted to feel hot and was perspiring freely.

He was helped into the car and taken to hospital where a diagnosis of gastroenteritis was made. He was noted to be slightly confused and had a temperature of 38.0°C. After discharge from hospital the next day (27 Dec.) JH was able to walk unassisted but on reaching home slept heavily the rest of the day. No detailed history of his activity during this period was available. On rising he was said to be unwell and grumpy but with no specific complaints.

At 1.00 a.m., December 28, he had some abnormal movements, fell out of bed and then had a grand mal convulsion. Following the fit he started vomiting but remained unconscious. Approximately 15 fits occurred over the following 3 hours after his readmission to hospital. He was unconscious until the early hours of December 29 when he started to ramble in an illogical manner and did not answer questions.

On December 30 he was reported to be occasionally rational but with intermittent periods of difficulty in concentration, confusion and visual disturbances (flashing lights). He complained of headache and pain in hips, thighs, knees and left wrists. He was unable to walk even with assistance. Examination of the blood and skull and chest X-rays were normal. A lumbar puncture produced clear CSF under elevated pressure with normal protein, glucose and chloride.

On January 2 a decision was made to fly him to the nearest adequate recompression facilities, 4000 kilometres away. An aircraft pressurized to ground level was used.

Seven days after the diving incident he arrived at the recompression chamber. Examination revealed a moderately obese man, confused and wandering in his story. Romberg's test showed a tendency to fall to the right side and there was marked incoordination in the left arm and leg. There was no nystagmus. Ophthalmoscopy revealed bilateral papilloedema, worse in the left eye. There were no other abnormalities detected on physical examination. With the Serial 7s test, he was unable to progress past 100–93. A score of 3 correct out of 12 was achieved on Raven's advanced progressive matrices.

Recompression on 100% oxygen to 3 ATA was dramatic. Within 3 minutes JH was asymptomatic and rational. Advanced progressive matrices revealed six correct.

Decompression was at the rate of 12 min/m. On reaching 2 ATA (10 m) his matrices score was eight correct and Serial 7s completed with only two mistakes.

Examination after recompression therapy revealed only mild papilloedema. Three hours later he had slight bilateral pectoral 'niggles', which responded to 100% oxygen.

Over the next few days he had occasional attacks of colicky abdominal pain and several episodes of melaena. Lumbar puncture, skeletal, chest and skull X-rays, and haematology were all normal 2 days later.

*Diagnosis:* DCS affecting neurological, musculoskeletal and gastrointestinal systems.

# Cardiorespiratory

Intravascular bubbles are more common in the venous system, and are associated with sudden or severe DCS. Although many of these bubbles may be trapped in the pulmonary capillaries, some may pass into the arterial circulation, either through the pulmonary plexus, a patent foramen ovale, a septal defect or a patent ductus arteriosus. The presence of gas bubbles in the blood may hamper microcirculation and produce both local hypoxia and generalized haematological sequelae.

## Local ischaemic effect

This may follow cerebral, coronary, renal or splenic occlusion etc. The result of these occlusions may be tissue ischaemia and infarction. The clinical manifestations will vary according to the organs involved. Specifically, an infrequent but troublesome cardiac manifestation of DCS is the development of a ventricular dysrhythmia, which may not respond to recompression therapy. It is not clear whether these all represent coronary emboli, or whether they result from extravascular bubbles interfering with the myoneural conducting mechanism of the heart.

## Pulmonary involvement ('chokes')

A small amount of bubble production may actually enhance the body's ability to expel nitrogen, when they become blocked in the pulmonary vascular bed, and diffuse into the alveolar spaces. As a general rule, however, it is probably safer that gas is transferred to the lungs in its dissolved form, and is then equilibrated with the alveolar gas pressures. After uneventful dives, bubbles may be entrapped in the lung circulation for an hour or two.

Clinical manifestations are noted when approximately 10% or more of the pulmonary vascular bed is obstructed. The effect of gas in the pulmonary vessels is to displace blood and inflate the lungs intravascularly. This may reflexly produce a shallow rapid breathing, due to the inflation of the vascular tree, and thereby reduce both alveolar ventilation and compliance. Pulmonary oedema develops.

Tachypnoea is significant. The initial symptom of chest pain is aggravated by inspiration, sometimes with an irritating cough which may be precipitated by cigarette smoking. Interference with the pulmonary circulation can result in a decrease in pulse rate and a decrease in blood pressure, progressing to circulatory collapse in severe cases.

The pulmonary effects usually appear early, and are able to be reduced by shallow respirations, oxygen inhalation or recompression. Without therapeutic intervention they are followed by either a rapid resolution (with pulmonary shunting of blood away from the obstruction and a loss of gas from the lung's vasculature by diffusion into the alveoli) or a progression of symptoms due to increased numbers of bubbles, vascular stasis and the blood/bubble interactions mentioned previously (see page 153). These may cause a deterioration in the clinical state irrespective of recompression and present as the well-recognized respiratory emergencies ('shock' lung syndrome, adult respiratory distress syndrome or ARDS, disseminated intravascular coagulation). Right heart failure may occur.

Investigations are often not possible, but electrocardiographic evidence of right axis deviation, high peaked P wave, and right ventricular strain may be found. Radiological evidence of pulmonary oedema may be detected.

## Post-decompression shock

In very severe cases, e.g. in explosive (very rapid) decompression or following grossly inadequate decompression, there may be a generalized liberation of gas into all vessels, resulting in rapid death. The presence of gas bubbles in the circulating blood results in a bubble/blood interaction which leads to all grades of vessel wall damage and haematological reactions from haemoconcentration to disseminated intravascular coagulation.

The effect of hypotension, combined with air, platelet and lipid emboli, causes secondary damage to capillaries, increased capillary permeability and extravasation of fluid into tissues. The signs and symptoms of hypovolaemic shock, such as haemoconcentration, postural hypotension, syncope, low urinary output etc., are not uncommon. Similar to the pulmonary manifestations, they are either resolved quickly or proceed ominously.

The consequences of both haemoconcentration and disseminated intravascular coagulation are discussed below.

## Coagulopathies and other laboratory findings

Certain biochemical and haematological abnormalities (the 'coagulation cascade') are often reported in association with decompression and DCS. A generalized stress response, from physical, environmental and psychological factors, may result in elevations of blood catecholamines, free fatty acids, isoenzymes, leucocytes and cortisol. A reduction in erythrocyte numbers is related to the aquatic environment and weightlessness. The additional influences of intravascular bubbles on these changes are not yet clarified. Abnormal red blood cells may be produced, with spiculated echinocytes originating at depth and becoming more marked with the development of DCS, from deep dives.

An increase in the erythrocyte sedimentation rate is noted in the latter stages of decompression from deep Heliox saturation dives and to a lesser degree from the more shallow air saturation dives. It is not directly related to depth or oxygen partial pressures.

Complement activation has been described with DCS and it is postulated that DCS produced by unstressful dive profiles may be predicted in some divers on the basis of this mechanism.

Biochemical changes are sometimes noted. There is a decrease in plasma cortisol associated with decompression and a decrease in serum sodium and blood lactate in DCS. Some of the reports of biochemical changes with DCS are suggestive of tissue damage. Decompression per se does not produce these enzymatic changes. With moderately severe DCS, serum enzymes will reflect the organs affected.

Decompression, and especially inadequate decompression, results in thrombocytopenia, increased fibrin formation and haemoconcentration. Many decompressions are associated with overt or 'silent' intravascular bubble formation. Blood reacts with bubbles as it does to other foreign bodies – with a deposition of protein (especially fibrinogen) and coalesced plasma lipids. The protein deposition is thrombogenic and attracts platelets, which aggregate around it and release clotting agents. With these developments, there is an associated drop in plasma lipids and circulating platelets. Hypovolaemia may result from a reduction in blood flow, or hypoxia, associated with the blood/bubble complex. Expansion of the intravascular volume, inactivation of the complement system and reduction in platelet adhesion and aggregation have been used therapeutically.

If the fibrin-clotting mechanism is activated, then all manifestations of disseminated intravascular coagulation may result. Once this cycle has commenced, the disease does not necessarily respond to recompression therapy. Thus, such cases may deteriorate even while at an initially adequate recompression depth. Attention to intravenous fluid replacement and correction of coagulation defects follows general medical principles, and may improve the recompression results.

## Long-term sequelae

The characteristic long-term sequelae include permanent neurological damage (as above), neuropsychological impairment (see Chapter 29) and dysbaric osteonecrosis (see Chapter 14).

US Navy divers who had DCS appeared to suffer a higher incidence of **hospitalization** for a variety of disorders, including especially headache and vascular disease, than controls.

Diving medicine, blessed with entrepreneurial talent, has suffered by being exposed to new technology, before its limitations have been appreciated by the more conservative general medical community. Nowhere is this more obvious than in the search for neuropsychological sequelae of high-pressure neurological syndrome and of DCS.

Most of the long-term **neuropsychological** problems involve conjecture and supposition, based on hearsay and theoretical postulates that require substantiation before any action. **Neurological** investigations are especially prone to enthusiastic misinterpretations. EEG abnormalities were very frequently reported, especially in uncontrolled series. Later on, variations in evoked cortical responses, somatosensory, visual and auditory, were fashionable. Computed tomography in cerebral lesions and magnetic resonance imagery in spinal lesions have not lived up to their earlier promise, in that they are usually not as sensitive as a clinical examination.

Neuropsychological tests have constituted a research minefield for well-meaning and enthusiastic amateurs (diving physicians and clinical psychologists). Positive results usually reflect a lack of appreciation of the personality characteristics of divers (influencing the manner in which they approach the tests), non-standardization of the conditions under which the investigations are performed (environmental, investigator capability, post-traumatic effects etc.) and finally a naïvety towards the limitations of the oversimplistic tests and the statistical interpretations (only one survey in the literature applied the Bonferroni adjustment to make allowance for the number of associations analysed).

Despite all this, there is still a clinical belief, with some research support, that short-term memory deficits and other neuropsychological manifestations follow neurological DCS.

Recently, Norwegians have claimed to show 'unidentified bright objects' in MRI studies, replicating the alleged effects of premature ageing. In the UK Calder and other pathologists have observed histopathological changes in the brain (usually of a non-specific or indefinite nature) and spinal cord (degeneration in the myelinated areas affecting both ascending and descending tracts, sensory fibres in the posterior columns and the tract of Lissauer) in divers who have died unrelated to diving exposure. Although implications should not be drawn at this stage, these findings deserve a thorough and controlled prospective investigation. The spinal cord damage appeared to be the more definite and extensive.

### Neuralgic pains

Occasionally there will be a continuation of severe pain, evidently from a persisting neurological abnormality and possibly similar to the phantom pains of amputation. When this happens there is usually a specific area involved, but the brachial or lumbosacral plexus areas seem vulnerable. Whether there is also spinal pathology, which produces similar syndromes, is unknown. The course is usually protracted, for months or years, and on the whole follows

clinically obvious neurological DCS, sometimes with sensory abnormalities, paraparesis or paraplegia.

### Miscellaneous

#### Aids

The problem of coping with an HIV-positive diver is becoming a source of concern, affecting both the diver and his companions. Neurological and neuropsychological manifestations have been demonstrated in asymptomatic HIV-positive subjects, with implications for diving judgements, diving accidents and management.

Disruption of the blood–brain barrier with CAGE and DCS presumably would increase the likelihood of conversion of an HIV positive to a neurological AIDS case.

Due to diving techniques, such as buddy breathing and the complications of resuscitation, cross-infection by HIV is a possibility. Resuscitation is more likely to be needed in hazardous activities, such as scuba diving.

Eight divers have developed **multiple sclerosis**, conjectured to be due to damage of the blood–brain barrier from intravascular bubbles.

**Retinal lesions** (see page 172), with low retinal capillary density at the fovea, microaneurysms and small areas of capillary nonperfusion, are related to DCS incidence.

Ocular **hyperuricosis** producing transient myopias and permanent nuclear cataracts are thought to follow hyperbaric exposure.

**Beau's** lines on fingernails have been described as a complication of saturation dives.

## Recommended reading

ADKISSON, G.H., HODGSON, M., SMITH, F. et al. (1989) Cerebral perfusion deficits in dysbaric illness. *The Lancet* ii, 119–122.

BECKMAN, E. (Ed.) (1975). *Man in the Sea Symposium. Clinical Studies on Commercial and Sport Divers*. University of Hawaii Publication.

DEMBERT, M.L., JEKEL, J.F. and MOONEY, L.W. (1984). Health risk factors for the development of decompression sickness among U.S. Navy divers. *Undersea Biomedical Research* **11**, 395–406.

DENNISON, W.L. (1971). *A Review of the Pathogenesis of Skin Bends*. US Navy Submarine Medicine Centre. Report 660.

DICK, A.P.K., VANN, R.D., MEBANE, G.Y. and FREEZOR M.D. (1984). Decompression induced nitrogen elimination. *Undersea Biomedical Research* 11, 369–480.

DICK, A.P.K. and MASSEY, E.W. (1984) *Neurological Injuries in Sport Divers*. Annual Scientific Meeting, Undersea Medical Society.

EDMONDS, C. (1986). *The Abalone Diver*. Victoria: National Safety Council of Australia.

EDMONDS, C. (1991). Peripheral neurological abnormalities in dysbaric disease. In *Neurological Dysbarism Workshop*, edited by T.J.R. Francis and D.J. Smith, in press.

ERDE, A. and EDMONDS, C. (1975). Decompression sickness; a clinical series. *Journal of Occupational Medicine* 17, 324–328.

FRANCIS, T.J.R., DUTKA, A.J. and HALLENBECK, J.M. (1990). In: *Diving Medicine*, edited by A.A. Bove and J.C. Davis, Chap 15. Philadelphia: Saunders.

FRANCIS, T.J.R, PEARSON, R.R., ROBERTSON, A.G. et al. (1988). Central nervous system decompression sickness. *Undersea Biomedical Research* 15, 403–417.

GOLDING, F.C., GRIFFITHS, P.D., HEMPLEMAN, H.V. et al. (1960). Decompression sickness during construction of the Dartford Tunnel. *British Journal of Industrial Medicine* 17, 167–180.

GORMAN, D.F., EDMONDS, C.W., PARSONS, D.W. et al. (1987). Neurological sequelae of decompression sickness. *Proceedings of 9th International Symposium on Underwater and Hyperbaric Medicine*. Bethesda, MA: Undersea and Hyperbaric Medical Society.

HALSEY, M.J. (Ed.) (1988). MRC Decompression sickness panel. Long term health effects working group. *Second International Symposium on Man In The Sea*, Hawaii.

HOW, J., WEST, D. and EDMONDS, C. (1976). Decompression sickness in diving. *Singapore Medical Journal* 17, 92–97.

KIZER, K.W. (1979). *Dysbarism in Paradise*. UMS North Pacific Chapter, Annual Meeting, Spring.

LANDOLT, J.P., MONEY, K.E., RADOMSKI, M.W. et al. (1984). Inner ear DCS in the squirrel monkey. *8th Underwater Physiology Symposium*. Bethesda, MA: Undersea and Hyperbaric Medical Society.

MEKJAVIC, I.B. and KAKITSUBA, N. (1989). Effect of peripheral temperature on the formation of venous gas bubbles. *Undersea Biomedical Research* 16, 391–401.

MOON, R.E., CAMPORESI, E.M. and KISSLOW, J.A. (1989). Patent foramen ovale and DCS in divers. *The Lancet* i, 513–514.

RIVERA, J.C. (1963). *Decompression Sickness Among Divers: An analysis of 935 cases*. USNEDU Research Report, pp. 1–63.

SLARK, A.G. (1962). Treatment of 137 cases of decompression sickness. *MRC Royal Naval Personnel Report* 63/1030.

*US Navy Diving Manual* (1986). Government Printing Office, Washington DC.

VANN, R.D. (1990). In: *Diving Medicine*, edited by A.A. Bove and J. C. Davis, Chap. 4. Philadelphia: Saunders.

WILMSHURST, P.T., BYRNE, J.C. and WEBB-PEPLOE, M.M. (1990). Relation between intraarterial shunts and decompression sickness in divers. *The Lancet* ii, 1302–1306.

WORKSHOP REPORT (1987). *Diagnostic Techniques in Diving Neurology*. Medical Research Council Decompression Sickness Panel, London.

# 13

# Treatment of decompression sickness

For every difficult problem, there is a simple
solution – but it is usually wrong

Meeghan

## Introduction

The ideal treatment will vary as the disease
varies. There is often little similarity between
the decompression sickness (DCS) syndromes.
Compare the following cases:

1. Saturation DCS as the diver very slowly
   approaches the surface.
2. The same diver subjected to an extreme
   excursion from saturation.
3. Inner-ear or helium-based DCS.
4. The cerebrovascular incident after a short
   bounce to 60 metres.
5. The joint bend developing hours after a
   long shallow dive.
6. The dramatic crises involving pulmonary,
   haematological and neurological systems
   after explosive decompression from saturation or from gross omitted decompression.
7. Respiratory symptoms followed by rapid
   development of spinal paraplegia.
8. The mild joint DCS of a shallow diver who
   has remained well within the established
   tables.

These cases cannot be optimally managed by
a single approach.

Even within any one organization there will
be a great variety in presentation and severity
of symptoms; the Hyperbaric Unit at Hawaii
treats cases similar to those in Australia
(because they cope with deep air diving by
civilian populations). The US Navy Experimental Diving Unit, when it was sited in
Washington DC, treated cases similar to those
of the Royal Naval Physiological Laboratories
at Alverstoke (saturation cases and Navy
divers who were adhering to, or testing,
decompression tables).

No wonder a variety of approaches developed, based on different clinical experiences. The therapy is also influenced by the facilities, and there is little similarity between the sophisticated technology of the hyperbaric complex at Duke University, North Carolina, and the welded steel cylinder improvised by a pearl diver in Darwin, Northern Australia. Some areas have many hyperbaric chambers, transfer under pressure facilities, hyperbaric ambulances, multi-compartment chambers etc. Others lack emergency transport and even basic communications.

For these reasons, it is wise to question the universal applicability of 'a scheme' or 'a flow chart' to treat all DCS cases. They may be of value for the typical cases in ideal situations and those that behave as expected. The complex and complicated cases – and there are many – in less than ideal environments, require greater assessment and skill.

The complete diving physician will collect all knowledge and all techniques, and apply them as he considers appropriate to the clinical state of the patient, utilizing whatever transport and recompression facilities are available to him.

> *Treatment of decompression sickness involves immediate recompression, followed by gradual decompression.*

## Recompression therapy

No-one who has seen the victim of compressed air illness, gravely ill or unconscious, put back into a chamber and brought back to life by the application of air pressure, will forget the extraordinary efficiency of recompression, or will be backward in applying it to a subsequent case of illness.

(Robert Davis, 1935)

The application of pressure (recompression) reduces the size of bubbles and usually the symptoms of DCS; decompression involves return to atmospheric pressure without the recurrence of symptoms. Recompression followed by a slow decompression as the bubble resolves is thus the basis for treatment. There are three problems to consider in deciding the precise form of the recompression therapy.

These are the depth required for therapy, the gas mixtures used and the rate of decompression. The gas mixtures and decompression rate are partly reliant on the depth of recompression.

The application of recompression therapy to various types of DCS requires an approach based on the dynamic nature of the disease, and a clinical approximation of what is happening to the tissue/ bubble/blood transfer of inert gas.

An integral part of assessing each case is in hypothesizing what type of tissue is involved, e.g. a 54-metre (180-feet) dive for 10 minutes will produce saturation of fast tissue – and the fastest tissue is blood itself. Thus, a rapid ascent from this dive is likely to produce 'fast tissue' DCS, and the systems most likely to be involved are the cerebral, respiratory and cardiovascular. All these have a rich vascular supply and are vulnerable to the effects of the venous and arterial gas emboli produced. A 30-metre (100-feet) saturation dive with a slow ascent is likely to result in a 'slow tissue DCS'. As a general rule, fast tissue involvement is less predictable and potentially more serious. Bubbles floating around the blood stream can be as damaging as they can be innocuous – depending on chance. The clinical sequence and the treatment requirements are usually predictable in a slow tissue DCS.

Some other general guidelines may be drawn, and these will influence the form of treatment to be selected. If a diver has developed DCS a considerable time before he presents for treatment, then it is likely that the tissues and the bubble have reached some sort of equilibrium, as regards the pressure of inert gas. Thus the diver is unlikely to deteriorate rapidly due to further expansion of the bubble (unless he is subjected to subatmospheric pressures such as in aircraft travel!). Under those conditions, it is wise not to aggravate the condition by further exposure to high pressures of inert gas, and it is reasonable to rely entirely on 100% $O_2$, either on the surface, in a recompression chamber to a maximum of 18 metres or in the water to a maximum of 9 metres. Thus the pressure gradient between the bubble's inert gas and the near zero pressure of inert gas in the arterial blood will result in a maximal eviction of the inert gas from the bubble, via the venous system. Consider two illustrative case histories: 13.1 and 13.2.

---

## CASE REPORT 13.1

A dive was made to 18 metres (60 feet) for 60 minutes on scuba. There had been no dives for a month prior to this. The isolated symptom of a left shoulder pain developed 5 hours after the dive and had been in existence for 24 hours prior to the diver presenting for medical treatment.

*Comment:* this is not only a mild case of DCS, it is not going to get significantly worse, if the patient avoids further exposure to hyperbaric conditions. By the time the medical assessment was made (29 hours' post-dive) the tissues will have equilibrated fully with the atmospheric pressure, and thus there will be no significant pressure gradient pushing nitrogen into the bubble. On the contrary, there will be a mild gradient in the opposite direction. The administration of 100% oxygen will enhance this gradient even more. Estimated pressures may be seen by reference to Figure 11.3 (a) and (c). In this type of case, to expose the diver to any treatment which could either aggravate his situation (treatment schedules that could result in air therapy tables being applied), or which could expose the patient to other complications (extended or deep oxygen therapy tables), seems injudicious and against the oslerian principle of *primum non nocere* (first, do no harm).

The authors' approach to such a mild case would be to attempt to relieve the patient's symptoms and perhaps to reduce the possibility of subsequent bone damage – although there is no definite evidence that this is possible with such delayed treatment. Treatment was successfully achieved by breathing 100% oxygen at 1 ATA for 6 hours (25 minutes' oxygen, 5 minutes' air intervals) but if safe conditions had permitted, the patient would have been subjected to oxygen recompression therapy at 9 metres' depth for 2.5–3 hours, and would not breathe air under pressures. These techniques are discussed later.

---

Causes for deterioration in a patient's clinical state, other than inadequate recompression, include disseminated intravascular coagulation and secondary tissue pathology, e.g. perfusion and re-perfusion damage, ischaemia, infarctions, haemorrhages, fluid and electrolyte changes etc.

Incomplete resolution of symptoms is more common with previous DCS, failure of compliance with decompression tables, physical activity and the number of ascents during the dive or 'treatments'. It is also more common with delayed treatment (when the easily reversible bubble becomes converted into other, less reversible, pathology) and with the increased nitrogen loading during or soon after air breathing.

Even with the most enthusiastic treatments, there will often be residual and variable symptoms which can be attributed to the sequelae of bubble damage to tissues. The skill is to differentiate this from the continued presence of bubbles, which necessitates further treatment. To reduce this bubble factor, these authors tend to be enthusiastic in their use of oxygen before, during and after early recompression therapy and reluctant to employ unnecessary air breathing under pressure.

---

*Anyone can easily achieve the therapeutic miracles . . . in DCS in over 95% of patients, when the problem is recognised and treated quickly. In a small proportion of the other cases it is the lack of response to well founded treatment; frustrating, tragic and defying compression; which demands all the knowledge and skill of the trained physician and scientist.*

*Robert C. Bornmann (1990)*

---

## CASE REPORT 13.2

Identical symptoms to case 13.1, with left shoulder pain. The main difference in the two presentations is that the left shoulder symptoms in case 13.2 followed 10 minutes after a 30-metre dive (100 feet) for 30 minutes with a rapid ascent and omitted decompression. The diver then presented for assistance immediately after the symptom developed.

*Comment:* a very different situation exists from case 13.1. Even assuming that the left shoulder pain is locomotor and not referred neurological or cardiac, the likelihood of progression of this case from the theoretical 'minor symptom' to a major case of DCS, is much higher. First, the symptom developed soon after the dive, thus it is likely to become worse. Secondly, more symptoms are likely to develop remembering that DCS manifestations continue to arise over the next 24 hours. Thirdly, the tissues surrounding the bubbles might well have nitrogen supersaturation pressures of almost 4 ATA. The bubble, existing on the surface, will have a nitrogen pressure of approximately 1 ATA, as the bubble is at the same ambient pressure as the body. Under these conditions, there will be a gradient between the tissues and the bubbles, increasing the size of the latter until the tissue gas tension becomes equated with the bubble gas tension.

The therapeutic approach to this diver is to recompress him to the maximum depth at which 100% oxygen can be used therapeutically, i.e. 18 metres (60 feet), and if a satisfactory response is obtained and maintained, to decompress him from that depth. Recompression treatment at 18 metres will not necessarily reverse the tissue-to-bubble nitrogen gradient and, if other more serious symptoms develop, it may be necessary to recompress him deeper on an inert gas/oxygen mixture – these authors would select a 30-metre 50% $O_2$, Nitrox or Heliox treatment schedule as the most valuable (e.g. Comex Cx30). At this depth there would be no tissue-to-bubble nitrogen gradient.

---

## Therapeutic recompression tables

### Basic concepts

DCS is an indication for recompression therapy. Serious DCS is a medical emergency which requires immediate recompression therapy.
   The guidelines of treatment are:

- Symptomatic therapy and transport on 100% $O_2$.
- Supportive and rehydration therapy.
- Early compression to reduce the bubble's size and damage.
- Replace the inert gas in the bubble with metabolizable gas and/or less soluble inert gas.
- Decompress slowly enough to prevent bubble expansion.
- Prevent recurrences with surface oxygen.

- Administer hyperbaric oxygenation treatments in severe (spinal/cerebral) cases with residuum.
- Avoid further aviation and diving exposure, until cured.

### Depth

In deciding the depth of recompression, there are three different approaches which may be made, and these are as follows:

1. Recompress to a pressure (depth) dependent upon the depth and duration of the **original dive**.
2. Recompress to a depth which produces a **clinically acceptable result**, and then tailor the gas mixtures for decompression from that depth.
3. Recompress to a predetermined fixed depth, i.e. according to **standard tables of recompression therapy**.

Only the third is in common practice, but each has some logic to it under certain circumstances. These are now elaborated further.

### Recompress to a pressure (depth) dependent upon the depth and duration of the original dive

This is not a particularly satisfactory technique, because it is designed to cope with the total quantity of gas dissolved in the body during the original dive, irrespective of its distribution. Because DCS is the clinical manifestation of a gas bubble lodged in a vulnerable area, it is necessary to recompress in order to reduce the size of that particular bubble, irrespective of the total quantity of inert gas dissolved in the body. This approach was best typified by the now defunct concept of treating aviator DCS merely by descent to ground level.

The one advantage of this approach, apart from its simplicity, is seen when a diver develops DCS very soon after surfacing from a deep dive. Under these conditions, a prompt return to the original depth will ensure that there is no tissue-to-bubble pressure gradient which could cause bubble growth at a lesser depth.

### Recompress to a depth producing a clinically acceptable result

This Australian technique is too complex (and unnecessary in most cases) for inexperienced therapists, because it requires an ability to predict the problems and prognosis from the dive profile, the sequence of events and the clinical presentation. It also needs the ability to mix and administer different gas combinations. The developments of recent years, allowing substitution of gas mixtures (Heliox, Nitrox) for air in many of the conventional tables, together with the introduction of gas mixture tables, have made the Australian tables less necessary.

Nevertheless, the freedom to be able to choose any depth, and then select an appropriate breathing gas, is invaluable in the delayed, atypical or very serious cases.

### Recompression to a predetermined fixed depth

This is according to standard recompression therapy tables (see Appendices II and IV). The standard tables of recompression clearly state the gas mixture to be used (usually air or oxygen). The application of the standard recompression tables produces relief in 90% of cases, if treatment commences within half an hour of the onset of symptoms. This proportion falls to 50% if the delay exceeds 6 hours. After a 12-hour delay, the results were poor. Standard air tables, oxygen tables and gas mixture tables are presented in the Appendices.

The **air tables** are of use when oxygen is unavailable or is contraindicated (e.g. due to toxicity problems, personnel limitations etc.). They may also be of value when the oxygen therapy tables have failed to produce a satisfactory response and where permanent disability is otherwise likely, or if the clinical state is life threatening. In the latter case, the extra reduction of the bubble volume may be all that is needed to re-establish blood flow in a marginal area. The tables include:

Short air tables: 1A, 2A (USN); 52, 53 (RN)
Long air tables: 3, 4 (USN) 54, 55, 71, 72, 73 (RN)
Saturation air tables: 7 (USN), Buhlmann 7A

The shallow air tables (30 metres or 100 feet) are only applicable to mild cases of DCS in which deterioration is not expected. These tables need less than 10 hours' decompression, compared to the other air tables which may extend to over 40 hours.

The conventional air therapeutic tables usually involve a depth of 165 feet or 50 metres. This was rationalized as being a depth beyond which further volume change would become insignificant, and at which the increase in nitrogen saturation of tissues becomes prohibitive by increasing subsequent decompression requirements. That depth was also consistent with the working medical attendants not being grossly incapacitated by nitrogen narcosis. The air Tables 1–4, of the *US Navy Diving Manual*, had their counterparts in most other navies. They were initially approved without being tested in DCS patients.

The Royal Navy have 70 metres as their maximum for air therapy tables; the USSR have 97 metres. Deep air tables (70 metres or more) may be unavoidable in serious cases which have not responded to the conventional air or oxygen tables. The protracted 50-metre air table (Table 4 USN) is notorious for producing DCS in attendants and therefore can be expected to make some patients worse. For this reason, there is a strong tendency to move away from its use to other options. These include substituting oxygen in the top 18 metres (60 feet), moving to Table 72 or the deep air tables of the Royal Navy, or the substitution of Nitrox or Heliox saturation tables.

The difficulties with air tables may include: prolonged decompression, aggravation of symptoms during ascent, nitrogen narcosis and DCS in the attendants, respiratory distress due to the increased density of air under pressure – especially if pulmonary involvement is already present. The results are often not good unless the symptoms are mild, recent and not produced from gross omitted decompression.

Many experienced clinicians are reluctant to use air tables because of the problems they bring and their dubious benefits.

The introduction of standard **oxygen tables** using 100% oxygen interspersed with air breathing gave far more flexibility and improved results. They include:

Shallow oxygen tables: Comex Cx12
Aust 9 (RAN 82)
Deep oxygen tables: 5, 6 (USN)
61, 62 (RN)

They can be extended and interchanged with the air tables at certain depths – mainly 9 metres and 18 metres. These tables became popular because of the improved results and the economy in time, needing only 2–5 hours. The physiological advantages are in the speed of bubble resolution and increased oxygenation of tissues and in countering some of the pulmonary arteriovenous shunting effects.

Disadvantages include the less immediate reduction in bubble size, i.e. to less than half the volume achieved with the 50-metre standard air tables, the fire hazard, oxygen toxicity, and the occasional intolerance of a distressed patient to oxygen or to a mask. Although the pressure gradient of nitrogen in the intravascular bubble-to-blood is increased with the oxygen breathing, if the diver has previously dived in excess of 18 metres, there could well be a positive gas pressure gradient from tissue-to-extravascular bubble during the early phase of recompression.

With the above qualifications, the use of oxygen tables has received world-wide acceptance as an alternative to the air tables. Apart from the improved results with the oxygen therapy tables, there is considerable flexibility by extending them at either the 18-metre (60-feet) or 9-metre (30-feet) depths.

A shallow oxygen table, valued by both French and Australian workers, allows for the treatment of mild cases and delayed cases, who have little likelihood of permanent disability. Here the patient is subjected to 12 metres (40 feet) or 9 metres (30 feet) on 100% oxygen, for periods of 2–3 hours respectively. Neither is as likely to produce oxygen toxicity as the standard oxygen tables, and they do include slower rates of ascent, thereby reducing the likelihood of both symptom recurrence and the 'oxygen-off effect'. Ascent on 100% oxygen at 12 min/metre (4 min/foot) is of considerable value during ascent from 9 metres (30 feet).

Whenever oxygen is used at atmospheric or greater pressures, attention must be paid to oxygen toxicity. Unless following established safe protocols, it is usually suggested that the oxygen parameters should not exceed those likely to result in neurological or pulmonary toxicity (see Chapter 18). In cases of potential disability, these risks may be acceptable.

Some **gas mixture tables** have also been used with great benefit, because they permit maximum oxygen usage without restricting the depths.

The advantages of depth and of high oxygen pressures together are used by the French, who recommended standardized tables with high oxygen/nitrogen mixtures, and the Australians who used whatever depth was necessary for a successful clinical result, and then administered the highest acceptable oxygen mixture (with helium or nitrogen) at that depth and during decompression.

Substitution of oxygen (at 18 metres or less) or high oxygen/nitrogen mixtures (at greater depths) during the conventional air tables was then introduced by both the Royal Navy and US Navy, to reduce the high failure rate of those air tables and to reduce the incidence of DCS in the attendants.

Helium has been substituted for nitrogen in the breathing gases for treatment of:

1. Helium DCS.
2. DCS from air breathing, especially if 100% $O_2$ cannot be used due to $O_2$ toxicity.
3. DCS refractory to treatment.
4. DCS during the recommended 'air' breaks of the oxygen tables.
5. Respiratory symptoms ('chokes'), at depth.

A frequent clinical observation is that DCS may be precipitated or worsened in a Heliox-breathing diver, when he transfers to air breathing during his ascent from saturation diving. This is difficult to understand by counterdiffusion principles, but it may be that the change to air breathing interferes with pulmonary dynamics (increasing the work of breathing and reducing gas mixing) because of the increased density, and that this may potentiate the decompression sickness by reducing helium elimination. Some workers have found that, in tissue, and specifically neurological tissue, oxygenation is less with the breathing of nitrogen/oxygen mixtures than with helium/oxygen mixtures at the same oxygen partial pressure.

The implication, in diving manuals and by many experienced clinicians, is that, if helium is available for treatment, it is preferable to air, either for the 'air breaks' in the oxygen tables or for the longer 'air' tables. This view does not have universal sanction yet, but is widespread. Also, air recompression has been used effectively to treat DCS in helium-breathing, non-saturation US Navy divers.

Heliox breathed on the surface has been shown to be as effective in removal of nitrogen bubbles in adipose tissue as oxygen. Nevertheless, until verified as safe in all tissues, if Heliox is to be used as a treatment gas for air DCS, it should probably only be given in conjunction with recompression therapy.

An additional technique of considerable value with air and helium tables, when there is no significant time factor involved and if the patient is severely affected, is the 12-hour or **'overnight soak'**. It may be of benefit for many reasons to halt all decompression for this prolonged time. Bubbles have a chance to resolve before Boyle's law comes into effect with decompression. Also tissue supersaturation of gas will become equilibrated with the ambient pressures. Last, but not least, medical and chamber personnel will be able to regroup and

reorganize from what can be a gruelling experience.

A prudent diving physician will advise non-experts to adhere to **strict treatment guidelines**, as depicted in the manuals, but retain his own flexibility to treat the cases which did not respond, or when the facilities may not be appropriate to apply the guidelines. It is for this reason that more than one set of treatment techniques is covered in this text.

---

*Standard oxygen therapeutic tables have the following advantages over the standard air tables:*

- *Economy of time*
- *Increased speed of bubble resolution (increased nitrogen gradient)*
- *Increased oxygenation of tissues*
- *Flexibility of combining with air tables*
- *Better results than air tables*

*Disadvantages include:*

- *Less immediate reduction in bubble size*
- *Oxygen toxicity*
- *Intolerance of patient to oxygen or mask*
- *Increased risk of fire*

---

**Saturation treatments** are applied when divers have developed DCS during or just after decompression from saturation exposures. Due to the extreme gas loads in 'slow' tissues, the contributions that this can make to developing bubbles, the presumed slow development of symptoms and the often excessive oxygen exposure, make the customary treatment tables inappropriate. In general, increased pressure is applied and the oxygen percentages are less. They may also be used after recompression to depth of relief in severe cases and when other tables have failed (see Chapter 36).

**Inner-ear DCS**, a great rarity with air diving, should only be diagnosed after considering the differential diagnosis. It is best treated with long oxygen tables, as used for other neurological DCS. It is rarely effective if delayed much longer than an hour.

**Hyperbaric oxygen therapy**, repeated daily, may be of value in severe and refractory cases. With spinal cord or cerebral damage, it is mandatory to continue with intermittent hyperbaric oxygen therapy until all subjective and objective improvement has ceased. These authors employ oxygen at 9–12 metres for 1–2 hours, then ascend at 3 min/metre, without air breaks, twice a day. Other regimes may be applied, but the use of repeated **diving therapeutic tables**, such as extended Table 6 (USN) with its hyperbaric 'air breaks', is illogical and has increased complications to both attendant and patient.

---

*In determining the therapeutic procedure the following should be remembered:*
- *The natural history of the disease*
  - *with increasing surface interval prior to symptoms, the less likely they are to worsen*
  - *neurological symptoms leave sequelae. Many others do not.*
- *The value of pressure*
  - *recompression to depth of dive will prevent bubble growth, and may hasten resolution*
  - *if air is required, decompression is made more difficult as nitrogen load is increased*
  - *with increasing duration of symptoms, the recompression depth effect is of less value*
- *The value of 100% oxygen, before during and after recompression*
  - *see pages 184, 185 and 189*
  - *intravascular bubbles do not develop with oxygen breathing, (especially at 2 ATA)*
  - *denitrogenation is maximized, reducing tissue bubbles*
  - *it reverses the development and the redevelopment of DCS*

---

## Cerebral arterial gas embolism (CAGE)

(See 'Air embolism' from pulmonary barotrauma (Chapter 9) and DCS (Chapters 11 and 12).)

The CAGE due to DCS has developed originally from venous gas emboli and therefore there must be a significant nitrogen load in the tissues to produce these emboli in the first instance. For this reason, the therapy tables often used for the CAGE from pulmonary barotrauma may not be adequate.

The pulmonary barotrauma cases, which are treated by an initial excursion to 50 metres (165 feet) before moving to the oxygen tables, are mainly from submarine escape training accidents, and have no significant nitrogen load in the tissues. Thus the extra nitrogen added by the excursion may be tolerable. This is not so with divers who already have so much nitrogen load that they developed DCS. The extra 15–30 minutes at 50 metres will add to this, and thus a 50-metre 'air' dip, followed by oxygen treatment tables, is not always safe for neurological DCS cases.

---

*Recompression tables specifically designed for the treatment of CAGE are not applicable to DCS cases. All the other CAGE regimes, including adjuvant therapy, are applicable.*

---

There is a recent tendency, based mainly on animal experimentation, to prefer the conventional oxygen tables to the 50-metre dip followed by the oxygen tables. This avoids the problems of the extra nitrogen load, but may not achieve the compression value of reducing the bubble to a size and frictional resistance that will allow the arterial pressure to force it through the arteriole into the capillary and venous system.

## Recompression facilities and transport

In large commercial operations, such as the North Sea oil fields, hyperbaric ambulances are available and are transportable by sea or air to onshore hyperbaric facilities. Transport by sea always introduces the complementary problems of motion sickness with electrolyte and dehydration abnormalities associated with vomiting.

Diving is frequently carried out in localities remote from major hospitals. Transportation of a sick patient requiring recompression therapy then becomes a major problem. Air transport may result in deterioration of the patient due to the further reduction in pressure, unless the patient is within a recompression chamber. As most aircraft are pressurized to about 2000 metres above sea level (0.8 ATA), flight will increase the size of gas bubbles. If the aircraft cannot be pressurized to 1 ATA,* the patient should not be transported at altitude, unless no other alternative is available, and time and speed are essential. Even a high mountain range can impose a threat if the diver is being moved by road. All these factors must be evaluated before deciding on the best means of transport of the patient to the chamber or vice versa.

One hundred per cent oxygen should be administered as immediate first aid and while transporting the patient to recompression facilities.

Recompression chamber treatment of a diver in a remote location can be expedited if an efficient transportation and treatment system has previously been established. There are two possibilities:

1. Treating the diver on location with oxygen and bringing a nearby portable recompression chamber to him. Once under pressure his danger may be diminished, but it still remains to treat him in the best chamber facility available. This portable recompression chamber should have compatible transfer under pressure facilities with other recompression chambers, for the transfer of both patients and attendants. It may then be moved to a more suitable chamber and the patient transferred.
2. Transporting the diver without compression direct to the treatment chamber.

The choice of system depends on the seriousness of the injury, the availability and type of recompression chambers and gas supplies, transport availability, and time and distance relationships. The initial treatment carried out by other divers on site will influence subsequent management.

It is important that a central experienced authority is responsible for decisions regarding treatment and transportation. This authority is best situated where the large definitive treatment chambers are located. The capability to transfer experienced staff and equipment to remote localities will prove of great value in the decision as to whether to treat on site or transport (see Chapter 33).

## Supportive and drug therapy

**General medical** treatment is required. This will vary according to the DCS manifestations, but will always include monitoring of the vital signs and repeated medical examinations.

**Positioning** of the patient with intravascular bubbles is somewhat contentious. The 'head-down' or Trendelenburg positions were originally used to divert emboli from the brain, by the effect of buoyancy. Arguments are now made for not assuming these positions, because the increased venous return causes increasing intracranial pressure, decreasing cerebral perfusion, aggravating the neurological pathology – as well as increasing the possibility of paradoxical gas embolism through a potentially patent foramen ovale (see page 167). For similar reasons, the legs should not be raised.

The patient should be supine or in the coma position and advised not to strain or perform Valsalva manoeuvres.

**Rehydration**, with a urinary output of 1–2 ml/kg per hour, should be achieved, preferably with electrolyte fluids. Dehydration from immersion and cold-induced diuresis may be aggravated by the haematological effects of DCS. This increases blood viscosity and reduces blood flow to the major organs. It needs urgent correction, orally or intravenously. Glucose and other carbohydrate fluids are avoided if other fluids are available.

**Urinary catheterization** will be required for most spinal DCS, as will careful skin and body maintenance.

**Monitoring** of electrocardiogram, electroencephalogram and electronystagmogram are sometimes indicated and should not cause difficulties in most chambers.

**Chest X-rays** can be performed through the ports or walls of many chambers, but this usually requires practice and pre-planning. Water aspiration and pulmonary barotrauma can both mimic and complicate DCS.

---

* Aircraft which can be pressurized to 1 ATA, while flying at an altitude of 5500 m (18 000 feet), include the C-130 Hercules, Boeing 707, 727, 737 and 747, DC-8 and DC-10, BAC-III and the Lear Jet.

**Arterial gases** are invaluable in severe cases, and **biochemical** and **haematological** studies can be performed on blood taken under pressure.

**Cardioversion** is rarely required, and can be performed in some specialized recompression facilities.

As an adjunct to recompression therapy, **drugs** and intravenous fluids may be used to correct some of the sequelae of DCS. Over the years there have been many such drug treatments recommended, but few have stood the test of time. They are often based on animal experimentation, usually specifically related to very rapid decompressions and often of more value if administered before the actual decompression accident, or at least very soon afterwards. There is a considerable degree of logic in the use of pharmacological agents to reduce platelet aggregation, microthrombi, haemoconcentration, neurological oedema etc. Although the logic is understandable, the clinical value is less than remarkable.

Reduction of the intravascular volume occurs with DCS and is often of clinical importance. In most cases it is probably worth while using **intravenous fluids** to expand the intravascular volume. Hartmann's solution, Ringer's lactate or physiological saline is preferable, until the serum electrolytes and plasma osmolarity can be determined. Intravenous colloids may be of value, and low-molecular-weight dextran in saline has been used in the past to prevent rouleaux formation, expand the blood volume rapidly and to reduce the likelihood of intravascular coagulation. There are occasional problems with its use. Glucose or dextrose may have harmful effects on cerebral pathology, and should be avoided if possible.

The use of **aspirin** (acetylsalicylic acid) has been widespread over many years. It is certainly a traditional form of analgesia, but may also have an influence on the haematological sequelae of DCS. It was recommended by the French workers, in the belief that, as an anticoagulant, it may reduce platelet clotting. Comex recommended an oral regime, whereas Fructus recommend the intravenous route – together with high doses of steroids.

There are more arguments against the use of aspirin than for it, in that the effects on an already haemorrhagic disease could be catastrophic – and haemorrhage in the gastrointestinal tract and brain have been the cause of some decompression deaths. Also, the likelihood of aggravating inner-ear or spinal cord haemorrhagic pathology is increased. It has a variety of other negative influences on susceptible individuals, such as bronchospasm and metabolic changes.

**Aminophylline**, probably with other sympathomimetic drugs, may be contraindicated in dysbaric diving accidents – and was removed from the North Sea medical packs. It results in the dilatation of the pulmonary vasculature and a profuse release of bubbles trapped in the pulmonary circuit, to enter the systemic circulation.

**Diazepam** (Valium) has also been recommended for use in DCS, when indicated. It may be of considerable value in reducing the incidence and degree of oxygen toxicity, especially in the serious cases which require extensive exposure to oxygen under pressure, during transport and after recompression therapy. It is also of considerable value in the occasional patient with a toxic–confusional state, because of the involvement of the neurological system from either DCS or air embolism. These patients can cause much concern, as well as being very difficult to handle in the recompression chamber, and may not tolerate the oronasal mask without a tranquillizer. In the latter circumstance, the dosage must be regulated according to the clinical state of the patient, but otherwise a 10 mg initial dose may be supplemented by 5 mg every few hours, without causing any significant drowsiness, respiratory depression or interference with the clinical picture.

Vestibular DCS may require suppressants, such as diazepam. Vomiting may require antiemetics.

**Lignocaine** (lidocaine) has been recommended in the same dosage as used for cardiac dysrhythmias, in both cardiac and cerebral DCS (see pages 167 and 175), on experimental grounds. It has complications and is an epileptogenic drug. Its value in DCS requires confirmation in clinical trials.

To reduce both cerebral and spinal oedema, mannitol and other diuretics have been used, as has the administration of **steroids**. These have not received general acceptance and, despite attempts, evidence of value is lacking. If dexamethasone is used then 16 mg is given intravenously, then 8 mg (i.v. or i.m.) 6-hourly

> *Supportive therapy in treatment of DCS may include:*
> - *Replacing fluids, improving micro-circulation and treating hypovolaemic shock*
> - *Diazepam to reduce confusional states and reduce oxygen toxicity, in serious cases*
> - *Urinary catheterization in cases of spinal DCS and/or severe shock*
> - *Treatments to improve cerebral blood flow and reduce cerebral and spinal oedema*

for 24 hours, 6 mg 12-hourly for 24 hours and 4 mg 12-hourly for 24 hours. It should be discontinued within 72 hours unless maintenance steroids are to be used. Others would recommend the use of hydrocortisone intravenously with a dosage of 1000 mg, as this is thought to produce a more dramatic response than the slower-acting dexamethasone.

Early research indicated that, if oxygen therapy tables are used, steroids should be avoided until the patient is at a depth of 9 metres or less, to reduce the aggravation of oxygen toxicity. Others claim that it does not affect oxygen toxicity and that this is less serious than the DCS disease. The consensus is now away from its routine use, as there is evidence that steroids cause more injury to hypoxic neurons and worsen morbidity and survival when given for oedema surrounding cerebral haemorrhage.

**Heparin** has been advocated because of its lipaemic clearing activity and its protective effect against platelet clumping. It was thought to be indicated in cases of disseminated intravascular coagulation which had no evidence of systemic infarction and bleeding. It is now rarely, if ever, used. Correction of specific coagulation defects seems a more logical approach to the rare problem of disseminated intravascular coagulation in DCS. It can be harmful following the haemorrhagic pathologies of the spinal cord, inner ear and other DCS manifestations.

Methods of **increasing vascular perfusion**, e.g. with vasodilator and prostaglandin active drugs, negative pressure breathing, lying down, and even warm water immersion, have been proposed.

Occasionally, a joint bend persisting after treatment may be relieved or cured by the temporary application of a **local increase in pressure** from a sphygmomanometer cuff.

## Surface oxygen administration

> *One area that has been relatively overlooked recently is the administration of oxygen at normobaric pressure.*
> *Albert R. Behnke, July 1990*

The administration of 100% oxygen, carried out by those trained to do so, will often relieve some of the patient's symptoms and may reduce the likelihood of others developing. It is particularly of value prior to subjecting the patient to altitude environments.

Oxygen has been demonstrated to:

- Enhance the inert gas elimination.
- Prevent venous gas emboli, as detected by Doppler.
- Reduce the size of inert gas bubbles.
- Prevent DCS developing.
- Treat developed DCS.
- Prevent recurrences of DCS.
- Possibly improve oxygenation of damaged tissues.

In one series, oxygen was shown to be an effective treatment for neurological DCS. Although this was a highly selected population, it did demonstrate the value of surface oxygen, given early and for some hours, in remote areas where recompression facilities are not readily available.

Although the value of administering 100% oxygen, with intermittent air breaks, is unquestioned, problems do arise with inexperienced personnel. Commonly, an inadequate mask is used, e.g. the Edinburgh or other plastic nosepieces which struggle to produce 40% oxygen in the inspiratory gas. Other risks involve the inflammable nature of oxygen and the development of oxygen toxicity.

Perhaps the most neglected aspect of the treatment of DCS is that instituted after recompression. An increasing awareness of the importance of 100% oxygenation for the patient during transit is often offset by the neglect of an apparently cured patient post-treatment. Most cases which respond well to recompression therapy, and especially to oxygen recompression therapy, will redevelop symptoms within a few hours of leaving the chamber. These are usually mild in nature, but may progress to require further recompression.

Information about mild symptoms may not be volunteered because the patient does not wish to undergo further recompression therapy, because he has lost contact with the diving medical specialists (having been transferred to a hospital bed), or perhaps because the patient has decided that the symptoms were significantly less severe and therefore less important than the original ones.

> *The administration of oxygen after recompression therapy reduces the incidence of recurrence and hence the need for further recompression.*

Possible and likely explanations for the recurring symptoms include not only the return to atmospheric pressure, but also the breathing of air which allows nitrogen access again to the tissues and permits the existing small bubbles to grow, as the nitrogen tension is transferred from blood to bubble. This sequence of events can either be prevented or reversed at an early stage by the reintroduction of 100% oxygen breathing. The excellent response to this therapy is only obtained if performed early.

If careful clinical monitoring is maintained on the patient after recompression therapy, the early re-emergence of a symptom can be rapidly corrected by the use of 100% oxygen – often within a few minutes. After 30 minutes or so, the patient returns to air breathing and the symptoms will often re-emerge, but more gradually than previously. One can almost titrate the oxygen administration against the natural increase in bubble size, and symptom development. Because of this, it is now common

practice to institute the 30 minutes air/30 minutes oxygen regime for 6–8 hours post-recompression therapy, to prevent deterioration of the patient's clinical state. This also implies a continuation of the regime of lung function tests to guard against the possible, but unlikely, development of further oxygen toxicity.

## Recurrence of symptoms

The fact that a therapeutic table has been promulgated by some authority does not make it effective, and there have been many modifications and deletions made to these tables during the professional lives of these authors.

As a good general rule, if symptoms recur during treatment, the management should be seriously questioned. Attention should be directed to ensure that there has been adequate recompression and supportive therapy, including correct positioning, rehydration etc. Medical reassessment of diagnoses should be made, considering:

- Pulmonary barotrauma and each of its clinical manifestations (Chapter 9)
- Complications of DCS, affecting target organs.
- Non-diving general medical diseases.

Nevertheless, DCS patients do sometimes deteriorate during recompression therapy. The composition of the breathing mixture should be confirmed, as should the efficiency of the mask seal.

Retrospective surveys of the effects of treatment tables, by statisticians, usually show fewer recurrences than are observed in practice, due to the deficiencies of recording and the lack of follow-up clinical assessments. Many of these surveys do not allow for the degree of decompression stress, the severity of disease and the delay in treatment. These lead to better treatment results reported with professional and navy divers' DCS than with civilians'.

One table (USN 4, RN 54) frequently caused DCS in attendants, who did not even have a nitrogen load to start with. It is difficult to understand how it could then improve patients, at the shallow stops. Oxygen is now used by both patient and attendant from 18 metres, to reduce this. The short 'air embolism' Table 5A, which many of us believed to be a contributor to deaths during treatment, has recently been removed from the *US Navy Manual*.

Frequently, symptoms will recur towards the end of, or just after, the air breaks in the oxygen tables. They also tend to redevelop during the ascents and within an hour or two after surfacing. It is for this reason that oxygen is continued or Heliox is substituted by some therapists during the designated 'air breaks' and after surfacing.

If similar and significant symptoms recur, it must be presumed to be a re-expansion of a bubble which was not completely removed – and treated accordingly.

Occasionally there may be other explanations, such as:

- The inflammatory tissue reaction to the bubble produced pathology.
- Lipid/platelet/fibrin deposits or emboli.
- Re-perfusion injury.
- Redistribution of gas emboli.

Only the last of these could be expected to respond to recompression therapy, and it would be a great coincidence if it were to reproduce the same symptoms as the original lesion.

Recurrences of the original symptoms or the development of other serious symptoms should be looked upon as due to inadequate treatment, or the aggravation of the problem by the re-exposure to nitrogen at depth or on the surface. Recurrence of symptoms requires surface oxygen (if mild), hyperbaric oxygenation or a conventional therapy table.

Paraesthesia and other symptoms developing while undergoing recompression therapy may well be due to the development of oxygen toxicity (see Chapter 18) and therefore are not necessarily an indication to extend the therapy.

It is not necessary to **recompress repeatedly** for minor and fluctuating symptoms, unless these have some ominous clinical significance. Minor residual musculoskeletal or peripheral nerve pathology is very common and chasing these symptoms to obtain a 'cure' becomes demoralizing and exhausting for both patient and attendants.

Both recompression and altitude exposure may affect these minor symptoms, presumably by affecting marginal ischaemia or nerve irrita-

bility from myelin sheath damage. Similar 'Will o' the wisp' symptoms occur in other neurologically damaged patients. Patients should be reassured that such minor symptoms – often developing for months after DCS – are not uncommon and do not require intervention.

## Underwater treatment

### Traditional in-water treatments

By far the most traditional of the non-chamber treatments of DCS is underwater recompression therapy. In this situation the pressure is exerted by the water, instead of a recompression chamber. Air supply is usually from compressors sited on the diving boat. Although this treatment is frequently ridiculed by those in the cloistered academic environments, especially when they are committed to elaborate recompression facilities, it has frequently been the only therapy available to severely injured divers, and has had many successes. This was certainly so in those remote localities such as Northern Australia, in the pearl fishing areas, where long periods were spent under water and standard diving equipment was used. Underwater air treatment continued to be used, in the absence of available recompression chambers.

The failure of DCS to respond to recompression therapy is often related directly to the delay in treatment. Sometimes chambers are not readily available. For this reason, underwater air recompression is currently used in Hawaii, with good results, within minutes of symptoms developing. This was also the experience of professional shell divers of Australia, at least until the underwater oxygen became available.

Despite the value of the underwater air recompression therapy, many problems are encountered with it. These are well recognized by both divers and their medical advisers. It is of interest that most diving medical textbooks do not mention this therapy at any stage.

The US and Royal Navy have occasionally tried to apply their standard air treatment tables to underwater conditions, with manifestly impractical depth and duration recommendations. Most of the underwater air treatments are more applicable than these. A typical example is that given by Sir Robert

Davis, in which the duration depends upon the depth required for relief of symptoms. Many regimes are makeshift, and are varied with experience.

The problems are as follows. Most amateurs or semi-professionals do not carry the compressed air supplies or compressor facilities necessary for the extra decompression. Most have only scuba cylinders, or simple portable compressors that will not reliably supply divers (the patient and his attendant) for the depths and durations required. Environmental conditions are not usually conducive to underwater treatment. Often the depths required for these treatments can only be achieved by returning to the open ocean. The advent of night, inclement weather, rising seas, tiredness and exhaustion, and boat safety requirements make the return to the open ocean a very serious decision. Because of the considerable depth required, hypothermia from the compression of wet suits become likely. Seasickness in the injured diver, the diving attendants and the boat tenders is a significant problem. Nitrogen narcosis produces added difficulties in the diver and the attendant.

The treatment often has to be aborted because of these difficult circumstances, producing DCS in the attendants, and aggravating it in the diver. Underwater air treatment of DCS is not to be undertaken lightly. In the absence of a recompression chamber, it may be the only treatment available to prevent death or severe disability. Despite considerable criticism from authorities distant from the site, this traditional therapy is recognized by most experienced and practical divers often to be of lifesaving value.

## Underwater oxygen therapy

The value of substituting oxygen for air, in the recompression chamber treatment of DCS, is now well established. The pioneering work of Yarborough and Behnke (1939) eventuated in the oxygen tables described by Goodman and Workman (1965). They received widespread acceptance and, with revisions and modifications, they are now incorporated into oxygen treatment tables of most navies.

The advantages of oxygen over air tables include: increasing nitrogen elimination gradients, avoiding extra nitrogen loads, increasing oxygenation to tissues, decreasing the depths required for the exposure time and improving the overall therapeutic efficiency. The same arguments are applicable when comparing underwater air and underwater oxygen treatment.

In 1970, this new option was applied to the underwater treatment of decompression sickness. It developed in response to an urgent need for management of cases in remote localities – remote in both time and distance from hyperbaric facilities. As a result of the success of this treatment, and its ready availability, it became known and practised, even when experts were not available to supervise it.

The physiological principles on which this treatment is based are well known and not contentious, although the indications for treatment have caused some confusion. As for conventional oxygen therapy tables, it was first applied mainly for the minor cases of DCS, but was subsequently found to be of considerable value in serious cases.

The techniques and equipment for underwater oxygen therapy were designed to make for safety, ease and ready availability, even in medically unsophisticated countries. It is now in widespread use in the Pacific Islands and the northern parts of Australia. It spread to the colder southern waters of Australia, where it is now used by abalone divers who sometimes dive in areas difficult to service by conventional transport.

It has also been included in certain diving manuals (Tables 81 and 82 in the *Royal Australian Navy Diving Manual*) and has been modified by allowing the use of oxygen rebreathing equipment, in the current *US Navy Diving Manual*. The French have had a very similar table (Comex 12) which was immediately applicable to underwater use, and some Italian groups claimed to have employed the full US Navy oxygen therapy tables under water – although how they managed this is not clear.

The original procedures and tables seem simpler and less likely to cause problems for the general diver population than these various alternatives.

**Hawaiian** commercial divers have included a **deep air 'dip'** prior to the underwater oxygen treatment, in an attempt to either force bubbles back into solution or to allow bubbles trapped in arteries to transfer to the venous system.

### Technique

Oxygen is supplied at maximum depth of 9 metres (30 feet), from a surface supply. Ascent is commenced after 30 minutes in mild cases, or 60 minutes in severe cases, if significant improvement has occurred. These times may be extended for another 30 minutes, if there has been no improvement. The ascent is at the rate of 12 min/metre (4 min/foot). After surfacing, the patient should be given periods of oxygen breathing, interspersed with air breathing, usually on a one hour on, one hour off basis, with respiratory volume measurements and chest X-ray examination if possible.

Whenever oxygen is given, the cylinder should be turned on and the flow commenced, before it is given to patients or divers.

### Equipment

No equipment should be used with oxygen if it is contaminated, dirty or lubricated with oil.

The equipment required for this treatment includes the following: a G size oxygen cylinder (220 cubic feet or 7000 litres). This is usually available from local hospitals, although in some cases industrial oxygen has been used from engineering workshops. Breathing this volume of oxygen at a depth varying between 9 metres (30 feet) and the surface is usually insufficient to produce either neurological or respiratory oxygen toxicity. A two-stage regulator, set at 550 kPa (80 lb/in$^2$) is fitted with a safety valve, and connects with 12 metres (40 feet) of supply hose. This allows for 9 metres' depth, 2 metres from the surface of the water to the cylinder and 1 metre around the diver. A non-return valve is attached between the supply line and the full face mask. The latter enables the system to be used with a semi-conscious or unwell patient. It reduces the risk of aspiration of sea water, allows the patient to speak to his attendants and also permits vomiting to occur without obstructing the respiratory gas supply. The supply line is marked in distances of 1 metre from the surface to the diver, and is tucked under the weight belt, between the diver's legs, or is attached to a harness. The diver must be weighted to prevent drifting upwards in an arc by the current.

A diver attendant should always be present, and the ascent controlled by the surface tenders. The duration of the three tables is 2 hours 6 minutes, 2 hours 36 minutes and 3 hours 6 minutes.

The treatment can be repeated twice daily, if needed.

### Overview

It was originally hoped that the underwater oxygen treatment would be sufficient for the management of minor cases of DCS, and to prevent deterioration of the more severe cases while suitable transport was being arranged. When the regime is applied early, even in the severe cases, the transport is often not required. It is a common observation that improvement continues throughout the ascent, at 12 min/metre. Presumably the resolution of the bubble is more rapid at this ascent rate than its expansion due to Boyle's law.

Certain other advantages are obvious. During the hours of continuous hyperbaric oxygenation, tissues become effectively denitrogenated. Bubbles are initially reduced in volume, due to the hyperbaric exposure and Boyle's law, and the resolution is speeded up by increasing the nitrogen gradient from the bubble. Attendant divers are not subjected to the risk of DCS or nitrogen narcosis, and the affected diver is not going to be made worse by premature termination of the treatment, if this is required. Hypothermia is much less likely to develop, because of the greater efficiency of the wet suits at these minor depths.

The site chosen can often be in a shallow protected area, reducing the influence of weather on the patient, the diving attendants and the boat tenders. Communications between the diver and the attendants are not difficult, and the situation is not as stressful as the deeper, longer, underwater air treatments or even as worrying as in some recompression chambers.

The underwater oxygen recompression treatment is not applicable to all cases, especially when the patient is unable or unwilling to return to the underwater environment. It is also of very little value in the cases where gross decompression staging has been omitted, or where the disseminated intravascular coagulation syndrome has developed. These authors would be reluctant to administer this regime where the patient has either epileptic convulsions or clouding of consciousness. Reference to the case reports reveals that others are less conservative.

One of the common comments in Australia is that this underwater treatment regime is applicable to the semi-tropical and tropical areas (where it was first used), but not to the southern parts of the continent, where water temperatures may be as low as 5°C. There are certain inconsistencies with this statement. First, if the diver developed DCS while diving in these waters, then he is most likely already to have effective thermal protection suits available to him. Also, the duration under water for the oxygen treatment is not excessive, and it is at a depth at which his wet suit is far more effective than at his maximum diving depth. If he is wearing a dry suit, the argument is even less applicable. The most effective argument is that it is used, and often very successfully, in these very areas.

Some claim that the underwater oxygen treatment is of more value when there are no transport facilities available. Initially this was also our own teaching, but with the logic that comes with hindsight, only a 3-hour gap is needed between the institution of underwater oxygen therapy and the arrival of transport, to be able to utilize this system. It is probably just as important to treat the serious cases early, even though full recovery is unlikely, than to do nothing and watch the symptoms progress during those hours.

There is no doubt, especially in serious cases, that transport should be sought while the underwater treatment is being utilized.

There has been a concern that, if this technique is available for treatment of DCS, other divers may misuse it to decompress on oxygen under water, and perhaps run into subsequent problems. This is more an argument in favour of educating divers, than depriving them of potentially valuable treatment facilities. With the same rationale, this argument could be used to prohibit totally all safety equipment, including recompression chambers, and thereby hope to circumvent all diving-related problems.

It has been argued that this treatment is unlikely to be of any value for those patients suffering from air embolism. Such may well be the case. The treatment was never proposed for this, and nor was it ever suggested that the underwater oxygen treatment can be used in preference to recompression facilities where they exist, or where they can be obtained. It is, however, possible that the treatment may be of value for cases of mediastinal emphysema, and perhaps even a small pneumothorax.

When hyperbaric chambers are used in remote localities, often with inadequate equipment and insufficiently trained personnel, there is an appreciable danger from both fire and explosion. There is the added difficulty in dealing with inexperienced medical personnel not ensuring an adequate face seal for the mask. These problems are not encountered in underwater treatment.

The underwater oxygen treatment table is an application, and a modification, of current regimes. It is not meant to replace the formal treatment techniques of recompression therapy in chambers. It is an emergency procedure, able to be applied with equipment usually found in remote localities and is designed to reduce the many hazards associated with the conventional underwater air treatments. The customary supportive and pharmacological adjuncts to the treatment of recompression sickness are in no way avoided, and the superiority of experienced personnel and comprehensive hyperbaric facilities is not being challenged. The underwater oxygen treatment is considered as a first aid regime, not superior to portable recompression chambers, but sometimes surprisingly effective and rarely, if ever, detrimental.

The relative value of current first aid regimes (underwater oxygen, an additional deep air dip and surface oxygen treatment) needs to be clarified.

## Use of underwater oxygen treatment

Because of the nature of this treatment being applied in remote localities, many cases are not well documented. Twenty-five cases were well supervised before this technique increased suddenly in popularity. Two such cases are described.

## CASE REPORT 13.3 (a 68-year-old male salvage diver)

Two dives to 30 metres (100 feet) for 20 minutes each were performed with a surface interval of $1\frac{1}{2}$ hours, while searching for the wreck of *HMS Pandora* about 100 miles from Thursday Island in the Torres Strait.

No decompression staging was possible, allegedly because of the increasing attentions of a tiger shark. A few minutes after surfacing, the diver developed paraesthesia, back pain, progressively increasing incoordination and paresis of the lower limbs.

Two attempts at underwater air recompression were unsuccessful when the diving boat returned to its base moorings. The National Marine Operations Centre was finally contacted for assistance.

It was about 36 hours, post-dive, before the patient was finally flown to the regional hospital on Thursday Island.

Both the Air Force and the Navy had been involved in the organization, but because of very hazardous air and sea conditions, and very primitive air strip facilities, another 12 hours would be required before the patient could have reached an established recompression centre (distance 3000 km, 2000 miles).

On examination at Thursday Island, the patient was unable to walk, having evidence of both cerebral and spinal involvement. He had marked ataxia, slow slurred speech, intention tremor, severe back pain, generalized weakness, difficulty in micturition, severe weakness of lower limbs with impaired sensation, increased tendon reflexes and equivocal plantar responses.

An underwater oxygen unit was available on Thursday Island for use by the pearl divers, and the patient was immersed to 8 metres' depth (the maximum depth off the wharf). Two hours were allowed at that lesser depth and the patient was then decompressed. There was total remission of all symptoms and signs, except for small areas of hypoaesthesia on both legs.

## CASE REPORT 13.4 (a 23-year-old female sports diver)

Diving with a 2000-litre (72 cubic feet) scuba cylinder in the Solomon Islands (nearest recompression chamber was 3500 km away and prompt air transport was unavailable), the dive depth was 34 metres (110 feet) and duration approximately 20 minutes, with 8 minutes' decompression. Within 15 minutes of surfacing she developed respiratory distress, then numbness and paraesthesia, very severe headaches, involuntary extensor spasms, clouding of consciousness, muscular pains and weakness, pains in both knees and abdominal cramps. The involuntary extensor spasms recurred every 10 minutes or so.

The patient was transferred to the hospital, where neurological DCS was diagnosed, and she was given oxygen via a face mask for 3 hours without significant change. During that time an underwater oxygen unit was prepared and the patient was accompanied to a depth of 9 metres (30 feet) off the wharf. Within 15 minutes she was much improved, and after 1 hour she was asymptomatic. Decompression at 12 min/metre was uneventful and the patient was subsequently flown by commercial aircraft to Australia.

## Medical attendants

General medical treatment is required during the recompression regimes. Patients should not be left unattended in recompression chambers, and especially while breathing increased oxygen concentrations.

First aid and resuscitation techniques are often required, as are accurate clinical assessments – and for these reasons it is desirable to have a trained medical attendant in the chamber. It may be necessary to consider the possibility of DCS occurring in the attendants, especially when the patient is subjected to oxygen or oxygen-enriched mixtures. The decompression regimes are based on the gas mixtures being breathed by the patient, and not the air being breathed by the attendants.

> *It is embarrassing to produce DCS in attendants during recompression therapy.*

With respect to general medical personnel, both paramedical and professional, it is essential that, wherever possible, the medical staff should be specifically trained in both hyperbaric problems and diving accidents. Where this is not possible, a direct communication is required between the clinical staff administering to the patient and an expert in diving medicine.

## Return to diving and flying

Following decompression accidents, unless changes are made to the exposures, the past is likely to be repeated – but with greater severity. We recommend that DCS cases may resume diving as follows

**Uncomplicated type 1 DCS if produced by exceptional DCS stress** (exceeding normally accepted dive profiles or ascent rates), the period before diving should be 4 weeks for humans, 3 weeks for pure-bred English Pointers.

**Uncomplicated type 1 DCS, unexpected** according to the dive profiles: period should be 4 weeks after:

1. Search for and remedy of any factors that increase susceptibility.
2. Exclusion of other diseases.
3. Addition of a depth/duration penalty for future diving, e.g. reducing the no-decompression times and ascent rates, and avoiding decompression, computer-controlled, repetitive and deep diving.

**Complicated type 1 DCS, neurological DCS and other type 2 DCS:**

1. Exclusion of other causes e.g. pulmonary barotrauma, cardiac shunts etc.
2. Follow-up with clinical assessments, neuropsychological tests, electroencephalography, somatosensory evoked cortical responses, brain imaging techniques, bone scans etc. until full recovery.
3. After these have been satisfactorily achieved, and at least a month has elapsed, scuba may be resumed in a very limited manner, e.g.
   (a) no-decompression dives with allowable bottom times halved;
   (b) maximum depth 15 metres (50 feet);
   (c) surface intervals in excess of 6 hours.
4. If sequelae persist and are stable after many months then, as long as the diver's psychological and physical fitness is not impaired, scuba diving may be permitted to 9 metres for short periods. Even this restricted diving is appreciated by yachtsmen, marine scientists and devotees.

Some groups permit type 1 DCS cases to return after a week, and type 2 DCS cases to resume after clearance of all symptoms. Others add the conditions that all investigations should be normal or that any clinical residuum should not make the diver permanently unfit.

Unfortunately, many divers are encouraged to believe that DCS is a totally correctable disease, despite experimental and autopsy findings to the contrary. Enthusiastic divers seek reassurance which may not be appropriate. Commercial expediency and countering of litigation may both motivate recommendations to return to diving, which are not in the patients' best interests.

For at least 4 days after the DCS patient appears 'cured' or 7 days after he has reached a plateau in his response to daily hyperbaric oxygen therapy (without hyperbaric air exposure), the patient may not be considered suitable for commercial **aviation transfer**. Earlier exposure not infrequently results in a recurrence of symptoms, as bubbles may persist without evidence after DCS or hyperbaric treatments (especially air tables or tables that employ 'air periods').

If the patient has to be transferred earlier, this should be carried out in an aircraft pressurized to ground level or while breathing 100% oxygen and after 2–4 hours' oxygen breathing at ground level.

Often aviation exposure causes minor symptoms in marginally ischaemic neurological states, including DCS, possibly because of hypoxia (altitude effect) or hypocapnia (hyperventilation induced) from breathing the rarified atmosphere.

## Acknowledgement

Acknowledgement is made to Dr E.D. Thalmann, USN, for his review of this chapter. Although he did not always agree with the contents, his criticisms and comments were immensely valuable and were often incorporated. His involvement does not imply that the chapter reflects his personal endorsement or *official* US navy policy.

## References and recommended texts

### Treatment

BARNARD, E.E.P. (1978). Use of oxygen and pressure as independent variables in the treatment of decompression sickness. *Proceedings Medical Aspects of Diving Accidents*, pp. 47–76. EUBS Publication.

BEHNKE, A.R. and SHAW, L.A. (1937). The use of oxygen in the treatment of compressed-air illness. *Naval Medical Bulletin Washington* **35**, 61–73.

CATRON, P.W., THOMAS, L.B., FLYNN, E.T. et al. (1987). Effects of helium/oxygen breathing during experimental decompression sickness following air dives. *Undersea Biomedical Research* **14**, 101–111.

DAVIS, R.H. (1962). *Deep Diving and Submarine Operations*. Surrey, England: Siebe Gorman & Co.

DICK, A.P.K., MEBANE, G.Y. and JOHNSON, J. (1984). *Early Oxygen Breathing for Scuba Injuries*. Annual Scientific Meeting, Undersea Medical Society.

DOUGLAS, J.D.M. and ROBINSON, C. (1988) Heliox treatment for spinal decompression sickness following air dives. *Undersea Biomedical Research* **15**, 315–322.

DUFFNER, G.J., VAN DER AUE, O.E. and BEHNKE, A.R. (1946). *The Treatment of Decompression Sickness*. USNMRI Research Project X-443, Report No 3.

EDMONDS, C., LOWRY, C. and PENNEFATHER, J. (1981). *Diving and Subaquatic Medicine*, 2nd edn. St Leonards, Australia: Diving Medical Centre.

KINDWALL, E.P., GOAD R.F., FARMER, J.C. LEITCH, D.R. and HALLENBECK, J.M. (1984). *The Physicians Guide To Diving Medicine*, Sections 5 and 6. New York: Plenum Press.

MILLER, J.N., FAGRAEUS, L. and BENNETT, P.B. (1978). Nitrogen-oxygen saturation therapy. *The Lancet* 169–171.

THALMANN, E.D. (1990). Principles of U.S. Navy recompression treatments for decompression sickness. In: *Diving Accident Management Workshop*, edited by P.B. Bennett and R. Moon. DAN/NDAA/UHMS.

UMS Workshop on Decompression Sickness Therapy (1979).

YARBOROUGH, O.D. and BEHNKE, A.R. (1939). The treatment of compressed air illness using oxygen. *Journal of Industrial Hygiene and Toxicology* **21**, 213–218.

### Therapy tables

BERGHAGE, T.E., VOROSMARTI, J. JR and BARNARD, E.E.P. (1978). An evaluation of recompression tables. *NMRI Report to US Navy*.

*COMEX Medical Book 11*, Bucksburn, Aberdeen.

*RN Diving Manual* (1970). London: HMSO.

*US Navy Diving Manual* (1989). US Government Printing Office, Washington DC.

# 14

# Dysbaric osteonecrosis

## Introduction

Infarction of areas of bone associated with exposure to pressure, be it in air or water, has been recognized since the turn of the century. A causal relationship with pressure exposure was first suggested by Twynam in 1888 in a case report of a caisson worker constructing the Iron Cove bridge in Sydney, although in retrospect the man appeared to be suffering from 'septic' necrosis.

In 1912, there were 500 cases of decompression sickness reported among the caisson workers on the Elbe tunnel at Hamburg, and 9 had bone changes. Bassoe, in 1913, suggested a relationship between initial joint 'bends' and subsequent X-ray evidence of bone atrophy and sclerosis. Taylor, in 1943, noted that several months elapsed between the hyperbaric exposure and the joint symptoms, and that shaft lesions are usually asymptomatic and may

be replaced by new bone. Osteonecrosis has been observed following caisson work at a pressure as low as 17 lb/in$^2$ (117 kPa) (less than 12 metres of sea water), and also for as short a time as 7 hours, divided into two shifts, at 35 lb/in$^2$ (242 kPa).

The first report of osteonecrosis in a diver appears to have been in 1941. It has been known to develop within 3 months of the diving exposure, and has occasionally resulted from 'once only' exposures.

Three of five men who escaped from the submarine *Poseidon*, in 1931 in the China sea after being at a depth of 38 metres for 2–3 hours, subsequently developed dysbaric osteonecrosis.

Aseptic necrosis of bone has even been described in diving lizards (mosasaurs) of the cretaceous period, although the association with diving may not be entirely relevant. Various names (Table 14.1) have been given to this disease but the term '**dysbaric osteonecrosis**' has gained precedence as it clearly distinguishes the causal relationship with pressure from the other myriad causes of bone necrosis.

**Table 14.1 Some synonyms for dysbaric osteonecrosis**

| |
| --- |
| Caisson arthrosis |
| Caisson disease of bone |
| Hyperbaric osteonecrosis |
| Barotraumatic osteoarthropathy |
| Avascular necrosis of bone* |
| Ischaemic necrosis of bone* |
| Aseptic necrosis of bone* |
| Diver's bone rot |
| Diver's crumbling bone disease |

* To be distinguished from other causes of bone necrosis.

# Incidence

Detailed studies of the incidence were not undertaken until the 1960s. Figures should be considered cautiously, because different radiological techniques and diagnostic criteria may have been used by the radiologists or physicians in each survey. Other factors influencing the results include the difficulty in obtaining adequate follow-up of workers of divers and the different decompression regimes followed.

For example, at the Clyde tunnel, only 241 **compressed air workers** were surveyed of a total of 1362 workers, 19% having lesions, half of which were juxta-articular. By 1972, the UK Medical Research Council Decompression Sickness Council Panel had X-rays of 1674 workers of whom 19.7% had positive lesions. Also, in 1972, a study by Jones and Behnke on the Bay Area Rapid Transit tunnelling project in San Francisco revealed no clinical or X-ray evidence of necrosis. All workers had pre-employment X-rays and those with lesions were excluded. The pressure ranged from 9 to 36 lb/in$^2$ (62–248 kPa) with only one decompression per day. However, the follow-up period was relatively short.

The incidence of this disorder reported in divers is exceedingly variable, ranging from 2.5% in the US Navy to a doubtful 80% in Chinese commercial divers. Some representative surveys are listed in Table 14.2. The lower incidences are reported in military series where strict decompression schedules are adhered to, as with many commercial diving operations. However, in the usually self-employed diving fishermen of Japan, Hawaii and Australia, the divers undertake relatively deep dives with long bottom times and, sometimes, with inadequate decompression. These divers appear to have the highest risk of all. There is a higher incidence among divers over the age of 30 years, which may reflect increased exposure rather than age per se.

The Medical Research Council Decompression Sickness Central Registry has X-rays for nearly 7000 professional divers and reports that there are only 12 cases of subchondral bone

**Table 14.2 Reported incidence of dysbaric osteonecrosis in divers**

| Report | Type of diver | Total no. | Percentage positive |
| --- | --- | --- | --- |
| Ohta and Matsunaga (1974)* | Japanese shellfish | 301 | 50.5 |
| Fagan and Beckman (1976) | Gulf coast commercial | 330 | 27 |
| Elliot and Harrison (1976) | Royal Navy | 350 | 4 |
| Harvey and Sphar (1976) | US Navy | 611 | 2.5 |
| Wade et al. (1978) | Hawaiian fishermen | 20 | 65 |
| Davidson (1981) | North Sea commercial | 4422 | 4.4 |
| Lowry et al. (1986) | Australian abalone | 108 | 25 |
| Kawashima and Tamura (1983)* | Japanese shellfish | 747 | 56.4 |

* The Kawashima and Tamura survey is an extension of the Ohta and Matsunaga survey and they have divers in common.

collapse, i.e. about 0.2%. Asymptomatic shaft lesions appeared in about 4%. The prevalence of crippling osteoarthritis requiring total joint replacement has been conservatively estimated at more than 2% in Australian abalone divers. The majority of cases in most series involve shaft lesions which have no long-term significance to health and well-being, except for the rare possibility of malignant change.

Earlier UK studies on professional divers indicated that lesions occurred significantly more among the older males who had longer diving experience, and also who had exposures to greater depths. Only 0.4% of the compressed air divers, who had never exceeded 50 metres, had these lesions. The helium-breathing divers who did not exceed 500 feet (150 m) had an incidence of 2.7% which rose to 7.6% if they had been deeper. There was a definite increase in incidence among saturation divers and those who had had decompression sickness. Approximately one-quarter of the lesions were of a serious nature, closely associated with joints.

Another UK study of caisson workers, with 2200 subjects, showed an incidence of dysbaric osteonecrosis of 17%. The lesions were more often in older men, with more exposure to pressure and also correlated significantly with decompression sickness. The incidence rose to 60% for those who had worked for 15 years in compressed air.

Although rare, several cases have been reported in aviators not exposed to hyperbaric conditions.

---

> *Dysbaric osteonecrosis is rare in recreational scuba divers who breathe compressed air at depths of less than 50 metres, and who follow the customary decompression tables.*

---

Whether the incidence of bone lesions is related more to the cumulative effects of hyperbaric exposures than to the statistical chance of a single event increasing with multiple exposures is unknown.

The incidence of avascular necrosis of bone, within the general population not exposed to hyperbaric environments, is also not clearly defined.

# Aetiology

The most common cause of aseptic necrosis of the femoral head is fracture of the neck of the femur. The necrotic lesions of high-dose steroid therapy, whilst being multiple and bilateral, often involve the articular surface of the knee and ankle joints, which is virtually never seen with dysbaric osteonecrosis. This variation in distribution suggests that the pathogenesis may be different, even if the pathology is identical. Aseptic osteonecrosis may occur idiopathically. It is also frequently reported in association with those diseases in which there is some disturbance of fat metabolism, e.g. diabetes mellitus, pancreatitis, alcoholism and cirrhosis, Gaucher's disease and hyperlipidaemia. Trauma and steroid administration are the most common associations.

It has been postulated that many of these conditions may lead to fat emboli and obstruct end arteries in rigid haversian canals of bone, leading to osteonecrosis. These fat emboli may arise from a fatty liver, coalescence of plasma lipoproteins, disruption of bone marrow or other fat tissue, or a combination of the above mechanisms.

There are many other conditions associated with a high incidence of aseptic necrosis:

- Decompression sickness or dysbaric exposure.
- Trauma (e.g. fractured neck of femur, dislocated hip and unrelated fractures).
- Alcoholism.
- Steroids (Cushing's syndrome and steroid therapy).
- Systemic lupus erythematosus.
- Occlusive vascular disease.
- Diabetes mellitus.
- Hyperlipidaemia.
- Liver disease (fatty liver, hepatitis, carbon tetrachloride poisoning).
- Gaucher's disease.
- Gout.
- Rheumatoid arthritis.
- Polycythaemia/marrow hyperplasia.
- Haemoglobinopathies (especially sickle cell).
- Sarcoidosis.
- Syphilis.
- Syringomyelia.

- Specific bone necrosis (Perthe's, Kienbock's, Freiberg's and Kohler's diseases).
- Radiotherapy.

The exact mechanism of the production of bone necrosis in association with hyperbaric exposure has not been fully elucidated. The most widely held belief is that it is due to the decompression phase and represents a delayed or long-term manifestation of **decompression sickness** (DCS). There is a definite relationship between dysbaric osteonecrosis and exposure to inadequate decompression, experimental diving and clinical decompression sickness.

There are, however, numerous variations on this theme. One theory is that the infarction is caused by **arterial gas emboli** produced during decompression. Certainly, 'silent' bubbles can be detected by Doppler techniques during clinically apparently safe decompression schedules. Several series show a relationship to either type 1 DCS or total DCS rather than type 2 (serious) DCS which are, perhaps, more likely to be associated with intra-arterial bubbles. There is also a relationship with 'inadequate' decompression and experimental diving.

Others propose that large amounts of nitrogen are taken up by the fat in bone marrow during longer pressure exposures. During or after decompression, gas is liberated from this fatty tissue and its expansion interferes with blood supply within the non-compliant bony tissue. Bubbles have been found in the large venous sinusoids in animal experiments on DCS at post mortem, and may well have obstructed venous outflow from marrow, leading to areas of infarction. Bubble formation within bony lacunae is also possible following decompression with destruction of osteocytes.

Changes secondary to intravascular bubbles, be they arterial or venous, may then take place – such as platelet clumping and intravascular coagulation causing further **vascular obstruction**. This is supported by the post-dive observation of increased platelet adhesiveness and decreased platelet count after certain dive profiles.

There may be a critical period of bone ischaemia after which pathological changes become irreversible. This may help to explain the somewhat 'hit or miss' nature of this disease.

It is possible that a number of factors may combine to produce necrosis in a given situation and that the aetiology is complex and multifactorial. Experimental evidence is available to suggest that both intravascular and extravascular aetiologies are consistent with the bone pathology, but a direct cause-and-effect relationship has not been proven. The 'silent bubbles', i.e. asymptomatic bubbles during or after decompression, are incriminated in those divers who have had neither DCS nor exposure to hazardous diving practices.

Other theories have been suggested to explain the pathogenesis of bone necrosis. Fat embolism, similar to the mechanisms described for other causes of aseptic necrosis, has also been postulated for dysbaric disease. It is thought that gas (nitrogen) bubbles may disrupt fatty tissue in marrow or elsewhere leading to intraosseous vascular occlusion, either directly or by the initiation of platelet aggregation and intravascular coagulation.

All embolism theories (gas, fat or other) do not adequately explain why other tissues do not appear to be embolized, and why the femur and upper end of the humerus are particularly affected.

**Oxygen toxicity** is another possible cause for dysbaric osteonecrosis. Several mechanisms have been postulated. One suggests that the local vasospastic reaction to high oxygen pressures leads to ischaemia. High oxygen pressures have been shown to cause swelling of fat cells, which may produce increased intramedullary pressure and ischaemia or, if insufficient to obstruct blood flow completely, could inhibit the clearance of gas from the marrow during decompression.

**Raised intramedullary pressure**, reported in aseptic necrosis areas in patients who had received high-dose steroid therapy, is also thought by some to be involved in the aetiology of dysbaric osteonecrosis. This latter concept, if proven correct, would have important implications regarding early active therapy.

An **osmotic** aetiology has also been suggested, incriminating the movement of water into or out of the bone, due to differential gas concentrations causing osmosis. Rapid pressure changes, especially during compression, are thought to be responsible for the large gas gradients. During the compression phase, a gradient exists for all inspired gases across the capillary wall, with the higher partial pressure on the intravascular side. Water would then move into the vascular compartment, and such water movements within the rigid bone structure are thought to lead to local bone ischaemia.

> *Dysbaric osteonecrosis is thought to be a long-term effect of inadequate decompression, i.e. decompression sickness.*

Various animal models have been developed to study the aetiology of dysbaric osteonecrosis because of the obvious difficulties in early detection and monitoring of such a capricious and chronic disease. A great deal of current research thus involves the experimental induction of bone necrosis in animals such as mini pigs and mice, but it is difficult to be convinced that these lesions are strictly comparable to those of divers and caisson workers. They nevertheless produce a model whereby pathophysiological, biochemical and radiological features may be correlated.

Any theory must account for the following observations:

1. Dysbaric osteonecrosis may follow a single exposure to pressure.
2. Although there appears to be a relationship between decompression sickness and dysbaric osteonecrosis, not all divers with dysbaric osteonecrosis have a history of decompression sickness.
3. Not all divers who suffer decompression sickness develop dysbaric osteonecrosis.
4. Not all divers at high risk develop dysbaric osteonecrosis.

The importance of establishing the mechanisms involved lies in the development of effective methods of both prevention and treatment.

## Pathophysiology

When examined histologically, the area of necrosis is usually much more widespread than evident radiologically. Necrosis is first recognized histologically by the absence of osteocytes in the bone lacunae. This probably starts within a few hours of infarction.

Revascularization then commences from areas of viable bone to form an area of vascular granulation tissue which extends into the infarcted area. Necrotic trabeculae are effectively thickened and strengthened by this new growth, and some lesions even disappear. The revascularization may be arrested before all areas of necrosis have been invaded. Continuing formation of new bone forms a zone of thickened trabeculae separated from necrotic bone by a line of dead collagen. This area of increased bone bulk is the first sign seen radiologically.

The necrotic trabeculae, not strengthened by the revascularization process, may eventually collapse under a load. It is at this stage that clinical symptoms, not necessarily related to recent hyperbaric exposure, may be noted. With lesions near articular cartilage, there is some flattening of the articular surface and, with further load stress, fractures appear in the subchondral bone. The underlying necrosis causes a progressive detachment of the articular surface from its bed. This process resembles that of late segmental collapse, as seen in ischaemic necrosis following fractures of the neck of the femur. Secondary degenerative osteoarthritis often develops in affected joints.

Cases of malignant fibrous histiocytoma, superimposed on dysbaric osteonecrosis, may develop in conjunction with the prolonged reparative process set in train by the necrosis.

## Clinical features

There may be a history of decompression sickness or repeated inadequate decompression leading to further investigation of diving-related pathology. Early lesions are usually asymptomatic and may currently be detected only by bone scintigraphy or radiological examination. However, there are reports of symptoms of persistent pain related to a joint prior to the development of X-ray changes.

Symptoms of pain and restricted joint movement, usually affecting the hip or shoulder joint, may develop insidiously over months or years and are due to secondary degenerative osteoarthritic changes.

Occasional atypical cases seem to have pain in the area of necrosis dating from the decompression sickness incident, with scintigraphic verification.

An increase of 50% in the total mineral content of the bone is necessary before it can be recognized as an area of increased density on the X-ray, and these changes may take 3–6 months from the time of initial insult. Radioactive isotope bone scans and magnetic resonance imaging (MRI) are proving useful in much earlier diagnosis.

> *X-ray lesions are usually found in the large long bones of the upper and lower limbs. These may be subdivided into juxta-articular, or head, neck and shaft lesions.*

There are two major sites for the lesions, separated because of the prognostic implications, which may be present alone or in combination. The lesions are classified as juxta-articular lesions and head, neck and shaft lesions.

### Juxta-articular lesions

These are also referred to as joint lesions or A lesions. These may cause symptoms and are potentially disabling. They are near weight-bearing joints where constant pressure is exerted, and may eventually result in collapse of the joint. The most common sites are the hips and shoulders. They predominate in caisson workers and divers working in undisciplined or experimental conditions. It has rarely been reported in other joints, e.g. the ankle.

### Head, neck and shaft lesions

Lesions away from the articular surface are also referred to as medullary or B lesions. They are usually asymptomatic and are seldom of orthopaedic significance. The most common sites are the shafts of the femur and humerus. They do not extend beyond the metaphysis or involve the cortex of the bone. The shaft is not weakened, pathological fracture being a rare complication. New bone replacement has been observed in these lesions. Their importance lies in that they may demonstrate that people with the lesions are at greater risk from further dysbaric osteonecrosis, although this has not yet been proven statistically.

In assessing the **radiological** diagnosis of these lesions, it is important to realize that the X-ray will show only a fraction of the total lesion, and that some bone necrosis areas revealed by scintigraphy (see page 210) never become apparent on the X-rays.

### Symptoms

Symptoms referable to juxta-articular lesions depend on the position and severity of the bone damage. Usually there is pain over the joint. This may be aggravated by movement and may radiate down the limb. There is often some restriction of movement, although a useful range of flexion may remain. In the shoulder, the signs are similar to those of a rotator cuff lesion, i.e. painful arc from 60° to 180° abduction with difficulty in maintaining abduction against resistance. The onset of pain may be precipitated by lifting heavy weights. Secondary degenerative osteoarthritis follows collapse of the articular cartilage, further reducing joint movement. The siting of these lesions is approximately in the ratio of femur:humerus, 1:2 to 1:3.

### Neoplasia

Malignant tumours of bone (usually fibrous histiocytoma) have been reported in cases of aseptic necrosis, many of which were asymptomatic. The risk appears greatest with large medullary lesions.

The danger of irradiation from X-rays contributing to neoplasia cannot be neglected. With good equipment and technique, the diver has one-third of the annual maximum recommended dose of body irradiation for one long bone series. This amount will increase with poor equipment, extra exposures, slower screens etc.

# Radiology and differential diagnosis

The main difficulty is in determining (1) whether the radiological lesion under examination is either a variant of normal bone structure or perhaps a minor dysplasia of bone, or (2) whether the osteonecrosis has a cause other than the dysbaric environment.

Early diagnosis is based on minor alterations in trabecular pattern of bone, resulting in abnormal densities or lucencies. Early detection of asymptomatic lesions may only be verified by serial radiological examinations, showing the progression of the lesion. As considerable skill is required in these assessments, they are best performed by independent observers from a specialized radiological panel, whose members then compare their written reports, to exclude subjective errors. This was well done in the UK where a central registry for cases and X-rays was sponsored as a government body (MRC). Lesions are classified as in Table 14.3. Such a classification is useful to compare results between different studies.

**Table 14.3 The UK MRC radiological classification of dysbaric osteonecrosis**

*A lesions (juxta-articular)*

A1 Dense areas with intact articular cortex
A2 Spherical opacities
A3 Linear opacities
A4 Structural failures
    a Translucent subcortical band
    b Collapse of articular cortex
    c Sequestration of cortex
A5 Secondary degenerative osteoarthritis

*B lesions (head, neck and shaft)*

B1 Dense areas
B2 Irregular calcified areas
B3 Translucent and cystic areas

The first decision to make is whether the bone is normal. Cysts and areas of sclerosis occur widely and sporadically in other diseases. Chance cortical bone defects must be eliminated and recognition of the normal **bone islands** is essential. These are dense areas of bone within the cancellous bone structure, but which are sharply defined, round or oval, with the long axis running parallel to the long bone, usually towards the ends of the bone. They have a normal trabecular pattern around them and have no clinical significance. They are thought to develop early in life. It was once believed that bone islands occurred more frequently in subjects exposed to hyperbaric environments, but this is no longer believed to be so.

Causes of radiological anomaly which may cause confusion in diagnosis include:

1. **Bone islands** (as above).
2. **Enchondroma** and other innocent tumours: these may calcify causing an opacity in the shaft of the long bone. Medullary osteochondroma may show foci of calcification which are more circular, whorled and in closer apposition than the foci of calcification of dysbaric osteonecrosis.
3. **Normal variants**: these include sesamoid bones, the shadow of the linea aspera and its endosteal crest.
4. **Osteoarthritis**: osteoarthritis, unassociated with juxta-articular dysbaric osteonecrosis, usually has a reduction of the joint space, with sclerosis of the underlying bone on both sides of the joint. In dysbaric osteonecrosis, the cartilage space is not narrowed unless osteoarthritis has supervened.

**Other causes of osteonecrosis**, not due to dysbaric exposure, must be excluded (see page 200). Both the radiological features and medical history are important in establishing the diagnosis. They should be rare in a fit, active diving population who had undergone medical assessment (see Chapter 35). Among the more important causes are:

1. **Trauma**: a history and its localization to one area may be relevant, but it has also been reported remote from multiple fractures.
2. **Alcohol:** a history of heavy consumption or other organ damage may be obtained.
3. **Steroid therapy**: the likelihood of this increases with the increased dose of steroid, the minimum being 10 mg prednisone or its equivalent per day for 30 days. Short courses of high-dose 'pulse' therapy have also been incriminated. It is especially noted with rhematoid arthritis, renal transplantation and asthma.

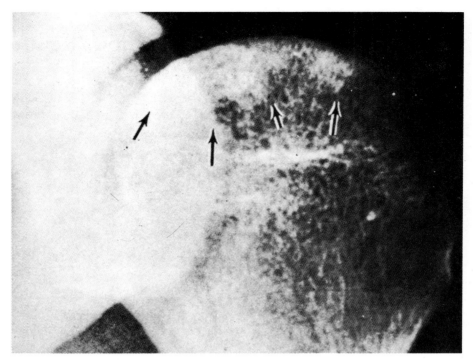

**Figure 14.1** A1 lesions: *dense areas*, with intact articular cortex. At the top of the humerus are two areas where the trabecular pattern is blurred. The edge of the cortex looks 'woolly'. These changes represent what Miles refers to as a wedge *infarct*

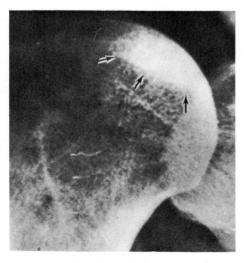

**Figure 14.2** A2 lesion: *spherical segmental opacity*. Originally called *snowcap lesion*, it may remain symptomless

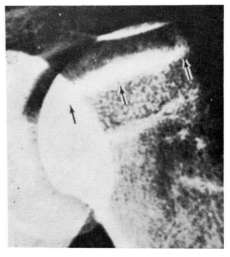

**Figure 14.3** A3 lesion: *linear opacity*. The dense line marked with arrows represents the lesion. The extremities of such linear opacities characteristically extend to the cortical margin

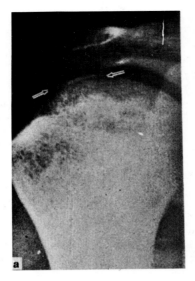
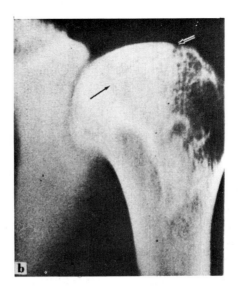

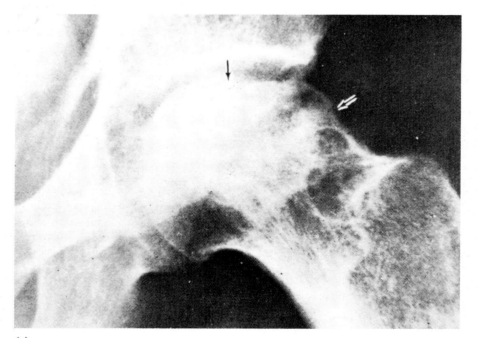

(c)

**Figure 14.4** A4 lesion: *structural failures*. (a) *Translucent subcortical band:* this lesion (between arrows) is sometimes called a *crescent sign*. Situated just under the articular cortical surface, the translucent line indicates that a sliver of the cortical surface is about to detach. (b) *Collapse of the articular cortex* or *subchondral depression*: tomogram shows a fracture line (arrows) developing between the sclerotic part of the bone above, which is being depressed into the humeral head, and surrounding bone cortex. (c) *Sequestration of the cortex:* a loose piece of dead articular cortex has been pushed into the body of the femoral head, causing the latter to appear flattened (arrows)

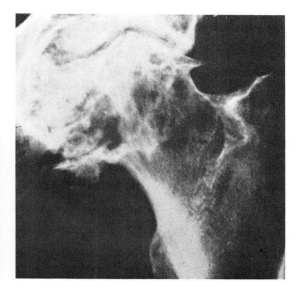

**Figure 14.5** A5 lesion: *osteoarthritis*. This condition can supervene on any lesion in which disruption of the articular surface has occurred. In ostenecrosis, the cartilage often remains viable so that a joint space of reasonable size often continues to be radiologically visible despite signs of severe osteoarthritis. The cartilage seems to persist even longer in caisson disease than in similar osteopathic conditions

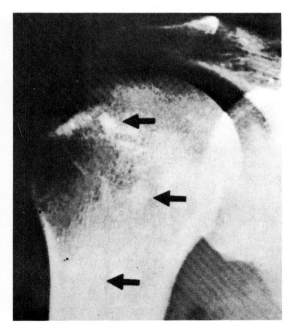

**Figure 14.6** B1 lesion: *dense areas*. These areas can be seen just at and below the junction of the humeral head and shaft. They are typical of the ostenecrotic lesions seen in such sites, and it is unlikely that they will ever cause disability

4. **Haemoglobinopathies**, sickle-cell anaemia, thalassaemia and other variants. Diagnosis is made by haematological investigations and by demonstrating lesions in the spine and skull.

5. **Specific bone diseases** – such as Perthe's disease (idiopathic aseptic necrosis affecting children), Kienbock's disease (spontaneous avascular necrosis of the carpal lunate), Freiberg's disease (second metatarsal, head). The osteochondroses of epiphyseal heads, such as Perthe's disease (hip) and Kohlers' disease (tarsal scaphoid), have specific age and clinical parameters.

6. **Systemic lupus erythematosus** is associated with a very high incidence of osteonecrosis of the hip, both with and without steroid therapy.

7. **Pancreatitis** and other pancreatic disorders.

8. **Radiotherapy** and radium therapy, leading to radiation necrosis.

9. Diseases of **lipid metabolism** or the liver: these include Gaucher's disease, fatty liver, carbon tetrachloride poisoning, hyperlipidaemia, diabetes etc.

10. Spontaneous or **idiopathic** avascular necrosis.

11. Other diseases, e.g. rheumatoid arthritis, gout, neurosyphilis, syringomyelia, alkaptonuria and arteriosclerosis.

The initial diagnosis of dysbaric osteonecrosis must be reasonably certain because it has serious implications to the professional diver. Solitary lesions especially require careful assessment, whereas multiple lesions make the diagnosis easier.

The radiological changes are relatively late manifestations. The first radiological signs may be noted within 3–6 months, but may take much longer – even years. The density usually increases, due to an overall increase in the amount of calcification present. Apparently, as a result of the reactive changes to the presence of dead tissue, new bone is laid down on the surface of the dead bone.

The pathological lesion may never produce radiological changes. Autopsy cases reveal that the pathological areas are often far more extensive than the radiological demarcation. Diagnostic radiological parameters include the following.

### Juxta-articular lesions (A lesions)

1. Dense areas with intact cortex (usually humeral head).
2. Spherical opacities (often segmental in humeral head)
3. Linear opacities (usually humeral head).
4. Structural failure showing as transradiant or translucent subcortical bands (especially in heads of femur and humerus), and often collapse of articular cortex with sequestration.
5. Secondary degenerative arthritis with osteophyte formation.

There is usually no narrowing of the joint spaces until later stages.

These lesions appear to be quite different from other causes of avascular necrosis.

### Head, neck and shaft lesions (B lesions)

1. Dense areas, usually multiple and often bilateral, commonly in the neck and proximal shaft of the femur and humerus. These must be distinguished from normal 'bone islands'.
2. Irregular calcified areas in the medulla. These are commonly seen in the distal femur, proximal tibia and the proximal humerus. They may be bilateral.
3. Translucent areas and cysts, best seen in tomograms of the head and neck of the humerus and femur.
4. Cortical thickening.

Emphasis is on minor variations of trabecular structure, and special radiographic techniques combined with skilled interpretation are required. Cylinder cone and tomography may be used. Computed tomography or bone scintigraphy may clarify a questionable area.

---

*Dysbaric osteonecrosis and pregnancy have certain features in common: there may be no awareness of the condition until it is too late; there is sometimes a degree of doubt regarding the aetiology; it cannot be detected radiographically until 3 months after the causal incident (and radiology is not a harmless procedure); it is feared much more than experienced; and precautionary techniques usually, but not always, work.*

---

## Other investigations

The value of the plain X-ray in early diagnosis is being questioned and other imaging techniques are being increasingly used.

### Bone scintigraphy ('bone scans')

This now has an established role in the early detection of bony reaction to osteonecrosis, before they are seen on X-rays. Any lesion which stimulates bone formation will be shown up as a 'hot spot' by the radioactive bone-seeking tracer, on the scintigram. [99m]Tc-labelled Osteoscan or [99m]Tc-labelled methylene diphosphonate (MDP) may be injected intravenously and serially imaged with a gamma camera. Following up the scintigraphy 'lesions' produced in animals as early as 2–3 weeks after decompression, with autopsy 3 months after the event, show that these lesions have a pathological counterpart of necrotic bone with osteogenesis – even though X-ray changes still had not developed in most cases.

Similar findings in humans with biopsy or radiological follow-up indicate that the 'hot spots' occur far earlier and are more numerous than the radiological changes. These 'hot spots' may resolve with no apparent changes radiologically or may disappear despite classic radiological disease.

Bone scintigraphy in early lesions is thus much more sensitive than radiology but has a low specificity, as any bone reparative reaction will be detected, no matter what the cause.

### Single position emission computed tomography (SPECT)

This is said to improve specificity, as sections can be obtained in three planes thus eliminating over- or underlying activity in a specific plane of reference. 'Cold' areas occurring immediately after occlusion of blood supply may be detected. SPECT can be performed immediately after the bone scan. It thus does not increase the radiation dose.

---

*Imaging techniques*
- *Plain radiography*
- *Scintigraphy*
- *Computed tomography*
- *Magnetic resonance*

---

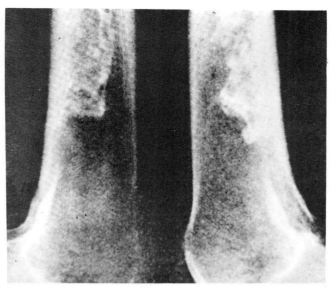

**Figure 14.7** B2 lesion: *irregular calcified areas*. This condition is commonly seen in divers. Sometimes the appearance is that of rather foamy areas in the medulla at the lower end of the femur, often with a calcified margin. Sometimes femoral lesions have a hardish scalloped edge around a translucent area. Endosteal thickening frequently accompanies these lesions.

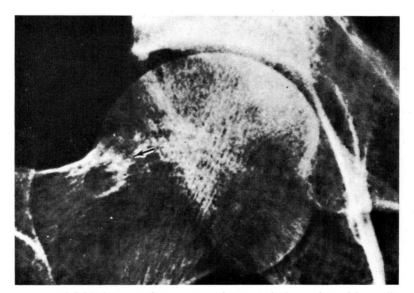

**Figure 14.8** B3 lesions: *translucent areas and cysts*. A single cyst (arrow) is usually seen in the femoral neck. Sometimes a line of small cysts appears at the point where the hip-joint capsule attaches to the femoral neck. These irregularities may also be found at the junction of the shoulder-joint capsule and humeral neck. Some believe that these multiple lesions are not osteonecrotic, but, rather, that they relate to past damage at the point of a capsule's insertion into the neck of a bone

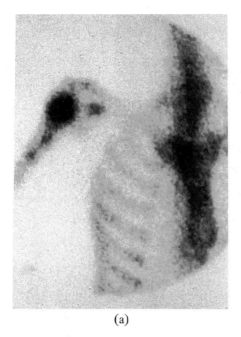

(a)

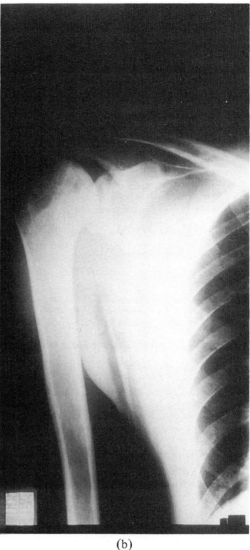

(b)

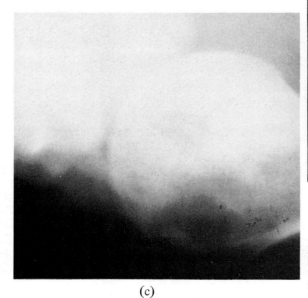

(c)

**Figure 14.9** (a) Qualitative scintigram using $^{99m}$Tc-labelled methylene diphosphonate (MDP) which shows a 'hot spot', i.e. increased concentration of technetium with increased up-take of MDP, in the right shoulder of a 38-year-old diver who had done a lot of deep bounce dives on Heliox. The great majority of these were experimental dives, although he has never had treatment for DCS and would only admit to the odd minor discomfort in a variety of joints after dives. Routine screening X-rays at this time showed a normal shoulder. (b) X-ray of the right shoulder 4 months after first scan. (c) Tomogram showing an A lesion under the articular surface. (Photographs courtesy of Dr Ramsay Pearson)

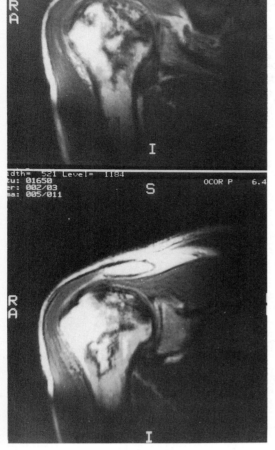

dth= 521 Level= 1184
tu: 01650
er: 002/03
ha: 005/011                    OCOR P    6.4

**Figure 14.10** MRI of right shoulder: on these slightly 'T1 weighted' images there is evidence of marked distortion of the marrow signal with areas of necrosis indicated by the dark signal. There is also cortical irregularity. This process involves the articular surface of the glenohumeral joint

## Computed tomography (CT)

This gives greater definition revealing both structural collapse and areas of new growth. CT scans may help in the diagnosis of early or doubtful changes on plain X-rays. It is essential if some of the surgical techniques, such as rotational osteotomy, are being contemplated.

## Magnetic resonance imaging (MRI)

This can detect necrosis of marrow fat within 2–4 days of the ischaemic episode and thus offers the best opportunity for early diagnosis.

MRI studies may indicate far greater necrosis than conventional plain radiography. MRI changes are not yet fully documented and the expensive equipment is not readily available.

It is possible that, with more experience of bone scintigraphy and MRI, treatment with surgery, hyperbaric oxygenation or other methods may be instituted within days of the lesions being provoked, in order to avoid the progression of the disease. This, however, remains experimental at this stage.

## Invasive investigations

Invasion investigations have been undertaken to aid in earlier diagnosis, and guide to therapeutic intervention.

These techniques include arteriography, intraosseous phlebography, intramedullary pressure measurement and core biopsy. The latter three are often combined in a technique described by Ficat as functional exploration of bone.

### *Arteriography*

This is generally non-contributory in investigating osteonecrosis, although selective, medial, circumflex, femoral artery catherization, with digital subtraction angiography, has demonstrated arterial occlusion in the early stages.

### *Functional exploration of bone*

This requires regional or general anaesthesia. The injection of contrast medium into a femoral head with osteonecrosis present is said to be extremely painful. Although some claim that intramedullary pressure elevation is an indication of osteonecrosis, others report a wide range of normal values.

## Prevention

**Early recognition** is imperative, and the following routine investigations are recommended for all professional divers exposed to frequent hyperbaric conditions at depths greater than 15 metres:

1. Baseline long bone X-ray and, if possible, bone scintigraphy examinations.
2. CT examination in doubtful plain X-ray findings, or to define extent of lesions.
3. Bone scintigraphy for any minor arthralgia or bursitis.
4. X-ray examination (baseline) and bone scintigraphy 1–2 weeks after DCS.
5. X-ray examination 6 months after decompression sickness.
6. MRI (if available) of demonstrated or suspected tensions.

**Follow-up surveillance** may be carried out by bone scintigraphy (after initial baseline X-rays). Although scintigraphy has a lower specificity, it detects changes earlier, is more sensitive and exposes the diver to less radiation. Follow-up long bone X-rays may be required if scintigraphy is not available.

The disease is rare in recreational scuba divers who follow decompression tables and use only compressed air to depths less than 50 metres. For these groups, unless there is a specific cause for concern, serial radiological investigation is certainly not warranted, because of the unnecessary irradiation hazards and expense.

The problem of what to do when confronted with an asymptomatic B lesion is not yet solved. If the B lesion is thought to be provoked by non-adherence to established diving tables, these should clearly be followed in the future. Under these conditions, it is assumed that the B lesion is induced because of excessive provocation. If the diver has adhered to normal decompression tables, then it is presumed that he is particularly predisposed to dysbaric osteonecrosis, and diving should be restricted to shallow depths. For example, the Royal Australian Navy restricts these divers to non-decompression dives, to a maximum depth of 18 metres, reduced duration and slower ascent rates. It is generally accepted that the need for decompression should be avoided, as should experimental or helium diving. Doubtful cases should be treated as if positive, until further radiological assessment clarifies the issue.

If a juxta-articular lesion is present, all exposure to compression should cease, although some authorities still permit diving with 100% oxygen. Such a patient should also avoid heavy work and sporting activities that may put unnecessary stress on the joint.

# Treatment

Although healing is seen histologically, the possibility of resolution of radiologically positive asymptomatic lesions is controversial. There is at least one case of aseptic necrosis of the hip (which may have been diving and/or steroid induced), which resolved symptomatically and showed MRI improvement with a long course of hyperbaric oxygen therapy. Nevertheless, the treatment of juxta-articular (A) lesions should be based on the fact that dysbaric osteonecrosis often progresses through the stages outlined below. The asymptomatic head, neck and shaft lesions require no active therapy.

## Surgical treatment

Surgical treatment of disabling aseptic osteonecrosis must be based on the aetiology, which may have a rational basis in dysbaric osteonecrosis, that is obviously absent in idiopathic disease. It should be borne in mind that attempts at curative treatment relate to idiopathic osteonecrosis. It is not known if extrapolation of that experience to dysbaric osteonecrosis is valid.

The majority of experience is with idiopathic osteonecrosis of the femoral head – the site at which osteonecrosis produced the most devastating disability, and also the most common site. Some procedures may also be applicable to the shoulder joint.

The type of treatment is determined by the staging of the disease process (as described by Ficat), the age of the patient and the joints involved.

## Staging

0 Asymptomatic, pre-radiological (i.e. high index of suspicion confirmed by raised intramedullary pressure or positive scan)
1 Symptomatic, pre-radiological
2 Symptomatic, radiological pre-destruction
3 Collapse of articular surface
4 Destruction of joint

## Curative treatment

### Core decompression

This has its advocates, but the value of the procedure is still questionable. If accepted, it is indicated for stage 0–2. The results are, as expected, better for the earliest stages.

### Vascularized fibular graft

This has been used for stage 0–2 disease, mainly that affecting the hip. The results are not known.

## Reconstructive treatment

When gross damage to the articular surfaces exists, reconstructive techniques offer the best chance of rehabilitation.

1. **Osteotomy** of the femoral neck, either rotation or wedge, endeavours to move the weight-bearing axis away from a localized necrotic area.
2. **Arthrodesis** is possible for a young patient, with destruction of one hip only.
3. **Arthroplasty** is indicated for 'end-stage' joints especially if the patient is old or the disease is bilateral. Total joint replacement has proved useful in replacing severely affected hip and shoulder joints. The concern about this form of surgery is that the life of the prosthesis is unknown as it is employed in a relatively young population with a long life expectancy.

# Radiological technique

1. Good definition of the trabecular structure of the bone is important.
2. The gonads must be protected from ionizing radiation in young divers by the use of a lead shield, although this may hinder interpretation.
3. The following projections are required:
   (a) an anteroposterial projection of each shoulder joint. A 30 × 25 cm film is recommended. The patient is placed in a supine position with the trunk rotated at an angle of approximately 45° to bring the shoulder to be radiographed in contact with the table. This arm is par-

tially abducted and the elbow is flexed. Centre 2.5 cm below the coracoid process of the scapula, and cone to show as much humerus as possible, bringing in the lateral diaphragms to show only the head and shaft of the humerus. This view should show a clear joint space, and the acromion should not overlap the head of the humerus;
   (b) an anteroposterior projection of each hip joint. A 30 × 25 cm film is recommended. The patient is placed in a supine position with the feet at 90° to the table top. The edge of the gonad protector should be as near the femoral head as possible, but not in any way obscuring it. Centre the cone over the head of the femur, i.e. 2.5 cm below the midpoint of a line joining the anterior, superior iliac spine and the upper border of the pubic symphysis;
   (c) an anteroposterior and lateral projection of each knee. An 18 × 43 cm film is recommended. Centre at the level of the upper border of the patella. The field should include the lower third of the femur and the upper third of the tibia and fibula.

# Acknowledgements

The authors are grateful to Drs S. Ruff and E. Murrell, of the Department of Orthopaedics, Royal North Shore Hospital, Sydney, for helpful advice in the preparation of this chapter. They also wish to acknowledge the Medical Research Council Decompression Sickness Panel, Professor Dennis Walder, University of Newcastle upon Tyne, Dr Ramsay Pearson of the Royal Navy, and Dr Greg Briggs of the Department of Radiology, Royal North Shore Hospital, Sydney, for permission to use the various illustrations.

# Recommended reading and references

CALDER, I.M. (1982). Bone and joint diseases in workers exposed to hyperbaric conditions. In: *Current Topics in Pathology*, edited by C.L. Berry. Heidelberg: Springer-Verlag.

CHRYSSANTHOU, C.P. (1978). Dysbaric osteonecrosis. *Clinical Orthopaedics and Related Research* **130**, 94–106.

DAVIDSON, J.K. (1989). Dysbaric disorders: aseptic bone necrosis in tunnel workers and divers. *Baillière's Clinical Rheumatology* **3**, 1–23.

DAVIDSON, J.K., HARRISON, J.A.B., JACOBS, P., HILDITCH, T.E., CATTO, M. and HENDRY, W.T. (1977). The significance of bone islands, cystic areas and sclerotic areas in dysbaric osteonecrosis. *Clinical Radiology* **28**, 381–393.

FICAT, R.P. (1985). Idiopathic bone necrosis of the femoral head. Early diagnosis and treatment. *Journal of Bone and Joint Surgery* **67B**, 3–9.

KAWASHIMA, M. and TAMURA, H. (1983). Osteonecrosis in divers – prevention and treatment. In: *Hyperbaric Medicine and Underwater Physiology*, edited by K. Shiraki and S. Matsuoka, Proceedings of IIIrd International Symposium of UOEH on Hyperbaric Medicine and Underwater Physiology (III UOEH Symposium).

KENZORA, J.E. (Ed.) (1985). Symposium on Idiopathic Osteonecrosis, October 1985. *Orthopedic Clinics of North America*.

KUIPERS, R.M., SCHARDIJIN, G.H.C, AGENANT, D.M.A., HOEFNAGEL, C.A. and HAMELYNCK, K.J. (1985). Early detection and treatment of avascular necrosis in divers. *Proceedings of European Undersea Biomedical Society meeting*, Göteborg.

LOWRY, C.J., TRAUGOTT, F.M. and JONES, M.W. (1986). Dysbaric osteonecrosis – a survey of abalone divers. In: *The Abalone Diver*, edited by C. Edmonds, pp. 50–62. Diving Medical Centre/National Safety Council of Australia Publication.

NEBAUER, R.A., KOGEN, R.L. and GOTTLIEB, S.T. (1989). Use of hyperbaric oxygen for treatment of aseptic bone necrosis. A case study. *Journal of Hyperbaric Medicine* **4**, 69–76.

TWYNAM, G.E. (1888). A Case of Caisson Disease. *British Medical Journal* **1**, 190–191.

WILLIAMS, E.S., KHREISAT, S., ELL, P.J. and KING, J.D. (1987). Bone imaging and skeletal radiology in dysbaric osteonecrosis. *Clinical Radiology* **38**, 589–592.

# 15

# Inert gas narcosis

## Introduction

Inert gas narcosis (IGN) refers to a clinical syndrome characterized by impairment of intellectual and neuromuscular performance and changes in mood and behaviour. It is produced by an increased partial pressure of inert gas. In compressed air exposure, these changes, which have been observed for over 100 years, are now known to be largely due to nitrogen. The effects are progressive with increasing depth but not with increasing time at the same depth. The word 'inert' indicates that these gases exert their effect without undergoing chemical change in the body, rather than inert gas in the physiological sense.

Similar effects have been described with other metabolically inactive gases such as the rare gases (neon, argon, krypton, xenon), hydrogen and the anaesthetic gases, although at different partial pressures. Xenon is 'anaesthetic' at sea level, but no narcotic effect due to helium has been demonstrated at currently attainable pressures. Inert gas narcosis may be considered as a state of impending general anaesthesia.

The 'inert' gas in compressed air is nitrogen and its effects are also called nitrogen narcosis, depth intoxication, 'narks', rapture of the deep (*l'ivresse des grandes profondeurs*), the latter term coined by Cousteau. The narcosis due to nitrogen places a depth limit to safe diving with compressed air at approximately 40–50 metres. Effective work at greater depth requires the substitution of a less narcotic respiratory diluent such as helium or hydrogen.

Unless otherwise indicated, the 'inert gas' is regarded as nitrogen, so that in compressed air exposure, the terms 'inert gas narcosis' and 'nitrogen narcosis' are interchangeable.

---

*Inert gas narcosis: depth intoxication; rapture of the deep; 'narks'; l'ivresse des grandes profondeurs; nitrogen narcosis.*

---

## History

The first recorded description of symptoms suggestive of air intoxication and related to hyperbaric exposure was by a Frenchman, Junod, in 1835, who reported 'thoughts have a peculiar charm and in some persons, symptoms of intoxication are present'. He was conducting research into the physiological effects of compression and rarefaction of air. J.B. Green in 1861 observed sleepiness, impaired judgement and hallucinations in divers breathing com-

---

### CASE REPORT 15.1

**Descriptions of divers about their experiences at between 250 and 300 ft – reported by Hill and Phillips (1932)**

'You notice the dark more although it may not be darker; the light is a comfort and company. You notice things more if there is nothing to do; I get comfort from seeing the fish, it takes your mind off everything else.'

When asked for a description, an old hand at diving gave the following account: 'You have to be more careful in deep water; in deep water you know that you are concentrating.' He described how you think of each heave as you turn a spanner. He said: 'If you go down with a set purpose it becomes an obsession; it will become the main thing and you will forget everything else.' He described how he thinks very deliberately; he says, 'I have finished my job, what shall I do next? – of course, I have finished and now I must go up'. He described how he was aware of every action: 'If my hand goes out I think of my hand going out.' He gave the following as an analogy: 'If I saw a thing of value, say half-a-crown, in the street, I would pick it up. Down below I would look at it and think, "What is that, shall I pick it up? Yes, I will pick it up" and then I feel my hand go out.'

'I left the ladder determined to get to the bottom; at 250 feet. I got a recurrence of the tingling and a feeling of lying on my back. I decided to rest a couple of minutes and then go on. I slid 10 feet and felt I was going unconscious. I made signals to be pulled up and kept repeating them. I lost the use of my limbs and let go everything. While hanging on to the rope I saw my own face in the front glass; it was outside the glass and looked all greenish; I was dressed in my shore-going suit. I heard the order, "Pull the diver up", again and again, as if someone in the suit was saying it. When I got to the DSDC I did not appreciate the oxygen as usual, I wanted fresh air.'

'Suddenly I came over rather "funny"; it was a distinct "different" feeling; I stood up, the tank wire in my right hand, and thinking it was a touch of $CO_2$, I began to breathe deep and hearty, thinking of course that in a couple of minutes I would be able to resume work. Then I seemed to go quite limp, a feeling of "no life or energy"; this was new and strange to me, whether it was a part of $CO_2$, I didn't know, because I had never experienced a real dose of $CO_2$; anyhow, after stopping and doing the drill for $CO_2$ I thought I would be alright, but suddenly something definitely seemed to – say – snap inside my head and I started to, what I thought, go mad at things.'

**Description of interview of above diver after an aborted deep dive**

Practically no hypnoidal effort was required to produce the horrors of that morning's dive, and the picture of stark, mad terror . . . . left an impression which is very difficult to describe. The impression was of sitting in the stalls and watching the acting of Grand Guignol. To such a pitch did he arouse his emotions that he clawed his face to remove the imaginary face-glass and tore his clothes which he mistook for his diving suit.

pressed air at 5.8 ATA, sufficient to warrant an immediate return to the surface. Paul Bert, in 1878, also noted that divers became intoxicated at great depth. In 1903, Hill and McLeod described impairment of intellectual functioning in caisson workers at 5.5 ATA pressure. Damant, in 1930, likened the mental abnormalities and memory defects observed in men at 10 ATA to alcoholic intoxication and postulated that it was caused by the high partial pressure of oxygen.

Hill and Phillips, in 1932, suggested that the effects may be psychological due to claustrophobia or perhaps due to impurities in the air from the compressors.

The Royal Navy appointed a committee to investigate the problems of deep diving and submarine escape, and their report in 1933 contained a section entitled 'semi-loss of consciousness'. Between 7 and 11.6 ATA divers answered hand signals but in many cases failed to obey them. After return to surface, they could not remember the events of the dive. It was noted that all divers regained full consciousness during the return to 1 ATA. The report also noted great individual variation in divers' reactions, but was unable to elucidate the problem.

It was not until 1935 that Behnke, Thomson and Motley proposed the now generally held theory of the cause of this compressed air intoxication. They stated that the narcosis was due to the raised partial pressure of the metabolically inactive gas, nitrogen. At a depth of 30 metres (4 ATA), compressed air produced a state of 'euphoria, retardation of the higher mental processes and impaired neuromuscular co-ordination'. This effect was progressive with increasing pressure so that at 10 ATA stupefaction resulted. Unconsciousness developed between 10 and 15 ATA. They also invoked the Meyer–Overton hypothesis to relate the narcotic effect to the high ratio of solubility of nitrogen in oil to water.

It was not long after this major breakthrough that Behnke and Yarbrough reported that the substitution of helium for the nitrogen in compressed air eliminated that narcosis.

The nitrogen partial pressure theory was not universally accepted. The 1933 Deep Diving Committee Report raised the possibility of carbon dioxide retention being implicated. Case and Haldane, in 1941, reported that the addition of carbon dioxide to compressed air worsened the mental symptoms, although up to 6% concentrations at 1 ATA had little mental effect. Bean, in 1947, demonstrated a reduction in arterial pH during compression and later also showed increased alveolar carbon dioxide concentrations. He explained these changes as being due to reduced diffusion of carbon dioxide in the increased density of the air. He postulated that carbon dioxide was an alternative cause of the depth narcosis. He was later supported by Seusing and Drube in 1961. Buhlmann (1961) felt that increased airway resistance led to hypoventilation and hypercapnia.

Rashbass (1955) and Cabarrou (1959) have refuted the carbon dioxide theory observing signs of narcosis despite methods to ensure normal alveolar carbon dioxide levels. Later work (Hesser, Adolfson and Fagaeus) showed that the effects of nitrogen and carbon dioxide are additive in impairing performance. Normal arterial carbon dioxide and oxygen levels, while breathing air and helium/oxygen at various depths, demonstrate the key role of nitrogen in the production of this disorder, and the relative insignificance of carbon dioxide. In relation to the Martini law, the carbon dioxide is analogous to the olive.

> *Martini's law: each 15 metre (50 feet) depth is equivalent to the intoxication of one Martini.*

## Clinical manifestations

Although there is marked individual variation in susceptibility to IGN, all divers breathing compressed air are significantly affected at a depth of 60–70 metres. The minimum pressure producing signs is difficult to define, but some divers are affected subjectively at less than 30 metres.

The higher functions, such as reasoning, judgement, recent memory, learning, concentration and attention are affected first. The diver may experience a feeling of well-being and stimulation similar to the overconfidence of mild alcoholic intoxication. Occasionally, the opposite reaction, terror, develops. This is more probable in the novice who is apprehensive in his new environment. Further elevation of the partial pressure of the inert gas results in impairment of manual dexterity and progressive deterioration in mental performance, automatisms, idea fixation, hallucinations and, finally, stupor and coma. Some divers complain of a restriction of peripheral visual field at depth (tunnel vision). They are less aware of potentially significant dangers outside their prescribed tasks (perceptual narrowing).

From a practical point of view, the diver may be able to focus his attention on a particular task, but his memory of what was observed or performed while at depth may be lost when reporting at the surface. Alternatively, he may have to abort his dive because of failure to remember instructions. Repetition and drills can help overcome these problems.

---

*Narcosis is aggravated by anxiety, cold, fatigue, sedatives, alcohol and other central nervous system depressant drugs.*

---

Some of the reported observations at various depths breathing compressed air are shown in Table 15.1.

The narcosis is evident within a few minutes of reaching the given depth (partial pressure) and is not progressive with time. It is said to be initially more pronounced with rapid compression (descent). The effect is rapidly reversible upon reduction of the ambient pressure (ascent).

---

*Nitrogen narcosis is characterized by:*
- *Increasing mental impairment with increasing depth*
- *Marked individual variation*
- *Effects are rapidly reversed on ascent*

---

Other factors have been observed to affect the degree of narcosis. Alcohol, fatigue, anxiety, cold, reduced sensory input, and arterial oxygen and carbon dioxide disturbances are interrelated in impairing the diver's underwater ability. In experimental conditions, with an attempt to control variables, alcohol and

**Table 15.1 Some observations on the effects of compressed air**

| Pressure (ATA) | Effects |
| --- | --- |
| 2–4 | Mild impairment of performance on unpractised tasks<br>Mild euphoria |
| 4 | Reasoning and immediate memory affected more than motor coordination and choice reactions<br>Delayed response to visual and auditory stimuli |
| 4–6 | Laughter and loquacity may be overcome by self-control<br>Idea fixation, perceptual narrowing and over-confidence<br>Calculation errors; memory impairment |
| 6 | Sleepiness; illusions; impaired judgement |
| 6–8 | Convivial group atmosphere; may be terror reaction in some; talkative; dizziness reported occasionally<br>Uncontrolled laughter approaching hysteria in some |
| 8 | Severe impairment of intellectual performance<br>Manual dexterity less affected |
| 8–10 | Gross delay in response to stimuli<br>Diminished concentration; mental confusion |
| 10 | Stupefaction<br>Severe impairment of practical activity and judgement<br>Mental abnormalities and memory defects<br>Deterioration in handwriting; uncontrollable euphoria, hyperexcitability; almost total loss of intellectual and perceptive faculties |
| > 10 | Hallucinogenic experiences<br>Unconsciousness |

hard work have been shown to enhance narcosis. Moderate exercise and amphetamines may, in certain situations, reduce narcosis. Other studies showed unpredictable or increased narcotic effects with amphetamines. Increased carbon dioxide and nitrogen tensions appear to be additive in reducing performance. Task learning and positive motivation can improve performance. Frequent or prolonged exposure produces some acclimatization, but this may, rather than true adaptation, be due to a reduction in psychological stress. A recent study (Rogers and Moeller, 1989) showed no behavioural adaptation after brief, repeated exposures to narcotic levels of hyperbaric air. However, air saturation diving allows for safer excursions to greater depths than is possible from surface-oriented diving.

> *Narcosis develops within minutes of reaching the depth and is not progressive with time.*

The pharmacological effects of drugs may be altered under pressure (see Chapter 31). Some of the more important interactions may be due to an additive effect of drugs affecting the central nervous system and IGN. Divers are therefore advised to avoid such drugs.

Direct injury to the diver due to high pressure of inert gas is unlikely at less than 10 ATA. The danger is rather a result of how the diver may react in the environment, under the narcotic influence of nitrogen. Impaired judge-

---

## CASE REPORT 15.2

### A personal description of nitrogen narcosis by Jacques Cousteau

We continue to be puzzled with the rapture of the depths, and felt that we were challenged to go deeper. Didi's deep dive in 1943 of 210 feet had made us aware of the problem, and the Group had assembled detailed reports on its deep dives. But we had only a literary knowledge of the full effects of *l'ivresse des grandes profondeurs* as it must strike lower down. In the summer of 1947 we set out to make a series of deeper penetrations.

. . . I was in good physical condition for the trial, trained fine by an active spring in the sea, and responsive ears. I entered the water holding the scrap iron in my left hand. I went down with great rapidity, with my right arm crooked around the shotline. I was oppressively conscious of the diesel generator rumble of the idle *Élie Monnier* as I wedged my head into mounting pressure. It was high noon in July, but the light soon faded. I dropped through the twilight, alone with the white rope, which stretched before me in a monotonous perspective of blank white signposts.

At 200 feet I tasted the metallic flavour of compressed nitrogen, and was instantaneously and severely struck with rapture. I closed my hand on the rope and stopped. My mind was jammed with conceited thoughts and antic joy. I struggled to fix my brain on reality, to attempt to name the colour of the sea around me. A contest took place between navy blue, aquamarine and Prussian blue. The debate would not resolve. The sole fact I could grasp was that there was no roof and no floor in the blue room. The distant purr of the diesel invaded my mind – it swelled to a giant beat, the rhythm of the world's heart.

I took the pencil and wrote on a board, 'Nitrogen has a dirty taste'. I had little impression of holding the pencil, childhood nightmares overruled my mind. I was ill in bed, terrorized with the realization that everything in the world was thick. My fingers were sausages. My tongue was a tennis ball. My lips swelled grotesquely on the mouth grip. The air was syrup. The water congealed around me as though I were smothered in aspic.

I hung stupidly on the rope. Standing aside was a smiling, jaunty man, my second self, perfectly self-contained, grinning sardonically at the wretched diver. As the

**Case report 15.2 (contd)**

seconds passed the jaunty man installed himself in my command and ordered that I unloose the rope and go on down.

I sank slowly through a period of intense visions.

Around the 264 foot board the water was suffused with an unearthly glow. I was passing from night to an imitation of dawn. What I saw as sunrise was light reflected from the floor, which had passed unimpeded through the dark transport strata above. I saw below me the weight at the end of the shotline, hanging twenty feet from the floor. I stopped at the penultimate board and looked down at the last board, five metres away, and marshalled all my resources to evaluate the situation without deluding myself. Then I went to the last board, 297 feet down.

The floor was gloomy and barren, save for morbid shells and sea urchins. I was sufficiently in control to remember that in this pressure, ten times that of the surface, any untoward physical effort was extremely dangerous. I filled my lungs slowly and signed the board. I could not write what it felt like fifty fathoms down.

I was the deepest independent diver. In my bisected brain the satisfaction was balanced by satirical self-contempt.

I dropped the scrap iron and bounded like a coiled spring, clearing two boards in the first flight. There, at 264 feet, the rapture vanished suddenly, inexplicably and entirely. I was light and sharp, one man again, enjoying the lighter air expanding in my lungs. I rose through the twilight zone at high speed and saw the surface pattern in a blaze of platinum bubbles and dancing prisms. It was impossible not to think of flying to heaven.

(From *The Silent World* by Jacques Cousteau)

---

ment can lead to an 'out-of-air' drowning sequence, with no other apparent cause of death found.

## Measurement of central nervous system effects

Although suitable and reliable indices of IGN are not yet available, the search continues. Such tests would be useful in: predicting individual susceptibility (diver selection); comparing the relative narcotic potencies of different respiratory diluents for oxygen; delineating the role of factors other than inert gas in producing depth intoxication; and monitoring the degree of impairment during practical tasks.

Attempts to quantify the effects of IGN can be roughly divided into two methods. The first is a psychological behavioural approach measuring performance on tasks such as mental arithmetic, memory, reaction time, manual dexterity. The second relies on observing a change in some neurophysiological parameter. Some representative studies will be discussed to illustrate points.

### Behavioural approach

The aspects of behaviour usually studied may be divided into three categories: **cognitive ability, reaction time** and **dexterity**. The cognitive functions are the most affected and dexterity the least. One early study measured the performances of 46 men on simple arithmetic tests; reaction time and letter cancellation were measured at pressures from 3.7 to 10 ATA. This demonstrated quantitatively the previously observed qualitative progressive deterioration with increasing pressure of compressed air. It also showed that individuals of high intelligence were less affected. The impairment was noted on arrival at the given pressure and was exacerbated by rapid compression.

Another study using simple arithmetic and tests of manual skill showed that narcosis was maximal within 2 minutes of reaching depth, and continued exposure did not result in further deterioration, but rather there was a suggestion of acclimatization. Muscular skill was much less affected than intellectual performance.

Other studies, involving reaction time, conceptual reasoning, memory and psychometric tests, showed progressive deterioration with increasing pressure.

> *Narcosis has been measured by tests of intelligence, practical neuromuscular performance, the electroencephalogram and alpha blocking, flicker fusion frequency, visual and auditory evoked responses.*

Some work on open water divers suggested a greater impairment of performance on manual tasks at depth when anxiety was present. Plasma cortisol and urinary adrenaline:noradrenaline (epinephrine:norepinephrine) excretion ratios were used to confirm the presence of anxiety noted subjectively. Divers were tested at 3 and 30 metres at a shore base and in the open sea. Intellectual functions, as assessed by memory test, sentence comprehension and simple arithmetic, showed evidence of narcosis in both 30-metre dives but the decrement was greater in the ocean dives. This may be due to the greater psychological stress in the open sea. These effects have not been reproduced in the laboratory.

Many of these tests have been criticized because the effects of motivation, experience and learning etc. are difficult to control. A card-sorting test using caisson workers showed some impairment at 2–3 ATA, especially in those who had relatively little exposure to pressure. However, with repeated testing, i.e. practice, this difference disappeared and no loss of performance was noted even deeper than 3 ATA. These experiments were repeated using 80 naval subjects at 2 ATA and 4 ATA breathing air and helium–oxygen mixtures. The only significant impairment was found at 4 ATA breathing air.

The effects of IGN on behaviour, as measured by the psychologist have been well reviewed by Fowler, Ackles and Porlier (1985). Human performance under narcosis is best explained using the 'slowed processing' model. Slowing is said to be due to decreased activation or arousal in the central nervous system, manifested by an increase in reaction time, perhaps with a fall in accuracy. Increases in arousal, such as by exercise or amphetamines, may explain improved performance. Manual dexterity is less affected than cognitive functioning because dexterity requires fewer mental operations and there is less room for cumulative slowing of mental operations (processes). Although memory loss and impaired hearing are features of narcosis, these effects are more difficult to explain (as yet) using the slowed processing model.

Studies of the subjective symptoms of narcosis have indicated that the diver can identify these symptoms and that they could relate the effect to the 'dose'. Euphoria, as described by 'carefree, cheerful' etc., is only one of these symptoms and may not always be present. Other descriptive symptoms such as 'fuzzy', 'hazy' (state of consciousness) and 'less efficient' (work capability), 'less cautious or self-controlled' (inhibitory state) may be more reliable indicators of effect on performance.

Behavioural studies have cast doubt on some traditional concepts of narcosis. True adaptation to narcosis has not been found in many performance tests. Where adaptation has been found, it is difficult to distinguish learned responses or an adaptation to the subjective symptoms as opposed to physiological tolerance. Carbon dioxide probably has additive and not synergistic effects in combination with nitrogen, and probably acts by a different mechanism. Behavioural studies have not been able, so far, to show potentiating effects on IGN of anxiety, cold, fatigue anti-motion-sickness drugs and other sedatives (except alcohol).

## Neurophysiological changes

Attempts have been made to confirm the subjective experiences and obtain objective evidence of performance decrement, with some neurophysiological parameter. The investigations included **electroencephalographic** records of subjects exposed to compressed air in chambers. Contrary to the expected findings of depression, features suggesting cortical neuronal hyperexcitability were noted at first. These included an increase in the voltage of the basal rhythm and the frequent appearance of low voltage 'spikes' elicited by stimuli which do not have this effect at 1 ATA. Experiments, in which the partial pressures of oxygen and nitrogen were controlled, showing that in compressed air these changes are due to the high oxygen partial pressure. If nitrogen–oxygen mixtures containing 0.2 ATA oxygen are breathed, these changes are absent. The depressant effects of nitrogen are then revealed. These consist of a decrease in the voltages of the basal rhythm and the appearance of low voltage theta waves.

**Blocking of electroencephalographic alpha rhythm** by mental activity can be observed in half of the population. The observation that there is an abolition of this blocking on exposure to pressure introduced the concept of 'nitrogen threshold'. It was found that the time to abolition of blocking was inversely proportional to the square of the absolute pressure ($T$ is proportional to $1/P^2$) for an individual, although there was marked variation between subjects. In some persons abolition of blocking was noted as shallow as 2.5 ATA, where no subjective narcosis was evident.

**Flicker fusion frequency** was investigated in an attempt to obtain a measurement that could be applied to the whole population. Subjects were asked to indicate when the flickering of a neon light, at a steadily increasing rate, appeared continuous. This is termed a 'critical frequency' of flicker. After a certain time at pressure, the critical frequency dropped. The same relationship, $T$ proportional to $1/P^2$, resulted.

A more direct measure of central nervous system functioning may be obtained by observing the effect of inert gas exposure on **cortical evoked potentials**. Evoked potentials are the electroencephalographic response to sensory stimuli. A depression of auditory evoked responses on exposure to hyperbaric air has been shown to correlate with the decrement in mental arithmetic performance under the same conditions. It was therefore concluded that auditory evoked response depression was an experimental measure of nitrogen narcosis. However, other work was unable to support this hypothesis and concluded that there is a complex relationship between hyperbaric oxygen, nitrogen narcosis and evoked responses.

Auditory evoked response as a measure of narcosis is criticized because of sound alteration with pressure and the ambient noise during hyperbaric exposure. Therefore **visual evoked responses** were utilized in an attempt to produce more reliable information. Visual evoked responses as a measure of nitrogen narcosis were studied in US Navy divers and the investigators concluded that there were reliable and significant differences in visual evoked responses, while breathing compressed air at depths, which were not apparent on breathing helium–oxygen. A further study using visual evoked responses during a shallow 2-week saturation exposure with excursion dives suggested that some adaptation to narcosis occurred, but was not complete. Reduction of frequency and amplitude of alpha activity when compared to pre- and post-exposure surface levels were also noted. Nevertheless, the value of current methods of measurement of IGN, by the use of neurophysiological changes, is questionable.

> *Nitrogen and inert gases do not undergo metabolic change in the body to exert their narcotic effect.*

# Aetiology

Inert gas narcosis is thought to be produced by the same mechanism as general anaesthesia with gases or volatile liquids. Psychological studies suggest that the behavioural effects of all inert gases which produce narcosis are identical. These agents are simple molecules with no common structural features and do not undergo chemical change in the body to exert their effect. This suggests that general physical methods must be involved and most research is based on the hypothesis that the mechanism is the same for all agents (unitary hypothesis of narcosis).

Most workers have tried to identify the physical nature of site of action by relating anaesthetic potency to the physical properties of the agents. Although obviously in the central nervous system, the exact cellular site of action of inert gases (and general anaesthetics) is yet to be determined.

## *Lipid solubility*

At the turn of the century, Meyer and Overton noted that there is a parallel between the solubility of an anaesthetic in lipid and its narcotic potency, i.e. the Meyer–Overton hypothesis. Later, Meyer and Hopf (1923) stated 'all gaseous and volatile substances induce narcosis if they penetrate cell lipids in a definite molar concentration which is characteristic for each type of cell and is approximately the same for all narcotics'. This means that the higher the oil–water partition coefficient the more potent the inert gas. The inert gas molecule is thus thought to be taken up by brain lipid and somehow interferes with cell membrane function. There are some discrepancies in this approach (Table 15.2), for example, although both neon and hydrogen have been shown to be narcotic, neon appears to be more so. Also, argon is about twice as narcotic as nitrogen but has a similar oil:water solubility ratio. There are also anomalies among the general anaesthetics, but, in general, the relationship is much closer than with other physical properties.

More recently, extensions of the lipid solubility hypothesis have been proposed by applying the **critical volume** concept. Narcosis is said to occur when the inert gas or anaesthetic agent causes a lipid portion of the cell (possibly the cell membrane) to swell to a certain volume. Thus, there is a lipid volume change which differentiates the anaesthetized from the unanaesthetized state. Other factors, in particular pressure compressibility of the lipid, will also affect their volume. That the narcotic effect can be reversed by application of increased hydrostatic pressure lends weight to this hypothesis.

## Molecular weight

It has been known for some time that the narcotic effect of the rare gases increases with their molecular weight. The prediction, from this correlation, that xenon would be anaesthetic at 1 ATA was proved to be correct. Attempts to explain this correlation suggest that, with increasing molecular weight, there is an increasing density, leading to carbon dioxide retention or inducing a histotoxic hypoxia. Measurements of blood and cerebral dioxide tension and cerebral oxygen utilization appear to disprove this explanation.

## Hydrate formation

The aqueous phase theories relate narcosis to the stability of the gas hydrates formed by anaesthetics in aqueous solution. This is essentially an ordered structure of the water molecules around the inert gas molecule. It differs from the lipid theories in that the anaesthetic molecule is associated with water molecules rather than lipid. These microcrystals of gas hydrate may hinder transmission of nerve impulses in the synaptic region. Unfortunately, some anaesthetic agents, e.g. ether and halothane, do not form hydrates. Helium does not form hydrates, but has not been shown to be narcotic at current diving depths. There is virtually no evidence to suggest that an aqueous phase of the central nervous system is the site of narcotic action, thus narrowing the search to hydrophobic regions.

## Physical theories

The physical theories, in general, support the concept that the site of action is a hydrophobic portion of the cell, the traditional view being that this is the cell membrane. Many studies

**Table 15.2 Narcotic potencies and physical properties of simple gases**

| Gas | Molecular | | Solubility in oil at 37°C | Molecular attraction (van der Waals constant) | Partition coefficient (oil:water solubility ratio) | Relative narcotic potency |
|---|---|---|---|---|---|---|
| | Weight | Volume | | | | |
| Helium | 4 | 2.370 | 0.015 | 0.0341 | 1.70 | 0.23 |
| Neon | 20 | 1.709 | 0.019 | 0.2107 | 2.07 | 0.28 |
| Hydrogen | 2 | 2.661 | 0.040 | 0.2444 | 3.10 | 0.55 |
| Nitrogen | 28 | 3.913 | 0.067 | 1.390 | 5.25 | 1.00 |
| Argon | 40 | 3.218 | 0.140 | 1.345 | 5.32 | 2.33 |
| Krypton | 83.7 | 3.978 | 0.430 | 2.318 | 9.60 | 7.14 |
| Xenon | 131.3 | 3.105 | 1.700 | 4.194 | 20.00 | 25.64 |

show that membranes are resistant to the effects of anaesthetics and other sites have been sought, such as the hydrophobic regions of proteins. Recent studies on the effects of anaesthetics on the light-producing enzyme luciferase in certain luminous bacteria suggest that the cellular enzymes may be the site of action and that the anaesthetics act by **competitive binding** to specific receptors. This site is thought to be a hydrophobic region of a cellular enzyme and thus does not conflict with the Meyer–Overton critical volume concept outlined above.

### Biochemical theories

Several biochemical theories have been advanced to explain narcosis/anaesthesia but these are not currently widely held. The Metabolic Theory of Quastel postulates that anaesthetics interfere with intracellular oxidation by preventing energy transfer from pyruvate to the cytochrome enzyme system.

It has also been suggested that the mechanism of narcosis may be ascribed to alteration in the function of neurohormone transmitters, such as noradrenaline, serotonin, dopamine etc. No definite evidence of this theory has been forthcoming. The application of pressure reverses the anaesthetic effect of many agents in most species, but not in certain invertebrates which lack glycine as a neurotransmitter. This has led to the suggestion that certain actions of anaesthetics may be enhanced by glycine and that pressure antagonizes these actions by an, as yet, undefined mechanism. Experiments with structurally similar drugs suggest that pressure acts by causing a conformational change in the receptor molecule inhibiting glycine binding. This may be more relevant to the high-pressure neurological syndrome (see Chapter 16), but an unravelling of the mechanism may also throw more light on the mechanism of general anaesthesia and thus inert gas narcosis. A combination of physical and chemical theories postulates that inert gas displaces oxygen from cells thus reducing available energy. This would cause a reduction of sodium pump activity and a delay of substrate transfer from capillary to neuron. Depression of central nervous system activity would then result.

### Neurophysiological theories

Neurophysiological explanations of the mechanism involve an effect on **axonal conduction** via ion transport disturbances or on **synaptic transmission**. There is little evidence for effects on axonal conduction. Whatever the mechanism, the polysynaptic reticular activating system, with its role in maintaining arousal, is probably a major site of action.

The above list is in no way comprehensive, but is included to show some of the approaches being made to understand the mechanism of inert gas narcosis and general anaesthesia.

## Prevention

In its simplest terms, this means avoidance of exposure to partial pressures of inert gas known to produce intoxication. In practice, safe diving on compressed air requires an awareness of the condition and its effect on performance and judgement at depths greater than 30 metres. The maximum depth limit for an air dive should be between 30 and 50 metres, depending on the diver's experience and the task to be performed. Safe diving at a greater depth requires the substitution of a less narcotic agent to dilute the oxygen, such as helium, neon or hydrogen.

Saturation at depths between 30 and 40 metres allows the development of adaptation. Excursion dives to greater depths can then be made with more safety and improved work performance. A conventional working dive to 100 metres would be inconceivable using air as the breathing medium. However, operational dives may be performed to 100 metres, if the excursion is from a saturated depth of 40 metres. At that depth, the diver becomes acclimatized to the nitrogen narcosis, with a progressive improvement of his job performance, approaching his 'surface' efficiency.

Currently, in deep diving the effect of IGN is avoided by substituting helium, or helium–nitrogen, as the diluent gases for oxygen. Oxygen cannot, of course, be used alone because of its toxicity at high pressure (see Chapter 18), but it can partially replace nitrogen in various Nitrox mixtures. Hydrogen is also being used as a substitute for nitrogen and would be ideal except for the formation of an explosive mixture with oxygen.

Factors other than narcosis may limit depth/pressure exposures for these gases, e.g. high-pressure neurological syndrome (see Chapter 16) or gas density (see Chapter 36).

The idea of liquid breathing (see Chapter 3) to avoid a respiratory diluent for oxygen remains a theoretical concept. The use of drugs to ameliorate narcosis has, as yet, no place in diving. Conversely, divers should be warned of the risks of taking central nervous system depressant drugs, which, in the diver, might include alcohol, antihistamines (in 'cold' and 'sinus' preparations) and anti-motion-sickness drugs.

## Acknowledgements

The authors wish to acknowledge Professor Peter Bennett, Director of the F.G. Hall Laboratory, Duke University for reviewing this chapter and making constructive criticism.

## Recommended reading and references

BEHNKE, A.R. Inert gas narcosis. In: *Handbook of Physiology: Respiration II*. American Physiological Society.

BEHNKE, A.R., THOMSON, R.M. and MOTLEY, E.P. (1935). The psychological effects from breathing air at 4 atmospheres pressure. *American Journal of Physiology* 112, 554–558.

BENNETT, P.B. (1966) *The Aetiology of Compressed Air Intoxication and Inert Gas Narcosis*. London: Pergamon.

BENNETT, P.B. and ELLIOTT, D.H. (1982). *The Physiology and Medicine of Diving and Compressed Air Work*. London: Baillière Tindall.

BIERSNER, R.J. (1987). Emotional and physiological effects of nitrous oxide and hyperbaric air narcosis. *Aviation Space and Environmental Medicine* 58, 34–38.

COUSTEAU, J.Y. (1954). *The Silent World*. London: The Reprint Society.

FOWLER, B., ACKLES, K.N. and PORLIER, G. (1985). Effects of inert gas narcosis on behaviour – a critical review. *Undersea Biomedical Research* 12, 369–402.

FOWLER, B., HAMILTON, K. and PORLIER, G. (1986). Effects of ethanol and amphetamine on inert gas narcosis in humans. *Undersea Biomedical Research* 13, 345–354.

FRANKS, N.P. and LIEB, W.R. (1984). Do general anaesthetics act by competitive binding to specific receptors? *Nature*, 310.

HALSEY, M.J. (1989). The molecular basis of anaesthesia. In: *Anaesthesia*, Vol. 1, edited by W.S. Nimmo and G. Smith. Oxford: Blackwell Scientific.

HILL, L. and PHILLIPS, A.E. (1932). Deep-sea diving. *Journal of the Royal Navy Medical Service* 18(3), 157–173.

MILLER, K.W., PATON, W.D.M., SMITH, D.A. and SMITH, E.B. (1973). The pressure reversal of general anaesthesia and the critical volume hypothesis. *Molecular Pharmacology* 9, 131–143.

ROGERS, W.H. and MOELLER, G. (1989). Effects of brief, repeated hyperbaric exposures on susceptibility to nitrogen narcosis. *Undersea Biomedical Research* 16, 227–232.

SMITH, E.B. (1984). The biological effects of high pressure: underlying principles. *Philosophical Transactions of the Royal Society of London. Series B: Biological Sciences* 304, 5–16.

SMITH, E.B. (1987). Priestley lecture 1986. On the science of deep-sea diving observations on the respiration of different kinds of air. *Undersea Biomedical Research* 14, 347–369.

# 16

# High-pressure neurological syndrome

## Introduction

The high-pressure neurological syndrome (HPNS), also called the high-pressure nervous syndrome, is a condition noted in deep diving. With divers breathing helium mixtures, it is noticeable from about 200 metres. The first effects are tremors, but the condition progresses to lapses of consciousness at depths in excess of 300 metres. In animals compressed to greater depths, convulsions and death occur. To date these have not been observed in humans.

HPNS is a complex phenomenon characterized by biochemical, clinical and electroencephalographic (EEG) changes. These parameters are affected by the gas composition, the rate of compression and the absolute pressure. HPNS appears to be ameliorated by gases having an anaesthetic or narcotic effect.

> *High-pressure neurological syndrome (HPNS) is noted in helium diving deeper than 200 metres.*

## History

Recognition of the effects of hydrostatic pressure as a limiting factor in diving physiology has a curious history, characterized in part by the reluctance of the scientific community to recognize pressure as an environmental influence per se.

In the 1880s, workers recorded abnormalities of excitement, disturbed locomotion and paralysis in marine animals exposed to high pressure environments. During the 1920s, a series of publications dealt with the effects of high hydrostatic pressures. Halsey cites a report published in 1936 where manifestations, which may have been HPNS, were reported in vertebrate animals. Most of these effects developed at pressures greater than 100 ATA. In the 1960s, investigators observed what we now call HPNS in humans. Several explanations were advanced for the effects observed.

Helium toxicity, narcosis, histotoxic effects of oxygen, and normoxic hypoxia were advanced to explain the early observations of tremors and performance impairment in humans. These were noted by British, French and American workers when divers were compressed to depths of 200–400 metres of sea water.

In 1965, at the Royal Navy Physiological Laboratories, coarse tremors involving the extremities or even the whole body, accompanied by nausea, vomiting, dizziness and vertigo, were observed during a series of deep chamber dives to depths of 200–250 metres. Bachrach and Bennett (1973) called this condition helium tremors. A considerable decrease was noticed in the subjects' ability to carry out fine movements, e.g. picking up ball bearings with tweezers and placing them in a tube of similar diameter.

In 1966, Brauer and his colleagues demonstrated similar changes in animals and showed that they could progress to generalized seizures. In 1968, a French dive to 363 metres was aborted after a few minutes at depth, because of the development of EEG changes, dizziness, nausea, confusion, somnolence and microsleep.

---

> *HPNS is the current limiting factor in deep diving.*

---

## Animal experiments

HPNS has been observed in all animals studied that have a central nervous system at least as complex as a flat worm. The results from fish demonstrated that the effect is not dependent on the elevated pressure of gas molecules and, in part, it is due to hydrostatic pressure.

With compression on Heliox mixtures, animals develop fine then coarse tremors. These proceed to localized myoclonic episodes and then to generalized clonic seizures (type 1 seizures). If compression is stopped, the animal will continue to show this seizure activity for as long as 12 hours. Reduction in pressure will relieve the symptoms. If compression is continued, then tonic–clonic (type 2) seizures may develop and proceed to death. The available data, from mice, suggest that type 1 and 2 seizures have different biophysical

causes. HPNS is reversible up to a certain stage, beyond the type 1 convulsion threshold.

The depth at which convulsions occur can be increased by using a slower rate of compression. The threshold of type 1 convulsions can be increased from 70 ATA to 100 ATA by slowing compression rate from 1000 ATA/hour to 10 ATA/hour. This effect is probably a combination of the compression effect with a compensation response to the pressure that takes time to develop. Acclimatization and loss of pressure tolerance have also been demonstrated. These responses are probably mediated by monoamine neurotransmitters.

The addition of nitrogen, hydrogen or nitrous oxide to oxygen–helium atmospheres significantly delays the onset of both convulsions and tremor. The anti-tremor effect is only about one-half as great as the anticonvulsant effect. The potency of these gases in alleviating the HPNS is directly proportional to their relative narcotic potency. Thus the tremor and convulsion thresholds with helium are unchanged where it is mixed with other gases producing isonarcotic atmospheres. This observation is consistent with the demonstration by Miller and associates (1973) of a reversal of anaesthesia by high pressures.

Increased hydrostatic pressure increases the excitability of the central nervous system, and this may be counteracted to some degree by the use of narcotic agents. This suppression of HPNS is unfortunately not as generalized as was first thought. These agents act differently on various aspects of the HPNS, and therefore a different clinical pattern develops if the HPNS is countered by nitrogen, barbiturates or ketamine. It could be that these agents, in suppressing HPNS, may also be reducing the pressure acclimatization.

Barbiturate anticonvulsants also significantly elevate the tremor and the convulsion threshold pressures, and may be synergistic with narcotic and anaesthetic gases.

---

> *The development of HPNS depends on the rate of compression, the absolute pressure and the composition of diluent gases.*

## Clinical effects

Bennett and McLeod (1984) characterize HPNS in humans as: dizziness, nausea, vomiting, postural and intention tremors, fatigue and somnolence, myoclonic jerking, stomach cramps, increased slow wave and decreased fast wave activity of the EEG, decrements in intellectual and psychomotor performance, and poor sleep with nightmares. The syndrome is enhanced by rapid compression and decreased by a slow rate of compression, with stages at interim depths to permit adaptation. Some divers appear to be more susceptible than others.

The **tremor** is thought to be an extension of the normal resting tremor, as both have a large component between 8 and 12 Hz. This differs from other tremors such as Parkinson's and cerebellar disease, which have a peak frequency of 3–8 Hz. The tremors of alcoholism, thyrotoxicosis and shivering due to cold also have a frequency of 8–12 Hz, but they are usually postural. In HPNS, the resting and an intention tremor tend to be of the same frequency. The intensity of the tremor is aggravated by rapid compression as well as pressure. There is a gradual return towards normal following the cessation of compression, but this may not reach a plateau despite prolonged bottom times, even in excess of 100 hours. Other neuromuscular disturbances include fasciculations and myoclonic jerks.

**Psychomotor tests** involving manual dexterity reveal a considerable performance decrement, correlated with the tremor, and averaging 1% for each 20 metres of depth. It gradually starts returning towards normal levels after $1\frac{1}{2}$ hours at a constant pressure.

**Dyspnoea** at depths in excess of 300 metres may be a manifestation of HPNS. It might be related to incoordination of the neuromuscular control of breathing, or involvement of the reflex control and feedback systems with a mismatch of afferent and efferent impulses. It can develop or intensify suddenly and it may be precipitated by exercise and/or increasing the pulmonary ventilation to close to the maximum voluntary ventilation. The distress is greater during inspiration, even though the increased gas density objectively restricts expiratory flow. Higher oxygen concentration does not affect this dyspnoea. The arterial gases and pH are usually normal.

This dyspnoea was ameliorated by reducing the HPNS with supplementary nitrogen which increases gas density. Thus, the relationship between inspiratory dyspnoea at depth and HPNS remains to be clarified. Recently, Flook and Fraser (1989) suggested that the condition is caused by compression of the trachea. The vocal folds are thought to act as an orifice that induces an increase in air velocity and causes a low pressure region. The induced pressure gradient may be sufficient to cause compression of the trachea.

---

*Clinical features:*
- *Tremor 8–12 Hz*
- *Fasciculations*
- *Myoclonic jerks*
- *Psychomotor performance decrement*
- *Dizziness, nausea, vomiting*
- *Impaired consciousness*
- *Dyspnoea?*

---

Results of **EEG studies** are conflicting. The most consistent observation is an increase in theta waves (4–7 Hz), from as shallow as 150 metres and increasing with depth. There is a parallel decrease in alpha waves (8–13 Hz) and overall activity. These changes do not develop immediately; once theta activity occurs it continues to increase for approximately 6 hours, regardless of whether compression has ceased. After this, it falls towards normal values over a further 12 hours.

The **evoked cortical responses** may also be altered during deep dives. A progressive decline in the auditory evoked response, by as much as 50% at 457 metres, has been observed. Somatic evoked responses increase in amplitude, but are accompanied by an increase in threshold for sensory stimulation. Visual evoked responses have not shown any consistent changes.

## Aetiology

Attempts have been made to identify a single cause of HPNS. Halsey (1982) presents evidence that tends to disprove causes that had been proposed in the past. These included an effect of temperature, gas-induced osmosis, a modified form of inert gas narcosis, and response to a metabolic disturbance or a neurological hypoxia or hypercapnia that is caused by the respiratory limitations imposed by increased gas density.

The best evidence suggests that HPNS is caused by a series of changes in cells, with effects on the nervous system. The changes observed in the nervous system include pressure-induced depression of synaptic transmission, probably as a result of decreased release of transmitter substances.

A series of pressure-induced changes in cell chemistry and physiology has been reported. The factors that caused them could also cause HPNS: erythrocyes become spherical; isolated muscle preparations develop more tension and eventually become rigid; some membranes become more permeable.

At the biochemical level, high pressure directly inhibits reactions that involve an increase in volume. It has been suggested that pressure could influence the reactions in glycolysis and those involving adenosine triphosphate.

## Amelioration of HPNS

In view of the possible causes of HPNS, it is unlikely that any set of conditions or treatments will totally prevent HPNS; however, several techniques have been shown to delay its development.

Both nitrogen narcosis and HPNS can be postponed or reduced by a judicious mixture of gases. This comprises a neurological stimulant, helium, and a neurological depressant, e.g. nitrogen. Hydrogen occupies an intermediate position between these two gases. Currently the most common combination is that of oxygen, helium and nitrogen (Trimix). At a fixed percentage of nitrogen and helium, the nitrogen narcosis tends partly to counter the HPNS. The advantages of added nitrogen include decreased cost, increased thermal comfort, a reduced distortion of speech and a reduction in the HPNS. The advantages of helium include a reduction in the narcotic effect, and a reduction in the work of breathing.

Compression to 220 metres in 20 minutes, with Heliox, induced signs and symptoms of marked HPNS. When nitrogen was added to

the Heliox, the same dive profile was performed without tremors or other manifestations of HPNS. Bennett and his team, who have conducted a long serious of Trimix dives, now use 5% nitrogen in their mixture.

Rostain and co-workers (1988) have reported good results using a mixture containing up to 55% hydrogen. One dive involved compressing the divers to 200 msw with Heliox then to 450 msw by adding hydrogen. During ascent, the hydrogen was removed from the mixture before the divers reached 200 msw. The narcotic and anti-HPNS effect of hydrogen was demonstrated during another similar dive. A change to Heliox at 450 metres induced HPNS; because the amount of oxygen in the hydrogen mixture was less than 2% there was no fire hazard. The divers in these dives appreciated the lower density of the hydrogen mixture compared to oxygen–helium. It is not yet known what will be the optimum amount of hydrogen, or if it will be generally favoured over Trimix.

It has recently been suggested that there may be a role for ketamine instead of using nitrogen in the gas mixture (Bennett, 1989). This would avoid increasing the density of the gas mixture.

Brauer has raised two possible problems: first the efforts to counter HPNS may only be countering type 1 HPNS. By avoiding type 1 HPNS, a situation may be created where the first sign may be type 2 HPNS; in animals this has been fatal. The second problem is that, in baboons, a new set of symptoms which may involve brain damage can be induced by delaying the development of HPNS (Brauer, 1984).

---

*HPNS can be delayed by:*
1. *Adding a narcotic gas, e.g. nitrogen, to the stimulant diluent, helium.*
2. *Reducing the speed of compression.*

---

Reduction in the speed of compression reduces the incidence and severity of HPNS. Divers who were compressed to 650 metres in 4.6 days were in better condition than divers who were compressed in about half the time. HPNS is also likely to be induced by compression at too great a rate from saturation depths. From 240 metres, excursions to 340 metres and

320 metres at rates of 8.2–8.5 m/min resulted in weakness and tremor but a slower rate of 5.2 m/min did not.

A potential problem is that agents which delay the onset of HPNS may also reduce the acclimatization to the stimulus that is causing the condition.

## Conclusion

HPNS is the major limiting factor in deep diving. Extrapolation from lower primates to humans suggests that human divers are approaching depths at which seizures may be anticipated. It is likely that, with the use of techniques described in this chapter, this depth limit can be increased. It is difficult to justify these dives on commercial grounds. The decompression time from 600 metres is unlikely to be reduced to less than 4 weeks. The oil industry, the major market for these diving skills, may prefer to use alternative methods to work at these depths.

## Acknowledgement

Dr Ralph W. Brauer, Director of the Institute for Research on the Interrelation of Science and Culture, Inc., Wilmington, North Carolina, USA, gave helpful criticism and assistance in reviewing this chapter.

## References and recommended reading

BACHRACH, H.J. and BENNETT, P.B. (1973). The high pressure nervous syndrome during human deep saturation and excursion diving. *Forsvarsmedicin* **9**, 490–495.

BENNETT, P.B. (1989). Physiological limitations to underwater exploration and work. *Comparative Biochemistry and Physiology* **93A**, 295–300.

BENNETT, P.B. and MCLEOD, M (1984). Probing the limits of human deep diving. *Philosophical Transactions of the Royal Society of London* **B304**, 105–117.

BRAUER, R.W. (1984). Hydrostatic pressure effects on the central nervous system: perspectives and outlook. *Philosophical Transactions of the Royal Society of London* **B304**, 17–30.

FAGEUS, L. (1981). Current concepts of dyspnoea at depth. In *Proceedings of the Seventh Symposium on Underwater Physiology*, edited by A. J. Bacherach and M.M. Matzen, pp. 141–149. Undersea Medical Society.

FLOOK, V. and FRASER, I.M. (1989). Inspiratory flow limitations in divers. *Undersea Biomedical Research* **16**, 305–311

HALSEY, M.J. (1982). Effects of high pressure on the central nervous system. *Physiological Reviews* **62**, 1341–1377.

LEMAIRE, C. and ROSTAIN, J-C. (1988). The high pressure nervous syndrome and performance. Collections *Impressions Hyperbares*.

MILLER, K.W., PATON, W.D.M., SMITH, R.A. and SMITH, E.B. (1973). The pressure reversal of general anaesthesia and the critical volume hypothesis. *Molecular Pharmacology* 131–143.

ROSTAIN, J.C., GARDETTE–CHAUFFOUR, M.C., LEMAIR, C. and NAQUET, R. (1988). Effects of $H_2$–He–$O_2$ mixture on the HPNS up to 450 msw. *Undersea Biomedical Research* **15**, 257–270.

SALZANO, J., CAMPORESI, E.M., STOLP, B., SALTZMAN BELL, H.W. and SHELTON, D. (1981). Exercise at 47 ATA and 66 ATA. In: *Proceedings of the Seventh Symposium on Underwater Physiology*, edited by A. J. Bachrach and M. M. Matzen, pp. 181–196. Undersea Medical Society.

# 17

# Hypoxia

## Introduction

Aerobic metabolism is much more efficient in the production of biological energy than anaerobic metabolism. For example, 1 molecule of glucose can be utilized to produce 38 molecules of the energy storage compound adenosine triphosphate (ATP). In the absence of oxygen, the conversion of 1 molecule of glucose to lactic acid produces only 2 molecules of ATP. Thus, anaerobic conditions drastically reduce the available energy. Cells of the brain, liver and kidney, which use large amounts of energy, are the first affected by hypoxia. Skin, muscle and bone are less vulnerable because of their lower energy requirements.

Dry air, at a barometric pressure of 760 mmHg, has an oxygen partial pressure of 160 mmHg. When inspired it becomes saturated with water vapour at body temperature. By this dilution the oxygen pressure drops to 150 mmHg. Alveolar gas has a lower partial pressure of oxygen than inspired air, the difference being proportional to the ratio of oxygen consumption to alveolar ventilation. Normal levels are in the region of 105 mmHg. The tension in arterial blood is slightly lower (100 mmHg) in healthy subjects due to venous admixture. After passage through the tissues the oxygen tension falls to approximately 40 mmHg in mixed venous blood.

Oxygen moves passively down partial pressure gradients from the lungs to the cellular level where it is utilized (Figure 17.1 and Table 17.1). The amount of oxygen stored in the body is limited as are the high energy phosphate bonds used to store energy. A person breathing air at sea level would hold the following amounts of oxygen (from Nunn, 1987):

| | |
|---|---:|
| In the lungs | 450 ml |
| In the blood | 850 ml |
| Dissolved in body fluids | 50 ml |
| Bound to myoglobin in muscle | ? 200 ml |
| Total = | 1550 ml |

Not all of this oxygen is readily available for utilization in vital tissues such as brain and heart.

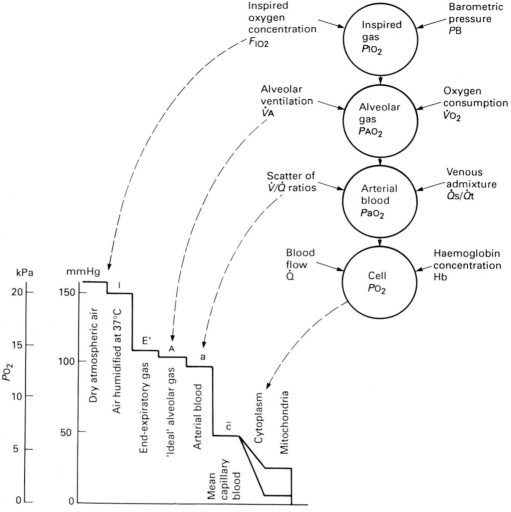

**Figure 17.1** The oxygen cascade: on the left is shown the cascade with $Po_2$ falling from the level in the ambient air down to the level in mitochondria, which is the site of utilization. On the right is shown a summary of the factors influencing oxygenation at different levels in the cascade. (Redrawn from J.F. Nunn (1987) *Applied Respiratory Physiology*, 3rd edn, London, Butterworths)

Basal oxygen consumption is of the order of 200 ml/min but in swimming and diving much higher values are possible (up to 3 litres/min). This explains why hypoxia develops so rapidly on cessation of pulmonary ventilation.

The delivery of oxygen to the cellular level requires an adequate inspired oxygen pressure, adequate lung function, adequate cardiac output and adequate functional haemoglobin for carriage.

Although impairment of aerobic metabolism of tissues is probably the ultimate mechanism of death in most fatal diving accidents, hypoxia, as the primary event, is uncommon in conventional scuba diving. It is much more likely in mixed gas and rebreathing equipment.

The diving disorders mentioned here are discussed more fully in appropriate chapters.

## Clinical features

The physiological associations of hypoxia in general medicine are well known and will not be discussed here.

Symptoms and signs of hypoxia in diving become obvious when the arterial oxygen tension drops below 50 mmHg. This corresponds to an inspired concentration at sea level of 8–10%. If the fall in oxygen tension is rapid, then loss of consciousness may be unheralded. With slower falls, an observer may note incoordination or poor job performance by the diver. Euphoria, over-confidence and apathy have also been reported. Memory is defective and judgement impaired, leading to an inappropriate or dangerous reaction to the emergency which may also endanger the diving buddy. The diver may complain of fatigue, headache or blurred vision.

---

*There are rarely any symptoms to warn the diver of impending unconsciousness from hypoxia.*

---

Hyperventilation may develop in some cases, but is usually minimal if the arterial carbon dioxide tension is normal or low.

There are marked individual differences in susceptibility to hypoxia. When combined with hypo- or hypercapnia, a milder hypoxia will impair mental performance. When the carbon dioxide is controlled, mental performance may not be severely impaired until the alveolar oxygen tension falls below 40 mmHg. Hypoxia may precipitate or exacerbate other pathological conditions, such as coronary, cerebral or other ischaemic lesions.

Cyanosis of the lips and nail beds may be difficult to determine in the peripheral vasoconstricted 'cold and blue' diver. Generalized convulsions or other neurological manifestations may be the first sign. Eventually, respiratory failure, cardiac failure and death supervene.

Diagnostic confusion may arise because some of the above manifestations are common to nitrogen narcosis, oxygen toxicity and carbon dioxide retention. The attending physician should also consider cerebral air embolism and decompression sickness should the above features develop during or after ascent of a diver breathing compressed gases.

## Classification

Hypoxia ('anoxia') has been classified into four types, i.e.

1. Hypoxic.
2. Stagnant.
3. Anaemic.
4. Histotoxic.

### Hypoxic hypoxia

This covers all conditions leading to a reduction in arterial oxygen (Figure 17.2). A better term would therefore be '**hypoxaemic** hypoxia'. This is the common form of hypoxia seen in diving. Causes of hypoxaemia, with examples related to diving, are the following.

### *Inadequate oxygen supply*

This is due to a decrease in oxygen pressure in the inspired gas, which may be due to an incorrect gas mixture or equipment failure. Carbon dioxide retention is not a feature of this hypoxaemia.

### *Alveolar hypoventilation*

This occurs where the amount of gas flowing in and out of functioning alveoli per unit time is reduced. It may be due to increased density of gases with depth, decreased compliance with drowning etc. The extreme example is breath-holding. There is associated carbon dioxide retention.

### *Ventilation–perfusion inequality and shunt*

Perfusion of blood past non-ventilated alveoli results in non-oxygenated blood moving into the systemic circulation (shunt). Lesser degrees of mismatching of perfusion and ventilation also result in arterial desaturation. This may be seen in near-drowning, salt water aspiration syndrome and pneumothorax. Inequality of ventilation and perfusion may also occur in pulmonary decompression sickness and pulmonary barotrauma. The carbon dioxide response is variable with ventilation–perfusion disorders, but mild hypocapnia is common if ventilation can be increased by the hypoxic drive.

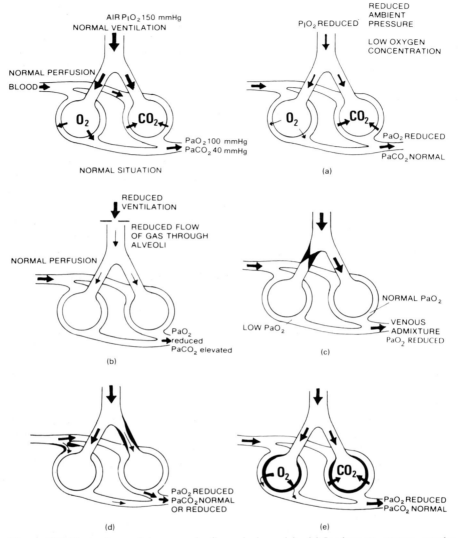

**Figure 17.2** Mechanisms of hypoxaemia (hypoxic hypoxia). (a) Inadequate oxygen supply; (b) alveolar hypoventilation; (c) perfusion of non-ventilated alveoli causing venous admixture; (d) ventilation–perfusion inequality; (e) diffusion defect. $PaO_2$ = arterial oxygen tension; $PaCO_2$ = arterial carbon dioxide tension; $PIO_2$ = inspired oxygen tension

### Diffusion defect

This is due to thickening of the alveolar–capillary barrier. This may add to the persistent and late hypoxia of near drowning, and pulmonary oxygen toxicity. Carbon dioxide retention is not characteristic of this hypoxaemia because it diffuses through the barrier much more rapidly than oxygen.

There is obviously a great overlap in the different mechanisms by which the various diseases produce hypoxaemia.

### Stagnant (or ischaemic) hypoxia

This is the term used to describe reduced blood perfusion of tissue, either regional or general. The extreme form is circulatory arrest. Syncope of ascent (see Chapter 32) is a transitory manifestation due to inadequate cardiac output. Reduced cardiac output may also be present in decompression sickness. Local ischaemia may result from gas bubbles or gas emboli arising in decompression sickness or pulmonary barotrauma. The localized ischaemia is the cause of many of the symptoms and signs in those disorders.

## Anaemic hypoxia

This refers to any condition in which there is a reduction in haemoglobin or in its capacity to carry oxygen. One cause is traumatic haemorrhage with restoration of blood volume with fluids. Carbon monoxide poisoning (see Chapters 20 and 37), where the formation of carboxyhaemoglobin reduces the oxygen-carrying capacity of the blood, is a possible danger with the use of compressed air. The capacity of haemoglobin to carry oxygen is diminished in the presence of alkalaemia, e.g. low arterial carbon dioxide tension, and hypothermia. At arterial oxygen tensions below 60 mmHg, the amount of oxygen given up to the tissue is greatly reduced.

## Histotoxic hypoxia

This refers to the situation where adequate oxygen is delivered to the tissues, but there is a failure of utilization within the cell. Carbon monoxide, as well as the action described above, poisons the cytochrome oxidase enzyme. Histotoxic hypoxia has also been postulated as a mechanism for inert gas narcosis (see Chapter 15) and oxygen toxicity (see Chapter 18).

## Hypoxia and diving equipment

Hypoxia due to inadequate inspired oxygen is due to improper use, or failure of, the diving equipment. It occurs mainly with the use of closed or semi-closed rebreathing apparatus. Of the following six causes only the first two mechanisms are possible with open-circuit scuba: (1) exhaustion of gas supply; (2) low oxygen concentration; (3) inadequate flow rates; (4) increased oxygen consumption; (5) dilution hypoxia; and (6) hypoxia of ascent.

### Exhaustion of gas supply

The 'out of air' situation remains a major cause of diving accidents despite training.

---

### CASE REPORT 17.1

Two commercial divers were engaged in making a 110 metre mixed gas dive from a diving bell. The purpose of the dive was to tie in a 6-inch riser. While one diver was in the water at depth working on the riser, the diving bell operator excitedly informed topside that the bell was losing pressure and flooding. The rack operator who was disconcerted by this information opened valves to send gas to the bell. Communication with the bell operator was lost. The diver who was in the water working on the riser was instructed to return to the bell which he did. When the diver arrived at the bell, he found the bell operator unconscious and lying on the deck of the bell. The diver climbed out of the water into the bell, took off his Kirby–Morgan mask, and promptly collapsed. When topside personnel realized that they had completely lost communications with the bell, they made ready the standby divers. The first standby diver was dressed, put on his diving helmet and promptly collapsed unconscious on deck. At this point the bell with the diver and the bell operator was brought to the surface with the hatch open and without any decompression stops. The divers were extricated from the bell and recompressed in a deck decompression chamber. Both the diver and the bell operator died in the deck decompression chamber at 165 feet of fulminating decompression sickness.

Examination of the rack showed that the rack operator had mistakenly opened a cross-connect valve which should have been 'tagged out' (labelled to indicate that it should not be used). This valve permitted 100% helium to be delivered to the diving bell and the standby divers, instead of the appropriate helium–oxygen breathing mixture.

*Diagnosis:* acute hypoxia and fulminant decompression sickness.

## Low oxygen concentration in the gas supply

Accidental filling of an air cylinder with another gas, such as nitrogen may result in unconsciousness. Low percentage oxygen mixtures (10% oxygen or less), designed for use in deep or saturation diving, would lead to hypoxia if breathed near the surface.

Rusting of scuba cylinders has reduced the oxygen content, leading to at least one fatality and several 'near misses'.

## Inadequate flow rates

Most rebreathing diving sets have a constant flow of gas into the counterlung (see Chapter 4 for explanation of this equipment). A set designed to use various gas mixtures will have a means of adjusting these flow rates. The flow rate should be set to supply enough oxygen for the diver's requirements, plus that lost through the exhaust valve. The higher the oxygen concentration, the lower the required flow rate, and vice versa. If an inadequate flow rate is set

---

### CASE REPORT 17.2

MB, a civilian diver, was asked to cut free a rope which was wrapped around the propeller of a diver's charter boat. Because of the very shallow nature of the dive (10 feet maximum), he used a small steel cylinder not often used by divers. After he entered the water, his diving partner noticed that he was acting in a strange manner and swam to him. At this point he was lying on the bottom and was unconscious but still breathing through his single hose regulator. The diving partner rescued the unconscious diver and got him on deck. His fellow divers prised the mouth piece from him and gave him cardiopulmonary resuscitation, and the diver promptly regained consciousness.

On analysis, the gas in the cylinder was found to be 98% nitrogen and 2% oxygen. There was sea water present in the interior of the cylinder, together with a considerable amount of rust.

*Diagnosis:* acute hypoxia due to low inspired oxygen concentration.

---

### CASE REPORT 17.3

AS was diving to 20 metres using a 60/40 oxygen/nitrogen mixture in a semi-closed rebreathing system. After 15 minutes he noted difficulty in obtaining enough gas. He stopped to try and adjust his relief valve and then suddenly lost consciousness. Another diver noticed him lying face-down on the bottom. He flushed the unconscious diver's counterlung with gas and took him to the surface, after which the set was turned to atmosphere, so that the diver was breathing air. He then started to regain consciousness, but was still cyanosed. He became aware of his surroundings and did not require further resuscitation. Equipment investigation revealed that carbon dioxide absorbent activity was normal but reducer flow was set at 2 litres/min instead of the required 6 litres/min. This would supply inadequate oxygen for the diver's expected rate of utilization.

*Diagnosis:* hypoxia due to inadequate gas flow rate.

for the oxygen mixture used, then the inert gas, e.g. nitrogen, will accumulate in the counter-lung. Low concentrations of oxygen will then be inspired by the diver.

### Increased oxygen consumption

Most rebreathing sets are designed for maximum oxygen consumptions between 1 and 2.5 litres/min depending on the anticipated exertion. Commonly the maximum oxygen uptake is assumed to be 1.5 l/min. Several studies have shown that divers can consume oxygen at much higher rates than expected from land studies. Values of over 2.5 l/min for 30 min and over 3 l/min for 10–15 min have been recorded without excessive fatigue. This may be due to the cooling effect of the environment and/or greater tissue utilization with increased amount of oxygen physically dissolved in the plasma. The values indicate that it is quite possible for the diver to consume oxygen at a greater than expected rate under certain conditions. In rebreathing sets, a hypoxic mixture could then develop in the counterlung due to accumulation of nitrogen (i.e. dilution hypoxia).

### Dilution hypoxia

This applies mainly to the oxygen rebreathing sets. It is due to the oxygen in the counterlung being diluted by nitrogen. The unwanted nitrogen may enter the system by three methods: first, into the gas supply; secondly, the diver may not clear the counterlung of air before use, thus leaving a litre or more nitrogen in it; thirdly, the diver may not clear his lungs prior to using the equipment, e.g. if he breathes into the set from full inspiration, he may add up to 3 litres of nitrogen to the counterlung. These dangers may also occur if the diver surfaces and breathes from the atmosphere, in order to report his activities, or for some other reason.

This dilution hypoxia is more dangerous if oxygen is only supplied 'on demand' (i.e. when the counterlung is empty), rather than having a constant flow of gas into the bag. As the diver continues to use up the oxygen, the nitrogen remains to distend the counterlung. Carbon dioxide will continue to be removed by the absorbent. Thus, the percentage of oxygen in his inspired gas falls as it is consumed. There is approximately 1 litre of nitrogen dissolved in the body, but the amount that would diffuse out into the counterlung to cause a dilution hypoxia would be a small contribution.

### Hypoxia of ascent

By one of the above mechanisms, the percentage of oxygen being inspired may drop to well below 20%. An inspired oxygen concentration of 10% can be breathed quite safely at 10 metres, as the partial pressure would still be adequate (approximately 140 mmHg). Hypoxia will develop when the diver ascends sufficiently to reduce this oxygen partial pressure to a critical level. It is therefore most likely to develop at or near the surface.

---

**CASE REPORT 17.4**

RAB was diving to 22 metres using a semi-closed rebreathing set with a 40/60 oxygen/nitrogen mixture. After 36 minutes he was instructed to ascend slowly. At approximately 3–4 metres he noted some difficulty in breathing but continued to ascend and then started to climb on board, but appeared to have some difficulty with this. When asked if he was well he did not answer. He became cyanosed around the lips and his teeth were firmly clenched on the mouth piece. On removal of his set and administration of oxygen he recovered rapidly but remained totally amnesic for 10 minutes. Examination of his diving equipment revealed that both main cylinders were empty and the emergency supply had not been used.

*Diagnosis:* hypoxia of ascent.

## Hypoxia and breath-hold diving

In a simple breath-hold, with no immersion or preceding hyperventilation, the breaking point (the irresistible urge to breathe) is initiated mainly by a rise in carbon dioxide level, and to a lesser extent by a fall in arterial oxygen. If the subject first breathes oxygen, he can hold his breath for longer. Hyperventilation also prolongs the length of the breath-hold by reducing the arterial carbon dioxide level. Other mechanical and psychological factors are also involved.

Pressure changes, initiated by diving or hyperbaric chamber operation, complicate the gas exchanges during breath-hold. During descent, the lungs are compressed and the partial pressures of oxygen and carbon dioxide both rise. The rise in oxygen partial pressure is beneficial in that more oxygen can be extracted from the alveolar air. The alveolar carbon dioxide partial pressure may be greater than that in the blood or the tissues, and so carbon dioxide excretion will be stopped or reversed, i.e. carbon dioxide will accumulate in the tissues and blood. The influx of carbon dioxide into the lungs during ascent is dependent on the circulation time and is relatively slow, so that with a rapid ascent the alveolar carbon dioxide level may be normal or even low on reaching the surface.

Although it is probably uncommon, blackout from hypoxia can occur during simple breath-hold dives without prior hyperventilation. It is more likely during **deep dives** where the increased oxygen tension delays the breaking point. During ascent from such a dive, severe hypoxia may develop with the decrease in alveolar partial pressure of oxygen due to the reduction in ambient pressure. Levels as low as 25–30 mmHg, with associated confusion and occasional blackouts, have been reported following dives to 27 metres.

**Hyperventilation** can lead to a marked reduction in alveolar and arterial carbon dioxide tension, to as low as 15 mmHg (hypocapnia). The alveolar oxygen may be increased to 140 mmHg. The period of breath-holding after the hyperventilation is prolonged because the main stimulus to breathing – arterial carbon dioxide tension – is reduced. This allows a breath-hold diver to remain submerged for a longer period of time. Consequently, the alveolar and arterial oxygen tensions can fall to lower levels than found without hyperventilation. If the oxygen tension falls sufficiently, unconsciousness will occur. This mechanism is a common cause of drowning in apparently healthy strong swimmers performing breath-hold dives.

---

> *Hyperventilation prior to breath-hold diving is a dangerous practice.*

---

The dangers of hyperventilation and breath-hold diving are illustrated in Figure 17.3. The diagram illustrates the point that, with prior hyperventilation, the time to reach the irresistible urge to breathe ('breaking point') is prolonged. This extra time may allow the blood arterial oxygen to fall to dangerous levels (hypoxic danger zone) (see Chapter 3 for physiological details).

## Hypoxia and deep diving

Animal experiments at great pressures are being regularly undertaken to determine the

**Table 17.1 Partial pressures of respiratory gases in normal resting humans at sea level**

| Partial pressure | Dry inspired air (mmHg) | Humidified tracheal air (mmHg) | Alveolar gas (mmHg) | Arterial blood (mmHg) | Mixed venous blood (mmHg) |
|---|---|---|---|---|---|
| $P_{O_2}$ | 159 | 149 | 104 | 100 | 40 |
| $P_{CO_2}$ | 0.3 | 0.3 | 40 | 40 | 46 |
| $P_{H_2O}$ | 0 | 47 | 47 | 47 | 47 |
| $P_{N_2}$ | 601 | 564 | 569 | 573 | 573 |

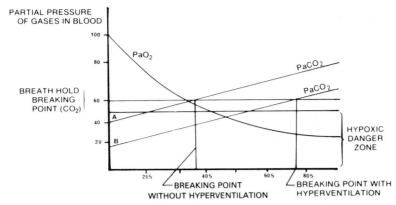

**Figure 17.3** A diagrammatic representation of changes in arterial oxygen and carbon dioxide levels with breath-holding. (A) Without preceding hyperventilation; (B) with preceding hyperventilation. (See Figure 3.4 for specific data)

limits of human exposure and thus ocean penetration. Ventilatory capacity is likely to be limited by restricted gas flow or increased work of breathing, both due to the effects of increased gas density.

Hypoxia might be expected, due to such factors as an increased 'diffusion dead space', caused by a slowed diffusion of alveolar gases or incomplete mixing of fresh inspired gases and alveolar gases despite adequate inspired oxygen pressure and overall pulmonary ventilation.

The **Chouteau effect** (a disputed concept) is an apparent clinical hypoxia despite normal inspired oxygen tension which, at least in goats, is rectified by a slight increase in the inspired oxygen tension (i.e. normoxic hypoxia).

Saltzman has an alternative explanation, suggesting that at greater than 50 ATA there is a decreased oxygen uptake, with decreased pH and increasing acidosis. Thus, there is a block in the utilization or transport of oxygen.

# Management

First aid management involves the basic principles of resuscitation, establishing an **airway**, ensuring that there is **ventilation** of the lungs and that the oxygenated blood is being **circulated** to the tissues. One hundred per cent oxygen should be administered as soon as possible. Further management depends on the aetiology of the hypoxia (see Chapter 33).

| | *First aid* |
|---|---|
| *Airway* | *Head extended, lower neck flexed, jaw forward* |
| | *Foreign material, secretions removed* |
| *Breathing* | *If breathing – 100% oxygen by mask* |
| | *If not breathing – mouth-to-mouth or mouth-to-nose respiration followed by IPPR (intermittent positive pressure resuscitation) with 100% $O_2$ when available* |
| *Circulation* | *If pulse absent – cardiac massage* |

## Hypoxic hypoxia

These cases should be given supplemental inspired oxygen or ventilated with 100% oxygen at whatever pressure is needed to ensure adequate arterial oxygen levels. Once these have been achieved, the pressure and percentage of oxygen can be progressively reduced while monitoring arterial gases or tissue oxygen by transcutaneous pulse oximetry.

## Stagnant hypoxia

The aim of therapy is to increase perfusion to the affected areas. This may require restoration of total circulatory volume as well as vasodilator drugs, and hyperoxygenation as a temporary measure.

### Anaemic hypoxia

Blood loss from trauma may require blood transfusion with packed red cells after crystalloid or colloid resuscitation. In the case of carbon monoxide poisoning, hyperbaric oxygenation may be life saving during the early critical period.

### Histotoxic hypoxia

This can only be treated by removing the toxic substance and using hyperoxygenation as a temporary measure.

In many cases there may be an **overlap** of different causes of tissue hypoxia and all should receive a high inspired oxygen concentration.

Recompression or hyperbaric oxygenation may be indicated as a temporary measure to allow the above regimes time to have an effect. (See Chapters 9, 11–13 and 21.)

### Methods of oxygen delivery

There are various devices or apparatus for the therapeutic administration of oxygen. Selection of the appropriate mode of administration depends on a number of factors:

1. Desired inspired oxygen concentration.
2. Need to avoid carbon dioxide accumulation.
3. Available oxygen (i.e. efficiency and economy).
4. Need to assist or control ventilation.
5. Acceptance of the method by the patient.

Various methods for the administration of oxygen are shown in Table 17.2. It is important to note that most plastic masks deliver less than 60% $FIO_2$ unless a reservoir bag is incorporated and this increases the risk of $CO_2$ retention.

**Table 17.2 Modes of oxygen therapy**

| Apparatus | Oxygen flow (l/min) | Concentrations (%) |
|---|---|---|
| Nasal catheters | 2–6 | 22–50 |
| Semi-rigid mask (e.g. MC, Edinburgh, Hudson, Harris) | 4–12 | 35–65 |
| Venturi-type mask (e.g. Ventimask, Accurox) | 4–8 | 24, 28, 35, 40, 50, 60 |
| Soft plastic masks (e.g. Pneumask, Polymask) | 4–8 | 40–80 |
| Ventilators | Varying | 21–100 |
| Anaesthetic circuits | Varying | 21–100 |
| Demand valves | Varying | 21–100 |
| Hyperbaric oxygen | Varying | Varying |

## Recommended reading

EDMONDS, C. (1968). *Shallow Water Blackout*. RAN School of Underwater Medicine Research Project Report, 8/68.

HONG, S.K. (1990) Breathhold diving. In: *Diving Medicine*, edited by A.A. Bove and J.C. Davis. Philadelphia: WB Saunders.

LANPHIER, E.H. (1967). Interactions of factors limiting performance at high pressures. In: *Proceedings of the Third Symposium on Underwater Physiology*, edited by C.J. Lambertsen. Baltimore, MA: Williams & Wilkins.

LANPHIER, E.H. and RAHN, H. (1963). Alveolar gas exchange during breathhold diving. *Journal of Applied Physiology* **18**, 471–477.

MILES, S. (1969). *Underwater Medicine*, 3rd edn. London: Staples Press.

NUNN, J.F. (1987). Oxygen. In: *Applied Respiratory Physiology*, 3rd edn. London: Butterworths.

SCHAEFER, K.E. (1965). Circulatory adaptation to the requirements of life under more than one atmosphere of pressure. In: *Handbook of Physiology*, Section 2, *Circulation*, Vol. III, pp. 1843–1873. Washington DC: American Physiology Society.

UNDERSEA AND HYPERBARIC MEDICAL SOCIETY (1987). *The Physiology of Breathhold Diving*. Undersea and Hyperbaric Medical Society Workshop.

# 18

# Oxygen toxicity

## Introduction

The normal partial pressure of oxygen in air is approximately 0.2 ATA. Although essential for survival, oxygen may become toxic at an elevated partial pressure. This may be due to a rise in the inspired oxygen concentration, an increase in the environmental pressure or a combination of both.

High inspired oxygen pressure has several physiological effects on the body which are not regarded as toxic effects. These include an increase in ventilation and decrease in alveolar and arterial carbon dioxide buffering tension ($P_{CO_2}$). This is due to a rise in central venous $P_{CO_2}$ due to the reduction in $CO_2$ capacity of haemoglobin (see Chapter 19) overcoming decreased carotid body excitation. Other physiological responses to high oxygen include vagally mediated bradycardia and vasoconstriction of intracranial and peripheral vessels.

There is a small rate-dependent fall in cardiac output.

In diving and diving medicine, toxicity is likely to be encountered in the following situations:

1. Closed and semi-closed rebreathing equipment.
2. Saturation diving.
3. Where oxygen is used to shorten decompression times.
4. Oxygen therapy for diving disorders.
5. Therapeutic recompression.
6. Accidental use of high oxygen mixtures instead of air.
7. Cases of respiratory failure requiring prolonged resuscitation (e.g. near drowning).

High oxygen partial pressures are known to produce retrolental fibroplasia in pre-term infants, and lung damage, convulsions, red cell suppression and cataracts in adults. In vitro, toxic effects on cells of many other organs have also been demonstrated. In diving, toxic effects on cells of the central nervous system and respiratory epithelium and endothelium are of prime importance and only these will be discussed in detail.

In both the central nervous system and lungs there is a latent period prior to the onset of toxicity. This delay before the onset of toxicity (Figure 18.1) enables high partial pressures to be used. The length of this latent period depends on the partial pressure of oxygen inspired.

---

*Development of oxygen toxicity depends on:*
- *Partial pressure of oxygen*
- *Duration of exposure*
- *Inter- and intra-individual variation in susceptibility*

---

## History

Oxygen was discovered in the latter half of the eighteenth century by Priestley and immediately excited interest as to its possible therapeutic effects. Priestley himself, in 1775, was among the first to suggest that there may be adverse effects of oxygen. He observed the rapid burning of a candle and speculated that 'the animal powers be too soon exhausted in this pure kind of air'. Later, in 1789, Lavoisier and Sequin demonstrated that oxygen at 1 ATA does not alter oxidative metabolism but did note a damaging effect on the lungs.

In 1878, Paul Bert published his pioneer work *La Pression Barometrique* in which he presented the results of years of study of the physiological effects of exposure to high and low pressures. He showed that, although oxygen is essential to sustain life, it is lethal at high pressures. Larks exposed to air at 15–20 ATA developed convulsions. The same effect could be produced by oxygen at 5 ATA. Bert recorded similar convulsions in other species and clearly established the toxicity of oxygen on the central nervous system.

In 1899, the pathologist J. Lorrain Smith noted fatal pneumonia in a rat after 4 days' exposure to 73% oxygen at atmospheric pressure. He conducted further experiments on mice and gave the first detailed description of pulmonary changes resulting from moderately high oxygen tensions (approximately 1.0 ATA) for prolonged periods of time. Smith was aware of the limitations that this toxicity might place on the clinical use of oxygen. He also noted that early changes are reversible and that higher pressures shortened the time of onset.

Although numerous animal studies were performed, evidence of the effect of high pressure oxygen on humans was sparse until the 1930s. In 1933, two Royal Naval Officers, Damant and Philips, breathed oxygen at 4

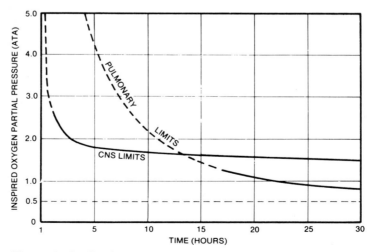

**Figure 18.1** Predicted human pulmonary and central nervous system tolerance to high pressure oxygen

ATA. Convulsive symptoms were reported at 16 and 13 minutes. Behnke then reported a series of exposures to hyperbaric oxygen. Exposure at 4 ATA terminated in acute syncope after 43 minutes in one subject and convulsions at 44 minutes in the other. At 3 ATA no effects were seen after 3 hours, but at 4 hours some subjects noted nausea and a sensation of impending collapse. At that time it was believed that 30 minutes' exposure at 4 ATA and 3 hours' exposure at 3 ATA were safe for men at rest.

Becker-Freyseng and Clamann, in 1939, found that 65 hours' exposure to 730 mmHg oxygen at normal atmospheric pressure produced paraesthesiae, nausea and a decrease in vital capacity. In 1941 Haldane reported a convulsion in less than 5 minutes at 7 ATA oxygen.

At the beginning of World War II, a number of unexplained episodes of unconsciousness were noted in divers using closed circuit rebreathing oxygen sets at what were considered safe depths. This prompted Donald, in 1942, to commence a series of experiments on oxygen poisoning. His observations in over 2000 exposures form the basis of current oxygen diving limits. Among the more important findings were the marked variation of tolerance and the aggravating effects of exercise and underwater exposure. He suggested a maximum safe depth for oxygen diving of 8 metres.

Donald also drew attention to Dickens' work on rat brain slices. Dickens showed that respiration of cortical cells was irreversibly poisoned by high pressure oxygen and felt that the primary effect was on sulphydryl groups of pyruvic oxidase, thus interfering with carbohydrate metabolism. Toxic effects were also noted on spinal cord, liver, testis, kidney, lung and muscle in decreasing order of sensitivity.

Research over the last 20 years has been primarily directed at elucidation of the mechanism of the toxicity. Workers have looked at such factors as the role of inert gas and carbon dioxide, blockage of airways and atelectasis, changes in lung surfactant, changes in cellular metabolism, inhibition of enzyme system and the role of the endocrine system. Recently, further efforts to delineate the pulmonary limits of exposure have been undertaken. This has become increasingly important with saturation diving involving prolonged stays under increased ambient pressure and the use of oxygen mixtures to shorten decompression time.

# Central nervous system toxicity
(the 'Paul Bert effect')

In diving, central nervous system (CNS) oxygen toxicity is more likely when closed or semi-closed circuit rebreathing sets are used, and is the factor limiting depth when oxygen is used. With compressed air, the effect of increased partial pressure of nitrogen (see Chapter 15) usually prevents the diver from reaching a depth and duration at which oxygen will become a problem. High oxygen pressures are used in therapeutic recompression for decompression sickness and air embolism. Therefore, the diving physician is more likely to encounter toxicity under these conditions.

> *The danger of convulsions prevents divers breathing 100% oxygen deeper than 10 metres in safety.*

### Clinical manifestations

A wide range of symptoms and signs has been described, the most dramatic of which is a grand mal type **convulsion**. Consciousness is maintained up to the time of convulsion and there are apparently no changes in the electroencephalogram prior to convulsion.

There is no satisfactory consistent warning of impending convulsions, but any unusual symptom should be considered. The following manifestations have been reported, singly and in combination: nausea, vomiting, lightheadedness, dizziness, tinnitus, vertigo, incoordination, sensations of impending collapse or uneasiness (dysphoria), facial pallor, sweating, bradycardia, constriction of visual fields, dazzle, lip twitching, dilatation of pupils, twitching of hand, muscular twitching elsewhere, hiccups, paraesthesiae (especially fingers), dyspnoea, retrograde amnesia, illusions, disturbance of special senses, hallucinations and confusion.

**Facial twitching** is a common objective sign in chamber exposures to oxygen greater than 2 ATA, and signifies an imminent convulsion. Lip twitching may be seen if a mouth piece is being used. Nausea, retching and vomiting are particularly noted after prolonged exposures between 1 and 2 ATA.

---

*CNS oxygen toxicity:*
- *Twitching (especially lips)*
- *Nausea*
- *Dizziness*
- *Dysphoria*
- *Convulsions*

---

The facial pallor is thought to be due to the intense peripheral vasoconstriction of hyperoxia and not necessarily a sign of cerebral toxicity. Similarly, the paraesthesiae in fingers and toes do not necessarily indicate an impending convulsion. They may persist for hours after exposure and may represent an effect on peripheral nerves of local vasoconstriction.

An important aspect of toxicity is the great **variation in susceptibility**. As well as the wide range of tolerance between individuals, there is marked variation in one person's tolerance from day to day. Therefore, in any one diver, the time to onset of symptoms cannot be related to a predictable depth or time of exposure. Despite this variation, the greater the partial pressure and the longer the time of exposure, the more likely is the toxicity to develop.

---

*Factors lowering threshold to CNS toxicity:*
- *Exercise*
- *Immersion in water*
- *Increased arterial carbon dioxide*

---

Exposure in water rather than in dry chambers markedly decreases the tolerance of oxygen. Many of the previously listed clinical features are much less apparent in the water, where convulsions are more often the first manifestation. A convulsion is much more dangerous under water because of the added complications of drowning and pulmonary barotrauma. Therefore, most authorities have set a maximum safe depth for pure oxygen diving at about 10 metres. Short dives may be safe at greater depths and prolonged ones at shallower depths (Table 18.1). Compression chamber exposure is considered to be less hazardous for an equivalent dive profile. Current decompression procedures, if performed in chambers, prescribe oxygen exposures at 18 metres (2.8 ATA).

Exercise has also been shown to hasten the onset of symptoms. Shallower maximum safe depths have been set for 'working' as opposed to 'resting' dives on oxygen. This observation is also of importance when oxygen is used to shorten decompression times in the water. Divers undergoing decompression should be at rest, e.g. supported on a stage – not battling swell, current and buoyancy to maintain constant depth.

A recent US Navy study indicated that divers whose core temperature dropped more rapidly during a closed circuit oxygen dive were more likely to develop symptoms of oxygen toxicity.

Carbon dioxide build-up during exercise has been suggested as a potentiating factor in producing convulsions. Increased inspired carbon dioxide tension may develop with inadequate absorbent systems and in poorly ventilated helmets and chambers, thus rendering the diver more susceptible to oxygen convulsions.

The role of inert gas in the exacerbation of oxygen toxicity has been suggested but still needs to be fully elucidated (see Chapter 15).

**Table 18.1 US Navy oxygen depth – time limits in water**

| Normal operations | | Exceptional operations | |
| --- | --- | --- | --- |
| *Depth in feet* (m) | *Time* (min) | *Depth in feet* (m) | *Time* (min) |
| 10    (3) | 240 | 30    (9) | 45 |
| 15    (4.6) | 150 | 35    (10.7) | 25 |
| 20    (6) | 110 | 40    (12) | 10 |
| 25    (7.6) | 75 | | |

> *A subject is much more likely to develop central nervous system oxygen toxicity exercising in the water than in a dry chamber at rest, at equivalent pressures.*

The frequency of presenting symptoms in 'wet' divers resting and working is shown in Table 18.2 from Donald's work. In all cases exposure continued until the first symptoms developed ('end-point').

**Table 18.2 Incidence of symptoms resulting from exposure to 'end-point'**

| | Incidence in | |
|---|---|---|
| | *388 resting divers to end-point in water (%)* | *120 working divers to end-point in water (%)* |
| Convulsions | 9.2 | 6.8 |
| Lip twitching | 60.6 | 50.0 |
| Vertigo | 8.8 | 20.8 |
| Nausea | 8.3 | 17.5 |
| Respiratory disturbances | 3.8 | 5.0 |
| Twitching of parts other than lips | 3.2 | 1.7 |
| Sensation of abnormality (drowsiness, numbness, confusion etc.) | 3.2 | |
| Visual disturbances | 1.0 | |
| Acoustic hallucinations | 0.6 | |
| Paraesthesiae | 0.4 | |

From Donald (1947).

---

## CASE REPORT 18.1

BL, a 20-year-old trainee naval diver, was taking part in air diving training to a depth of 21 metres. He was using surface supply breathing apparatus (SSBA), which consists of a demand valve and a hose to the surface connected to large cylinder via a pressure regulator adjusted according to the depth. After approximately 20 minutes, he was signalled with a tug on the hose to return to the surface because the cylinder was running low. He remained in the water at the surface while his hose was connected to another cylinder and then recommenced his dive. Some 12 minutes into the second dive BL's surface attendant noted that there were no surface bubbles. The instructor told the attendant to signal BL via the hose tug system. There were no answering tugs on the line. The standby diver was then sent into the water to check BL. He found BL floating a metre off the bottom with his demand valve out of his mouth. He was brought rapidly back to the diving boat and CPR resuscitation was commenced using a portable oxygen resuscitator. After some time, probably about 15 minutes, the small oxygen cylinder of the resuscitator was noted to be low so one of the group was instructed to connect the resuscitator to the emergency large oxygen cylinder. The oxygen cylinder was then found to have a line already attached to it – BL's SSBA! BL failed to respond to intense resuscitation carried on for more than 2 hours.

*Diagnosis:* death due to central nervous system oxygen toxicity (presumably convulsions).

---

### CASE REPORT 18.2

AM and his buddy, military divers, were practising night-time underwater ship attack using closed circuit 100% oxygen rebreathing sets. While approaching the ship, they exceeded the maximum safe depth to avoid being spotted by lights, and had to ascend to the ship's hull (depth 9 metres). While escaping from the ship, AM had difficulty in freeing his depth gauge and, when he finally did examine it, discovered he was at 19 metres. He started to ascend and remembers '2–3 jerkings' of his body prior to losing consciousness. The buddy diver noted that AM 'stiffened' as he lost consciousness and then started convulsing, which continued while being brought to the surface. Total time of dive was 28 minutes. At the surface, he was pale with spasmodic respirations and the lug on the mouth piece had been chewed off. Artificial respiration was administered. AM was incoherent for 20 minutes and vomited once. A headache and unsteadiness in walking persisted for several hours after the incident. An electroence-phalogram 3 days later was normal. (The buddy diver was exhausted on surfacing, felt nauseated and was unable to climb into the boat, but recovered quickly.)

*Diagnosis:* central nervous system oxygen toxicity.

---

Convulsions, which may be the first manifestation of toxicity, are indistinguishable clinically from grand mal epilepsy. A review of neurological toxicity in US Navy divers showed convulsions were more likely to be the presenting feature in inexperienced divers breathing oxygen, compared with trained divers. It is inferred that some of the so-called premonitory symptoms may be due to suggestion rather than oxygen. Of 63 divers, 25 had convulsions as the first clinical manifestation, 10 had focal twitching, and 13 more progressed to convulsions despite immediate reduction of partial pressure. A more recent study revealed nausea as the most common manifestation, followed by muscle twitching and dizziness.

The following description of a typical fit has been given by Lambertsen, who performed much of the original work in the USA on this subject.

The convulsion is usually but not always preceded by localized muscular twitching, especially about the eyes, mouth and forehead. Small muscles of the hands may also be involved, and incoordination of diaphragm activity in respiration may occur. After they begin, these phenomena increase in severity over a period which may vary from a few minutes to nearly an hour, with essentially clear consciousness being retained. Eventually an abrupt spread of excitation occurs and the rigid tonic phase of the convulsion begins. Respiration ceases at this point and does not begin again until the intermittent muscular contractions return. The tonic phase usually lasts for about 30 seconds and is accompanied by an abrupt loss of consciousness. It is followed by vigorous clonic contractions of the muscle groups of head and neck, trunk and limbs, which become progressively less violent over about 1 minute. As the incoordinated motor activity stops, respiration can proceed normally. Following the convulsion, hypercapnia is marked due to accumulation of carbon dioxide concurrent with breath-holding. Respiration is complicated by obstruction from the tongue and by the extensive secretions which result from the autonomic component of the central nervous system convulsive activity. Because the diver inspired a high pressure of oxygen prior to the convulsion, a high alveolar oxygen tension persists during the apnoea. The individual remains well oxygenated throughout the convulsion. Due to the increased arterial carbon dioxide tension, brain oxygenation could increase the breath-holding period. This is in contrast to the epileptic patient who convulses while breathing air at sea level.

The **latent period** before the onset of toxic symptoms is inversely proportional to the inspired oxygen tension. It may be prolonged by hyperventilation and interruption of exposure, and shortened by exercise, immersion in water and the presence of carbon dioxide.

The 'oxygen off-effect' refers to the unexpected observation that the first signs of neurological toxicity may appear after a sudden reduction in inspired oxygen tension. Also, existing symptoms may be exacerbated. The fall in inspired oxygen pressure is usually the result of removing the mask from a subject breathing 100% oxygen in a chamber. It may also occur when the chamber pressure is reduced, or when the diver surfaces. It has been postulated that the sudden drop in cerebral arterial oxygen tension in the presence of persisting hyperoxic-induced cerebral vaso-constriction results in cerebral hypoxia in a brain already impaired by oxygen poisoning.

Typical grand mal epilepsy has been observed up to several hours after exposure to high oxygen pressure. It has been suggested that there may be a relationship between the manifestations of latent epilepsy and oxygen exposure. In hyperbaric oxygen therapy, known epileptics have convulsed at less than expected pressure exposure.

Some animal experiments have shown that older animals and male animals are more susceptible to poisoning, but this has not been conclusively demonstrated in humans.

The major differential diagnosis of neurological toxicity is cerebral air embolism (CAGE) producing neurological features. After reducing the oxygen partial pressure, recovery is to be expected from oxygen toxicity.

## Pathology

No pathological changes in the central nervous system directly attributable to oxygen toxicity have been observed in humans. Animal experiments with intermittent or continued exposure cause permanent neurological impairment with selective grey matter and neuronal necrosis (the John Bean effect). By light and electron microscopy, two types of changes have been reported in studies in rats at 8 ATA oxygen. Type A lesions are characterized by pyknosis and hyperchromatosis with vacuolization of the cytoplasm in scattered individual neurons. Type B lesions consist of lysis of the cytoplasm and caryorrhexis, in specific areas, such as in the reticular substance of the medulla, the pericentral area of the cervical spinal grey matter, the ventral cochlear nuclei, the maxillary bodies and the inferior colliculi.

Pharmacological control of convulsions and pulmonary oedema does not alter the findings. Severe exposure eventually leads to haemorrhagic necrosis of the brain and spinal cord but

---

### CASE REPORT 18.3

TL was using a semi-closed circuit rebreathing apparatus rigged for 60% nitrogen. After 17 minutes at 22 metres, he suddenly noted a ringing noise in his head. He flushed through his set, thinking his symptoms were due to carbon dioxide toxicity. He then noted that his surroundings were brighter than usual, and decided to surface.

On surfacing he was noted to be conscious but pale and panting heavily. He moved his mouth piece and while being brought on board 'went into a convulsion, where his whole face changed shape, his eyes rolled up into his head, his face turned a dark colour and his body began to cramp'. He recovered within 3–4 minutes and 30 minutes later there was no abnormality on clinical examination.

Equipment examination revealed that the emergency oxygen cylinder was nearly empty, i.e. that he had used 64 litres of 100% oxygen in addition to approximately the same amount of 60% oxygen. The oxygen in his breathing bag would therefore have approximated 80% and the inspired oxygen tension 2.4 ATA. The carbon dioxide absorbent was normal.

*Diagnosis:* central nervous system oxygen toxicity.

even single exposures (30 minutes at 4 ATA) produce ultrastructural changes in anterior horn grey matter.

## Aetiology

Oxygen has an effect on the regulation of blood flow, tissue oxygenation and energy metabolism in the brain. These effects are pressure dependent and are involved in the development of toxicity. The precise mechanism of oxygen toxicity is unknown. There are a great many sites at which oxygen acts on metabolic pathways or on specific cellular functions. Rather than causing an increase in metabolism, as suggested by early workers, hyperoxia has been demonstrated to depress cellular metabolism.

In vitro studies on isolated enzymes and tissue preparations have shown many enzymes are inactivated by high pressure oxygen, particularly those containing **sulphydryl** groups (–SH). It is postulated that adjacent –SH groups are oxidized to form disulphide bridges (–S–S–) thus inactivating the enzyme. The oxidation may be due to oxygen free radicals (see below). Enzymes containing –SH groups, and known to be susceptible, include glyceraldehyde phosphate dehydrogenase (a key enzyme in glycolysis), the flavoprotein enzymes of the respiratory chain and the enzymes involved in oxidative phosphorylation. The suppression of a metabolic pathway may result in accumulation of a metabolite and in this way cause toxicity.

> *Enzymes containing sulphydryl groups are particularly susceptible to high pressure oxygen.*

The **oxygen free radical** theory of toxicity is widely accepted as an explanation at the molecular level. The increased formation of partially reduced oxygen products by hyperbaric oxygenation is thought to be responsible for the cellular toxicity. These 'free radicals', such as superoxide anion and hydroxyl radical, produced in excess may lead to cellular structural damage or enzyme inactivation. Antioxidants such as glutathione and disulfiram have been shown to offer some protection.

The molecular disturbance produced by the free radicals is thought to then affect cellular metabolic function or neurotransmitter function (see also Aetiology of pulmonary oxygen toxicity).

**Gamma-aminobutyric acid** (GABA) is known to be a transmitter at central nervous system inhibitory nerve synapses. One of the demonstrated consequences of enzymatic changes induced by hyperoxia is a reduction in the endogenous output of GABA. This decrease is thought to produce the convulsions by allowing uncontrolled firing of excitatory nerves. Agents which raise brain levels of GABA appear to protect against convulsions. Lithium, which has been useful in the treatment of manic depressive psychosis, has proved to be effective in inhibiting convulsions in rats. It was also shown to prevent the decrease in brain GABA which normally precedes the convulsions.

> *Changes in brain GABA levels appear to be involved in neurological toxicity.*

The sites at which oxygen exerts its effect may involve: cell membranes and their function, 'active transport' membranes, synaptic transmission, mitochondria or the cell nuclei.

**Increased tissue carbon dioxide** levels have been proposed as a cause of the toxicity. At greater than 3 ATA oxygen, oxyhaemoglobin is not reduced on passing through capillaries and so is not available for the carriage of carbon dioxide as carboxyhaemoglobin. Therefore carbon dioxide cannot be eliminated by this route. The resultant increase in brain carbon dioxide tension has proved to be small (2.5–6 mmHg). An equivalent rise is caused by breathing 6% carbon dioxide and does not cause convulsions in the presence of a normal partial pressure of oxygen, but the slight rise in $P_{CO_2}$ may reduce the cerebral vasoconstrictive effects of hyperoxia.

**Exercise** and carbon dioxide inhalation predispose to convulsions and hyperventilation protects against them. Carbon dioxide may play a role in lowering seizure threshold both at the cellular level and by influencing cerebral blood flow, and hence the 'dose' of oxygen delivered to the brain.

Thyroid and adrenal **hormones** enhance, and hypophysectomy and adrenalectomy, reduce susceptibility in animals. Adrenergic blocking drugs, some anaesthetics, GABA, lithium, magnesium and superoxide dismutase have a protective effect. Adrenaline, atropine, aspirin, amphetamine and pentobarbital are among a host of agents that enhance toxicity.

Light, noise and other stressful situations also affect CNS tolerance. Thus the general stress reaction, and more specifically adrenal hormones, may have a role in enhancing CNS (and pulmonary) toxicity.

## Prevention

Prevention of cellular changes by administration of drugs is not yet possible. In animal experiments, many different pharmacological agents have been shown to have a protective effect against toxic effects of oxygen. The agents include disulfiram, glutathione, lithium, iso-nicotinic acid, hydrazide, gamma-aminobutyric acid and sympathetic blocking agents. None of these agents is in prophylactic clinical use at present. Prevention of convulsions by anaesthetics of anticonvulsant agents removes only this overt expression of toxicity and damage at the cellular level will continue. The only current, safe approach is to place limits on exposure. These limits depend on the partial pressure of oxygen, the duration and the conditions of exposure (such as 'wet dive' or in a dry chamber, at exercise or rest).

The Royal Navy and Royal Australian Navy place a limit for pure oxygen diving of 9 metres for a resting dive and 7 metres for a working dive. The US Navy relates the duration of exposure to the depth (see Table 18.1).

The US Navy requires divers to undergo a test exposure of 30 minutes at 60 feet breathing 100% oxygen to eliminate those who are unusually susceptible. This does not take into account the marked variation in individuals from day to day, but certain individuals can be demonstrated to be excessively oxygen sensitive.

An awareness of levels at which toxicity is likely, and close observation for early signs such as lip twitching, should reduce the incidence of convulsions. If early signs are noted, the subject should signal his companion, stop excessive exertion and hyperventilate.

In therapeutic recompression tables, periods of air breathing are used to interrupt the exposure to high levels of oxygen and thus reduce the likelihood of toxicity. If the decompression illness is very serious, and the risks of oxygen toxicity are acceptable alternatives, diazepam (Valium) may be used to reduce the toxicity effects.

In chamber therapy, most therapeutic tables do not prescribe 100% oxygen deeper than 2.8 ATA. Intermittent exposure delays the onset of toxicity. It has been suggested that the rate of recovery is greater than the rate of development of cellular changes leading to toxicity.

At least in hyperbaric oxygen patients certain preventive measures have reduced the incidence of convulsions. Oxygen-breathing divers and hyperbaric workers are advised to avoid:

1. Exposure while febrile.
2. Drugs that increase tissue $CO_2$, e.g. opiates, carbonic anhydrase inhibitors.
3. Aspirin and steroids.
4. Fluorescent lights.
5. Stimulants such as caffeine (e.g. coffee).

## Treatment

Treatment is the management of a grand mal convulsion. The initial aim is basically to avoid physical trauma associated with the convulsion. A padded tongue depressor to prevent tongue biting may be useful in a chamber.

In the water, the diver should be brought to the surface only after the tonic phase of the convulsion has ceased. The same action is indicated in compression chambers, but with allowance made for decompression staging. If it is against the interests of the patient to ascend, it is usually a simple matter to reduce the oxygen in his breathing mixture.

Anticonvulsants may be used in exceptional circumstances. Phenytoin has been successfully used to stop convulsions in a patient with cerebral air embolism being treated with

**Table 18.3 The use of oxygen in recompression therapy**

### IF OXYGEN INTOLERANCE OCCURS OR IS ANTICIPATED

(A) Halt ascent, remove mask at once, maintain depth constant
(B) Protect a convulsing patient from injury due to violent contact with fixtures, deckplates or hull, but do not forcefully oppose convulsive movements
(C) With a padded mouthbit protect the tongue of a convulsing patient
(D) For non-convulsive reactions, have patient hyperventilate – with chamber air for several breaths
(E) Administer sedative drugs upon direction of a medical officer
(F) 15 minutes after the reaction has entirely subsided resume the schedule at the point of its interruption
(G) If the reaction occurred at 18 metres, on the 135 minute schedule, upon arrival at 9 metres switch to 285 minute schedule (15 minutes air – 60 minutes oxygen, 15 minutes air – 60 minutes oxygen

### OXYGEN REACTIONS – SYMPTOMS

Twitching (fasciculations or tremors) of facial muscles and lips, nausea, dizziness and vertigo, vomiting, convulsions, anxiety, confusion, restlessness and irritability, malaise, disturbances of vision and narrowing of visual fields, incoordination, tremors of arms or legs, numbness or 'tingling' of fingers or toes, fainting, spasmodic breathing

### OXYGEN ADMINISTRATION ROUTINE PRACTICES

(A) Ensure patient is as comfortable as possible
(B) Patient at complete rest
(C) Ensure snug face-mask fit
(D) Follow air–oxygen schedule closely
(E) Be alert for signs or symptoms of reactions
(F) Patient to take a few deep breaths every 5 minutes during treatment

After *US Navy Diving Manual* – Rules and Routines for administration of oxygen.

hyperbaric oxygen. Diazepam is also very effective.

## Pulmonary toxicity

(the 'Lorrain Smith effect')

Pulmonary toxicity is not a problem in normal short duration oxygen diving. It assumes importance in saturation and long chamber dives and especially where high partial pressures of oxygen are inspired, such as in therapeutic recompression. Prolonged exposures to partial pressures as low as 0.55 ATA (such as in space flight) have been found to produce significant changes.

> *The wide variation of tolerance among different species invalidates extrapolation of animal studies to humans.*

In animals, pulmonary oxygen poisoning causes progressive respiratory distress, leading to respiratory failure and finally death. Early signs in humans are similar to those in animals. In patients receiving high concentrations of oxygen therapeutically, it is sometimes difficult to distinguish between the conditions for which the oxygen is given and the effects of the oxygen itself (e.g. shock lung, respiratory distress syndrome).

## Clinical manifestations

As in neurological toxicity, the factors affecting the degree of toxicity are **partial pressure of inspired oxygen, duration of exposure** and **individual variation** in susceptibility. In one study of exposure to 2.0 ATA oxygen, some subjects experienced symptoms at 3 hours whilst one was symptom free for 8 hours.

The earliest **symptom** is usually a mild tracheal irritation similar to the tracheitis of an upper respiratory infection. This irritation is aggravated by deep inspiration which may produce a cough. Chest tightness is often noted, then a substernal pain develops which is also aggravated by deep breathing and coughing. The cough gets progressively worse until it is uncontrollable. Dyspnoea at rest develops and, if the exposure is prolonged, is rapidly progressive. The higher the inspired oxygen pressure, the more rapidly do symptoms develop and the greater the intensity.

Physical **signs**, such as râles, nasal mucous membrane hyperaemia and fever have only been produced after prolonged exposure in normal subjects.

---

*Pulmonary oxygen toxicity:*
- *Chest tightness*
- *Cough*
- *Chest pain*
- *Shortness of breath*
- *Fall in vital capacity*

---

Although **chest X-ray** changes have been reported, there is no pathognomonic appearance of oxygen toxicity. Diffuse bilateral pulmonary densities have been reported. With continued exposure, irregularly shaped infiltrates extend and coalesce.

There is a 10% fall in residual volume in normal subjects breathing 100% oxygen at sea level after about 10 minutes, presumably due to the loss of the splinting effect of nitrogen.

The measurement of **vital capacity** is one monitor of the onset and progression of toxicity, although it is less sensitive than the clinical symptoms. Reduction in vital capacity is usually progressive throughout the oxygen exposure. The drop continues for several hours after cessation of exposure and many occasionally take up to 12 days to return to normal. Because measurement of vital capacity requires the subject's full cooperation, its usefulness may be limited in the therapeutic situation. It has been used to delineate pulmonary oxygen tolerance limits in normal subjects – this is shown in Figure 18.2 which relates partial pressure of oxygen to duration of exposure. The percentage fall in vital capacity is plotted.

The size of the fall in vital capacity does not always indicate the degree of pulmonary toxicity as measured by other lung function tests, such as lung volumes, static and dynamic compliance, and diffusing capacity for carbon monoxide.

Certain subjects, especially at higher inspired oxygen pressures (2.5 ATA), demonstrate a rapid fall in vital capacity. The recovery after exposure is also more rapid than that after an equal vital capacity decrement produced at a lower oxygen pressure for a longer time. This rapid onset and reversal are said to be related to an interaction of neurological and pulmonary toxicity.

## Pathology

The pathological changes in the lung as a result of oxygen toxicity have been divided into two types: acute and chronic, depending on the inspired pressure of oxygen.

**Acute** toxicity is caused by pressures of oxygen greater than 0.8 ATA. It has been subdivided into exudative and proliferative phases. The exudative phase consists of a perivascular and interstitial inflammatory response and alveolar oedema, haemorrhage, hyaline membranes, swelling and destruction of capillary endothelial cells and destruction of type I alveolar lining cells. This phase was the type described by Lorrain Smith. Progression of the disease leads to the proliferative phase which, after resolution of the inflammatory exudate, is characterized by proliferation of fibroblasts, and type II alveolar cells. There is an increase in the alveolar–capillary distance. Pulmonary capillaries are destroyed and some arterioles become obstructed with thrombus.

The **chronic** response usually follows inspired oxygen tensions between 0.5 and 0.8 ATA for longer times. It is characterized by

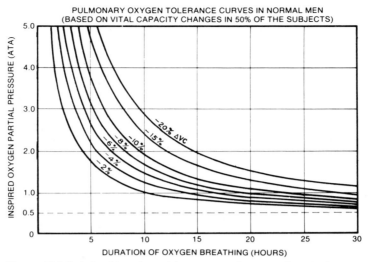

**Figure 18.2** Relationship of partial pressure of oxygen breathed, and duration of exposure, to degree of pulmonary oxygen damage

hyperplasia of type II cells, replacing type I cells and progressive pulmonary fibrosis, especially affecting alveolar ducts rather than alveolar septa. These features are also found in the adult respiratory distress syndrome (shock, drowning, trauma) for which high oxygen tensions are given. Whether oxygen actually causes the damage in these situations or exacerbates the condition by interacting with the initial pulmonary damage is not clear.

A consequence of these effects on pulmonary physiology is to increase ventilation–perfusion mismatching. Obstruction of arterioles will result in an increase in deadspace.

## Aetiology

It is likely that there are many factors which act in combination to produce toxic changes in the lungs. These may be direct effects on pulmonary cellular metabolism, or indirect due to a sequence of events set in train by oxygen causing changes at extrapulmonary sites. Similar **enzyme changes**, as described in the aetiology of neurological toxicity, have also been described in pulmonary toxicity.

As in CNS oxygen toxicity, it is likely that many of the acute pulmonary changes are brought about by **oxygen free radicals**. These radicals are intermediates formed in many cel-

lular biochemical enzyme-catalysed reactions. Superoxide anion ($O_2^-$) is formed when oxygen ($O_2$) accepts a single electron and hydrogen peroxide two electrons. The final reaction is the acceptance by oxygen of four electrons to form water or stable hydroxyl anion. Superoxide and peroxide can react to form the hydroxyl radical ($\cdot$OH). All these species of oxygen are referred to as oxygen radicals and are highly oxidative.

Cells have a system of enzymes to scavenge these radicals called the tissue antioxidant system. Two of these enzymes, superoxide dismutase and catalase, are involved in maintaining adequate supplies of reduced glutathione (containing sulphydryl groups) to deal with the free radicals. Hyperoxia may cause this system to be swamped and the excess free radicals may then produce cell damage. Examples of unwanted oxidation reactions are peroxidation of lipid in cell membranes and protein sulphydryl oxidation causing cross-linking. Nevertheless, the exact cellular site of action is still uncertain.

The characteristic feature of chronic pulmonary oxygen toxicity is pulmonary fibrosis. In animal studies, paraquat, bleomycin and ozone have all been noted to produce pulmonary fibrosis. These agents are known to produce oxygen free radicals. This further supports the belief that oxygen toxicity involves free radicals.

Further evidence for the role of the super-oxide and hydroxyl free radicals is the demonstration by electron paramagnetic resonance of their increased production in pulmonary endothelial cells.

**Atelectasis** is a frequently described change in aviation pathology and is due to absorption collapse of alveoli during 100% oxygen breathing. This has also been suggested as a contributory mechanism to oxygen toxicity in divers. Although absorption collapse has been demonstrated, it is not an initiating factor, as toxicity develops in the presence of inert gas. If the inert gas is at narcotic levels, it actually enhances the onset of toxicity. Human studies show no difference in the progression of pulmonary oxygen toxicity when comparing pure oxygen or diluted oxygen at the same partial pressure.

**Endocrine** studies show that hypophysectomy and adrenalectomy protect against hyperoxia. ACTH and cortisone reverse this effect and, when given in normal animals, enhance toxicity (see also aetiology of CNS toxicity).

Several observations suggest a role of the **autonomic nervous system** in modifying the degree of toxicity. Adrenergic blocking drugs reduce the severity of toxicity as does bilateral adrenal medullectomy. Convulsions have been shown to hasten the onset of pulmonary oxygen toxicity in some animal studies. This may be related to an activation of the sympatho-adrenal system during convulsions. Lithium inhibits the development of lung oedema in rats exposed to high pressure oxygen. Lithium also decreases the sensitivity of humans to infused noradrenaline, thus providing a clue to the mechanism of its action.

**Carbon dioxide** retention is not now thought to be a prime contribution to this toxicity, but related changes in acid–base balance may modify the syndrome of pulmonary toxicity. These modifying influences may act via neurogenic and endocrine mechanisms. Very high levels of inspired carbon dioxide actually protect against pulmonary damage.

## Prevention

No specific therapy is available which can be used clinically to delay or modify the pulmonary damage caused by hyperoxia. Intermittent exposure may delay the onset of toxicity.

When toxicity is apparent, the oxygen partial pressure should be reduced. It is therefore important to be aware of the earliest signs of the syndrome.

The monitoring of vital capacity is thought by some to be a useful indicator of the progression of toxicity. The maximum acceptable reduction in vital capacity is dependent upon the reasons for the exposure. Although a 20% reduction may be acceptable in the treatment of severe decompression sickness, a 10% reduction would cause concern under operational diving conditions.

The degree of oxygen toxicity equivalent to a 2% decrease in vital capacity is completely reversible, asymptomatic and very difficult to measure under ordinary circumstances. With the elevated pressures of oxygen used in the treatment of serious diseases, such as severe decompression sickness or gas gangrene, it may be reasonable to accept a greater degree of pulmonary toxicity in order to treat the patient. The primary requirement of any therapy is that the treatment should not be worse than the disease.

The degree of pulmonary toxicity which produces a 10% decrease in vital capacity is associated with moderate symptoms of coughing and pain in the chest on deep inspiration. This degree of impairment of lung function has been shown experimentally to be reversible within a few days. It is suggested that a 10% decrement in vital capacity be chosen as the limit for most hyperbaric oxygen therapy procedures.

> *Intermittent rather than continuous exposure to high oxygen pressure delays the onset of both neurological and pulmonary oxygen toxicity.*

Periodic hyperinflation of the lungs is recommended in an attempt to delay atelectasis. The adherence to proposed pressure-duration limits for pulmonary oxygen toxicity is advised. This is difficult where extended durations and changing partial pressures of oxygen are involved.

Methods for calculating cumulative pulmonary toxicity have therefore been devised, and probably have a role in prolonged decompression and hyperbaric oxygen therapy. One of these is the contentious, but sometimes valuable, unit of pulmonary toxicity dosage at 1 ATA (UPTD). Although it has not received universal acceptance, it is at least a genuine attempt to measure the dose administered – as opposed to the actual response, which is assessment either clinically or by respiratory function testing.

At 1 ATA, by definition, 1 minute of breathing oxygen produces 1 UPTD. This is a 'unit' of oxygen toxicity causing damage to pulmonary tissue. It is a very theoretical concept, and must not be presumed to be reliable in all clinical situations. It is nevertheless sometimes of value to predict the extent of pulmonary damage with complicated recompression therapy regimes.

The UPTD can be calculated by knowing the degree of oxygen exposure and extracting the UPTD from specially constructed tables, or by a simple arithmetic calculation.

A UPTD of 615 will produce a degree of pulmonary toxicity roughly proportional to a 2% decrease in vital capacity. A UPTD of 1425 will produce a degree of oxygen toxicity equivalent to a 10% decrement in vital capacity. As greater exposure may not be reversible, the latter UPTD limit is chosen as the extreme for most hyperbaric oxygen therapy procedures.

Studies in mice have demonstrated that hyperoxia induces hypothermia and that hypothermia, rather than being protective, aggravates pulmonary oxygen toxicity.

As discussed in the prevention of neurological toxity, many drugs have been shown to be effective in animal experiments. They will probably have a role in the future in the prevention of pulmonary and other oxygen toxicity.

## Other manifestations of oxygen toxicity

It has been suggested that oxygen, although essention for survival of aerobic cells, should be regarded as a universal cellular poison. Nevertheless, in other organs receiving a high blood flow such as heart, kidney and liver, no toxicity has yet been detected in humans. It may be that CNS and pulmonary toxicity preempt its development in other organs.

Oxygen, in space flight exposures, has been shown to have a deleterious effect on **red blood cells** manifested by abnormal cell morphology and/or a decrease in circulating red blood cell mass. This may be due to depression of erythropoiesis, inactivation of essential glycolytic enzymes by oxidation of –SH groups or damage to red cell membranes resulting from peroxidation of membrane lipid. There have also been occasional reports of **haemolytic** episodes following hyperbaric oxygen exposure, but these seem to be related to individual idiosyncrasies such as specific enzyme defects.

Animal investigations of pulmonary toxicity have revealed hyperoxic activation of the intrinsic **coagulation** syndrome and consumptive coagulopathy. Chronic daily exposures of 600 UPTD/day can produce a syndrome of fatigue, headache, dizziness and paraesthesiae in operational divers.

Oxygen at high pressure causes constriction of **retinal vessels**. Many studies have also shown a reversible peripheral visual field constriction in humans and occasional case reports show transient unilateral loss of vision. Retinal exudates and scotomata have been reported. Retrolental fibroplasia may develop in premature infants breathing 60% oxygen.

Animal studies have demonstrated death of visual cells and retinal detachments on exposure to from 0.9 to 3 ATA oxygen. It has been suggested that these findings are due to intense vasoconstriction with resultant lack of nutrient flow rather than to a direct toxic effect of oxygen.

Other disorders which may be affected by the vasoconstriction include Raynaud's phenomenon and Buerger's disease, and migraine in adults. Possible closure of the patent ductus arteriosus has been proposed in the fetus exposed to increased oxygen.

Irreversible changes in the cornea and lens of guinea-pigs occur after exposure to 3 ATA oxygen for between 4 and 16 hours.

Some patients receiving hyperbaric oxygen therapy have been reported to develop myopia and/or cataracts. **Myopia** is an immediate response due to reversible changes in the lens but **nuclear cataracts** develop 6 months to a year later after multiple exposures.

**Serous otitis media** has been noted in aviators exposed to high concentrations of oxygen. It is due to absorption of oxygen from the middle ear. A syndrome related to the middle ear has been described in US Navy divers breathing 100% oxygen from semi-closed and closed circuit diving equipment. The symptoms were fullness, popping or crackling sensation in the ear, and a mild conductive hearing loss. On examination the most common finding was fluid in the middle ear. The syndrome was first noted after rising from a night's sleep, not immediately after the dive itself, and disappeared rapidly. There was no suggestion of barotrauma.

It is likely that, as more sensitive methods of detection are used, evidence of oxygen toxicity in many other cells and organs will be noted.

One of the theories of the aetiology of **dysbaric osteonecrosis** (see Chapter 14) suggest that it may be another manifestation of oxygen toxicity. Oxygen is said to cause a swelling of the fat cells of the bone marrow thus occluding its blood supply.

## Recommended reading

BALENTINE, J.D. (1983). *Pathology of Oxygen Toxicity*. New York: Academic Press.

BEAN, J.W. (1945). Effects of oxygen at increased pressure. *Physiolog Reviews* **25**, 1–147.

BERT, P. (1878). *La Pression Barometrique (Barometric Pressure)*. Reprinted in 1943 in *Researches in Experimental Physiology*. Columbus, Ohio: College Book Company.

BUTLER, F.K. and KNAFEL, M.E. (1986). Screening for oxygen intolerance in US Navy Divers. *Undersea and Biomedical Research* **13**, 91–98.

BUTLER, F.J.K. and THALMAN, E.D. (1986). Central nervous system oxygen toxicity in closed circuit scuba divers 11. *Undersea Biomedical Research* **13**, 193–223.

CLARK, J.M. (1982) Oxygen toxicity. In: *The Physiology and Medicine of Diving*, edited by P.B. Bennett and D.H. Elliott, pp. 200–238. London: Baillière Tindall.

CLARK, J.M. and LAMBERTSEN, C.J. (1971). Pulmonary oxygen toxicity: A review. *Pharmacology* **23** (2).

CLARK, J.M. and LAMBERTSEN, C.J. (1971). Rate of development of pulmonary oxygen toxicity in man during oxygen breathing at 2.0 ATA. *Journal of Applied Physiology* **30**, 739–752.

CLARK, J.M., GELLAND, R., FLORES, N.D., LAMBERTSEN, C.J. and PIGARELLO, J.B. (1987). Pulmonary tolerance in man to continuous oxygen exposure at 3.0, 2.5, 2.0 and 1.5 ATA in predictive studies. *Ninth International Symposium on Underwater and Hyperbaric Physiology*, Undersea and Hyperbaric Medical Society, Bethesda, MD.

COTES, J.E., DAVEY, I.S., REED, J.W. and ROOKS, M. (1987). Respiratory effects of a single saturation dive to 300m. *British Journal of Industrial Medicine* **44**, 76–82.

DONALD, K.W. (1947). Oxygen poisoning in man. *British Medical Journal* **1**, 667–672, 712–717.

ECKENHOFF, R.G., DOUGHERTY, J.H., OSBORNE, S.F. and PARKER, J.W. (1987). Progression of the recovery from pulmonary oxygen toxicity in humans exposed to 5 ATA air. *Aviation, Space and Environmental Medicine* **58**, 658–667.

FISCHER, C.L. and KIMZEY, S.L. (1971). Effects of oxygen on blood formation and destruction. *Proceedings of the Fourth Symposium on Underwater Physiology*. New York: Academic Press.

GELFAND, R., CLARK, J.M., LAMBERTSEN, C.J. and PISAROLLO, J.B. (1987). Effects on respiratory homeostasis of prolonged, continuous hypoxia at 1.5 to 3.0 ATA in man in predictive studies. *Ninth International Symposium on Underwater and Hyperbaric Physiology*. Undersea and Hyperbaric Medical Society, Bethesda, MD.

GILLEN, H.W. (1966). Oxygen convulsions in man. *Proceedings of the Third International Conference on Hyperbaric Medicine*. National Academy of Sciences, Washington DC.

HART, G.B. and STRAUSS, M.B. (1987). Central nervous system oxygen toxicity in a clinical setting. *Ninth International Symposium on Underwater and Hyperbaric Physiology*. Undersea and Hyperbaric Medical Society, Bethesda, MD.

JAMIESON, D. and CARMODY, J. (1989). Low temperature worsens mammalian oxygen toxicity. *Aviation, Space and Environmental Medicine* **60**, 639–643.

LAMBERTSEN et al. (1987). Definition of tolerance to continuous hyperoxia in man: An abstract report of predictive studies V. *Ninth International Symposium on Underwater and Hyperbaric Physiology*. Undersea and Hyperbaric Medical Society, Bethesda, MD.

PALMQUIST, B.M., PHILPSON, B. and BARR, P.O. (1984). Nuclear cataract and myopia during hyperbaric oxygen therapy. *British Journal of Ophthalmology* **68**, 113–117.

PISARELLO, J.B., CLARK, J.M., LAMBERTSEN, C.J. and GELFAND, R. (1987). Human circulatory responses to prolonged hyperbaric hyperoxia in predictive studies V. *Ninth International Symposium on Underwater and Hyperbaric Physiology*. Undersea and Hyperbaric Medical Society, Bethesda, MD.

SMALL, A. (1984). New perspectives on hyperoxic pulmonary toxicity – a review. *Undersea Biomedical Research* **11**, 1–24.

STADIE, W.C., RIGGS, B.C. and HAUGAARD, N. (1944). Oxygen poisoning. *Americal Journal of the Medical Sciences* **207**, 84–114.

STRAUSS, M.B., SHERROD, L. and CANTRELL, R.W. (1973). Serous otitis media in divers breathing 100% oxygen. Presented at Annual Scientific Meeting, Aerospace Medical Association, May 7–10.

TORBATI. D. (1987). Oxygen and brain physiologic functions: A review. *Ninth International Symposium on Underwater and Hyperbaric Physiology*. Undersea and Hyperbaric Medical Society, Bethesda, MD.

US NAVY DIVING MANUAL (1988).

WEAVER, L.K. (1983). Phenytoin sodium in oxygen-toxicity-induced seizures. *Annals of Emergency Medicine* **12**, 38–41.

WRIGHT, B.W. (1972). Use of the University of Pennsylvania Institute for Environmental Medicine procedure for calculation of cumulative oxygen toxicity. *US Navy EDU Report* 2–72.

ZWEIER, J.L., DUKE, S.S, KUPPASAMY, P., SYLVESTER J.T. and GAHRIELSON, E.W. (1989). Electron paramagnetic resonance evidence that cellular oxygen toxicity is caused by the generation of superoxide and hydroxyl free radicals. *FEBS Letter* **252**, 12–16.

# 19

# Carbon dioxide toxicity

## Introduction

Carbon dioxide ($CO_2$) is normally present in the atmosphere in a concentration of 0.03–0.04% volume of dry air. This represents a partial pressure of 0.23–0.30 mmHg. It is one of the products of metabolism of protein, carbohydrates and fats produced in mitochondria in roughly the same volume as oxygen is consumed;

$$C_6H_{12}O_6 + 6O_2 = 6CO_2 + 6H_2O + energy$$

The resultant $CO_2$ has to be transported from the tissues by the circulation and eliminated by exhalation from the lungs. The normal $CO_2$ tension in arterial blood ($Pa_{CO_2}$) is 40 mmHg and for mixed venous blood is 46 mmHg, these values being a balance between production and excretion. $CO_2$ in the alveolar gas is in equilibrium with that leaving the pulmonary capillaries. The alveolar partial pressure ($PA_{CO_2}$) is therefore also 40 mmHg. After mixing with deadspace gas the partial pressure of $CO_2$ in the expired gas is about 32 mmHg.

$CO_2$ is the most potent stimulus to respiration. The central medullary chemoreceptors in the brain are stimulated by increases in arterial $CO_2$ and pH. In normal conditions, adjustments in ventilation keep the arterial and alveolar $CO_2$ partial pressure remarkably constant. The peripheral chemoreceptors (carotid and aortic bodies) are primarily responsive to hypoxaemia but also respond to increases in hydrogen ion and $CO_2$ concentration.

The solubility of $CO_2$ is about 20 times that of oxygen so there is considerably more $CO_2$ than oxygen in simple solution. $CO_2$ is transported in the blood in both plasma and red cells. In each 100 ml of arterial blood, 3 ml are dissolved, 3 ml are in carbamino compounds (with haemoglobin and plasma proteins) and 44 ml are carried as bicarbonate ($HCO_3^-$).

At rest, approximately 5 ml $CO_2$ per 100 ml blood are given up from the tissues and liberated in the lungs. About 200 ml $CO_2$ are produced and excreted per minute. If this $CO_2$ is retained in the body (e.g. due to rebreathing) the $Pa_{CO_2}$ will climb at the rate of 3–6 mmHg/min.

With exercise, much larger amounts of $CO_2$ are produced. The working diver can produce over 3 litres of $CO_2$ per minute for short periods, and 2 litres per minute for over half an hour, usually without serious alteration in $Pa_{CO_2}$ (due to a concomitant increase in lung ventilation).

In diving, although the environmental pressure is increased, the arterial and hence alveolar $CO_2$ tensions should be maintained at approximately 40 mmHg. This is because the number of molecules of $CO_2$ produced, and therefore the alveolar $P_{CO_2}$ is independent of the depth. The alveolar $P_{O_2}$ and $P_{N_2}$ increase with depth. Therefore the alveolar $CO_2$ percentage decreases.

> *Whereas 40 mmHg carbon dioxide partial pressure represents 5% of the alveolar air on the surface, it is only 1% of the alveolar air at a depth of 40 metres (5 ATA).*

With a constant rate of $CO_2$ production the alveolar, and hence arterial, $CO_2$ tension is inversely proportional to the alveolar ventilation, to which must be added the tension of $CO_2$ in the inspired gases. This is shown in the following equation:

$$P_{ACO_2} = \frac{kV_{CO_2}}{Va} + P_{ICO_2}$$

where

- $P_{ACO_2}$ is alveolar partial pressure of carbon dioxide
- $k$ is a conversion factor to convert conditions at STPD (standard temperature and pressure dry) to BTPS (body temperature and pressure saturated)
- $V_{CO_2}$ is the carbon dioxide production in litres/min STPD
- $Va$ is the alveolar ventilation in litres/min BTPS
- $P_{ICO_2}$ is the inspired carbon dioxide partial pressure

Alterations in $Pa_{CO_2}$ have widespread effects on the body, especially on the respiratory, circulatory and nervous systems. Apart from the hypocapnia produced by hyperventilation prior to breath-hold diving (see Chapters 3, 17 and 32), the more frequent derangement in diving is **hypercapnia**, an elevation of $CO_2$ in

blood and tissues. This may be an **acute** effect, or **chronic**. Where hypercapnia produces pathophysiological changes dangerous to the diver, the term '$CO_2$ toxicity' (or $CO_2$ poisoning) is used.

**Table 19.1 Abbreviations**

| | |
|---|---|
| $CO_2$ | Carbon dioxide |
| $P_{CO_2}$ | Partial pressure of $CO_2$ |
| $P_{ICO_2}$ | Inspired $CO_2$ partial pressure or tension |
| $Pa_{CO_2}$ | Arterial $CO_2$ tension (or pressure) |
| $P_{ACO_2}$ | Alveolar $CO_2$ tension |
| $P_{O_2}$ | Partial pressure of oxygen |
| $P_{N_2}$ | Partial pressure of nitrogen |

## Acute hypercapnia

### Causes

Excluding asphyxia and drowning, there are four main mechanisms of 1 carbon dioxide toxicity in diving:

1. **Failure of absorbent system**, e.g. in closed or semi-closed rebreathing appratus, submarines, saturation complexes etc.
2. **Inadequate ventilation of an enclosed environment**, e.g. in standard dress or other helmet diving and compression chamber diving where flushing is required to remove $CO_2$.
3. **Inadequate pulmonary ventilation**, e.g. in deep diving where the work of breathing dense gases is greater, or with increased resistance from the equipment.
4. **Contamination** of breathing gases by $CO_2$.

With all these causes, $CO_2$ toxicity is much more rapid when the diver is exercising and producing large amounts of $CO_2$.

> *Carbon dioxide toxicity is most commonly encountered in divers using closed or semi-closed rebreathing equipment. It is also seen where there is inadequate ventilation of an enclosed space such as a helmet, recompression chamber or submarine.*

In diving operations that rely on recycling of respiratory gases, the most common method of $CO_2$ removal uses the reaction between alkali

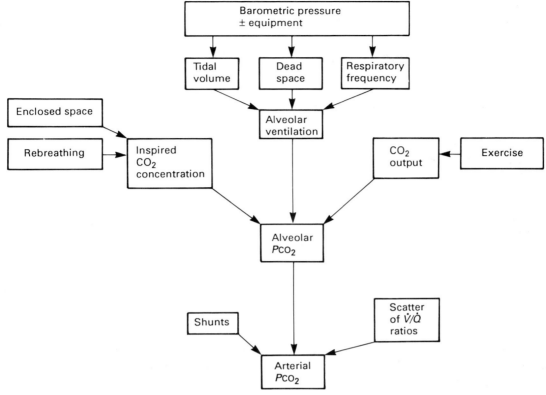

**Figure 19.1** Some factors which influence $P_{CO_2}$. (Adapted from J.F. Nunn, *Applied Respiratory Physiology*, 3rd edition, 1987, Butterworths)

metal hydroxide reagents (Protosorb, Sodasorb, Baralyme etc.) and carbonic acid:

$$H_2O + CO_2 \rightarrow H_2CO_3$$
$$H_2CO_3 + 2NaOH \rightarrow Na_2CO_3 + 2H_2O$$
$$Na_2CO_3 + Ca(OH)_2 \rightarrow 2NaOH + CaCO_3$$

Other techniques, some still being developed, include cryogenic freeze-out of $CO_2$ with liquid air or oxygen, molecular sieves, electrolytic decomposition into carbon and water, and the use of peroxides and superoxides which generate oxygen while removing carbon dioxide.

### Failure of the absorbent system

This failure in rebreathing sets may be due to the following causes.

### Inefficiency of absorbent material

This may be due to large granule size, low environmental temperature, low alkali content, low water content or sea water contamination.

### Equipment design faults

The canister should be of adequate size and adequate length compared to cross-sectional area. It should be insulated against extreme temperature changes. The design should prevent 'channelling' of gases through the absorbent. In circuit rebreathing equipment, the gas space between the absorbent granules should exceed the maximum tidal volume, so that there is time for absorption during the next part of the respiratory cycle. In pendulum rebreathing equipment, excessive functional deadspace between the diver's mouth and the canister causes him to inhale more expired $CO_2$.

### Operator error

$CO_2$ build-up may result if the diver fails to pack his canister properly with active absorbent, undertakes excessive exertion or exceeds the safe working life of the set.

### Inadequate ventilation of the environment

In helmet and recompression chamber dives, there must be a sufficient volume of gas supplied to flush the enclosed system of $CO_2$. In the same way that alveolar $P_{CO_2}$ is dependent on alveolar ventilation, the level of $CO_2$ in the enclosed space is inversely proportional to the ventilation of that space. When corrected to surface volumes, this means progressively greater amounts of gas must be supplied as the diver or chamber goes deeper.

### Inadequate pulmonary ventilation

At depth this is primarily due to the increased density of the respired gases. This causes an increased resistance to gas flow, both in the breathing apparatus and in the diver's own airways. Tight wet suits, harnesses and buoyancy compensators further restrict thoracic movement. An increased workload is thus placed on the diver's respiratory muscles. The extent to which this load is overcome varies greatly among divers, but there is often some elevation of the alveolar $P_{CO_2}$.

Significant exercise ($O_2$ uptake $> 60\%$ of maximal) under water always produces an elevation of $P_{a_{CO_2}}$ and is sometimes marked ($P_{a_{CO_2}} > 60$ mmHg) with concurrent symptoms. With increasing depth, a progressively greater amount of energy is required to rid the body of the same amount of $CO_2$. This is another reason for the substitution of lighter gases for nitrogen in deep diving. Even with lighter gases, the increased work of breathing is likely to limit the depth human beings can reach. Much current research is designed to define these limits.

The relevance of $CO_2$ retention in the **conventional open-circuit scuba** diving is not clear.

It is known that different regulators produce varying degrees of resistance to ventilation, with consequent retention. This will also rise with the increased breathing resistance due to inadequate maintenance of the regulator, or the deposition of foreign bodies and salt particles. Maintaining regulator performance to an acceptable performance level can be extremely difficult. The level of $CO_2$ retention is usually minor and does not lead to $CO_2$ toxicity. It does, however, increase with exposure to depth, and with low scuba cylinder pressure driving the gas through the regulator.

Perhaps more important than the consistent but mild $CO_2$ retention with scuba diving, is the occasional atypical subject who responds inadequately, either under pressure or on the surface, to raised $CO_2$ levels. It may be that these divers progressively elevate their $CO_2$ levels, as an alternative to increasing their ventilation, with the increased resistance to breathing. Under these conditions, it is theoretically possible that $CO_2$ toxicity, to the stage of unconsciousness, may eventuate.

Certain individuals have been shown to have a markedly reduced ventilatory response to elevated $P_{a_{CO_2}}$, including divers who have had otherwise unexplained episodes of loss of consciousness. In some cases the $CO_2$ toxicity combines with nitrogen narcosis to produce unconsciousness, but in others the depth is too shallow to expect significant nitrogen narcosis.

### Contamination

Some buoyancy vests are fitted with a $CO_2$ cartridge to inflate the vest in an emergency. A diver who, in a panic situation, then breathed this gas would rapidly develop $CO_2$ toxicity.

In cave diving, gas pockets may form under the roof. A diver may be tempted to remove his regulator and breathe in this gas which, not being replenished, will gradually accumulate $CO_2$. Such a diver may then develop toxicity.

### Clinical features

These depend on the rate of development and degree of $CO_2$ retention. They vary from mild compensated respiratory acidosis, detected only by blood gas and electrolyte estimations, to rapid unconsciousness with exposure to high inspired $P_{CO_2}$. Although $CO_2$ is a respiratory

## CASE REPORT 19.1

The diver was a healthy man who, during the course of a night dive to about 16 metres in cold but relatively still water, became disoriented, developed a headache and became nauseated and giddy. He signalled his companions and went to the surface uneventfully, but after 5 minutes at the surface he began vomiting. He was nauseated and dizzy, and a severe headache continued until he went to bed and to sleep about 1 hour later. The next day he felt drowsy, unable to concentrate, and generally 'not too sharp'. He had recently recovered from 'a virus' and was tired before the dive. He did not have any particular trouble equalizing ear pressure on descent. He commented that he had let go of his diver's light momentarily and that the brief period of darkness seemed to precipitate the episode.

About 2 weeks after the initial episode, the diver was feeling well and made a dive to about 18 metres. He had the same odd feelings (dizziness, disorientation etc.) at depth as before but this time without headache and nausea. Neither time had he experienced any symptoms that directly implicated the ears. He recalled an episode the year before when he had similar symptoms at 150 feet and had been very seasick returning to shore in the boat.

Laboratory measurement at rest and in both tethered swimming and on the treadmill were unremarkable except for end-tidal and arterialized venous $P_{CO_2}$ values as high as 49 mmHg during moderate work. Overall, the pulmonary function laboratory had seen only one healthy athlete whose $P_{CO_2}$ values exceeded those of this diver.

*Diagnosis:* possible $CO_2$ toxicity due to inadequate pulmonary ventilatory response to rising $Pa_{CO_2}$. Perhaps more detailed attention should have been paid to the ears and ENGs performed.

Authors' note: CL found this '$CO_2$ report' after some searching. CE suggested that it be moved to Chapter 27 or 28, and claimed that the only time he had seen $CO_2$ toxicity in scuba divers was when he inflated his BC with a $CO_2$ cartridge and then tried to breathe it down. A nasty acid taste it had too. The rarity of verifiable cases is indicative of the doubts surrounding the validity of the diagnosis.

---

stimulant, most of its effects are related to the acidosis it produces and are neurologically depressant.

At 1 ATA, a typical subject breathing air to which 3% $CO_2$ has been added doubles his respiratory minute volume. There is no disturbance of central nervous system function. A 5–6% $CO_2$ supplement may cause distress and dyspnoea accompanied by an increase, mainly in tidal volume but also in respiratory rate. There is a concomitant rise in blood pressure and pulse rate. Mental confusion and lack of coordination may become apparent. A 10% inspired $CO_2$ eventually causes a drop in pulse rate and blood pressure and severe mental impairment. A 12–14% level will cause loss of consciousness and eventually death by central

respiratory and cardiac depression if continued for a sufficient time ($Pa_{CO_2}$ greater than 150 mmHg). A 20–40% inspired $CO_2$ level rapidly causes midbrain convulsions, extensor spasm and death.

These effects will occur at progressively lower inspired concentrations with increasing depth, because toxicity depends on partial pressure, not inspired concentration.

If the inspired $CO_2$ is allowed to increase gradually (as might occur with a rebreathing set with failing absorbent), the following sequence is observed on land. The subject notices hyperpnoea, dizziness, unsteadiness, disorientation and restlessness. There is sweating of the forehead and hands, and his face feels flushed, bloated and warm. Respiration is increased in both depth and rate. Muscular fasciculation, incoordination and ataxia are demonstrable. Jerking movements may occur in the limbs. The subject becomes confused, ignores instructions and pursues his task doggedly. Gross tremor and convulsions may appear. Depression of the central nervous system may lead to respiratory paralysis and eventually death if not discontinued.

Under water, the diver may not notice sweating and hot feelings, due to the cool environment. Incoordination and ataxia are much less obvious because movements are slowed through the dense medium and the effect of gravity is almost eliminated. Hyperpnoea may not be noted by the diver performing hard work or engrossed in a task. With the rapid development of hypercapnia, there may be no warning symptoms preceding unconsciousness. During the recovery period, the diver may remember an episode of lightheadedness or transitory amblyopia, but these occupy only a few seconds and there is therefore insufficient time to take appropriate action.

A throbbing frontal or bitemporal headache may develop during a slow $CO_2$ build-up or after a rapid one.

> *An exercising diver in the water may have little warning of carbon dioxide toxicity prior to becoming unconscious.*

If the diver is removed from the toxic environment prior to the onset of apnoea, recovery from an episode of acute $CO_2$ toxicity is rapid and he appears normal within a few minutes. He may complain of nausea, malaise or severe headache for several hours. The headache does not respond to the usual analgesics or ergotamine preparations.

Carbon dioxide retention enhances nitrogen narcosis (see Chapter 15) and renders the diver more susceptible to oxygen toxicity (see Chapter 18). Conversely, there is evidence that nitrogen narcosis does not exacerbate $CO_2$ retention by depressing ventilatory response. The hyperoxia of depth may slightly reduce ventilatory drive. It is also believed that $CO_2$ increases the possibility of decompression sickness by increasing tissue perfusion and by increasing red blood cell agglutination (see Chapter 11).

---

### CASE REPORT 19.2

JF was doing a compass swim using a closed circuit 100% oxygen rebreathing set at a maximum depth of 5 metres. He had difficulty keeping up with his companion, noticing that his breathing was deep and the air seemed very hot. He ventilated his counterlung with fresh oxygen but still had breathing difficulty. Just prior to being called up after 33 minutes in the water, his companion noted that he 'got a new burst of speed, but kept adding more gas to his counterlung'.

On reaching the tailboard of the boat, JF complained that he was nearly out of gas. His eyes were wide, his face flushed, his respirations panting and spasmodic. He then collapsed and stopped breathing. His face mask was then removed and he was given mouth-to-mouth respiration, then 100% oxygen as respiration returned. He was unconscious for 10–15 minutes and headache and amnesia extended for several hours after the dive.

Oxygen percentage in the counterlung was 80% and the activity time of the absorbent was reduced to 32 minutes (specification 61 minutes). The canister plus absorbent from JF's set was placed in another set and a fresh diver exercised in a swimming pool using this set. He was unable to continue for more than 5 minutes, due to a classic $CO_2$ build-up.

*Diagnosis:* $CO_2$ toxicity.

## Prevention and treatment

Familiarizing divers who use rebreathing sets with the syndrome under safe control conditions has been suggested so that appropriate action can be taken at the first indication. In the water there may be no warning symptoms, so this method cannot be relied upon. It may be of some value in alerting the divers to the problem. Divers should be drilled to report any unusual symptoms.

The ideal prevention is by $CO_2$ monitoring and an alarm system to warn of rising levels. At present, this is practical for recompression chambers, habitats, submarines etc., but not for self-contained rebreathing apparatus.

If $CO_2$ levels are not monitored, then attention must be paid to such factors as adequate ventilation of chambers, avoidance of hard physical work, keeping within the safe limits of the absorbent system etc. Even with these precautions, accidents will still happen.

It must be remembered that the percentage of $CO_2$ in the inspired gas becomes increasingly important as the pressure increases. Although 3% $CO_2$ in the inspired air at the surface produces little effect, at 30 metres (4 ATA) it is equivalent to breathing 12% on the surface and would be incapacitating. At very great depth, minimal percentages of $CO_2$ could be dangerous.

The diver using underwater rebreathing apparatus should be well trained in the immediate action to be taken when $CO_2$ toxicity is suspected. He should stop and rest, thus reducing muscular activity. At the same time he should signal his diving partner, as assistance may be required and unconsciousness may be imminent. Either the diver or his companion should flush the counterlung with fresh gas, ditch his weights and surface by using positive buoyancy. In deep diving, it may be necessary to return to a submersible chamber. On arrival at the surface or submersible chamber, the diver should immediately breathe from the atmosphere.

First aid treatment simply requires removal from the toxic environment. Maintenance of respiration and circulation may be necessary for a short period. $P_{CO_2}$ and pH return to normal when adequate alveolar ventilation and circulation are established.

## Chronic hypercapnia

The need for defining tolerance limits to $CO_2$ for long exposures is becoming increasingly important with the development of saturation diving, the use of submersibles and extended submarine patrols (see Chapter 39).

Marked adaptation to exposure to inspired $CO_2$ levels between 0.5% and 4% has been demonstrated. This adaptation is characterized by an increased tidal volume and a lower respiratory rate. There is a reduction in the ventilatory response to the hypercapnia produced by exercise.

Biochemically, there is a reversal of the initial increase in hydrogen ion concentration, a rise in the plasma bicarbonate and a fall in the plasma chloride, i.e. a mild compensated respiratory acidosis. There is a slight rise in arterial carbon dioxide tension. These latter changes are almost complete in 3–5 days' exposure, although there is a significant reduction in the ventilatory response in the first 24 hours. There is also a rise in serum calcium and other mineral changes.

While at rest, the average diver can tolerate a surface equivalent of up to 4% inspired $CO_2$ ($P_{ICO_2}$ of 30 mmHg), without incapacitating physiological changes. During exercise, alveolar ventilation does not increase sufficiently to prevent a significant degree of $CO_2$ retention as shown by an elevation of arterial $P_{CO_2}$. This loss of the ventilatory response to $CO_2$ (of the order of 20% in submariners) may also be of great significance in the saturation diver, particularly during exercise. Many saturation diving operations have the chamber $CO_2$ limit set at 3.5 mmHg, which is high enough to produce the above changes.

## Recommended reading

BARLOW, H.B. and MACINTOSH, F.C. (1944). Shallow water blackout. R.N.P. 44/125 Report prepared for the Subcommittee on Underwater Physiology of the Royal Naval Personnel Research Committee.

BEHNKE, A.R. and LANPHIER, E.H. (1965). Underwater physiology. In: *Handbook of Physiology*, Section 3, *Respiration*, Vol. 11, edited by Wallace O. Fenn and Herman Rahn. American Physiological Society, Washington DC.

CLARK, J.M., SINCLAIR, R.D. and LENOX, J.B. (1980). Chemical and non-chemical components of ventilation during hypercapniac exercise in man. *Journal of Applied Physiology* **48**, 1065–1076.

EDMONDS C. (1968) Shallow water blackout. *Royal Australian Navy School of Underwater Medicine Report*, 10/68.

FAGRAEUS, L. (1981). Current concepts of dyspnea and ventilatory limits to exercise at depth. *Seventh Symposium on Underwater Physiology*. Underwater Medical Society.

GELFAND, R., LAMBERTSEN, C.J. and PETERSON, R.E. (1980). Human respiratory control at high ambient pressures and inspired gas densities. *Journal of Applied Physiology* **48**, 528–539.

LANPHIER, E.H. (Ed.) (1980). *The Unconscious Diver: Respiratory Control and Other Contributing Factors*. U.M.S. Workshop.

LANPHIER, E.H. (1982). Pulmonary function. In: *The Physiology and Medicine of Diving and Compressed Air Work*, 3rd edn, edited by P.B. Bennett and D.H. Elliott, London: Baillière Tindall.

LANPHIER, E.H. (1988). Carbon dioxide poisoning. In: *Case Histories of Diving and Hyperbaric Accidents*, edited by C.L. Waite. Undersea and Hyperbaric Medical Society.

LEITCH, D.R. (1977–78). Living with carbon dioxide. *Transactions of the Medical Society of London* **94**, 32–37.

MacDONALD, J.W. and PILMAIS, A.A. (1981). Carbon dioxide retention with underwater work in the open ocean. *Seventh Symposium on Underwater Physiology*. Undersea Medical Society.

MILES, S. (1957). Unconsciousness in Underwater Swimmers. R.N.P. 57/901. Report prepared for the Subcommittee on Underwater Physiology of the Royal Naval Personnel Research Committee, Oct. 1957.

MORRISON, J.B., FLORIO, J.T. and BUTT, W.S. (1981). Effects of $CO_2$ insensitivity and respiratory pattern on respiration in divers. *Undersea Biomedical Research* **8**, 209–217.

NUNN, J.F. (1987). Carbon dioxide. In: *Applied Respiratory Physiology*, 3rd edn. London: Butterworths.

SCHAEFER, K.E. (1982). Carbon dioxide effects under conditions of raised environmental pressure. In: *The Physiology and Medicine of Diving and Compressed Air Work*, 3rd edn, edited by P.B. Bennett and D.H. Elliott. London: Baillière Tindall.

SINCLAIR, R.D., CLARK, J.M. and WELCH, B.E. (1971). Comparison of physiological responses of normal man to exercise in air and in acute and chronic hypercapnia. In: *Proceedings of the Fourth Symposium on Underwater Physiology*, edited by C.J. Lambertsen. New York: Academic Press.

# Breathing gas contamination

## Introduction

Death of a diver due to breathing a contaminated gas mixture is an uncommon event. Despite this, we should all be aware of the causes of contamination and methods of prevention and treatment. With advanced compressor technology and better quality control, such accidents should become even rarer.

## Air compressors

The most common compressor designs for diving use are high pressure systems. They take in air at atmospheric pressure and compress it to about 200 ATA. The air is then stored in scuba cylinders before being used by the diver. Some commercial divers use low pressure compressors which are connected to a large volume storage and to a hose that supplies the diver. The more common high pressure unit will be considered in this section.

If the air was compressed in one step there would be several problems. The gas would become very hot; large amounts of condensation would form when the gas cooled; it would be difficult to design a seal to prevent air leakage round the large pistons required. Due to these problems most compressors compress the air in three or four stages.

The basic design of a three-stage system is shown in Figure 20.1. In each stage the gas is compressed by a piston that moves up and down in a cylinder with inlet and outlet valves. In the first stage, the air is compressed to about 8 ATA. It is then cooled and the pressure falls to about 6 ATA. When the gas cools water vapour will tend to condense. This is drained off along with any oil that has mixed with the air during first-stage compression. The second stage of compression raises the pressure to about 40 ATA. Again the air is cooled and more water is condensed out. The final stage compresses the air to the pressure required for the storage tanks or scuba cylinders. A four-stage compressor differs from the three-stage one shown only in that there are four stages and smaller steps in each stage.

The cylinder, piston and valves in each stage of the compressor are smaller than the preced-

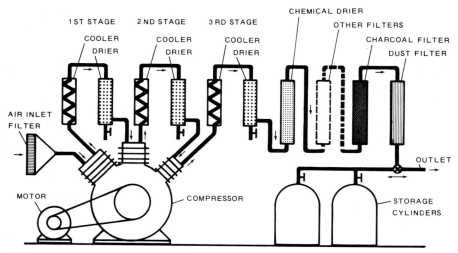

**Figure 20.1** Diagram of three-stage compressor

ing ones because the volume of gas decreases in accordance with Boyle's law. In the example above, if the volume of the first-stage cylinder is 1000 ml, to match the pressures given, the second stage needs to be less than 200 ml and the third stage about 25 ml.

The moisture which condenses is the water vapour in the air that was compressed. If the relative humidity of the air entering the compressor were 50%, condensation would occur when the air pressure increased to 2 ATA (if the temperature remains constant). It is difficult and expensive to remove water from compressed air by chemical means. Due to this, it is common practice to have a spring-loaded valve after the final stage. It only opens to discharge air when the compressor outlet pressure has built up to a set value that is higher than the working pressure of the storage cylinders. This increases the amount of water that will be removed by condensation. As an extreme example, consider the discharge valve being set at 400 ATA and the cylinders filled to 200 ATA – without any other drier the air going to the cylinders will have a relative humidity of 50%.

A refrigeration system is sometimes used to increase condensation from the air. Both a high outlet valve pressure and refrigeration will increase the removal of any other contaminants that condense with or in the water.

There is a divergence of opinion on what should be used to lubricate compressors. Oil

vapour or combustion products can contaminate the air. Some experts advocate synthetic oils, others advocate natural oils. Given the conflict of opinion, the manufacturers' instructions are probably the best guide to selecting the lubricant.

Attempts have been made to design a compressor that does not need lubrication. Another option is to use water as coolant and lubricant. Neither approach has won general acceptance.

Compressors range in size from small units which can be carried by one or two people, to large units which need a large motor and weigh several tonnes.

## Sources of contaminants

Compressed air is the only breathing gas used by most divers. Any contaminant in it may have been in the air prior to compression, added during compression because of some fault in the compressor system, or present or generated within the storage system.

There are many potential contaminants in air, particularly if compressed in an industrial area. Carbon monoxide and nitrogen oxides are components of polluted city air, in levels that may be toxic. They may also get into the compressed air if the compressor is driven by, or operated near, an internal combustion machine which produces these compounds.

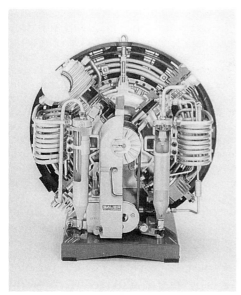

**Figure 20.2** A portable four-cylinder Bauer Air Compressor in which some components have been cut away to show the internal design. To reduce the size of the compressor, the cylinders are arranged in a radial pattern. The spiral coils are to cool the air between stages of compression; cooling is aided by a fan attached to the far side of the unit. Contaminants are removed from the compressed air by chemicals in prepared packs which go into the two cut-away vertical cylinders in front of the compressor

High temperatures ('hot spots') and high pressures within the compressor produce an ideal environment for contaminants to form. Both these factors promote chemical reactions and hence the production of contaminants. If an unsuitable lubricating oil is used in the compressor, it may produce oil vapour, break down to produce volatile hydrocarbons, or burn and form carbon monoxide. The same trouble can also result if the compressor overheats, causing 'cracking' (oil breakdown) or 'flashing' (oil combustion). The air becomes contaminated with volatile hydrocarbons or combustion products such as carbon monoxide and nitrogen oxides.

> *Contaminants in compressed gas may have been present in the gas prior to compression, added during compression or resident in the storage system.*

Some divers believe that using an electric compressor prevents carbon monoxide contamination. It removes one common cause of carbon monoxide – that of the driving motor exhaust. It does nothing to reduce the other external or internal sources of carbon monoxide. This can develop suddenly, or intermittently. Carbon monoxide can be in the air being compressed, i.e. outside the source, such as the exhaust of a nearby vehicle. Carbon monoxide can be produced when oil in the cylinder of the compressor overheats. Other hydrocarbons may also be formed. The excessive heat may be due to irregularities in the cylinder, rings or piston, causing increased friction.

Overheating may also be produced by poor design or maintenance of the compressor:

1. Restriction of the compressor intake, e.g. dirty filter, excessive length, or inadequate cross-sectional area of intake, or a kinked intake hose. Under these conditions, the compressor must compensate for the restricted intake with a high compression ratio.
2. Leaks between the compressor stages, via piping, loose fittings or head gaskets, or around the piston, will also require higher final stage compression ratios.
3. Leakage around the valves between the compressor stages.
4. General or local overheating beyond the compressor's design limits. Any inequality or impairment of the cooling system can cause this, and result in overheating

> *'I have an electric compressor, so I can't get carbon monoxide poisoning'* – Nonsense

Oil may contaminate the compressed air cylinder or the compressor, by passing around the piston rings. This is most likely when the rings are damaged, or if the air intake is restricted in any way as above; even a hand being placed over the inlet may have a similar effect.

Air contamination from residues within the storage vessel or bottle is not common. Residues of cleaning and scouring materials and scale formed by rusting can contribute vapour or dust if the cleaning operation is not conducted properly, or if the cylinder or storage vessel is allowed to deteriorate. Water may be introduced into bottles if they are left open after use.

The lubricants used on regulators and reducers can contaminate small amounts of air. A diver may taste the lubricant in his regulator and fear his air is contaminated. Only lubricants approved for use in breathing systems and high pressure oxygen should be used. Krytox, a grease produced by E.I. Du Pont, is approved by several authorities for these uses.

The most difficult source of contamination to isolate is intermittent inlet contamination. For example, an Australian firm had an air compressor inlet on the roof. On isolated occasions their air was contaminated with organic chemicals. Only after much work and customer dissatisfaction was the source identified. A factory several hundred metres away sometimes used spray painting equipment. With the right wind direction fumes would blow across the compressor inlet.

The gases used in mixture diving are generally prepared from gases purified by liquefaction. This reduces the risk of contamination because most of the potential impurities are readily separated by their higher boiling points. In using mixtures prepared for deep diving, problems can result because of the great pressure at which the mixtures are used. This will increase the risk of toxicity because of the higher environmental pressures and the higher partial pressures of contaminants. For example, at 1 ATA a carbon dioxide concentration of 2% in inspired air has little effect. At 5 ATA a carbon dioxide concentration of 2% may cause unconsciousness as would 0.2% at 50 ATA.

There is a possibility of increasing the concentration of trace contaminants when using recycled and reclaimed gases for deep diving operations and submarines. The chemicals that are not removed in the purification process can accumulate with recycling until they reach a level that causes a problem. For this reason a screening gas analysis programme is highly desirable.

> *With an increase in depth, and hence partial pressure of contaminants, toxicity will increase.*

**Table 20.1 Air purity standards**

|  | *British Sub-Aqua Club* | *Australian Standards (CZ 2299 – 1979)* | *US Navy Diving Manual (1988)* |
|---|---|---|---|
| Oxygen (%) | 21 + 0.5 | 20–22 by vol. | 20–22 by vol. |
| Carbon dioxide (%) | 0.03 max. (300 p.p.m.) | 900 mg/m$^3$ max | 0.1 max. (1000 p.p.m.) |
| Carbon monoxide | 10 p.p.m. max | 11 mg/m$^3$ max. | 0.002% max. (20 p.p.m.) |
| Oil (mg/m$^3$) | 1 max. | 1 max. (cylinder 12 MPa) | 5 max. (particulates + oil) |
| Nitrogen oxides | < 1 p.p.m. | – | – |
| Water | No condensation above 40°F, 5°C | 100 max. (cylinder 12 MPa) | – |
| Odour and taste | Nil | Not objectionable | Not objectionable |
| Hydrocarbons other than methane | – | – | 25 p.p.m. |

# Gas purity standards

Standards have been prepared, specifying the composition and the maximum concentration of contaminants in breathing air and for gases used in deep diving. Greater purity is demanded for gases used in deep diving because of the effect of greater pressures. The US Navy, the British Sub-Aqua Club and the Australian Standards Association specifications for dry breathing air are shown in Table 20.1. They are similar to most other standards for breathing air.

Review of the specifications could lead to the opinion that most specified limits are rather conservative. Safety margins are incorporated for two reasons: first, the standards are based on extrapolation of the effects of the contaminants in isolation at 1 ATA. This might not be entirely valid for contaminants in combination at high pressures. Secondly, a safety margin will help to allow for any deterioration in the air quality between tests.

It is important to note that these specifications are only a list of the maximum concentrations of some common impurities. Air might meet these specifications and still contain toxic substances. For example, acrolein, a toxic product from frying food, can occur in toxic concentrations if the compressor is near a galley, or the dive school is near a fish café.

A greater variety of contamination problems occurs in caisson work and recompression chamber operation, especially if therapeutic or research equipment is used in the chamber. Because exposure times are generally greater in chambers, the toxic contamination has more time to exert its effect. Toxic substances which may easily be present include: mercury from manometers etc., especially if damaged; ammonia or Freon, from leaking air conditioning plants; anaesthetic residues and other vapours from pharmaceutical preparations.

In avoiding toxicological problems in chambers, the basic rule must be 'if in doubt, leave it out'. Useful guidelines are available with reference to experience gained with chronic exposures in spacecraft and nuclear submarines.

The reasons for listing the components shown in Table 20.1 and the concentrations specified are outlined below.

## Oxygen

The concentration of oxygen is close to the range expected for clean dry air. Any significant deviation from these levels would, if the nitrogen concentration was elevated, increase the risk of decompression sickness, narcosis or hypoxia. If the oxygen concentration was increased, the risk of oxygen toxicity, and fire hazards in hyperbaric chambers, would increase. The oxygen may be elevated by connecting to a bulk oxygen supply; this may be accidental. On other occasions, it has been deliberate in the misguided belief that increasing oxygen concentration will increase the endurance available from a cylinder.

Professional diving organizations sometimes increase the oxygen concentration to reduce the decompression times required. The National Oceanic and Atmospheric Administration in the USA has sponsored the development of tables based on this premise.

## Carbon dioxide

A specified carbon dioxide level of 0.03% means that at 10 ATA the partial pressure of carbon dioxide would still be well below that required to cause any physiological effect. The British and Australian standards are probably too strict because the USN maximum limit of 0.1% would not be toxic to the depth limits of compressed air diving and would be easier for compressor operators to meet. The American level is a relaxation from the previous figure of 0.05%. The carbon dioxide level, even if it is within the specification used, should be considered in relation to the level in the ambient air. An excess may indicate lubricant breakdown or contamination from an external source.

## Carbon monoxide

This toxic gas reacts with haemoglobin to form carboxyhaemoglobin. The affinity of haemoglobin for carbon monoxide is about 200 times as great as its affinity for oxygen. This affinity also results in very slow elimination of carbon monoxide after the carbon monoxide is removed from the gas supply. The result of the formation of carboxyhaemoglobin is that this haemoglobin cannot carry oxygen. If sufficient haemoglobin reacts with carbon monoxide the subject will develop hypoxia. This effect is aggravated by a shift of the oxygen–haemoglobin dissociation curve to the left. This means that tissue hypoxia will be accentuated. The formation of carboxyhaemoglobin will also interfere with the transport of carbon dioxide by preventing its combination with haemoglobin. Carbon monoxide also has a toxic effect at the cellular level, and this may be more significant clinically.

The frequently described cherry-red colour of these victims is an unreliable clinical sign, especially with cardiorespiratory impairment.

Table 20.2 shows the percentage carboxyhaemoglobin produced in the blood as a result of breathing various amounts of carbon monoxide in air at 1 ATA. Some of the effects noted in a subject with a normal haemoglobin level are included. Similar effects can be produced by breathing weaker concentrations for longer. Exertion, and increased ventilation, will hasten the development of symptoms. Subjects with a low haemoglobin level are more susceptible to carbon monoxide poisoning.

The concentrations in this study are considerably greater than the maximum carbon monoxide level – 10 or 20 p.p.m. specified. A limit of 100 p.p.m. is a suggested maximum level for industrial workers exposed for up to 8 hours a day. For divers breathing air, the higher partial pressure of oxygen tends to protect against the effects of increased carbon monoxide partial pressure while at depth. The toxic limits of carbon monoxide at depth and how they are modified by varying ambient and oxygen partial pressures have not been established.

It would be expected that divers are at greatest risk as they surface and lose the protection offered by increased transport of oxygen in plasma. This protection occurs at depth when the partial pressure of oxygen in inspired air is elevated. For excursion air diving, the standards offer a safety margin in that 20 p.p.m. of carbon monoxide would not cause a serious danger at 10 ATA even if there was no protection from the increased partial pressure of oxygen. This has been shown by the US Navy accepting this concentration instead of the 10 p.p.m. previously required.

A lower maximum carbon monoxide concentration is needed for deep and saturation divers. This is because the exposure times are longer. Also, the oxygen partial pressure is usually limited to approximately 0.4 ATA, so the protection from an elevated oxygen pressure is reduced.

## Oil

Oil, occurring as a mist of vapour, can cause compressed air to have an unpleasant odour and taste. Its direct, toxic effects in normal people are not known except that, in high concentrations it can cause lipoid pneumonia. In some people low concentrations of oil vapour can trigger asthma. Condensed oil, especially if combined with solid residues, can cause malfunctions in some types of equipment.

**Table 20.2 Percentage carboxyhaemoglobin produced in the blood as a result of breathing various amounts of carbon monoxide in air at 1 ATA**

| Carbon monoxide concentration (p.p.m.) | HbCO (%) | Effect |
| --- | --- | --- |
| 400 | 7.2 | Nil |
| 800 | 14.4 | Headache, dizziness Breathlessness with exertion |
| 1600 | 29 | Confusion, Collapse on exertion |
| 3200 | 58 | Unconsciousness |
| 4000 | 72 | Profound coma |
| 4500 | 81 | Death |

---

**CASE REPORT 20.1**

An experienced diver dived in an area subject to tidal currents. He planned to dive at slack water and anchored his boat a short time before the low tide. The hookah compressor was correctly arranged with the inlet upwind of the exhaust and the dive commenced. After an hour at 10 metres the diver felt dizzy and lost consciousness but was fortunately pulled aboard by his attendant and revived.

*Diagnosis:* carbon monoxide poisoning, confirmed by blood analysis.

*Explanation:* as the tide turned, so did the boat. This put the compressor inlet downwind of the motor exhaust. The carbon monoxide from the exhaust was drawn into the compressor inlet and breathed under pressure by the diver.

---

ment. The other major medical problem with oil is that it can decompose into hydrocarbons and possibly toxic compounds of carbon, nitrogen and sulphur depending on the oil composition.

Some compressed air standards distinguish oil from other hydrocarbons and specify maximum limits for each. Most hydrocarbons in high pressure areas can be serious fire hazards. Some have other undesirable effects, such as being carcinogenic. The maximum level specified would appear to be well below that needed to cause any of these effects.

### Water

The control of water vapour is designed to protect the equipment more than the diver. Many people find compressed air unpleasantly dry. The dryness and cooling from the expansion both tend to trigger asthma in people with hyperreactive airways.

The standard is designed to reduce corrosion damage in equipment by limiting the amount of water present. A low water concentration is also needed to prevent condensation and ice formation when diving in cold water. For these purposes, the BSAC standard is barely adequate. Other standards require a dew point as low as −40°C, to prevent moisture formation and corrosion in high pressure cylinders.

Water condensation can also impair the efficiency of the filters used to remove other contaminants. Deaths have been reported from diving with steel cylinders containing water. Rusting occurs if these are left unused

for long periods. The process consumes oxygen and leaves a mixture that causes death from hypoxia. The other problem is that the rusting process weakens the cylinder and may cause it to become an unguided missile if the gas rapidly discharges. Deaths have been caused by flying cylinders.

### Solid particles

These have to be controlled to protect the diver and his equipment. The effect of the particles depends on their size and composition. Particles such as pollen can cause hay fever and asthma in susceptible divers. Other particles have various undesirable physiological effects depending on their size and composition. Any dust which causes coughing could be particularly hazardous, especially for a novice diver.

In diving equipment, abrasive particles such as mineral dust would accelerate wear on the equipment by abrasive erosion. Soluble particles such as salt crystals can accelerate corrosion by promoting electrolysis. Organic dust can also contribute to a fire hazard. There have been cases of filters breaking down, letting material through and contributing particles of filter material to the air supply.

### Nitrogen dioxide and nitrous oxide

Some of the oxides of nitrogen, nitrogen dioxide in particular, are intensely irritating, especially to the lungs, eyes and throat. Symptoms can occur when the subject is exposed to gas with a concentration of nitrogen dioxide greater than 10 p.p.m. At lower concentrations the initial symptoms are slight, and may not be noticed, or may even disappear. After a latent period of 2–20 hours further signs, which may be precipitated by exertion, appear. Coughing, difficulty in breathing, cyanosis and haemoptysis accompany the development of pulmonary oedema. Unconsciousness usually follows. The maximum level, 1 p.p.m., is also the maximum allowed level for 24-hour exposure in other standards. If the effect is increased with pressure then 0.1 p.p.m. may be a more appropriate limit. In industrial cities this level is often exceeded.

Nitrous oxide is an anaesthetic agent, but only at high concentrations. A low concentration of nitrous oxide is specified because, if nitrous oxide is generated within the compressor, a precursor, nitric oxide, must have been formed. Nitric oxide can also be converted to nitrogen dioxide at higher pressures and temperatures. Therefore a compressor which adds nitrous oxide to the air being compressed can also form nitrogen dioxide.

### Odour and taste

These are controlled to avoid the use of air that is unpleasant to breathe. It is also a back-up for the other standards because, if the air has an odour, it contains an impurity.

## Prevention of contamination

Contamination should not occur if clean dry air is pumped by a suitable, well-maintained compressor into clean tanks. Any deviation from this will lead to the risk of contamination.

> *Prevention of contamination involves the use of suitable well-maintained compressors, adequate filters, clean tanks and regular analysis of the gas.*

Filtering will be necessary to remove any contaminants introduced by compression. It will also be needed if the air compressed comes from a polluted area. Water removal will be needed in most situations. The choice of filtering agents and the frequency of the replacement of materials is a specialized field of engineering and should be considered with experts in the field. The following methods and agents are commonly used.

1. Silica gel, to remove water vapour.
2. Activated alumina, to remove water vapour.
3. Activated charcoal, to remove oil mist and volatile hydrocarbons.
4. Activated zeolites, and molecular sieves, to remove oil and water.
5. Reverse flow or centrifugal filters, to remove solids and large liquid drops.
6. Hopcalite, a mixture of chemicals that oxidizes carbon monoxide.
7. Sodium hydroxide (or soda lime) to remove carbon dioxide.
8. Cryogenic cooling, to remove impurities with a higher boiling point, normally water and carbon dioxide.

A Modess pad, used by some abalone divers to collect excess water, oil and solid particles, is not satisfactory for this use.

Some companies incorporate several filtering agents into a cartridge, simplifying the servicing of the compressor.

## Treatment

For most of the conditions caused by contaminated air, the first step is to replace the contaminated air supply. Rest, breathing 100% oxygen and general first aid measures may be required. In more severe cases resuscitation may be needed.

Serious cases of carbon monoxide toxicity benefit from hyperbaric oxygen therapy. This improves oxygenation of the patient's blood and aids the elimination of carbon monoxide by raising the alveolar and arterial partial pressures of oxygen, causing the displacement of carbon monoxide from carboxyhaemoglobin (see Chapter 37).

Treatment of nitrogen dioxide toxicity requires rest in all cases. This may prevent the condition progressing. If the exposure was thought to be due to a toxic concentration, or if the patient develops further symptoms, then 100% oxygen is indicated. If pulmonary oedema develops, then this should be managed appropriately.

## Detection of contamination

The accurate assessment of the concentration of contaminants is best left to specialists, such as air pollution analysts. The following tests will give the user a reasonable assessment of air quality. Some of the tests should not be used for samples where a death or legal action may be involved. This is because they require large amounts of air to achieve an imprecise answer.

For most compressor operators, the purchase of an indicating tube gas analyser system is a sound investment. These are made by Mine Safety Apparatus, Auer, Drager, Bendix and other firms. The devices operate by passing a metered volume of air through a glass tube filled with chemicals. These chemicals react with the contaminant and cause a colour change. A scale on the tube indicates the amount of contaminant present in the sample. Tubes from different makers cannot be mixed because the tube systems use different flows and volumes of gas.

The oxygen concentration may be checked using an oxygen electrode, analyser or indicator tube.

Carbon dioxide concentration can be measured using an indicating tube or a variety of chemical and physical techniques. Infrared absorption is the technique most commonly used.

Oil and dust can be determined by filtering and weighing, the increase in the dry weight indicating the weight of oil and dust. A solvent such as hexane may be used to dissolve the oil, the remaining weight being particulate matter.

This procedure requires an accurate balance because a full cylinder (2000 litres, 72 cubic feet) should contain less than 2 mg of oil. An indication of the presence of oil can be obtained by directing a jet of air on to a clean sheet of white paper and then examining the paper under ultraviolet light. The oil drops will fluoresce.

Nitrogen oxides may be detected using indicating tubes. These may also be used for detection of water vapour, but a method involving a measurement of the dew point is more suitable.

Combinations of gas chromatography and msas spectrometer systems are often needed to get an accurate identification of trace contaminants. They need a competent operator and a large stock of reference samples to give a satisfactory service. Laboratories involved with air pollution may be able to provide these facilities.

## Recommended reading

BLOOM, J.D. (1972). Some considerations in establishing diver's breathing gas purity standards for carbon monoxide. *Aerospace Medicine*.

HUNTER, D. (1975). *The Diseases of Occupations*, 4th edn. London: English Universities Press.

MORROW, P.E. (1975). An evaluation of recent $NO_x$ toxicity data and an attempt to derive an ambient air standard for $NO_x$ by established toxicological procedures. *Environmental Research* **10**, 92–112.

STANDARDS ASSOCIATION OF AUSTRALIA (1979). AS2299: Rules for Underwater Air Breathing Operations, Sydney.

*US Navy Diving Manual* (1988). NAVSEA 0944-LP-001 -9010, vol. 43, pp. 633–636.

ZANELLI, L. (1972). *The British Sub Aqua Club Diving Manual*.

# 21

# Drowning

## Introduction

Drowning is defined as the death of an air-breathing animal due to immersion in fluid. This term has been loosely used to refer to incidents in which recovery occurs; however, the terms 'near drowning' and 'the salt water aspiration syndrome' seem more appropriate for these cases. When patients lose consciousness, but subsequently recover, the term 'near drowning' is applicable. When symptoms are not severe enough to classify as near drowned, another term, 'salt water aspiration syndrome', is better employed. Although in most cases of drowning and near drowning fluid is aspirated into the lungs, in about 10–15% the lungs are 'dry'. The term 'submersion' is also used in the literature to refer to a drowning or near-drowning event.

Distinction is also made between warm water and cold water drowning and between fresh and salt water drowning. The term 'secondary drowning', which refers to a patient who initially survives but later succumbs due to a complication of aspiration during submersion, is best avoided.

The incidence of death by drowning cannot be estimated accurately, as two of the largest and most densely populated countries do not submit statistics to the World Health Organization. It is probably between 5 and 6 per 100 000 persons. It is greater in Japan, with its numerous small islands and its dependence on the fishing industry. No records exist of the number of near drownings.

> The incidence of drowning is 5–6 per 100 000 persons per year with an over-representation of young males.

Drowning is second only to motor vehicle trauma as a cause of accidental death in Australia and the USA. There is an over-representation of young males in most drowning series, and there is a predictable age distribution for specific drowning accidents. Most swimming pool deaths occur in the very young, surf deaths mostly in teenagers and young adults, deaths among boatmen and fishermen are in the whole adult range, and bathtub drownings are in either the very young or the very old. Alcohol consumption is involved in a high proportion of adult male drownings. This may be due to:

- Injudicious risk taking.
- Reduced capacity to respond to a threatening situation.
- Loss of heat due to peripheral vasodilatation.
- Interference with the laryngeal reflex.
- An increased tendency to vomit.
- An increased incidence of suicidal intentions.

Plueckhahn's series of drowning deaths revealed that alcohol was present in the blood at a concentration greater than 0.08 g/100 ml in none of the female but in 37% of all male victims. In 51% of those men in the 30–64 age group, blood alcohol levels were greater than 0.15 g/100 ml. The legal limit for safe driving is 0.05 g/100 ml.

---

*'Bacchus hath drowned more men than Neptune.' Old English proverb, reconfirmed by Plueckhahn*

---

Hyperventilation prior to breath-hold diving is a common cause of drowning in otherwise fit individuals who are good swimmers, but it is difficult to document statistically.

The treatment at the scene of the accident is often of little ultimate consequence in many accidents, but in drowning it will often determine whether the victim lives or dies. The standard of first aid and resuscitation training of the rescuers therefore influences outcome.

The temperature of the water and thus the degree of hypothermia may also be a factor. Poorer results are achieved in warm bath water drownings.

Whether the drowning occurs in sea or fresh water may have some influence on the prospects of recovery, and on the biochemical and pathological abnormalities of drowning. The chances of recovery from potentially fatal immersion in salt water appear to be better than in fresh water.

Other factors which influence outcome include: the presence of chlorine and other chemicals and foreign bodies, the aspiration of stomach contents, the subsequent development of haemolysis, renal failure, coagulopathy, respiratory infection etc.

In so-called 'dry' drowning, the patient either succumbs to hypoxia or, if rescued in time, makes a rapid recovery. When fluid aspiration occurs, as it usually does, there is a gradation between drowning, near drowning and the salt water aspiration syndrome. The differences relate to the degree of aspiration and the body's response to it. There is no clear-cut distinction between the near drowning and the salt water aspiration syndromes as there is a spectrum of severity between the comatose near-drowning patient and the diver who appears to have a mild, transitory, post-dive, inflammatory/respiratory disorder.

Death may occur during immersion, soon after or with delayed complications.

---

*The clinical findings of human drowning do not reflect the experimental observations in animal experiments.*

---

Spectacular recoveries have been recorded in patients who have been subjected to total submersion for extended periods of time. Case reports of submersion for 26, 30 and 40 minutes are in the medical literature, with many other similar causes known to clinicians experienced in this field. The explanations for such results include the following:

1. Hypothermia is produced by both submersion in cold water and also by inhalation of cold water. In one Australian series, the body temperature of near-drowned children averaged 31°C (88°F). The hypothermia is thought to protect the central nervous system from the effects of hypoxia. Due to the relatively increased surface area, hypothermia is more likely in the young, in

**Table 21.1 Some contributing factors to drowning**

Panic
Lack of supervision of children
Alcohol (especially adult males)
Illegal drugs
Suicide, murder
Inability to swim
Trauma (especially head or neck injury)
Exhaustion
Hypothermia
Hyperventilation and breath-hold diving
Medical catastrophe
   seizure
   cardiac arrhythmia
   myocardial infarction
   cerebrovascular accident
   hypoglycaemia
Scuba divers – all the above, plus
   'out of air'
   overweighted
   entrapment
   inert gas narcosis (nitrogen narcosis)
   gas toxicities (CO, $CO_2$, $O_2$)
   pulmonary barotrauma of ascent

whom most of the recoveries after pro-longed submersion have occurred.

2. With laryngeal spasm, a reservoir of gas is retained within the lungs from which oygen can be extracted and into which carbon dioxide can be discharged. Even in cases in which fluid does enter the lungs, the effect of gravity makes it unlikely that a great deal of the gas will be replaced by fluid, unless the victim is in the head and face upwards position.

3. The diving reflex (see Chapter 3) is more active in small children. This reflex allows for bradycardia, oxygen conservation and a shunting of oxygenated blood to the vital organs, especially the heart and brain. The diving reflex is stimulated by the effect of cold water on the skin of the face and permits the prolonged submersion of many of the diving mammals. In humans it is present in a rudimentary form, but has been disputed as a protective mechanism.

4. Even with fluid in the lungs there is still some exchange of gases, both oxygen and carbon dioxide, between the blood stream and the alveolar contents. This is quite different from the more usual 'cardiac arrest' situation.

The outcome of the treatment of near drowning is unpredictable. Physical signs of decorticate rigidity, which would carry an ominous prognosis in adults, may be followed by apparently full recovery in young children. Alternatively, a good early response to treatment may be followed by severe cerebral dysfunction. Nevertheless, several indicators give a guide to the prognosis:

1. The duration of submersion.
2. The presence of hypothermia (especially prior to final submersion).
3. Neurological status on hospital admission, i.e. those who are conscious usually do well.
4. Cardiac arrest not responding to initial first aid increases the chance of poor outcome.
5. Spontaneous respiration after initial resuscitation suggests a better outcome.

It is often difficult to determine the exact cause of death after immersion in water.

Drowing while scuba diving at depth is less dramatic. It is often slower. A partial air supply, diving training and nitrogen narcosis may result in a no-panic progression to hypoxia and unconsciousness.

# Near drowning

## Clinical

The *sequence of events* which occur immediately before death from drowning includes:

1. Initial submersion: this may be followed by immediate breath-holding. The duration of the breath-holding depends on several factors – general physical condition, exercise, prior hyperventilation, psychological reactions etc.
2. Fluid aspiration: eventually the rising arterial carbon dioxide tension ($Pa_{CO_2}$) compels inspiration. Laryngeal spasm may follow if aspiration occurs. While laryngospasm is maintained, the lungs may remain dry. Water is often swallowed and aspiration of fluid or vomitus may complicate the situation.
3. Progressive hypoxaemia leads to loss of consciousness and eventually arrhythmias and circulatory arrest may follow. In most cases there is involuntary aspiration of fluid due to diaphragmatic contraction. In about 10% of cases, there is no fluid in the trachea

probably due to marked laryngeal spasm caused by the parasympathetic reflex response to fluid in the larynx. Hypoxaemia still occurs, due to lack of ventilation. The cardiac responses are usually due to the hypoxaemia at which time hypoxic brain damage is also likely to be developing. The ultimate outcome thus depends on the time of rescue and the efficacy of resuscitation.

The effects of near drowning are multiple, but the initial and primary insult is to the **respiratory system** with hypoxaemia being the inevitable result.

Clinical features include: dyspnoea; retrosternal chest pain, increased with inspiration; blood-stained, frothy sputum; tachypnoea and cyanosis; pulmonary crepitations and, occasionally, rhonchi. Respiratory function abnormalities include decreases in peak expiratory flow, vital capacity, compliance and ventilation–perfusion ratio, causing persisting hypoxaemia despite resuscitation.

Initial chest X-rays may be normal, or show patchy opacities or non-cardiogenic pulmonary oedema. Significant hypoxia may, nevertheless, be present with a normal chest X-ray. Complications may include pneumonitis, pulmonary oedema, bronchopneumonia, pulmonary abscess and empyema. Severe pulmonary infections with unusual organisms leading to long-term morbidity have been resported.

**Central nervous system** effects of hypoxia include impairment of consciousness, convulsions, and focal cerebral damage consistent with hypoxia and cerebral oedema. The level of consciousness ranges from awake or blunted to comatose with decorticate or decerebrate responses.

**Cardiovascular manifestations** are also largely the result of hypoxaemia on the heart, with cardiac arrest (which may or may not respond to initial resuscitation) not uncommon. After rescue and resuscitation, supraventricular tachycardias are frequent but various other dysrhythmias may occur. When the hypoxic/acidotic insult has been severe, hypotension and shock may persist despite reestablishment of cardiac rhythm. The central venous pressure may be elevated due to right-sided heart failure or elevated pulmonary vascular resistance rather than volume overload. Left ventricular filling pressures (esti-

mated by pulmonary artery catheter 'wedge' pressure – PAWP) may indicate low intravascular volume. Cardiac output and mixed venous oxygen tension may also be low, indicating hypoperfusion.

**Multisystem** failure may develop secondary to the hypoxaemia, acidosis and resultant hypoperfusion. Decreased urinary output occurs initially but occasionally renal failure due to acute tubular necrosis develops. Haemoglobinaemia, coagulation disorders and even disseminated intravascular coagulation may also complicate the clinical features.

**Laboratory** findings include: decreased arterial oxygen with variable arterial carbon dioxide tensions; metabolic with respiratory acidosis, haemoconcentration; leucocytosis; increased lactic dehydrogenase; occasional elevated creatinine; haemolysis, indicated by elevated free haemoglobin. Serum electrolytes are usually within the normal range.

> *The arterial oxygen tension is always low but the carbon dioxide tension may be low, normal or elevated.*

Recovery from near drowning is usually complete; however, residual neurological deficiencies may persist, either in the form of mental impairment or extrapyramidal disorders. They seem more common in warm water drownings of children – as exemplified by the near drownings of infants in bath tubs.

Mild cases of aspiration may develop a characteristic disorder – the salt water aspiration syndrome – and are usually misdiagnosed as an infection. This is described later.

### Treatment

The stages of treatment are shown in Figure 21.1.

### *Basic life support*

The efficacy of prompt initial measures in support of the respiratory and circulatory systems greatly influences the eventual outcome. Treatment begins with rescue and removal from the water. Assisted breathing

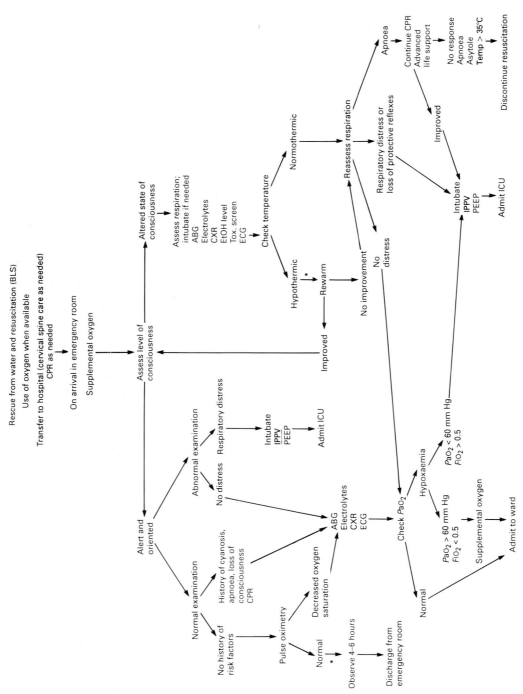

**Figure 21.1** Summary treatment algorithms for near drowning. ABG = arterial blood gas; BLS = basic life support; CMV = continuous mandatory ventilation; CPR = cardiopulmonary resuscitation; CXR = chest X-ray; ECC = external cardiac compression; EtOH = alcohol; $FiO_2$ = fractional inspired oxygen; ICU = intensive care unit; IPPV = intermittent positive-pressure ventilation; PEEP = positive end-expiratory pressure. * Coffee break. (Adapted with permission from K.N. Shaw and C.A. Briede (1989) Submersion injuries: Drowning and near drowning. *Emergency Medical Clinics of North America*, **16**, 72)

should be started as soon as possible even in the water. Aquatic cardiac compression has been described for scuba divers, but is not widely accepted and may cause further delay before effective cardiopulmonary resuscitation (CPR) is instituted.

The victim should be rapidly assessed for level of consciousness and injury. Movement should be with the head in a neutral position if cervical spinal injury is suspected. If CPR (Table 21.2) is required, the patient should be turned supine on a firm, flat, level surface with the head not higher than the thorax. Further help should be sought immediately, if possible.

**Table 21.2 Basic life support in near drowning**

*Airway*
1. **Assessment** – determine unresponsiveness
2. Call for **help**
3. **Position**
     Victim ? neck injury
     Rescuer
4. **Clear airways**
     Foreign material in pharynx
     Head-tilt/chin-lift
     Jaw-thrust (better for neck injury)

*Breathing*
5. **Assessment** – ear to mouth to determine absence of breathing
6. **Rescue breathing**
     Mouth to mouth or mouth to nose
     2 full breaths, assess response, then 12 breaths/minute

*Circulation*
7. **Assessment**
     Determine absence of carotid pulse
     Take 5–10 seconds and up to 1 minute if hypothermic
8. **External cardiac compression**
     Rate 80/min
     Up to 100/min if two-person CPR
9. Call for **help**
     Special equipment
     Paramedics
     Hospital transport

## Airways

Foreign particulate matter causing upper airway obstruction should be removed manually or later by suction. Obstruction of the upper airways by the tongue and epiglottis is the usual situation in the unconscious patient. Two methods are used to overcome the obstruction. **Head-tilt/chin-lift** is accomplished by pushing firmly back on the patient's forehead and lift-

ing the chin forward using two fingers under the jaw at the chin. The soft tissues under the chin should not be compressed and, unless mouth-to-nose breathing is to be employed, the mouth should not be completely closed. **Jaw-thrust** describes the technique of forward displacement of the lower jaw by lifting it with one hand on either side of the angles. Unless cervical spine injury is suspected, this technique is best combined with head-tilt.

Time should not be wasted in clearing water from the lower airways as only a small amount of water is usually aspirated. Fresh water is rapidly absorbed into the circulation and salt water leads to pulmonary oedema where the fluid is at the alveolar level and will continue to form despite attempts at removal.

If airway obstruction is encountered, which does not respond to normal airway management, the Heimlich manoeuvre (sub-diaphragmatic thrust) has been suggested. However, it should be used with caution and never as a first step, because of the risk of regurgitation of gastric contents and rupture of the stomach.

## Breathing

Respiration can be assessed by placing one's ear over the victim's mouth while looking for chest movement, listening for air sounds and feeling for the flow of expired air. If breathing is absent, mouth-to-mouth or mouth-to-nose breathing is instituted. Initially two full breaths of expired air, with an inspiratory time (for the victim) of 1–1.5 seconds are recommended. For adults an adequate volume to observe chest movement is about 800 ml. If no chest movement is seen and no air detected in the exhalation phase, the head-tilt or jaw-thrust manoeuvres should be revised. Failing that, further attempts at clearing the airway with the fingers (only if unconscious!) or possibly the Heimlich technique should be undertaken.

With mouth-to-mouth respiration, the rescuer pinches the nose, closing it gently between finger and thumb. Mouth-to-nose rescue breathing may be more suitable in certain situations, such as when marked trismus is present or when it is difficult to get an effective seal (injury to mouth, dentures etc.).

The rate of rescue breathing should be about 12 per minute (1 every 5 seconds) with increased rate and decreased volume in the very young.

### Circulation

If no carotid pulse is detected external cardiac compression (ECC) should be commenced after two initial 'breaths'. Up to a minute may be required in the hypothermic individual to determine pulselessness. Although it is possible that ECC could precipitate ventricular fibrillation in a hypothermic individual, if in doubt it is safer to commence ECC than not.

Higher rates of compression are now recommended with higher outputs achieved at 90–100/min compared to the traditional 60/min standard. Controversy still exists over the mechanism of flow in external compression with evidence for the older 'direct compression' model being challenged by the 'thoracic pump' theory. Abdominal binding, interposed abdominal compression, simultaneous compression–ventilation have all been proposed because there is evidence in animal studies of improved cerebral and coronary blood flow.

Cardiac compression should be performed with the patient supine on a firm surface. The legs may be elevated to improve venous return. The heel of the hand should be placed with the long axis in line with the sternum. The lower edge of the heel of the hand should be about two fingers above the xiphisternum (i.e. compression is of the lower half of the sternum). The second hand should be placed over the first and the compression of the sternum by about 4–5 cm in the adult should be in the vertical plane. To obtain this the rescuer's elbow should be straight with the shoulders directly over the sternum. A single rescuer may only be able to achieve rates of 80/min because of fatigue, but if several rescuers are present, it may be possible to maintain higher rates.

> *One rescuer: 2 breaths then 15 compressions (at 80 – 100/min). Two rescuers: 1 breath then 5 compressions (at 100/min with 1–1.5 second pause at end of the fifth).*

A regional organized emergency medical service (e.g. paramedics) who carry specialized equipment such as oxygen, endotracheal tubes, suction and intravenous apparatus should be activated, if available, but, in any case, the patient should be transferred to hospital as soon as possible. The early administration of oxygen by a suitable positive pressure apparatus, by people trained in its use, may be the critical factor in saving a life. For this reason it should be carried on all dive boats.

### Hospital treatment

This is subdivided into (1) initial emergency room management and (2) continuing intensive care.

### Emergency room management

The severity of the case determines the appropriate care. In mild cases oxygen administration and/or observation for 8–12 hours may be all that is required. Most patients who are asymptomatic with normal spirometry and chest X-ray at 4 hours post-incident, will not subsequently deteriorate. Patients who are obviously hypoxaemic or have respiratory symptoms or disturbed consciousness may deteriorate further. One series suggested that 15% of patients who were conscious on arrival at hospital subsequently died.

Patients who are unconscious and/or severely hypoxic on arrival should be intubated and ventilated despite the presence of spontaneous ventilation. Muscle relaxants may be required and steps should be taken to avoid gastric regurgitation and further pulmonary soiling. A nasogastric tube should then be inserted and the stomach emptied.

Concurrent with the resuscitation measures, attempts to establish the cause of drowning should be made. A careful search for any other injuries, such as cranial or spinal trauma, internal injuries and long bone fractures should be made. If the cause of drowning is not obvious, evidence of cerebrovascular accident, myocardial infarction, seizure or drug abuse should be sought. In the scuba diver, other diving disorders such as pulmonary barotrauma may have initiated or complicated the drowning.

The prime goal of therapy is to overcome the major derangement of hypoxia with its subsequent acidosis. The aim is to produce a $Pa_{O_2}$ of of above 70 mmHg. This may be achieved by administration of oxygen by mask in mild cases, but most will require more aggressive therapy with intermittent positive pressure ventilation (IPPR) with a high fractional inspired oxygen.

High ventilatory pressure may be required to obtain adequate tidal volume. Progress should be monitored by serial arterial blood gas (ABG) determinations and percutaneous pulse oximetry.

Hypoxaemia persists in the near-drowned victim due to the pathophysiological changes previously described and its resultant gross ventilation–perfusion mismatch. These changes do not return to normal for several days in most cases and much longer in the severely affected.

The institution of positive end-expiratory pressure (PEEP) with either IPPR or spontaneous ventilation, i.e. continuous positive airway pressure (CPAP), will decrease the pulmonary shunting and ventilation–perfusion mismatch and increase the functional residual capacity thus resulting in a higher $Pa_{O_2}$. Nebulized bronchodilator aerosols may be employed to control bronchospasm. Fibreoptic bronchoscopy can be used to remove suspected particulate matter. Endotracheal suction should not be used frequently to aspirate fluid because it will exacerbate pulmonary oedema and hypoxaemia.

If cardiac arrest is diagnosed, the rhythm should be rapidly determined and defibrillation and/or intravenous adrenaline (epinephrine) administered. Other dysrhythmias should be appropriately treated if they have not responded to correction of hypoxia and restoration of adequate tissue perfusion. Due to the fact that, in this situation, acidosis develops prior to cardiac arrest, large doses of bicarbonate (1–2 mmol/kg) may be required to reverse the acidosis. The use of bicarbonate remains controversial and some clinicians may prefer to hyperventilate the patient in order to permit a respiratory compensation for the metabolic acidosis.

Some patients have been found to be markedly hypoglycaemic and an association with alcohol intoxication, physical exhaustion and hypothermia has been noted. Blood glucose can be rapidly estimated along with blood gases on arrival at hospital and intravenous glucose therapy instituted where appropriate. Untreated hypoglycaemia may aggravate the hypoxic brain lesion.

Hypothermia (see Chapter 22) may complicate near drowning and may lead to difficulties in diagnosing cardiac arrest. When in doubt, CPR should be instituted and continued at least until the patient is warmed. Emergency room management of hypothermia depends on the severity and low reading thermometers are essential as severe hypothermia may otherwise be overlooked. Insulation, heating blankets and/or radiant heat may be sufficient but, in severe cases, cardiopulmonary bypass has been instituted. Hyperthermia should be avoided.

Circulatory support may be required to provide adequate perfusion of vital tissues. The maintenance of effective cardiac output may require the correction of hypoxia, arrhythmias and hypovolaemia. Cardiac output may be depressed by IPPR and PEEP, but will usually be restored by volume augmentation. If the patient has not rapidly resumed a good cardiac output and tissue perfusion as indicated by blood pressure, pulse, blood gases and urine output, careful fluid administration and/or inotropic support will be required.

Although central venous pressure is a useful adjunct, it may not give a true indication of hypovolaemia or failure especially in primarily non-cardiogenic pulmonary oedema. Therefore a Swan–Ganz pulmonary artery catheter giving information on left heart filling pressure (PAWP), cardiac output (CO) and mixed venous oxygen content may be invaluable in guiding fluid administration and inotropic support. Colloids may be more useful than crystalloids as fluid replacement. As a general rule, fluid restriction should be initiated and blood volume maintained with concentrated albumin. Diuretics (frusemide or furosemide, 1.0 mg/kg) have been advocated where overhydration is suspected. In most cases a urinary catheter should be passed and hourly urine output measured as an indication of renal perfusion and function. Infusion of dopamine in a 'renal' dose may help avert the development of acute renal failure.

Electrolyte status is usually not a problem initially, but any abnormality should be corrected. Acidosis is almost invariably present, but usually responds to hyperventilation alone, although bicarbonate infusion may be required to help restore cardiac function and thus, in turn, tissue perfusion. The mainstay of therapy is the maintenance of a high tubular flow. Some also advocate alkalinization of the urine.

Steroids have been shown to be of no benefit for the pulmonary lesion, but have still been advocated by some as part of an aggressive regime to control the cerebral oedema which develops after an hypoxic insult. They have not been shown to improve neurological outcome and may, in fact, be deleterious by increasing the risk of infection.

Prophylactic antibiotics have not been shown to be of benefit and should probably only be given where clinically indicated, guided by sputum and blood cultures.

### Continuing intensive therapy

The general principles of intensive therapy are followed but with special emphasis on respiratory function. The following clinical measurements should be regularly monitored:

1. Observations of pulse, blood pressure, temperature, respiratory rate, tidal and minute volume, inspiratory and PEEP pressures, electrocardiogram, pulse oximetry, urinary output and, where indicated, PAWP, CVP, CO via a pulmonary artery catheter.
2. Estimations of arterial blood gas and acid–base status, haemoglobin, packed cell volume, white cell count, serum and urinary electrolytes, serum haemoglobin and haptoglobin levels, serum osmolarity, serum creatinine, urea, glucose, proteins and coagulation status.
3. Regular chest X-ray examination to detect atelectasis, infection, pneumothorax etc.
4. Serial estimations of respiratory status, by measuring airway pressures and compliance, are useful in monitoring progress. In the less severely ill patient, bedside spirometry to estimate $FEV_1$ (forced expiratory volume in 1 second) and VC (vital capacity) are useful guides to recovery.

The optimal level of PEEP is that which produces the best arterial oxygen tension ($Pa_{O_2}$) at the lowest fractional inspired oxygen concentration ($FI_{O_2}$) and with the least haemodynamic disturbance. In combination with IPPR, this is usually about 5–10 cmH$_2$O. The $FI_{O_2}$ is reduced as much as possible to avoid pulmonary oxygen toxicity. Patients with IPPR

tend to retain salt and fluids so water intake should be reduced to about 1500 ml/day with a low sodium content. In such patients, fluid overload has a disastrous effect on pulmonary function.

The role of high frequency ventilation has not yet been fully established. Prolonged ventilatory support may occasionally be required, especially in cases of fresh water drowning and the continuing management is similar to other causes of (adult) respiratory distress syndrome (ARDS). Modes of ventilation, which allow some spontaneous breathing, have been found useful by some authors as they minimize the haemodynamic effects of IPPR. Also the patients tolerate the ventilator better (less sedation, relaxants) and are easier to wean off ventilatory support. Others have found self-triggered or pressure-supported ventilation more satisfactory.

Central nervous system function should be assessed clinically and by electroencephalography. Intracranial pressure (ICP) monitoring has been advocated in severe cases with prompt therapy for any sudden rises.

Hyperpyrexia commonly follows near drowning and its effect on oxygen consumption may be deleterious on a damaged brain. External cooling, antipyretic agents and perhaps pharmacotherapy to prevent shivering may be indicated. Barbiturates and relaxants may be required to control continuing hyperexcitability and rigidity.

An aggressive regime to improve cerebral salvage, allowing recovery of injured cerebral cells and preventing further deterioration, has been advocated. The regime involves initial hydration then fluid restriction, paralysis and hyperventilation, deliberate hypothermia, barbiturate coma and corticosteroids. So far, this regime has not been shown to improve outcome and indeed hypothermia may be deleterious because of a suppressed response to infection. Barbiturates and hyperventilation may have a role where there is raised ICP because without treatment survival is highly unlikely. Even so the prognosis for those with raised ICP is poor.

### Death

Treatment will always vary depending on the severity of the condition and the response to resuscitative measures; however, some effort should be made to continue until unequivocal signs of death are present.

Unresponsive coma, areflexia, fixed dilated pupils or absent corneal reflexes are not in themselves diagnostic signs of death. Patients with all these signs have made complete recoveries.

---

*Recovery has followed prolonged immersion (up to 55 minutes) with few sequelae. It is possible that many have perished from premature termination of resuscitative measures.*

---

## Prevention

The prevention of non-diving drownings will depend very much on the population being considered.

Mothers should be present and vigilant at all times while the baby is bathing. This is also relevant to older children who have episodes of unconsciousness from any cause, commonly epilepsy. Bath accidents in older children are more likely to result from boisterous games and resultant head injuries. Where there are swimming pools, fish ponds or other water containers, there must be protective fences with self-locking gates with a child-proof lock, and at a height that will prevent young children from entry.

As the child becomes older, he will be involved in more sporting activities which predispose to drowning accidents. The value of swimming training programmes and 'drown-proofing' techniques, cannot be overstressed. This is especially important in the countries where swimming is not a common social activity and therefore not frequently taught. While engaged in water sports and boating, life-jackets should be worn and should support the child's head well above the water level. The most important factor is adequate parental control and observation. Where a group of children are swimming together, many local authorities will insist upon experienced 'life-savers', trained in both aquatic skills and first aid. In most socially well-organized countries, instruction of school children, as well as their mothers and other adults, in the first aid technique of mouth-to-mouth respiration is now available.

The importance of avoidance of alcohol in association with aquatic pursuits should be stressed. An education programme, similar to those employed in 'drink–drive' campaigns, particularly targeting adult males, may be effective.

Drowning is a complication of diving. It is also the final common pathway of many or most severe diving accidents, and a pathological obfuscation of these accidents. The safety measures used in diving should prevent these accidents and should prevent drowning being a sequel to them.

## Pathology

Certain external characteristics of drowned victims are common, although these are more specific for immersion than for drowning (see Chapter 34). These include evidence of pale, wrinkled, 'washerwoman's' skin; post-mortem decomposition; lacerations and abrasions from impact with rocks, coral, shells, motor boats and their propellers; and post-mortem injuries from aquatic animals, from the nibbling of the extremities, ears, nose and lips due to crustaceans and fish, to the large tearing wounds of sharks and barracudas. The presence of large quantities of white, pink or overtly bloody froth in the mouth, nose and airways is more specific for drowning as opposed to immersion.

If the victim was alive during his descent to the seabed, it is likely that all entrapped gas spaces will show evidence of barotrauma of descent. Thus, if he wore a face mask, then the conjunctiva may be haemorrhagic. If he wore a dry suit, then linear skin bruising is possible. Haemorrhages may be observed in the victim's sinuses, mastoids and middle ears. The latter may be diagnosed either by otoscopy or autopsy exploration of the temporal bones, and may be mistakenly interpreted as a specific sign of drowning, instead of barotrauma, by pathologists not versed in the effects of hyperbaria. Sea or fresh water may be detected in perforated middle ears, sinuses, respiratory passages and stomach.

Biochemical tests designed to verify drowning as the cause of death have received unwarranted enthusiasm. The Gettler test, using a difference of 25 mg NaC1 per 100 ml plasma or serum from each side of the heart during an autopsy performed within 12 hours of death, is not always accurate. Comparison of the plasma total solids and/or specific gravities from each side of the heart is more reliable. The specific gravity of plasma is less in the left atrium than in the right in many drownings. A specific gravity greater in the right atrium is supportive evidence that death occurred prior to immersion. Magnesium concentration in the vitreous humour is said to give some idea of the duration of immersion in sea water.

There is often considerable venous congestion of the viscera, especially the brain, kidneys and other abdominal organs. Hypoxic cerebral necrosis and acute renal tubular necrosis, with blood pigment casts, are both described. The cerebral oedema and other changes are thought to be secondary to the low arterial oxygen levels, i.e. secondary to the pulmonary manifestations.

The lungs are heavy, oedematous and may be haemorrhagic, with pink or white froth occupying the airways, and even the stomach. Other cases have vomitus aspirated into the airways. In cases of fresh water drowning, fluid in the lungs may be less obvious and, if a considerable delay has occurred between aspiration of fluid and death, the lungs may be dry. Interstitial emphysema may be noted both on the pleural surface and in the mediastinum. Petechial haemorrhages may also be seen under the pleura, probably due to overdistension of the lungs.

Sand, marine organisms, algae and diatoms may be observed in the lungs. The extension of diatoms into the liver, vertebrae and elsewhere is strongly suggestive of drowning or at least sea water aspiration, as a contributory cause of death. This suspicion is supported further by identification and matching of the diatoms in the deceased to those in the marine environment in which the death occurred. The test requires careful interpretation.

Histological changes in the lungs are said to be helpful in differentiating fresh water from salt water drowning. In the former, overdistension of the lungs produces an 'aqueous emphysema' and there are endothelial changes, mitochondrial swelling and alveolar disruption. In the latter, there is swelling and vacuolation of cells, a perivascular neutrophilic infiltration and increased numbers of peroxidase-positive granules. The picture represents a chemical pneumonitis, varying with the salinity of the water, the presence of other irritants, and the duration between exposure and autopsy.

# Salt water aspiration syndrome

A review of diving illnesses in the Royal Australian Navy demonstrated that the most common diving syndrome, other than upper respiratory tract barotrauma, was a severe, rapidly developing, short lasting, systemic disorder.

The records suggested that the dominant characteristic was rigors or shivering. It was more common in the colder months and tended to present late in the day – a few hours after diving had stopped. Many of the patients were admitted to hospital, often with a provisional diagnosis of pneumonia, and had a dramatic response to antibiotic treatment, with complete resolution by the following morning! Pharmacologically, the response was too rapid to be attributed to the antibiotics given, so a subsequent group of patients had treatment withheld, and the cure was just as dramatic.

A prospective enquiry was then carried out into the next 30 cases which presented for treatment, and their symptomatology was documented. Concurrent 'volunteers' were encouraged to aspirate sea water and the symptoms they developed were consistent with the clinical series. The following observations were made.

## *Immediate symptoms*

On specific interrogation, a history of aspiration was given by 27 (90%) of the cases. Often this was not causally associated by the patient with the subsequent events. Over 90% noted an immediate post-dive cough, with or without sputum. Only in the serious cases was the sputum heavily blood stained, frothy and copious.

This condition, which is associated with the aspiration of small amounts of salt water during diving, may occur due to inexperience, while buddy-breathing training, or due to a faulty regulator. In some cases the aspiration occurred on the surface, after the diver had removed his regulator. At that time, navy regulators did not have purge valves. Novices were trained in buddy breathing during their first dive, which was in the open ocean. This led to a greatly increased incidence of sea water aspiration.

## Latent period

This followed the initial symptoms, and was a characteristic and striking feature of the syndrome. It occurred in 83% of the cases, with an average duration of 2 hours and a range of up to 15 hours. The distribution was skewed with an extremely long latent period in a small number of cases. This long latent period was especially noted with those cases which had respiratory symptoms coinciding with a resumption of normal activity after sleep. The latent period was absent in the more severe cases, although even with these there was a marked worsening of symptoms during the first hour or two.

The latent period was a remarkably constant feature and is experienced as either an asymptomatic interval, or a period of static symptoms preceding an intensification. It was typically of 1–2 hours' duration. It was also an occasional feature of near drowning. It is explicable by the osmotic accumulation of fluid diluting the salt water inhaled, spread of this fluid within the lung spaces and the alteration to surfactant function.

Precipitation of respiratory symptoms by movement and aggravation during positive pressure respiration is also understandable on this basis. A drop in vital capacity was interpreted as the clinical reflection of an overall drop in compliance seen in the Colebatch–Halmagyi (1962) near-drowning animal model. The blood gas analyses which were performed were also consistent with this model.

## Incidence of symptoms

The following symptoms were noted, after the latent period:

| Symptoms | Percentage |
|---|---|
| Rigors, tremors or shivering | 87 |
| Anorexia, nausea or vomiting | 80 |
| Hot or cold sensations | 77 |
| Dyspnoea | 73 |
| Cough | 67 |
| Sputum | 67 |
| Headaches | 67 |
| Malaise | 53 |
| Generalized aches | 33 |

## Respiratory symptoms

Following the latent period, symptoms of dyspnoea, cough, sputum and retrosternal discomfort on inspiration were noted. In the mild cases, respiratory symptoms persisted for only an hour, whilst in the more severe cases they continued for days. The respiratory rate roughly paralleled the degree of dyspnoea. Respiratory stimulants appeared to aggravate the dyspnoea and tachypnoea.

Physical examination of the chest revealed evidence of crepitations or rhonchi, either generalized or over-localized areas, in about half the cases. Rarely, the rhonchi were high pitched and similar to that of obstructive airway disease. Signs usually disappeared within the first 24 hours.

Administration of 100% oxygen was reliably effective in relieving respiratory symptoms and removing cyanosis when this was present.

X-ray of the chest revealed areas of patchy consolidation, or a definite increase in respiratory markings, in about half the cases. These usually cleared within 24 hours, but remained for up to a week in severely affected cases. X-rays taken after the incident and repeated within a few hours sometimes showed a variation of the radiological abnormality.

Respiratory function tests of $FEV_1$ and VC, when performed over the first 6 hours, showed an average drop of 0.7 litre in both measurements. These values usually reverted after this time, although the abnormality could persist in a lesser form for up to 24 hours. Even those patients who had no respiratory symptoms demonstrated a reduction in lung volumes. Blood gases revealed $Pa_{O_2}$ levels of 40–75 mmHg with low or normal $Pa_{CO_2}$ (breathing air). (see Case report 23.2, page 310.)

The individual's airway reactivity may influence the severity of this syndrome. Clinical provocation tests to detect incipient asthma in non-diving populations have demonstrated severe reductions in respiratory volumes (a litre or more) in some subjects who are made to inhale aerosol sprays with 15 ml of hypertonic physiological saline (3.5%). The presence of marine organisms and particulate matter may also contribute to the airway responsiveness.

## Generalized symptoms

The patients complained of being feverish in most cases. Malaise was the next most prominent feature. Headaches and generalized aches through the limbs, abdomen, back and chest were important in some cases, but usually not the dominant symptoms. Anorexia appeared the rule. Objectively, the temperature was increased in half the cases, up to 40°C (mean 37.8°C, s.d. 0.6), and the pulse rate was elevated (mean 102/minute, s.d. 21), over the first 6 hours.

Gross shivering, similar in most cases to a rigor, and in some cases to generalized fasciculation, was a common feature of this syndrome. It was precipitated or aggravated by exposure to cold, exercise or breathing 10% oxygen (a procedure not recommended!). It was relieved by administration of 100% oxygen. It occurred especially in those exposed to cold because of duration and depth of dive, clothing worn and environmental conditions during the dive and subsequently.

Some patients realized that relief from their symptoms may be obtained by either hot water baths or showers, or lying in a very warm bed.

The signs and symptoms usually reverted to normal within 6 hours, and rarely persisted beyond 24 hours, unless the case was of considerable severity. In some, there was an impairment of consciousness, including a transitory mild confusion (three cases), syncope on standing (two cases) and unconsciousness (two cases). The latter could, more correctly, be considered as near drowning.

The rather prominent manifestation of shivering is not readily explained. The shivering occurs concurrently with the pyrexia, which also takes an hour or two to develop. The 2-hour delay between leaving the cold water environment and experiencing this symptom is paradoxical. A report on shivering in otherwise healthy men was made by Bullard. He demonstrated that men exposed to cold conditions were more likely to shiver if, concurrently, they were exposed to mild hypoxia. The likelihood of hypoxia was supported by the clinical observation of cyanosis in some of these patients and verified by arterial gas estimations. The rigors or shivering in this series may thus be due to the combination of hypoxia (aspiration) and cold (immersion).

Haemoglobin, haematocrit, ESR and electrolytes remained normal. The white cell count was usually normal, although a mild leucocytosis (not in excess of 20 000 per $mm^3$) was noted in a few cases, with a moderate polymorphonuclear increase and a shift to the left.

Lactic dehydrogenase estimations revealed a mild rise in some cases X-ray and lung volume changes are described above.

## Differential diagnosis

The above observations served to focus on an illness which mimicked a severe respiratory infection and developed soon after a dive. It is often claimed that a mild upper respiratory infection is likely to result in a rapid deterioration, due to the spread of infection immediately following a dive. This belief is countered by the fact that most divers, during their very rigorous training, develop evidence of such an infection or of bronchitis, and continue to dive without ever consulting a medical officer. The paradox now appears to be resolved with the description of this syndrome. Differentiation between the salt water aspiration syndrome and an acute infection can be made from the history of aspiration, serial chest X-rays and spirometry, and a knowledge of the natural history of the diseases. In the first few hours of this syndrome, the possibility of pneumonia causes considerable anxiety.

In the differential diagnosis of the salt water aspiration syndrome, the possibility of other occupational diseases of divers must be considered:

1. Decompression sickness, with cardiorespiratory or joint manifestations. If there is any question regarding the possibility of cardiorespiratory symptoms of decompression sickness ('chokes'), recompression therapy is mandatory. Decompression sickness should be considered with subjects who use scuba or surface supply breathing apparatus and conduct deep or repetitive diving. This diagnosis is unlikely in the above series, because in no case did the depth/duration figures approach those from which decompression is required, but it must be considered in civilian diving practice. The specific joint pains and abnormal posturing characteristic of 'bends' is quite unlike the

vague generalized muscular aches involving the limbs and lumbar region seen with this syndrome. The rapid beneficial response to the inhalation of 100% oxygen in the salt water aspiration syndrome is of diagnostic value. Chest X-ray, lung function and blood gas analyses may be used to confirm the diagnosis. Decompression sickness responds rapidly only to recompression therapy. The natural history of the two disorders, except for the occurrence of a latent period, is quite dissimilar.

2. Pulmonary barotrauma: serious cases of pulmonary barotrauma result in pneumo-thorax, air emboli and surgical emphysema occurring suddenly after a dive. In minor cases of pulmonary barotrauma, confusion with the aspiration syndrome may arise. In these cases, the diagnosis and treatment of the former must take precedence over the latter, until such time as the natural history, chest X-ray, spirometry and blood gas ana-lysis show the contrary.

3. The effects of cold and immersion are usually maximal at, or very soon after, the time of rescue. The clinical features are only likely to be confused with the salt water aspiration syndrome when both conditions exist.

4. Key West scuba divers' disease: this and other infective disorders due to the use of contaminated regulators and mouth pieces, may cause some confusion. Fortunately, these illnesses usually take longer to de-velop (24–48 hours), and to respond to therapy. There is thus very little clinical similarity in the sequence and duration of the clinical signs.

## Treatment

Most of the clinical manifestations of this dis-order respond very rapidly to the administra-tion of oxygen and rest. Warming the patient may be of equal symptomatic benefit, but in general no other regime is required. There is a possibility that some of the clinical manifesta-tions may not be due merely to the aspiration of water, but to the body's (and specifically the respiratory tract's) response to aspirated or-ganisms, foreign bodies or irritants carried to the lungs with the sea water aspiration.

# Research

## Animal experiments

Most of these studies were performed in dogs or sheep where water was instilled into the intubated trachea under anaesthesia. The res-ults may be summarized under several head-ings.

### Biochemical disturbances

### Fresh water drowning

Large volumes of fluid can pass across the alveolar membranes into the circulatory system. This haemodilution depends on osmosis and the immediate effects may include lowered haematocrit, serum protein specific gravity and electrolytes (especially sodium, cal-cium and chloride). There may be an increase in the serum potassium due to acidosis and osmotic haemolysis. The latter causes an increased concentration of total serum haem-oglobin with an absence of haptoglobins, and this may result in haemoglobinuria. Hyper-volaemia and increased central venous pres-sure (CVP) is usually transitory.

> *In animal experiments, fresh water drown-ing causes haemodilution due to passage of fluid along an osmotic pressure gradient from the lungs into the blood. Salt water drowning causes haemoconcentration due to passage of fluid along an osmotic pres-sure gradient from blood into the hypertonic sea water in the alveoli.*

### Salt water drowning

Sea water has an osmotic pressure approxi-mately 3.5–4 times that of blood and conse-quently there is movement of fluid from the circulatory system into the pulmonary air spaces. Subsequent haemoconcentration may be accompanied by an increase in haematocrit, serum protein specific gravity and electrolytes (sodium, potassium, calcium, magnesium and chloride). These increases are usually only marked if large volumes of sea water have been aspirated. There is a reduction in size of red

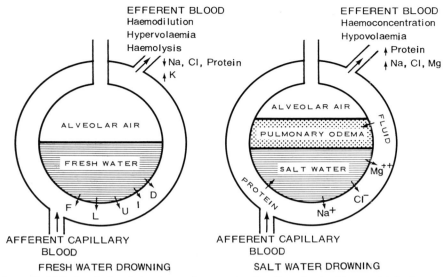

**Figure 21.2** Biochemical and circulatory changes after flooding of animal lungs with fresh and salt water.

blood cells, due to osmosis. Pulmonary oedema is marked. The hypovolaemia may persist for variable periods.

### Circulatory disturbances

With the rapid onset of hypoxia, hypercapnia and acidosis during drowning, the following cardiovascular effects are noted:

1. Increased CVP with a dilatation of the right ventricle. If small amounts of fluid are aspirated these changes soon revert to normal; however, if large amounts of fluid, especially fresh water, are aspirated, then the CVP may remain elevated for a considerable period.
2. Initial bradycardia with transient hypertension, followed by hypotension and arrhythmias. The type of dysrhythmia varies with the species of animal studied and may include premature atrial and ventricular ectopic beats, atrial tachycardia, ventricular tachycardia, variable degrees of heart block and ventricular fibrillation (especially in the case of fresh water drowning).
3. Death may be the result of cardiac asystole or ventricular fibrillation, which may be precipitated by electrolyte disturbances or by hypoxia.

### Respiratory disturbances

These effects vary with the type and amount of fluid aspirated, and include the following.

### Marked decrease in lung compliance

Compliance refers to volume change per unit ventilatory pressure applied. This decrease signifies an increased elastic resistance of the lung, which must be overcome by increased ventilatory pressures. The aspiration of 2–3 ml $H_2O$ per kg body weight causes a reduction in lung compliance to 10% of its normal value. Hence, an increase in inspiratory effort is required to maintain ventilation. It is thought that this change in compliance may be related to surfactant activity at the fluid–membrane interface within the alveoli. The partial removal of surfactant by sea water causes alveolar collapse and the development of pulmonary oedema. As fluid accumulates in the alveoli and other air passages, due to the osmotic gradient, ventilation is further reduced. Fresh water appears to destroy or alter surfactant; consequently, alveolar collapse may occur. If surfactant activity is not restored uneven ventilation will result, despite increased ventilatory pressures. It is also possible that the pulmonary oedema which also occurs in fresh water drowning may, if sufficient water aspiration has occurred, be partly the result of an overloading of the circulation and subsequent congestive heart failure. A secondary consideration may also include airway closure following reflex stimulation of the parasympathetic nervous system by fluid aspiration.

---

> *Aspiration of fluid causes a marked fall in lung compliance.*

---

### A decrease in arterial oxygen pressure

It has been shown that this may fall to less than 50% of normal, soon after the aspiration of 2–3 ml $H_2O$ per kg body weight. The degree of hypoxaemia appears to be directly related to the volume and tonicity (which is much greater with sea water) of the fluid aspirated, and may be sufficient to cause loss of consciousness. After the aspiration of a small amount of fluid, the hypoxaemia may rapidly reverse with treatment; however, it may persist for long periods if a large amount of fluid, especially sea water, has been aspirated. There appear to be different mechanisms responsible for the development of hypoxaemia after salt water aspiration. The main reason for the fall in arterial oxygen tension is the development of a marked ventilation–perfusion inequality due to the perfusion of both sea and fresh water aspiration. The difference lies, however, in the reason for the non-ventilation of the alveoli. With fresh water aspiration, these alveoli collapse after serious alteration to or destruction of pulmonary surfactant. Salt water not only results in alveolar collapse subsequent to partial removal of pulmonary surfactant, but in the collection of fluid (pulmonary oedema) in the alveoli and other air passages.

Other features which contribute to the hypoxia include:

1. Increased airway resistance.
2. Diffusion defects, which may develop as a result of damage to the alveolar capillary membranes after aspiration pneumonitis, pulmonary oedema or secondary infection.
3. Reduced alveolar ventilation: the arterial carbon dioxide level ($Pa_{CO_2}$) may remain normal or low with small amounts of aspirated fluid, but may be increased if larger amounts of sea water are involved.

### Increased pulmonary arterial pressure

This is probably a result of increased vascular resistance accompanying hypoxic pulmonary vasoconstriction. Dilatation of the right ventricle follows. This is unlike those cases in which death is the result of asphyxia, when the left ventricle is dilated.

### Pulmonary oedema

Exudate into the alveolar spaces occurs rapidly, especially in salt water drowning. Much foaming of the aspirated fluid results, with the production of copious frothy red sputum.

## Clinical series

There are no pathognomonic signs of drowning, as the post-mortem results of immersion and drowning are often similar. Post-mortem findings are variable and little attention has been paid to the time relationship between ante-mortem disturbances, death and autopsy. This may account in part for the differences observed between animal studies and human drowning, but the volume of aspirated fluid is probably more important.

The findings in several large series of human drownings and near drownings were as follows:

1. No cases of clinically significant haemodilution in either fresh and salt water drownings were noted.
2. Severe electrolyte shifts were rare.
3. Haemolysis, haemoglobinaemia and haemoglobinuria were uncommon.
4. Cardiac arrest in the field often responded to initial resuscitation. Ventricular fibrillation was recorded only on one occasion, and this was after fresh water aspiration. Supraventricular tachycardias were quite common.
5. Death sometimes followed seemingly good initial recoveries.
6. Severe acidosis was uncommon.
7. Pulmonary oedema was noticed in the majority of cases, but this appeared to bear

little relationship to the nature of the fluid aspirated.

8. Patients who arrived in hospital conscious and with a normal chest X-ray usually survived. Patients with fixed dilated pupils usually died. Otherwise, severity of chest X-ray findings and level of consciousness did not correlate with ultimate survival.

The lungs of 10% of victims of drowning are dry when seen at post-mortem examination. It is postulated that this may result either from reflex laryngospasm preventing fluid entry, or from removal of the water from the lungs by osmosis between the times of aspiration and autopsy.

Why are the biochemical changes reported in animal experiments not usually observed in human 'near drowning'? Why do the respiratory changes outweigh all others in significance in the acute stages of management? In human near drowning what is the difference between salt and fresh water?

The answers to these questions lie in the volume of fluid aspirated. In animal experiments large volumes (of the order of 11–20 ml/kg are administered to anaesthetized animals. Certainly, electrolyte and haemoglobin changes corresponding to these volumes of aspirate are very rarely seen in humans except in the extremely hypertonic Dead Sea. It is likely that in humans these volumes are not compatible with survival. Significant alteration in respiratory mechanics and marked hypoxaemia occur with volumes as low as 2.2 ml/kg in animals, and these changes simulate the human clinical picture.

Animal experiments suggest that the surfactant in the alveoli is denatured by fresh water and that the type II alveolar cells responsible for the manufacture of surfactant are also severely injured and take considerable time to regenerate. In salt water aspiration, this is not so and, even though the initial pulmonary oedema is greater (osmotic effect), the long-term effect is less. If there is any significant difference in humans between salt and fresh water near drowning, it is probable that in the 'equivalent' salt water case the hypoxia and respiratory derangements are initially worse but recovery is relatively rapid. In contrast, the fresh water case may not appear as serious at first but may have a more prolonged, stormy recovery period.

# Recommended reading and references

COLEBATCH, H.J.H. and HALMAGYI, D.F.J. (1962). Reflex airway reaction to fluid aspiration. *Journal of Applied Physiology* **17**, 787–794.

CONN, A.W. and BARKER, G.A. (1984). Fresh water drowning and near drowning – an update. Canadian Anaesthatists' Society Journal **31**(3), 538–544.

EDMONDS, C. (1970). A salt water aspiration syndrome. *Military Medicine* **135**(9).

HEIMLICH, H.J. and PATRICK, E.A. (1988). Using the Heimlich manoeuvre to save near drowning victims. *Postgraduate Medicine* **84**(2), 62–67, 71–73.

HOWLAND, J. and HINGSON, R. (1988). Alcohol as a risk factor for drownings: a review of the literature (1950–1985). *Accident Analysis and Prevention* **20**(1), 19–25.

KIZER, K.W. (1982). Aquatic rescue and in-water CPR. *Annals of Emergency Medicine* **11**, 166.

KIZER, K.W. (1983). Resuscitation of submersion casualties. *Emergency Medical Clinics of North America* **1**, 643–652.

MODELL, J.H. (1971). *The Pathophysiology and Treatment of Drowning and Near Drowning.* Springfield, IL: Charles C. Thomas.

MODELL, J.H. (1986). Treatment of near drowning: is there a role for H.Y.P.E.R. therapy? *Critical Care Medicine* **14**, 593–594.

NEAL, J.M. (1985). Near drowning. *Journal of Emergency Medicine* **3**, 41–52.

ORLOWSKI, J.P. (1987). Drowning, near drowning, and ice-water submersions. *Pediatric Clinics of North America* **34**, 75–92.

ORNATO, J.P. (1986). Special resuscitation situations: near drowning, traumatic injury, electric shock and hypothermia. *Circulation* **74**(6, Pt 2), IV23–26.

PEARN, J. (1977). Neurological and psychometric studies in children surviving fresh water immersion accidents. *The Lancet* **i**, 7–9.

PLUECKHAHN, V.D. (1984). Alcohol and accidential drowning. *Medical Journal of Australia* **2**, 22–25.

PRATT, F.D. and HAYNES, B.E. (1986). Incidence of secondary drowning after salt water submersion. *Annals of Emergency Medicine* **115**, 1084–1087.

SIMCOCK, A.D. (1989). The resuscitation of immersion victims. *Applied Cardiopulmonary Pathophysiology* **2**, 293–298.

# 22

# Cold and hypothermia

## Introduction

Immersion in cold water causes a complex response in the subject. In some cases the exposure may be rapidly fatal due to the cold shock. If he survives this period, a diver may still not be able to perform his tasks because of a loss of dexterity.

If exposure to conditions in which the heat loss from the body is greater than the heat production continues, then body temperature falls and the diver becomes hypothermic. In all except the warmest seas, most divers need assistance to maintain the balance between heat production and heat loss to the water. In temperate climates, the wet suit provides adequate insulation. In colder climates a dry suit, which provides more insulation, may be required. Under more extreme conditions the diver and his breathing gas may need supplementary heating.

Failure to maintain heat balance results in a fall in body temperature. If this is mild, 1–2°C, the diver feels cold and may shiver. This may affect delicate manual tasks. A continued loss of heat results in the body temperature falling to a level where the diver is incapable of looking after himself, and is liable to drown. At still lower body temperatures, death occurs even when drowning is prevented.

Hypothermia is a common cause of death in association with maritime accidents. None of the 1498 people who entered the water after the sinking of the 'Titanic' survived. Although many could swim and had life-jackets, few lived longer than 40 minutes. Almost all in the life-boats were saved. Figure 22.1 shows the relationship of expected survival time to water temperatures.

The temperature of the oceans ranges from −2 to 30°C. In most regions the annual range of temperature in open ocean is less than 10°C.

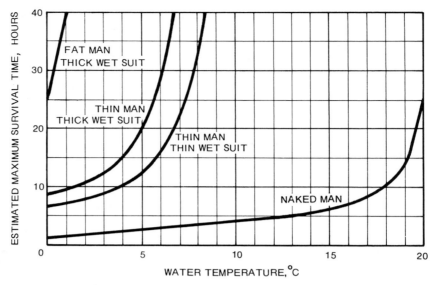

**Figure 22.1** Survival expectancy related to water temperature

This narrow range is caused by the high heat capacity of water which damps down the seasonal change in temperature. This stable thermal environment is predictable enough to allow for appropriate precautions to be taken when exposing people to it.

Cooling occurs because water is a good conductor, and has a high specific heat. Water conducts heat approximately 25 times as rapidly as air. The amount of heat required to raise water temperature is about 1000 times that required for an identical quantity of air.

> *Water is a much better conductor of heat than air.*

Insulation reduces heat loss, and may be required for survival during prolonged exposure to water temperatures of less than 32°C. The water temperature at which extra insulation is required depends on the internal insulation and the heat production the diver can maintain.

Hypothermia is one of the major limitations to deep diving in the cold seas, such as those of the North Sea and off-shore Alaskan oil fields. Similar temperatures are experienced by amateur divers diving in the waters off northern Europe and North America. It is far less of a problem for divers in the Indo-Pacific, Middle East and Central American areas.

Some suspect physiological and pathological data on the effects of hypothermia were obtained in the Nazi experiments on humans during World War II. The other tragic source of data was the experiences with shipwrecks and plane crashes during World War I and World War II. The realization that hypothermia was probably the most common cause of death of sailors during World War II lead to the development of covered inflatable life rafts and exposure suits which give better protection in cold water.

Newer information comes from the management of clinical cases of hypothermia and observations made during induced hypothermia in surgical procedures on neurological and cardiac patients. Other workers are interested in the physiological responses to immersion and the development of better protection for divers and for people who may suddenly be dropped in the sea. This group includes sailors, fishermen and occupants of aircraft flying over water.

In this chapter, the accent is on the clinical features, prevention and treatment of hypothermia as encountered by the diving physician.

Little consideration is given to the chronic hypothermia that develops in the elderly and malnourished in cold climates, because this causes different responses and requires somewhat different management.

There is an area of possible overlap between rapid-onset and chronic hypothermia, i.e. in the water temperature zone where the body can initially maintain core temperature. Hypothermia would develop when the energy sources have been depleted. Beckman and Reeves, in 1966, planned to immerse 24 subjects up to the neck in a 24°C bath for 12 hours. This should not have induced severe hypothermia but only 6 subjects completed the immersion. Two were withdrawn with mild hypothermia, 2 suffered nausea associated with hypoglycaemia and 13 had severe cramps. Information on the appropriate management of such cases is not available.

> *The correct management of cases with mild hypothermia and associated symptoms caused by prolonged exposure to cool water is unclear.*

# Initial reactions to immersion

Until recently, the initial responses to cold water immersion have not been well explained; in many cases, good swimmers have died within a few metres of safety after short periods of immersion. Some workers postulated that these deaths were caused by inhaling water, others suggested a cardiac aetiology. The Royal Navy studies in this area have been recently reviewed by Tipton (1989). He provides a logical system to explain these fatalities. Within the first 3 minutes, a complex series of changes is initiated. He divides them into several groups which are summarized below.

## Cardiovascular responses

There is an immediate increase in rate of about 20 beats/min and an increase in cardiac output. It is accompanied by an increase in blood pressure. There is a rapid fall in peripheral blood flow as a consequence of vasoconstriction. These factors are probably sufficient to

explain some of the sudden deaths. Subjects with coronary disease are obviously at risk because of the increased cardiac workload. Not only is the workload increased but the tachycardia will impair coronary blood flow. The second group at risk are those with arterial disease. The hypertension may trigger vessel rupture and death from a cerebrovascular incident.

## Respiratory responses

The initial gasp on entering cold water may be followed by uncontrollable hyperventilation. There may be a ten-fold increase in ventilation but three- to four-fold increases are more common. This response can rapidly lead to water inhalation and drowning, and this is more likely to occur in rough water or where there is a period in which the head is immersed. The victim cannot hold his breath, so even a good swimmer may aspirate water.

A less obvious problem is that the hyperventilation causes hypocapnia. Tipton cites a study where the arterial carbon dioxide fell 12 mmHg after an iced water shower for 1 minute. He suggests that this fall could cause enough reduction in cerebral blood flow to explain the disorientation and clouding of consciousness that has been noted.

Increased ventilation can trigger bronchoconstriction in asthmatics. In normal subjects, there is an inspiratory shift in end-expiratory volume so that the subject is breathing close to his or her total lung capacity. This will rapidly induce fatigue and is an inefficient form of respiration.

Figure 22.2 presents a more complete version of possible cold shock responses.

If the subject survives the initial immersion, the responses tend to return to normal. Hypothermia will start to develop. It may also develop in subjects who have had a less dramatic immersion.

> *Immersion in cold water usually causes:*
> - *Tachycardia*
> - *Hypertension*
> - *Hyperventilation*

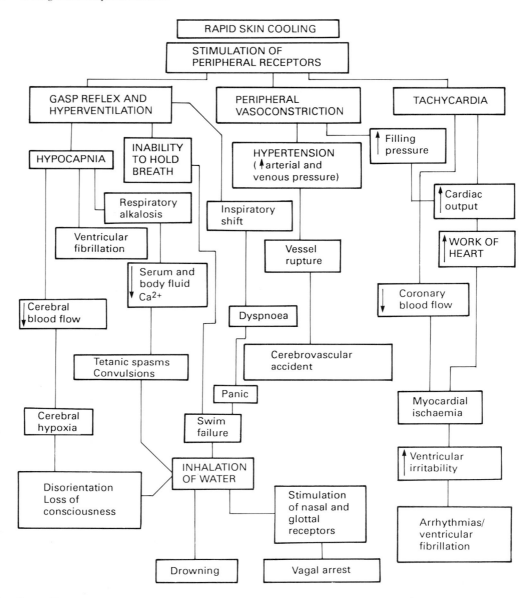

**Figure 22.2** A more complete version of possible cold shock responses. ↑ increase; ↓ decrease. (Adapted from Tipton, 1989)

# Signs and symptoms of hypothermia

The effects of hypothermia in humans are variable and may be complicated by those of immersion. The degree of hypothermia depends on environmental and physiological factors. Environmental factors include the water temperature and flow, the duration of exposure, the insulating materials present (fabrics, fat, grease etc.) and the gas mixture employed. Physiological factors include somatotype, activity during exposure, the degree of cold adaptation, and the use of drugs such as

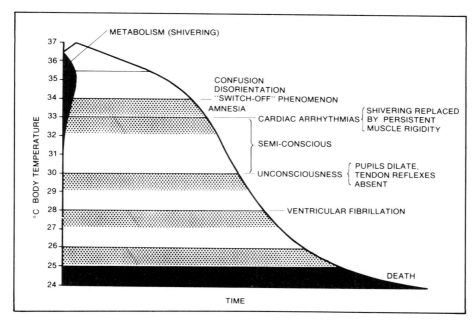

**Figure 22.3** Clinical features of acute hypothermia: the curve represents the behaviour of body temperature during cold water immersion, with associated clinical features at various body temperatures

alcohol or marijuana which either induce vasodilatation or prevent the adaptive mechanisms of vasoconstriction.

With rare exceptions, the lethal lower limit for humans is 23–25°C (rectal). The effects of hypothermia are set out below.

### Mild hypothermia

The core temperature is in the range 33–35°C. The victim will be handicapped by the cold but should be breathing and fully conscious. He will be probably be shivering and experience local reactions including the sensation of coldness in the extremities. Numbness occurs as the peripheral sensory nerves are affected. The vasoconstriction, particularly in combination with immersion, leads to a diuresis which can cause dehydration.

Difficulty in performing coordinated fine movements, due to motor nerve involvement, may result in a dangerous situation in which the diver cannot effectively manage either his task or his equipment. This loss of control may become a problem in divers with normal body temperature.

The other major danger is that lethargy and sluggish reactions may lead to accident or drowning. Other local reactions such as immersion foot and frostbite are more applicable to general and military medicine than to diving medicine.

### Moderate hypothermia

With a core temperature between 30°C and 33°C, the diver will be slow to respond or unconscious. Shivering usually persists to the lower end of the range when it is replaced by muscle rigidity. Heart rate and cardiac output fall. The electrocardiogram (ECG) may show prolonged Q–T intervals and the QRS complex may develop a terminal complication known as a J wave. Nodal rhythm, atrioventricular block or atrial fibrillation can develop. Respiratory frequency falls with the reduction in tissue oxygen needs.

Many of the maritime cases of hypothermia succumb at this stage as they are generally no longer able to contribute to their rescue, to keep swimming or even to keep their heads above water.

### Severe hypothermia

The victim will have a core temperature below 30°C. He will be unconscious or semi-conscious and shivering may be replaced by muscle rigidity that can be confused with rigor mortis. Respiration and pulse may be depressed or not detectable, and respiration may be reduced to 1–2 gasps/min. Below 30°C there is a high risk of ventricular fibrillation. Any electrical activity on the ECG or electroencephalogram (EEG) is evidence of continued life. In particular, bizarre ECGs should not be considered artefacts. In a field situation, the pupillary light reflexes may be helpful but their absence is not evidence of death. The chilled brain has a greatly increased tolerance to circulatory arrest – 25 min at 25°C. The Alaskan dictum 'do not assume a patient is dead until he is warm and dead' may lead to many unsuccessful attempts at revival but this is preferable to any unnecessary deaths.

---

*Clinical phases of progressive hypothermia:*

| | |
|---|---|
| 1. Mild | 35–34°C |
| 2. Moderate | 33–30°C |
| 3. Severe | < 30°C |

---

## System review

### Cardiovascular system

The initial response to immersion in cold water has been discussed above. Later, as temperature falls, the force of ventricular contraction is reduced; this leads to a reduction in blood pressure, heart rate and cardiac output. Ultimately, cardiac arrest may occur at approximately 13°C (rectal). Various arrhythmias are common – atrial fibrillation at approximately 30°C, and ventricular fibrillation usually below 25°C. The blood becomes more viscous and, because hypothermia reduces the effective release of oxygen from haemoglobin, tissue hypoxia may develop. Any blood gas measurements should be interpreted with respect to the patient's low body temperature.

Movement of the throat, limbs or chest during rescue or resuscitation may trigger ventricular fibrillation in a hypothermic heart.

If the skin temperature falls below about 10°C, the function of the smooth muscles controlling vasoconstriction may be impaired and vasodilatation occurs. This leads to a local increase in temperature and restoration of vasoconstriction. This cold intermittent vasodilatation accelerates the rate of temperature fall.

The effects of hypothermia on gas transport are complex. Cold decreases the blood flow to most areas and this could be expected to decrease gas uptake. However, cooling increases the solubility of gases and the amount of gas transported to a tissue at elevated partial pressures.

A further complication is the effect of rewarming after a dive where the increase in temperature decreases the solubility of inert gases. This could trigger gas release and cause decompression sickness. These symptoms could also be the result of returning neural function in a tissue that already has free gas in it.

### Central nervous system

With a core temperature below 35°C, there is an impairment of speech, fixation of ideas, sluggish reactions and mental impairment. Depersonalization, amnesia, confusion and delirium are possible. Unconsciousness may develop at about 30°C and by 27°C most reflexes are lost. Exposure to cold initially causes reflex hyperventilation; however, with hypothermia, the respiratory centre is depressed, and this contributes to hypoxia and acidosis. There is also a rare form of sudden apnoea following cold water stimulation of cutaneous receptors.

Hypothermia may sometimes serve a valuable protective function because the harmful effects of reduction of cerebral blood flow are mitigated by a reduction in metabolic rate. At 30°C the blood supply to the brain can be stopped for 10 minutes without neurological damage. Some of the successful and dramatic resuscitations reported in the medical literature may be explained by hypothermic protection.

### Gastrointestinal system

There is some slowing of intestinal activity, and retardation of the rate of destruction of bacteria. Paralytic ileus may develop in cases of severe hypothermia.

### Renal system

Cold and immersion cause an increase in central blood volume and diuresis. Hyponatraemia and hypovolaemia may follow. As the temperature falls further, cardiac output and hence glomerular filtration are reduced, resulting in a decreased urinary output. Acidosis results from both lactic acid accumulation and respiratory depression. Lysis of red blood cells may result in cold haemoglobinuria.

### Liver

There is a decrease in liver function – probably a direct temperature effect on enzyme kinetics. As a consequence metabolites such as lactate may accumulate. Drugs accumulate because their clearance is slowed or stopped.

---

*A chilled liver may not metabolize drugs.*

---

### Locomotor

Shivering is a heat-producing response to cold. It mainly affects the large proximal muscles, but also causes a loss of coordination and difficulty in the performance of fine tasks. There is also a loss of muscle power. Swimming ability is decreased, with increasing discomfort and fatigue. Apathy and euphoria may combine with the fatigue, stopping the diver from taking appropriate action for his rescue.

### Cutaneous reactions

Any prolonged immersion results in softening and swelling of the skin, rendering it susceptible to injury and infection. This so-called 'washerwoman's skin' is characterized by soft ridges, especially over the tips of fingers and toes, where there is a large surface area to mass ratio.

In cold water, there may be a sudden release of histamine in susceptible persons causing cold or allergic urticaria. In some cases, the skin rapidly becomes hot, red and oedematous. Symptoms may occur during or after exposure. Occasional deaths have been reported (see Chapter 30).

Cold-induced vasodilatation of the peripheral vessels has been discussed. In very cold water this does not stop the skin freezing. Freezing will occur at approximately $-0.53°C$. Since the freezing point of sea water is $-1.9°C$, it is only possible for skin to freeze when immersed in sea water near this temperature.

## Prevention of immersion shock and hypothermia

Immersion shock can be reduced by wearing protective clothing which attenuates the stimulus. Cold habituation will also condition the subject. These factors can also be used in the prevention of hypothermia.

The insidious effects on the diver's performance should not be ignored because the cold may cause him to make avoidable errors.

---

*The following preventive measures have been used or proposed:*
- *Wearing insulating fabrics or coatings*
- *Increasing the body deposits of subcutaneous fat*
- *Reducing exercise in the water and assuming a position to minimize the surface contact area*
- *Acclimatization to cold, over long periods*
- *Careful desensitization, which may reduce cold urticaria*

---

Hypothermia may be delayed or prevented after maritime accidents. The following advice may assist people in these circumstances:

- Wear a wet suit or a survival suit to reduce heat loss.
- If wearing a life jacket, try to adopt a spheroidal position (fetal position) with the head out of the water, and the legs pulled up to the chest and the arms wrapped round the legs. This may increase the survival time by 50%. Drown-proofing, where the victim rests with head under water between breaths is not advocated because of the increased heat loss from the head.

- Do not swim unless very close to safety; groups of survivors should remain huddled tightly together to conserve heat (and to give the rescuers a larger target to identify).
- Wear clothing to reduce heat loss, in particular a hood or some other protection on the head is important in conserving heat.
- Avoid or delay immersion if any other options are feasible.

A diver is in a better situation than others as he knows he will be entering the water and can plan for it. During diving activities, it is common to use protective clothing. The insulation offered by wet suits diminishes as the depth increases. Dry suits are generally preferred to wet suits for colder, deeper or longer dives.

The insulating efficiency of these materials is demonstrated by a comparison of the effects of subjects immersed in water at 4–5°C. Without the protection, about 50% will die within 1 hour. In the same water temperature the core temperatures of divers wearing neoprene foam wet suits will only fall 1°C in 6 hours.

Various techniques of diver warming have been utilized. They include the use of electrical and chemical energy and hot water supplies, to warm the diver's body and his breathing gases. These methods assume greater importance with deep diving because of the lower water temperature and the use of helium or hydrogen in the breathing mixtures. These gases have high thermal conductivity, causing increased heat loss and the likelihood of hypothermia.

Heat loss during immersion is much greater from certain body surfaces than others. These include skin over active muscles and areas of the body with little subcutaneous fat. At water temperatures of 5°C or less, about half the total heat loss from a diver in a wet suit takes place through the head, if it is without protection.

As a general rule, water temperatures of 20–30°C leave an unprotected diver normothermic, less than 20°C produce hypothermia and more than 35°C may lead to hyperthermia.

There is also a risk of **hyperthermia** caused by wearing a suit which gives very effective insulation on the surface while waiting to dive, particularly if the diver is in the sun or he exercises.

# Treatment of immersion shock and hypothermia

It is important to obtain a measurement of the victim's temperature if this is possible. In most facilities a rectal temperature can be obtained. It may be less than the true core reading. In facilities where hypothermia casualties are expected, the tympanic membrane is probably a better site as it reflects core temperature more closely.

A victim of immersion shock may respond to normal resuscitation techniques. The casualty may be suffering from cardiac failure, a cerebrovascular accident or drowning. Hypothermia is also possible if rescue has been delayed.

In milder cases of hypothermia, removal from the cold environment, protection from wind, the use of blankets and body-to-body contact in a sleeping bag are all remedies that have worked.

Shivering restores body heat if heat loss is prevented. Heat loss from the head should be minimized, as should evaporative heat loss from wet clothing. Two large plastic bags, one over the victim's body and one over an insulating layer such as a sleeping bag have been recommended. This prevents evaporative cooling as well as avoiding the need to strip the wet clothes from the survivor. In conditions where evacuation would involve further cooling, it is often better to revive the patient before moving him.

With more severe degrees of hypothermia, the treatment depends on the facilities available. The victim probably will not be shivering and has little heat production. Movement may sometimes trigger ventricular fibrillation, and active treatment can result in aggravation of core hypothermia and/or hypotension (see later).

The specific treatments of serious hypothermia include the following.

## First aid and resuscitation

In cases of hypothermia associated with immersion, it is best to keep the patient horizontal during, and following, removal from the water. A rescue basket, a stretcher or a double strop system, with one loop lifting the patient under the arms and another under the knees, can be used. This prevents a sudden fall in blood pressure that can occur with the loss of hydrostatic pressure on the legs.

There have been cases where the patient was alive and responsive in the water, but apparently dead by the time he reached a rescue helicopter after being lifted in a vertical position. This shock reaction is thought to be caused by blood pooling in the legs.

Care must be taken to avoid any unnecessary manipulation of the throat. For example, the use of a sucker can cause reflex vagal slowing of the heart and is liable to precipitate ventricular fibrillation. The airways must be clear, but if suction is necessary, it must be done with the greatest care. It is also important not to give cardiac massage or artificial ventilation just because the spontaneous rates are slow, as sudden over-ventilation and/or trauma to the heart are again liable to precipitate fibrillation. Even manipulation of the limbs can cause arrhythmias, probably by cooling the heart with cold blood from the periphery.

> *The pulse may be difficult to detect in a hypothermia casualty.*

The only circumstance in which cardiac massage and artificial ventilation are likely to be beneficial in hypothermia is when the heart has stopped or is in ventriculation fibrillation. If drowning has also occurred, then normal CPR takes precedence over the management of hypothermia. Cases of hypothermia or drowning and hypothermia will normally need rewarming before normal cardiac function can be restored, and rewarming can correct the abnormality. Therefore it is probably unwise to treat any electrocardiographic abnormalities except asystole until temperature has returned to normal.

Correction of fibrillation by drugs or defibrillation is not generally effective while the core temperature remains below 30°C. The use of drugs is also contraindicated because they will not be metabolized until the victim has been warmed, by which time they may not be needed.

A ventilator with a heater and humidifier is needed to prevent respiratory heat loss.

### Hospital care

The victim with severe hypothermia will need hospital care during and after his rewarming. The choice of rewarming method will depend on the skills and equipment available. Some of the options are outlined below. Intravenous fluids should be warmed. The use of solutions containing lactate should be avoided because the hypothermic liver will not metabolize lactate.

Physiological saline, or 5% glucose if the patient is hypoglycaemic, is suggested. Administration of 500 ml at once, then 100 ml/h, is a simple guide to overcome haemoconcentration and possible shock as the peripheral vessels expand.

It is important not to treat any abnormalities of blood chemistry unless the blood sample is a reliable one, preferably taken from a central vein, and with all temperature corrections made.

Thick bronchial secretions or aspirated gastric contents may require suction; this requires care to prevent developing arrhythmias. After rewarming, antibiotics should be used to prevent the development of respiratory infections.

## Methods of rewarming

Most victims of mild hypothermia will recover if put into a hot bath and disturbed as little as possible. This seems to be the best rewarming treatment that can be given in a small hospital. An initial water temperature of 36°C, to reduce the pain response and risk of atrial fibrillation, and then an increase over 5–10 minutes to 40–42°C, until the rectal temperature is above 33°C, has been recommended.

Limbs should be placed in an elevated position, outside the bath. Often a temporary degree of hypotension accompanies vasodilatation, but usually the elevation of the limbs is sufficient to counteract this. The position also reduces core cooling with cold blood from the extremities during the initial stages of rewarming.

---

### CASE REPORT 22.1

IQ was undergoing a diving course in winter. Following an uneventful dive to 10 metres for 20 minutes he joined the rest of the course members in a surface swim. After 15–20 minutes he was noted by his instructor to have stopped using his hands. He was told to return to the boat but showed no evidence of response. Soon after this, he submerged twice and required assistance. Back on board he looked pale and exhausted. He was confused, shivering, incoherent in speech and uncoordinated in movement. When the boat was returning to shore, he was placed near the engine and massaged, but did not improve. He was then given a hot drink and hot shower. When seen by a doctor 30 minutes later, his temperature was 34.8°C orally and 35.0°C per rectum. He appeared a dull grey ashen colour, was only able to walk with assistance and was still confused and amnesic. He was placed in a hot bath with arms and legs out and gradually improved over the next hour as his body temperature returned to normal. Chest X-ray and $FEV_1/VC$ measurements had not changed. Several hours later he was asymptomatic.

---

In a small hospital which is not prepared for cases of hypothermia, as well as on a small boat, the hypothermia may have to be treated without even the assistance of a low reading clinical thermometer. The diver can be left in his wet suit and immersed in warm water until he is asymptomatic and has started to sweat. Removal of the wet suit is an unnecessary and possibly dangerous manipulation. However, its presence helps protect the patient against pain from the hot water and hypotension from peripheral pooling of blood.

In these conditions, the use of active treatment must be weighed against the risk of possible complications from the rapid rewarming. Some workers advocate less rapid rewarming if monitoring equipment is not available. This allows the body more time to initiate its normal corrective responses to any disturbed biochemical parameters. This is probably the better approach for a victim who has had a long period of immersion. A glucose infusion may be indicated.

The common reaction, to have a hot shower, is far less effective. It may also be dangerous as the diver feels he has recovered before he has been adequately rewarmed.

**Active core rewarming** has been achieved by haemodialysis, intragastric irrigation, peritoneal dialysis and extracorporeal circulation, all utilizing a system of warming the perfused fluid. Of these, extracorporeal circulation from the femoral artery to vein is the most common and has given good results. King and Hayward

(1989) consider venoarterial warming with complete cardiopulmonary bypass to be the method of choice. This restores perfusion and oxygenation as well as warming.

Central venous infusion of warmed fluids may increase the temperature of the thoracic viscera. Care must be taken not to induce hyperpyrexia with active core rewarming. Warming of the humidified inspiratory gases to 38°C is recommended.

The use of low power microwave radiation, based on the same principle as the microwave oven, is being used experimentally. This technique offers considerable potential benefits because it could allow the heating of selected areas of organs from the exterior. It could be possible to warm the liver, then the aortic blood and so rewarm the body with less fear of complications than with current techniques.

## Recommended reading and references

BECKMAN, E.L. and REEVES, E. (1986). Physiological implications as to survival during immersion in water at 75°F. *Aerospace Medicine* **37**, 1136–1142.

KING, G. and HAYWARD, J.S. (1989). Hypothermia and drowning. *Medicine International*, 2964–2967

POZOS, R.S. and WITTMERS, L.E. (Eds) (1983). *The Nature and Treatment of Hypothermia*. Minneapolis: The University of Minnesota Press.

TIPTON, M.J. (1989). The initial responses to cold-water immersion in man. *Clinical Science* **77**, 581–588.

# 23

# Infections

## Introduction

A variety of pathogenic organisms may be encountered through contact with water. Infection associated with swimming or diving may be acquired in a number of ways. Water-borne pathogens may enter the body through intact or damaged skin, or mucous membrane. Portals of entry include eyes, ears, nose, throat, lungs, gastrointestinal or genitourinary tracts. The infection may remain localized to the site of entry or progress to severe, systemic disease.

The bacterial flora of water is determined by such factors as its proximity to human habitation, the content of organic matter, pH, temperature, light, salinity, oxygenation and rainfall. Some bacteria are found naturally in water, others are periodically washed into water from soil and others favour the artificially created environments of swimming pools, spas, baths and aquaria.

The exact mode of penetration of the organism into a body site depends on the interplay of a number of factors involving water, pathogen and host. For example, divers may lose the bacteriostatic benefits of cerumen, normal flora and acidic pH in the external ear with repeated immersion, thus predisposing to external-ear infections. Factors affecting host defences to permit infection by aquatic micro-organisms include trauma, aspiration and immunosuppression.

Marine bacteria were, until recently, thought not to cause infections in humans. In the last 25 years, these organisms have been isolated from a variety of human infections. Such pathogens may be acquired through trauma from coral, rock or marine animal spines, teeth or shell, or from ingestion or aspiration of water.

The morbidity resulting from diving with certain pre-existing infections is perhaps more important and certainly more common than infections directly due to swimming or diving. These infections are mainly those affecting the respiratory system and both cause and complicate barotrauma (see Chapters 9 and 10).

---

*Upper respiratory infections render the sufferer liable to barotrauma of sinuses and/or middle ear, due to blockage of equalizing air passages.*

---

Lower respiratory infections, where there is likely to be bronchospasm, mucus plugs and obstruction of smaller airways, are dangerous particularly if a flap valve arrangement exists. Gas can enter the alveoli distal to the 'valve' during descent, but is trapped as it expands on ascent. Possible sequelae are those of pulmonary barotrauma – pulmonary tissue damage, mediastinal emphysema, pneumothorax or air embolism, depending on the escape route of the expanding gas.

It has been suggested that spread of respiratory infections is enhanced by diving, and this does appear to be clinically so in some cases. Sharing of regulators may be a mechanism. Alternatively, many divers claim that a dive is a good way of 'cleaning the sinuses' of mucus resulting from a mild inflammation. Saline irrigations have a good reputation among sinusitis sufferers.

Infections acquired through immersion in an aqueous environment may be classified according to the specific aetiological infecting organism, or the organ or system primarily or secondarily affected. In this chapter, infections will be discussed according to the apparent site of entry.

---

### AQUATIC INFECTIONS

- *Aetiological organism*
- *Portal of entry*
  — *skin*
  — *gastrointestinal*
  — *respiratory*
  — *other*
- *Disease*
  — *localized*
  — *systemic*

---

*Pseudomonas folliculitis*, associated with spas and hot tubs, and mycobacterial infection,

associated with swimming pools and fish tanks, are also discussed as they may help in the understanding and treatment of other water-acquired infections.

Special problems of infection control arise in the closed environments of saturation chambers, undersea habitats, submarines and hyperbaric facilities.

Drugs taken to prevent or treat infection (e.g. malaria, sexually transmitted disease) and their possible adverse side effects for divers are discussed in Chapter 31.

## Aetiology and pathogenesis

Infections associated with the marine environment and aquatic activities are not uncommon. This is due to increasing use of water for recreational activities and also, unfortunately, increased sewage pollution of oceans and inland waterways.

Infecting organisms are usually bacteria, but protozoa, viruses, fungi and helminths may also be involved. Sea water contains many bacteria known to be potentially pathogenic for humans (Table 23.1).

The outcome of exposure to water-borne organisms depends on a number of factors. Factors relating to the organisms themselves include the causal organism, inoculum size and virulence. Host factors include site of inoculation, gastric acidity (for gastrointestinal infection) and host immunity. Interaction between the organism and host factors determines the outcome of exposure, i.e. whether infection occurs and, if it does, whether mild or severe disease results.

Many water-borne organisms which were previously considered non-pathogenic or of doubtful pathogenicity, have been implicated as definite pathogens – some causing severe, even fatal, disease. Certain species may be associated with disease more often. For example, *Aeromonas sobria* and *Aeromonas hydrophila* cause most clinically significant aeromonas infections. Severe invasive disease due to non-cholera vibrios is most commonly identified with *Vibrio vulnificus*. It can cause overwhelming septicaemia with rapid progression to death within 48 hours. Production of virulence factors by bacteria (e.g. cytolysins, proteolytic enzymes) may be seen with some

**Table 23.1 Potentially pathogenic bacteria found in sea water**

| | |
|---|---|
| *Acinetobacter lwoffi* | *Mycobacterium marinum* |
| *Actinomyces* species | *Neisseria catarrhalis* |
| *Aeromonas hydrophilia* | *Plesiomonas shigelloides* |
| *Aeromonas sobria* | *Proteus mirabilis* |
| *Alcaligenes faecalis* | *Pseudomonas aeruginosa* |
| *Bacillus cereus* | *Pseudomonas putrefaciens* |
| *Bacillus subtilis* | *Pseudomonas* species |
| *Clostridium botulinum* | *Salmonella enteriditis* |
| *Edwadsiella tarda* | *Serratia* species |
| *Enterobacter aerogenes* | *Staphylococcus aureus* |
| *Enterobacter* species | *Staphylococcus citreus* |
| *Enterococcus faecalis* | *Staphylococcus epidermidis* |
| *Erysipelothrix* species | *Streptococcus* species |
| *Escherichia coli* | *Vibrio alginolyticus* |
| *Flavobacterium* species | *Vibrio cholera* |
| *Klebsiella pneumoniae* | *Vibrio parahaemolyticus* |
| *Micrococcus sedentarius* | *Vibrio vulnificus* |
| *Micrococcus tegragenus* | |

organisms and correlate with invasiveness and pathogenicity.

Host factors may potentiate the development of infection. The skin is a most effective barrier to infection. Inoculation of organisms below the skin surface by penetrating injuries, or coincident with an apparently trivial abrasion or laceration, commonly enables environmental organisms to establish clinical infection which would otherwise not occur. Severe or even fatal infections due to *Vibrio vulnificus* predominantly occur in immunosuppressed persons, e.g. chronic renal disease, liver disease or immunosuppressive therapy. A particularly strong relationship is seen with haemochromatosis. Severe infections in normal individuals are not common, but do occur frequently enough to cause concern.

In the external ear and elsewhere in the body, environmental factors such as prolonged immersion resulting in skin maceration or high humidity aid bacterial penetration even through intact skin. Bacteria have been shown to survive longer in moist skin and may then gain entry following relatively minimal integumentary damage. The softened macerated skin of immersion is, of course, more prone to damage from minor trauma.

The type of trauma may be extensive, with infection to be expected, or minimal such as in fish handler's disease, coral cuts etc.

Infection may also enter through the mucosa of eyes or respiratory tract such as otitis media, sinusitis, or pneumonia following near drowning.

Gastrointestinal infection may follow immersion due to aspiration of water containing pathogenic organisms (see page 313).

For gastrointestinal infections, the size of inoculum is especially important. For example, an inoculum of less than $10^4$ bacteria is unlikely to cause significant infection or disease in normal hosts. An exception to this is infections due to *Shigella* species which may occur with ingestion of as few as 10–100 organisms. Gastric acidity is an important host defence. In people on antacids or with achlorhydria, the infective dose of organisms is considerably lower.

Severe infections have occurred following consumption of shellfish, oysters and fish contaminated with marine organisms, but this is outside the scope of this work.

## Clinical syndromes

Aquatic-derived infections are categorized according to the apparent site of entry of the organism. Some specific organisms are also discussed. The order is not meant to imply incidence or importance , nor is the list to be regarded as complete.

### Skin

Integumentary trauma is a common association of aquatic activities, be they recreational or occupational. Although potential pathogens may be present either in the water or the skin, many marine infections arise because the pathogen is part of the normal flora of the agent producing the trauma, such as fish spines or sea shells. In this context, various species of marine vibrios are frequently involved.

A vivid illustration of the potential for introduction of infection is a study of the teeth of a great white shark, which were found to harbour potentially pathogenic species of *Vibrio, Staphylococcus* and *Citrobacter*.

Gas gangrene has been reported following contamination of wounds received in a plane crash in the Everglades and also following shark attack.

Wounds suffered in or out of the water, including ulcerations due to poor fitting fins, are notoriously slow to heal in divers who spend considerable time in the water. Secondary infection is common and is aided by softening and maceration of the skin due to immersion, and also by swimming in contaminated water. Organisms isolated may be found in sea water or are normal human skin flora. They include *Staphylococcus, Streptococcus, Enterobacter, Pseudomonas, Bacillus*.

*Aeromonas hydrophila* and *Aeromonas sobria* wound infections have followed diving in polluted waters. *Aeromonas* can cause severe progressive wound infections with cellulitis leading to osteomyelitis.

A prolonged period of time out of the water with frequent dressings with antibiotic powder of ointments may be required to achieve healing. Prompt drying after immersion may be of prophylactic value.

---

*Secondary infections of cuts and abrasions, fin ulcers, otitis externa and minor upper respiratory infections, such as sinusitis and otitis media, are the most common infections encountered in divers.*

---

## Vibrio infections

The genus *Vibrio* (Gram-negative bacillus) tends to live in marine or brackish water. As well as cholera, several species of *Vibrio* cause infection in humans. All are indigenous to marine environments and are natural flora of shellfish. They thrive in warmer temperatures.

*Vibrio vulnificus* is an especially invasive organism and severe infections with septicaemia have resulted from marine trauma, especially from shellfish or crabs, but also from aspiration of sea water, gastroenteritis and aquatic sexual intercourse.

Patients succumbing to this infection may have underlying disease, such as diabetes, liver disease, renal failure, or be immune suppressed (e.g. renal transplant patients). The patient may present with fever, chills, headache, myalgia; bullous skin lesions may develop as may hypotension and shock.

**Table 23.2 Pathogenic marine vibrios causing wound and other infections**

| | |
|---|---|
| *V. vulnificus* | Septicaemia, pneumonia, meningitis, endometritis, peritonitis, gastroenteritis |
| *V. parahaemolyticus* | Otitis, conjunctivitis, osteomyelitis |
| *V. alginolyticus* | Epidural abscess, otitis, pneumonia |
| *V. damsela* | Septicaemia |
| (non 01) *V. cholerae* | Otitis |
| *V. cholerae* | Cholera |

Disseminated intravascular coagulation and respiratory distress syndrome have also been described due to *V. vulnificus*.

---

*Vibrio infections should be suspected in any patient presenting with fever, shock, wound infections or pneumonia where there is a recent history of immersion in salt water.*

---

Other vibrios, such as *Vibrio alginolyticus*, have also been seen in marine wound infections, but do not seem to be as invasive as *Vibrio vulnificus*. Nevertheless, a case of epidural abscess due to this organism has been reported, presenting 3 months after an open head injury incurred diving in sea water (see case report). *Vibrio damsela* wound infection has followed injury from a stingray barb.

**Clinical presentations** also include gastroenteritis, cellulitis, faciitis, septic thrombophlebitis, vasculitis, conjunctivitis, and otitis externa and media.

**Diagnosis** follows a high index of suspicion, Gram stain and culture of wounds and blood.

**Treatment** may require extensive surgical débridement and tetracycline administration prior to confirmation of the organism by Gram stain and culture. Gentamicin or one of the third generation cephalosporins, such as ceftriaxone, or a fluoroquindone, such as ciprofloxacin, may also be indicated, and may also be used in severe infections prior to obtaining antibiotic sensitivities.

### Coral cuts

Corals frequently cause lacerations and abrasions to inexperienced divers. These injuries may initially appear minor in nature, but because of foreign material such as pieces of coral, nematocysts, infected slime etc., they often become inflamed and infected.

### Clinical features

The laceration, usually on the hand or foot, causes little trouble at the time of the injury. Some hours later there may be a 'smarting' sensation and a mild inflammatory reaction around the cut. This may be due to the presence of discharging nematocysts. In the ensuing 1–2 days, local swelling, erythema and tenderness develop around the site. Usually this abates in 3–7 days.

Occasionally, an abscess or ulcer will form and discharge pus. This can become chronic, and osteomyelitis of the underlying bone has been reported. Cellulitis and/or lymphadenitis often accompanies the acute stage. Fever, chills, arthralgia, malaise and prostration occur

---

## CASE REPORT 23.1

A 20-year-old male struck his forehead on a submerged object while diving off a platform along the coast of Guam. He sustained an 8-cm laceration and lost consciousness for 2 min after the incident. The laceration was repaired, and X-rays were taken revealing a comminuted fracture of the frontal bone extending through the frontal sinus, with minimal depression of the fragments. A computed tomography scan showed the fracture site but no other evidence of intracranial pathology.

The patient underwent frontal craniotomy with exenteration of the frontal sinus and realignment of the frontal bone fragments 3 days after the accident. Bacterial cultures of the subdural and epidural spaces were negative. The patient did well postoperatively but did experience cerebrospinal fluid rhinorrhea.

The patient remained asymptomatic for 3 months until intermittent fever and headache developed. A repeat computed tomography scan revealed a displaced frontal fracture site as well as a large epidural fluid collection. Physical examination was completely normal other than the bony defect. Laboratory studies showed only that spinal fluid cultures were negative.

In the operating room, osteomyelitis of the frontal bone was noted. The entire frontal plate of involved bone was excised. A 25-ml collection of purulent material was recovered from the epidural space. Gram stain of this material revealed pleomorphic, curved, Gram-negative rods.

The aerobic culture of the epidural space and frontal bone tissue revealed heavy growth of *V. alginolyticus* in a pure culture.

The patient was treated with a 4-week course of intravenous chloramphenicol at a dosage of 50 mg/kg per day without complication. The patient recovered without neurological sequelae and was discharged without medication other than phenytoin for seizure prophylaxis. The patient was seen in follow-up 6 months later and was completely asymptomatic.

(From Opal and Saxon, 1986)

in some cases, probably reflecting the systemic effects of a severe bacterial infection. *Erysipelothrix rhusiopathiae* may be involved in the infection. Healing may take months to years if complications ensue.

### Treatment

The wound should be thoroughly cleaned with an antiseptic and all foreign material removed (e.g. with a soft brush). The wound should then be dressed with antibiotic powder or ointment several times daily. Tetanus prophylaxis is advisable. Cellulitis, lymphangitis etc. indicate the need for a broad-spectrum systemic antibiotic (e.g. ampicillin, erythromycin, tetracycline), after a swab is taken for culture and sensitivity. In such cases, bed rest, elevation of the affected limb and other general supportive measures will also be required.

### Prevention

Coral cuts can be avoided by the use of protective clothing, gloves and swim fins with heel covers, and prompt treatment of minor abrasions. Good training in buoyancy control for divers will also prevent damage to the coral.

### Erysipelothrix infections (erysipeloid)

Infections due to the Gram-positive bacillus *Erysipelothrix rhusiopathiae* or *insidiosa* are found world wide. Abrasions due to contact with fish, shellfish, meat or poultry may lead to the infection which is usually limited to the skin. In the marine context, this organism is involved in crayfish poisoning, coral poisoning, seal finger, whale finger and fish handler's disease.

### Clinical features

There is a history of skin injury which may appear to heal during a 1- to 7-day latent period. Then a sharply defined purplish-red area spreads outward from the injury site. There is associated itch, pain or burning sensation. Oedema develops and adjacent joints become stiff and painful. Regional lymphadenitis or systemic manifestations such as endocarditis have been reported but are rare.

Secondary infection may result in abscess formation.

### Prevention and treatment

All small marine cuts and injuries should be treated actively with antiseptic solutions. Definite lesions are best treated with local antibiotic powder or ointment and systemic penicillin or tetracycline.

### Otitis externa

Although otitis externa (see also page 363) occurs without indulging in aquatic activities, swimming increases the risk about three to five times.

In divers, external-ear infection is one of the most common and troublesome infections. Aetiological or aggravating factors include: hot, humid conditions such as in tropical climates, standard dress diving or recompression chambers; retention of fluid within the external auditory canal following immersion, particularly in contaminated water; exostoses, which are common in swimmers and divers, predispose to retention of cerumen, epithelial debris and water; local trauma, e.g. attempts to remove cerumen; dermatological conditions, such as seborrhoea, neurodermatitis and eczema.

The bacterial flora is usually mixed with *Staphylococcus aureus*, *Pseudomonas* and *Proteus* species predominating. Less commonly, diphtheroids, *Escherichia coli*, *Streptococcus faecalis*, *Aspergillus niger* and *Candida albicans* are found.

> Pseudomonas *species are the most common bacteria found in marine-acquired otitis externa.*

Prolonged exposure to water changes the healthy ear flora from Gram-positive cocci and diphtheroids to Gram-negative bacilli, and this change often precedes the acute symptoms of otitis externa. In such divers, *Pseudomonas aeruginosa* is probably the most frequently associated organism in otitis externa.

*Pseudomonas, Escherichia* species and fungi are the most common pathogenic organisms in saturation diving environments, where there is commonly a high ambient temperature and relative humidity.

Other marine bacteria causing otitis externa include *Achromobacter xylosoxidans, Escherichia coli, Enterobacter* and *Klebsiella* species, *Myobacterium marinum, Proteus* and *Vibrio* species.

### Clinical features

The infection may be either circumscribed (furuncle) or diffuse. Symptoms include itching or pain in the ear made worse by jaw movements and traction on the tragus. Examination reveals localized tenderness, moist debris in an oedematous external canal, and a possible conductive hearing loss. Regional lymphadenopathy and, rarely, a purulent discharge may be present. Divers may complain of vertigo due to obstruction of one canal.

### Treatment

Management consists of analgesia with topical and/or oral analgesics, and gentle cleaning of the canal. This should be followed by antibiotic–steroid ointments, which should completely fill the canal or be impregnated in a wick, or regularly applied antibiotic drops. Antifungal agents are often included in these preparations. Systemic antibiotics may be required. Severe or unresponsive cases should have culture and sensitivity tests to aid antibiotic therapy. Diving should cease until the condition has cleared.

### Prevention

Recurrence may be prevented by the use of olive oil drops prior to diving, or perhaps with spirit drops following the dive to ensure adequate drying. The prophylactic use of 2% acetic acid in aluminium acetate twice a day and after immersion has been shown to reduce the incidence of otitis externa during saturation dives which otherwise approaches 95%. Glacial acetic acid 5% in propylene glycol is also very effective. The use of oil-based antibiotic–steroid ear drops may be needed in refractory cases.

## Pseudomonas aeruginosa *dermatitis*

This condition, also known as 'splash rash', is usually seen after exposure to whirlpools, spas and hot tubs, but has also been described after swimming pool exposure.

A papulopustular eruption develops some 8–48 hours after exposure to a recirculating water environment. The lesions may be pruritic or even tender and usually occur on axillae, groin, trunk and buttocks. Fever and malaise may develop as may regional lymphadenopathy. Otitis externa, keratoconjunctivitis and urinary infections have also been described.

The condition is usually self-limiting in 1–2 weeks, but pustules or abscesses may recur for several months. Cultures of skin lesions and environmental source reveal the same serotype of *Pseudomonas aeruginosa*.

Prevention requires improved disinfectant and filtering systems and regular water testing.

Treatment is usually symptomatic, but, in severe cases, systemic antibiotics may be required.

## Tinea

**Tinea pedis** dermatophytosis, due to a *Trichophyton* species or *Epidermophyton floccosum*, is common in swimmers and divers due to such factors as moist environment, bare feet on wet decks and floors of communal showers etc. It is usually of nuisance value only, but secondary infection may lead to lymphangitis and lymphadenitis.

Treatment involves potassium permanganate soaks in the acute phase followed by the application of antifungal agents such as undecyclenic acid 5% with zinc undecyclenate 20%, tolnaftate 1%, or triacetim 15%.

Previously asymptomatic **pityriasis versicolor** due to *Malassezia furfur* will become obvious in swimmers and divers because of their exposure to sunlight when the small patchy areas fail to tan evenly.

Treatment is usually sought for cosmetic reasons only, and include fungicides: sodium thiosulphate, selenium sulphide 2.5%, Whitfield's ointment etc. Although this eradicates the infection, the areas of discoloration may persist for many months.

### Plantar warts

Outbreaks have been associated with heated swimming pools.

### Mycobacterium marinum *infections*

This acid-fast bacillus *M. marinum* (previously also called *M. balnei*) is the cause of cutaneous granulomata that have been called 'swimming pool granuloma' or 'swimmer's elbow'. *M. marinum* is also known to occur in sea water. This organism may gain entry to the skin via an abrasion from a swimming pool wall or ship's hull. Granulomata usually develop on elbows, knees or hands. There is one report of the infection following the bite of a dolphin and it has also been noted in tropical fish tank enthusiasts (fish-fancier's finger). Immunosuppressed individuals appear to be particularly susceptible.

#### Clinical features

The granulomata usually develop over bony prominences, i.e. sites of abrasion. The onset is noted 3–4 weeks after the predisposing injury (8 weeks in the case of the dolphin bite). They may develop as discrete red papules covered with fine scales and may be large enough to be fluctuant. Aspiration may then reveal thick pus. The papules or cysts may become indurated or even ulcerate. Spontaneous resolution can occur in 1–2 years but cases have been documented for 45 years. There is no evidence of systemic involvement.

#### Diagnosis

This is by punch skin biopsy of the ulcer and demonstration of the organism either by direct staining (acid-fast) or culture on Lowenstein–Jensen media at 30–33°C. Growth takes up to 3 weeks. Skin testing with tuberculin is positive in 85% of cases.

#### Treatment

Drug therapy should be guided by response to in vitro sensitivity tests. Infections have responded to treatment with trimethoprim–sulphamethoxazole, minocycline and tetracycline, which are less toxic than previously used antituberculous drugs. The use of local warmth may be beneficial and it has been suggested that the infection is confined to the skin because of the inability to grow at body core temperature.

The value of surgical excision or curettage is controversial, but may be required if the infection has extended to deep tissues such as tendon sheaths or muscle.

#### Prevention

These measures include adequate chlorination of swimming pools, smooth tiles and, in the case of divers, protective gloves and clothing.

### Schistosome dermatitis

This condition, also known as 'swimmer's itch', bathers' itch and marine dermatitis, is likely to be contracted near the surface of the water. It is due to penetration of the skin by the cercaria of non-pathogenic schistosome cercaria. The cercaria is the larval developmental stage in the lifecycle of the fluke. The organism is found in certain fresh or brackish lakes and swamps where a suitable ecological niche exists.

The lifecycle of the organism involves shore-loving birds and various gastropod molluscs such as snails of the sea shore. The adult fluke is a parasite and lives in the mesenteric vessels of vertebrates, including water birds. The fluke lays its eggs and these pass into the bird's gut, and faeces, and are deposited in the lakes which the birds inhabit. They hatch in the water, becoming young miracidiae, which then spend most of their life in the body of the water snails. In the water snails, the miracidiae develop into free swimming larvae called cercariae and these are capable of penetrating the skin of wading birds – or humans. If the cercariae enter the birds, then the life cycle starts anew. If it penetrates the skin of humans, it dies, due to an active foreign body reaction it induces in human tissue, and the disease may then become manifest.

#### Clinical features

Humans become involved accidentally in this cycle. Children playing in shallow water near weedbeds harbouring the snails are at risk. The cercariae are able to penetrate human skin but not blood vessels. This penetration causes a prickling sensation while in the water or soon after leaving it, and is thought to be a mechanical irritation.

The pruritus subsides to return a day later with increasing intensity in association with an erythematous papular eruption. There may be some associated inflammatory swelling. The rash is present for about one week and then fades leaving a brown pigmentation that persists for some time. The degree of reaction varies greatly, previous exposure causing hypersensitivity to develop in many subjects. The foreign protein of the dead cercariae causes antibody production. This antige-antibody reaction occurs at the site of each dead larva and is responsible for the itchy papules. It is important to note that lesions will only occur on parts of the body that have been exposed to water.

### Prevention

This is best obtained by the use of protective clothing and by vigorous rubbing of any exposed areas immediately after leaving the water. Dimethylphthalate is of value as a repellent. Prevention may also be achieved by clearing swamps of weeds which harbour the snail.

### Treatment

This is symptomatic (e.g. calamine lotion).

### Schistosomiasis

Schistosomiasis (bilharzia) is similar to the above with skin being the portal of entry. Humans are the definitive host to pathogenic schistosomes. **Schistosomiasis japonica** was described in the Phillippines in World War II in US servicemen. It is also endemic in the Yangtse river area of China. *S. haematobium* and *S. mansoni* occur in Africa, the Middle East and South America. The infection is derived from contact (bathing or swimming) with infected water. Following skin penetration, severe central nervous system involvement may develop with *S. japonicum*. Transverse myelitis has been reported with *S. mansoni* in Africa. Praziquantel is normally the drug of choice.

Schistosome infestations cannot be contracted from salt water or properly chlorinated swimming pools.

### Gastrointestinal tract

Gastrointestinal infection may result from ingestion of contaminated sea water while swimming. The most severe form with severe, profuse watery diarrhoea and dehydration and prostration is caused by *Vibrio cholerae*. Non-cholera *Vibrio* species, found in sea water, can cause gastroenteritis with nausea, vomiting, diarrhoea, fever and abdominal pain.

Other bacteria also found in water, and associated with gastroenteritis, include *Bacillus cereus*, *Escherichia coli*, *Salmonella* species and *Campylobacter jejuni*.

Typhoid and paratyphoid have been reported to follow swimming or bathing in contaminated water. Hepatitis has been contracted following ingestion of shellfish, but hepatitis and polio have not been reported following immersion in infected water.

### *Leptospirosis*

Human infection with **leptospirae** usually result from ingestion of water or food contaminated with these spirochaetes. Less often the organism gains entry via a break in the skin or mucous membrane. A number of epidemics from swimming in fresh water have been reported. Rats, swine, dogs and cattle are the principal sources of infection. Certain species, e.g. *Leptospira icterohaemorrhagiae*, *L. canicola*, *L. pomona* or *L. australis*, may predominate in a given geographical area.

### Clinical features

The incubation period of 1–2 weeks is followed by a sudden onset of fever, malaise, myalgia, conjunctival injection and headache. This period, during which the spirochaetes are present in the blood, is followed by organ involvement particularly of the liver (jaundice) or kidney (renal failure). There may also be meningism (benign aseptic meningitis), nausea and vomiting. The disease may persist for up to 3 weeks.

### Treatment

Antibiotics such as penicillin or tetracycline have some therapeutic effect if used early in the infection. Complete resolution of the disease process is possible.

### Prevention

This is by avoidance of exposure to potentially contaminated water, rodent and other host control, and possible vaccination of dogs to reduce contamination.

## Respiratory tract

### Otitis media

This infection is not nearly as common as otitis externa but may occasionally complicate middle-ear barotrauma (see Chapter 10), especially when the latter follows an acute upper respiratory infection (URTI). The most commonly involved organisms are haemolytic streptococci, pneumococci or staphylococci. These or other mixed flora gain entry to the middle ear via the eustachian tube or less commonly through a perforation of the tympanic membranes due to the middle-ear barotrauma or blast injury. The presence of water, fluid or blood provides a culture medium. Clinical features and management are similar to those of other causes of otitis media except that it is noted 4–24 hours after diving. Otitis media following severe middle-ear barotrauma can usually be prevented by systemic antibiotics.

### Sinusitis

Acute sinusitis is also a recognized infection in divers. The aetiology, clinical course and bacteriological findings are similar to those of otitis media. It sometimes follows sinus barotrauma (see Chapter 10).

Chronic sinusitis is a possible long-term occupational disease of divers. Orbital cellulitis, with the infection extending from the sinus, has also been observed – and is a medical emergency requiring intensive antibiotic therapy.

### Pharyngoconjunctival fever

This is an acute illness caused by several types of **adenovirus**. It has an incubation period of 5–9 days and is characterized by fever, malaise, pharyngitis, cervical lymphadenopathy, cough, conjunctivitis and sometimes diarrhoea. Outbreaks of pharyngoconjunctival fever have been reported in swimmers. Similar viruses are probably often involved in swimming pool conjunctivitis epidemics. No serious morbidity and no deaths have been reported.

---

## CASE REPORT 23.2

AM had been diving intermittently for some years. He had mild symptoms of an URTI but was able to equalize his ears satisfactorily and so went ahead with the planned dive. He was unable to descend beyond 5 metres because of pain in both ears and inability to autoinflate. After surfacing, the pain subsided but otoscopic examination revealed grade III aural barotrauma in the right ear and grade II in the left. Two hours after the dive, he developed increasingly severe pain in the right ear which was accompanied by tinnitus and later pyrexia. On examination his temperature was 38.2°C and the tympanic membrane appeared lustreless and erythematous with an outward bulge. Audiometry revealed a mild conductive hearing loss in the right ear. The administration of antibiotics and decongestants resulted in symptomatic improvement in 24 hours. Seven days later the appearance of both tympanic membranes was normal, as was the audiogram.

*Diagnosis:* otitis media complicating middle-ear barotrauma.

**Treatment** is symptomatic and **prevention** is achieved by adequate chlorination of swimming pools.

### Primary amoebic meningoencephalitis

This severe, often fatal, illness is caused by an amoeboflagellate *Naegleria*. This protozoan organism is found in fresh water and prefers warmer temperatures, being found more frequently in natural or industrial thermal waters. The organism cannot survive long in a marine environment.

*Naegleria* species gain entry to the central nervous system via the mucosa of the nasopharynx and the cribriform plate. The amoeba then multiplies in the meninges and olfactory bulbs and eventually elsewhere in the brain. Cases have been reported from Australia, Belgium, Czechoslovakia, the UK, New Zealand and the USA. It is likely that many others have been diagnosed as acute pyogenic meningitis with failure to demonstrate the infecting organism.

### Clinical features

The presentation is similar to that of acute pyogenic meningitis, the patient being in good health prior to the sudden onset of frontal headache, mild fever and lethargy, sometimes associated with sore throat and rhinitis. The headache and pyrexia progress over 3 days with vomiting, neck rigidity, disorientation and coma. The cerebrospinal fluid changes are those of bacterial meningitis, usually under increased pressure. The coma deepens, and death in cardiorespiratory failure supervenes on the fifth or sixth day of the illness. A high index of suspicion and absence of the expected pathogenic bacteria in the cerebrospinal fluid raises the diagnosis. This is confirmed by observing the motile amoebae in a plain wet mount of fluid.

Pathological findings at post-mortem examination reveal a slightly softened, moderately swollen brain, covered by hyperaemic meninges. There is a purulent exudate over the sulci and in the basal subarachnoid cisterns. Small, local haemorrhages are seen in the superficial cortex, but the olfactory bulbs are markedly reddened and in some cases haemorrhagic and necrotic. On microscopic examination, there is a mild fibrinopurulent meningeal reaction and amoebae may be seen in the exudate. The degree of encephalitis varies from slight amoebic invasion and inflammation to complete purulent, haemorrhagic destruction. The nasal mucosa is severely ulcerated and the olfactory nerves are inflamed and necrotic. There is no evidence of amoebic invasion elsewhere in the body.

> *Meningoencephalitis caused by the amoeba* Naegleria *may result from swimming or diving in contaminated water.*

### Treatment

There is a high mortality. Amphotericin B is the drug of choice, in high dosage intravenously and small doses intraventricularly. It has resulted in some cures. Concurrent miconazole and rifampicin have also been used.

### Prevention

Pollution of waterways by sewage and domestic waste water must be controlled if this disease is to be prevented. Swimming and diving should be avoided in potentially contaminated water especially if the water or environmental temperature is high.

### Key West scuba divers' disease

This syndrome was described in classes at the US Navy's Scuba training establishment at Key West, Florida. It was reported to occur 36 hours after first use of one particular type of scuba regulator and it was noted in several students at each new course.

### Clinical features

The disease is characterized by the onset of malaise, anorexia, myalgia, fever, often greater than 38°C, headache and substernal tightness. One death has been attributed to this condition. Apart from these features, physical examination, chest X-ray, urine examination, throat and blood cultures for bacteria are negative. Viral studies are also non-contributory. The illness subsides spontaneously in 72 hours. Continued use of the same regulator does not result in recurrence of the illness unless there is an intervening period without diving.

A multitude of organisms, including mainly *Pseudomonas* and *Fusarium*, has been found on the low pressure diaphragm and interior of the corrugated air hoses of the twin-hose regulators. Decontamination of these parts appears to prevent the illness.

### Salt water aspiration syndrome

This condition, which is due to aspiration of small amounts of salt water during diving, mimics an acute respiratory infection (see Chapter 21). It bears some resemblance to Key West scuba divers' disease. It is not thought to be an infectious disease but is included because of its importance in differential diagnosis. It usually resolves without antibiotic therapy.

### Near drowning and pulmonary infection

During recovery from aspiration of both fresh and sea water, some patients develop severe infections of the lungs. This is one of the many possible reasons for the delayed hypoxia seen in such patients. Post mortems performed on those who die more than 12 hours after near drowning often show evidence of bronchopneumonia or multiple abscesses. However, the changes are often those of an irritant pneumonitis rather than infection (see also Chapter 21).

Although in many cases it may be difficult to determine whether the infection was acquired in hospital, there have been numerous reports where organisms causing pneumonia have also been isolated from the drowning site. Such organisms include *Pseudomonas putrefaciens*, *Klebsiella pneumoniae*, *Pseudomonas aeruginosa*, *Pseudomonas pseudomallei*, *Chromobacterium violaceum*, *Aeromonas*, *Vibrio vulnificus*, *Pseudallescheria boydii* (fungus). Some of these primarily pulmonary infections have also developed septicaemia and metastatic abscesses.

Microscopy and culture of sputum or tracheal aspirate should be performed regularly and appropriate antibiotic therapy instituted.

### Other sites

### Eye

Keratoconjunctivitis due to *Pseudomonas* has been reported following similar exposures to

---

**CASE REPORT 23.3**

AS, aged 21 years, had been passed as medically fit (normal chest X-ray, $FEV_1$ 4.4/VC 5.1 litres) on the day of commencing his refresher diving course. His first dive was to 15 metres for 30 minutes. His demand valve was leaking and he was unable to clear the water from it. He felt well after surfacing except for a slight cough. Ninety minutes later he began to feel unwell with malaise, shivering and hot and cold sensations. His cough increased, productive with white frothy sputum, and he noticed mild breathlessness. He was also nauseated and vomited once.

On examination 2 hours after the dive he was pale, temperature 38.2°C, pulse 120/min, BP 140/90, respiratory rate 28 min. There were coarse bilateral chest crepitations. $FEV_1$ had dropped to 3.4 l and his VC to 3.8 l. Arterial blood $Po_2$ was 61 mmHg and $Pco_2$ 34 mmHg. Chest X-ray showed patchy consolidation in the right cardiophrenic region, right middle lobe and left base. He was given 100% oxygen by mask with gradual improvement in symptoms. Four hours after the dive his temperature was 38.0°C, pulse 104, respiratory rate 22/min, $FEV_1$ 3.7 l and VC 4.0 l. Removal of oxygen resulted in a return of symptoms, especially shivering.

Thirteen hours later he was asymptomatic, chest clear and other observations normal. Within 24 hours his chest X-ray and respiratory function tests were normal.

*Diagnosis:* salt water aspiration syndrome.

those resulting in pseudomonas folliculitis previously discussed.

Conjunctivitis due to *Chlamydia* has also been reported following swimming in certain lakes.

Keratitis due to *Acanthamoeba* has been associated with exposure of the eye to contaminated water (e.g. hot tubs) especially in wearers of contact lens. This organism is ubiquitous in aquatic environments and more cases may be expected. Treatment is oral ketoconazole and topical miconazole or neomycin or propamidine isethionate. Surgery such as keroplasty or even enucleation may be required.

### Genitourinary tract

*Vibrio vulnificus* has been previously discussed as a cause of severe wound infections contaminated by infected water, and gastroenteritis from consumption of raw shellfish. A case of endometritis following sexual intercourse while swimming in sea water known to harbour *V. vulnificus* has been reported, again indicating the virulent nature of this organism (see Case report 23.4).

Treatment should include tetracycline, aminoglycoside, or a third-generation cephalosporin such as ceftriaxone.

Pseudomonas urethritis has been reported following immersion in whirlpools or spas.

## Special environments

### Swimming and diving in polluted waters

Ingestion of polluted drinking water has long been known to pose the risk of hepatitis, typhoid, cholera, dysentery and other gastrointestinal diseases. With the greater worldwide awareness of increasing environmental pollution has come an awareness that the swimmer or diver may also be exposed to the risk of these and other infections.

In coastal waterways close to large population centres, the water may be heavily contaminated with a wide range of organisms, but especially faecal coliforms and streptococci, *Salmonella* spp., and entero- and rotaviruses.

'Coliform counts' are used as indication of water quality and the US Environmental Pro-

---

### CASE REPORT 23.4

A 32-year-old woman presented with a 24-hour history of severe pelvic pain described by the patient as 'worse than having a baby'. She also complained of right lower quadrant pain, low back pain, frequent urination with burning and constant cramping. Upon physical examination the patient appeared to be 'toxic' with a temperature of 38.4°C. Her lungs were clear and her abdomen was non-tender. Upon pelvic examination, there were no external lesions, but a non-bloody, purulent vaginal discharge was noted. The uterus was also very tender. An intrauterine device which had been in place for 1 year was removed through the cervix and sent to the microbiology laboratory for aerobic culture.

The patient initially received $4.8 \times 10^6$ U benzylpenicillin (penicillin G) in divided doses intramuscularly. She also received oral doxycycline, 100 mg per day for 14 days. Two days later she was much improved with little discomfort.

After isolation of *V. vulnificus* from this unusual site (endocervix), the patient was interviewed as to possible sources of exposure to this marine bacterium. The patient had not eaten any seafood in the 2 weeks before the onset of symptoms. However, about 18 hours before the onset of pelvic pain she had been swimming in Galveston Bay and had engaged in sexual intercourse while in the water.

*V. vulnificus* has repeatedly been isolated from Galveston Bay with a peak incidence during periods of warm temperatures and moderate salinities.

(From Tison and Kelly, 1984)

tection Agency (EPA) recommends that safe recreational water should contain not more than 200 faecal coliforms per 100 ml. High coliform counts correlate with the presence of pathogens such as *Salmonella*, *Shigella* and *Aeromonas*, but not so well with pathogenic viruses.

High faecal streptococcal counts in marine recreational water have been associated with various illnesses and the US EPA sets a limit of 35 colony-forming units/100 ml for safe exposure.

Viruses (especially enteric) can enter the marine environment in massive quantities in urban sewage disposal and are not all destroyed by normal sewage treatment processes. Some can survive for long periods of time in sea water and may be associated with

enteric disease among swimmers (especially children). Enteric and respiratory viruses shed directly into water from bathers may be a source of infection. One report suggested an association between water quality and gastroenteritis in swimmers at several US beaches. Polio vaccine viruses, adenoviruses and Coxsackie virus have been recovered from sewage-affected coastal water.

Professional divers may have to work in severely polluted water. Wet suits and normal masks provide little protection to the skin or gastrointestinal tract. Full hoods and occlusive dry suits may be required in such situations.

Table 23.3 lists pathogenic organisms isolated from polluted waters. Their role in the production of disease in swimmers and divers requires further epidemiological studies.

**Table 23.3 Potentially pathogenic micro-organisms isolated from polluted waters**

| *Gram-negative bacteria* | *Gram-positive bacteria* |
|---|---|
| Coliforms | *Staphylococcus* |
| | *Streptococcus* |
| *Escherichia coli* | *Bacillus* |
| *Klebsiella* | |
| *Enterobacter* | |
| *Citrobacter* | |
| *Edwardsiella* | |
| | |
| *Legionella pneumophila* | *Viruses* |
| | |
| *Campylobacter* | Enteroviruses |
| Gastroenteritis virus | |
| *Serratia* | Reovirus |
| | Adenovirus |
| *Proteus* | Hepatitis A virus |
| | |
| Oxidase positive group | |
| | |
| *Aeromonas* | *Protozoa* |
| *Plesiomonas* | |
| *Pseudomonas* | *Entamoeba* |
| *Chromobacter* | *Giardia* |
| *Yersinia* | *Acanthamoeba* |
| *Vibrio cholerae* | *Naegleria* |
| *V. parahaemolyticus* | *Hartmanella* |
| *V. alginolyticus* | |
| Group F 'vibrio-like' organisms | |
| Lactose (+) 'vibrio-like' organisms | |
| | |
| Anaerobes | |
| | |
| *Bacteroides* | |
| *Clostridium* | |
| *Fusobacterium* | |
| *Eubacterium* | |

Note: this list does not imply that all of these micro-organisms are present in any given body of water.

## Enclosed environments

The human–microbe–environment relationship is both subtle and complex. A change in any one of the elements may have substantial effects on the others.

An increasing problem in the closed environments in undersea **habitats, submarines** and **hyperbaric facilities** is contamination by microorganisms (see also Chapters 36 and 38). Cross-infection of divers through the use of common equipment, diving practices, such as buddy breathing, and the inhabitating of small enclosures, aggravate these problems. The concentration of pathogenic organisms may lead to an increased rate of skin, respiratory and systemic infection.

Whenever a group of people or animals live together in close proximity for days or weeks, they undergo an initial period of illnesses. After recovering from these infections, they are then immune to subsequent infections, as long as they live in isolation with their antigenic peers. They are, however, extremely susceptible to infections from exogenous sources, or when the period of isolation ends and they re-establish contact with outside personnel. Such examples are seen with the Polaris submarine crews, people living in Antarctica etc. This is readily explained by the limited sources of infection.

Other interesting changes in saturation complexes may be found because of the effects of pressure, temperature, gas changes and relative humidity on the survival, selectivity and transport mechanisms of micro-organisms. It was found that humidities in the region of 50% were the most detrimental to air-borne bacteria; however, this may not be applicable to marine organisms transported mechanically from the marine environment, which may assume a predominant role in the air flora of submersible habitats. In less-controlled saturation systems, with high humidities, there may be a greatly increased propensity to infection.

The specific changes from Gram-positive organisms to the Gram-negative *Pseudomonas* and *Proteus* spp. was referred to on page 306 (otitis externa).

## Hyperbaric effects

Oxygen under high pressure is of value in treating certain infections and may be life or limb saving in cases of clostridial gas gangrene. It has also been of value in the treatment of chronic osteomyelitis and other infections (see Chapter 37).

Oxygen under pressure may have a multitude of effects on the human–microbe–environment interaction.

Pulmonary oxygen toxicity is thought to impair antibacterial defence mechanisms and thus cause increased susceptibility to infections, particularly of the respiratory tract.

Oxygen and pseudomonas infection appear to be additive in damaging the lung to produce the adult respiratory distress syndrome.

Enhancement of viral infection by hyperbaric oxygen has been demonstrated in cell cultures, by an acceleration of virus maturation and production of abnormally high yields or faster host cell destruction. These effects do not depend on continual exposure during the infectious cycle, and therefore may be applicable to all types of hyperbaric exposures. The change appears to be produced by changes in the membrane of the cell and lysosomes.

Experimental studies on rats exposed to 100% oxygen at 3 ATA for 15 minutes prior to being infected with Coxsackie virus, demonstrate an inhibition of the interferon activity, a greater virus proliferation and less leakage of lysosome enzymes, together with increased host mortality.

Another group of viruses which have a common pattern of latency or chronic infectivity has received increased attention. These are the 'slow viruses' and are those implicated in neoplastic aetiology, such as the oncoma- and herpes viruses. In these circumstances, the viral elements may be triggered by the hyperbaric oxygenation. A similar, but related, interest is being kindled in the effects of hyperbaria on the carcinogenicity of other toxicants.

The effect of the hyperbaric environment on HIV-infected persons is as yet unknown.

Hyperbaric changes in physiology of the host have been inferred from tissue cultures. There appear to be alterations in cell permeability, and metabolism of amino acids and ribonucleic acid precursors. The divers' steroid levels are increased, both in saturation and brief diving excursions, increasing susceptibility both to bacterial and viral infections.

There does seem in some cases to be a tendency to impede the host's reaction, together with increased susceptibility to infection. Organisms may change, both in incidence and activity, when associated with a hyperbaric environment. Deep diving or a hyperbaric helium environment can increase the resistance to penicillin of *Streptococcus pneumoniae* and *Staphylococcus aureus*. Hyperbaria also seems to increase the effects of some antibiotics, e.g. in increasing permeability of tetracyclines into cerebrospinal fluid.

The above information remains patchy, selective and incomplete. The area is a productive field for future developments – especially if the research encompasses in vivo experiments and does not reflect merely the microbe–environment duet.

## Acknowledgements

The authors are grateful to Drs R. Pritchard and B. Hudson of the Department of Microbiology, Royal North Shore Hospital, for reviewing this chapter.

## Recommended reading and references

BARROW, G.I. and HEWITT, M. (1971). Skin infection with *Mycobacterium marinum* from a tropical fish tank. *British Medical Journal* 2, 505–506.

BELL, J.A. et al. (1955). Pharyngoconjunctival fever. Epidemiology of a recently recognized disease entity. *Journal of the American Medical Association* 157, 1083–1092.

BIRCH, C. and GUST, I. (1989). Sewage pollution of marine waters: the risks of viral infection. *The Medical Journal of Australia* 4(18), 609–610.

BUCK, J.D., SPOTTE, S. and GADBAW, J.J. (1984). Bacteriology of the teeth from a great white shark: potential medical implications for shark bite victims. *Journal of Clinical Microbiology* 20, 849–851.

CABELLI, V.J., DUFOUR, A.P., McCABE, L.J. et al. (1982). Swimming-associated gastroenteritis and water quality. *American Journal of Epidemiology* 115, 606–616.

CHANG, W.J. and PIEN, F.D. (1986). Marine-acquired infections. Hazards of the ocean environment. *Postgraduate Medicine* 80(4), 30–32, 37, 41.

DWORZACK, D.L., CLARK, R.B. and PADJITT, P.J. (1988). New causes of pneumonia, meningitis, and disseminated infections associated with immersion. *New Challenges from Infectious Diseases. Infectious Disease Clinics of North America* 2(3), 615–633.

EDMONDS, C. (1989). *Dangerous Marine Creatures.* Sydney: Reed.

FLOWERS, D.J. (1970). Human infection due to *Mycobacterium marinum* after a dolphin bite. *Journal of Clinical Pathology* 23, 475–477.

GREGORY, D.W. and SCHAFFNER, W. (1987). Pseudomonas infections associated with hot tubs and other environments. *Infectious Diseases Clinic of North America* 1 (3), 635–648.

GUSTAFSON, T.L., BAND, J.D., HUTCHESON, R.H. and SCHAFFNER, W. (1983). Pseudomonas folliculitis: an outbreak and review. *Reviews of Infectious Diseases* 5(1), 1–8.

HANSON, P.G., STANDRIDGE, J., JARRETT, F. and MAKI, D.G. (1977). Freshwater wound infection due to *Aeromonas hydrophila. Journal of the American Medical Association* 238, 1053–1054.

HILL, M.K., and SANDERS, C.V. (1988). Localised and systemic infection due to *Vibrio* species. *New Challenges from Infectious Diseases. Infectious Disease Clinics of North America* 2(3), 687–707.

HUGH, T.B. and COLEMAN, M.J. (1981). 'Fish fancier's finger' tropical fish tank granuloma. *Medical Journal of Australia* 13, 614–615.

HUMINER, D., PITLIK, S.D., BLOCK, C. et al. (1986). Aquarium-borne *Mycobacterium marinum* infection – report of a case and review of the literature. *Archives of Dermatology* 122, 698–703.

INSLER, M.S. and GORE, H. (1986). Pseudomonas keratitis and folliculitis from whirlpool exposure. *American Journal of Ophthalmology* 101(1), 41–43.

JACOBSON, J.A. (1985). Pool-associated Pseudomonas aeruginosa dermatitis and other bathing-associated infections. *Infection Control* 6, 398–401.

JOHNSTON, J.M. and IZUMI, A.K. (1987). Cutaneous Mycobacterium marinum infection ('swimming pool granuloma'). *Clinics in Dermatology* 5(3), 68–75.

JOSEPH, S.W., DAILY, O.P., HUNT, R.J. SEIDLER, D.A. and COLWELL, R.R. (1979). Aeromonas primary wound infection of a diver in polluted waters. *Journal of Clinical Microbiology* 10, 46–49.

KELLY, M.T. and AVERY, D.M. (1980). Lactose-positive Vibrio in seawater: a cause of pneumonia and septicemia in a drowning victim. *Journal of Clinical Microbiology* 11, 278–280.

KUEH, C.S.W. and GROHMANN, G.S. (1989). Recovery of viruses and bacteria in water's off Bondi beach: a pilot study. *Medical Journal of Australia* 4(18), 632–638.

LESSNER, A.M., WEBB, R.M. and RABIN, B. (1980). Vibrio alginolyticus conjunctivitis: first reported case. *Archives of Ophthalmology* 103, 229–230.

MAKINTUBEE, S., MALLONEE, J. and ISTRE, G.R. (1987). Shigellosis outbreak associated with swimming. *American Journal of Public Health* 77(2), 166–168.

McCOOL, J.A., SPUDIS, E.V., McLEAN, W., WHITE, J. and VISVESVARA, G.S. (1983). Primary amebic meningoencephalitis diagnosed in the emergency department. *Journal of the Annals of Emergency Medicine* 12(1), 35–37.

OPAL, S.M. and SAXON, R. (1986). Intracranial infection by *Vibrio alginolyticus* following injury in salt water. *Journal of Clinical Microbiology* **23**, 373–374.

PHILPOTT, J.A. et al. (1963). Swimming pool granuloma, a study of 290 cases. *Archives of Dermatology* **88**.

PITLIK, S., BERGER, S. and HUMINER, D. (1987). Nonenteric infections acquired through contact with water. *Reviews of Infectious Diseases* **9**, 54–63.

PORTER, J.D., RAGAZZONI, H.P., BUCHANON, J.D., WASKIN, H.A., JURNEK, D.D. and PARKIN, W.E. (1988). Giardia transmission in a swimming pool. *American Journal of Public Health* **78**, 659–662.

SAUSKER, W.F. (1987). *Pseudomonas aeruginosa* folliculitis ('splash rash'). *Clinical Dermatology* **5**(3), 62–67.

SEIDLER, R.J., ALLEN, D.A., LOCKMAN, H., COLWELL, R.R., JOSEPH, S.W. and DAILY, O.P. (1980). Isolation, enumeration and characteristics of Aeromonas from polluted waters encountered in diving operations. *Applied Environmental Microbiology* **39**, 1010–1018.

SEYFRIED, P.L., TOBIN, R.S., BROWN, N.E. and NESS, P.F. (1985). A prospective study of swimming-related illnesses. II. Morbidity and the microbiological quality of water. *American Journal of Public Health* **75**, 1071–1075.

SHUVAL, H.I. (1986). The transmission of virus disease by the marine environment. *Thalassogenic Diseases, UNEP Regional Seas Reports and Studies*, No. 79.

SIMS, J.K. (1984). Dangerous marine life. In: *The Physician's Guide to Diving Medicine*, edited by C.W. Shilling, C.B. Carlson and R.A. Mathias. New York: Plenum Press.

SIMS, J.K., ENOMOTO, P.I., FRANKEL, R.I. et al. (1983). Marine bacteria complicating seawater near-drowning and marine wounds: a hypothesis. *Annals of Emergency Medicine* **12**, 212–216.

STRAUSS, M.B. and DIERKER, R.L. (1987). Otitis externa associated with aquatic activities (swimmer's ear). *Clinical Dermatology* **5**(3), 103–111.

TACKET, C.O., BARRETT, T.J., MANN, J.M., ROBERTS, M.A. and BLAKE, P.A. (1984). Wound infections caused by *Vibrio vulnificus*, a marine vibrio, in inland areas of the United States. *Journal of Clinical Microbiology* **19**, 197–199.

THOMAS, P., MOORE, M., BELL, E., FRIEDMAN, S., DECKER, J., SHAYEGANI, M. and MARTIN, K. (1985). Pseudomonas dermatitis associated with a swimming pool *Journal of the American Medical Association* **253**, 1156–1159.

TISON, D.L. and KELLY, M.T. (1984). Vibrio vulnificus endometritis. *Journal of Clinical Microbiology* **20**, 185–186.

# 24

# Dangerous marine creatures

## Sharks

### General

The majority of the 350 species of sharks are marine inhabitants, but many will enter estuaries, and some will travel far up rivers, while a few are fresh-water species. Most live in the relatively shallow waters off the major continents or around islands, and inhabit the temperate or tropical zones.

Some, such as the great white shark, are pelagic species and, although they are poikilo-thermic, they have adapted to colder ocean temperatures. In other species, the activity of the shark may be more related to the environmental temperature. Shark attacks tend to be more frequent when the water temperature reaches 20°C or more, possibly because of these reasons and possibly because of the increased frequency of humans bathing in warm water.

Even though Australia is renowned as one of the most dangerous areas in the world for shark attack, there is an average of only one

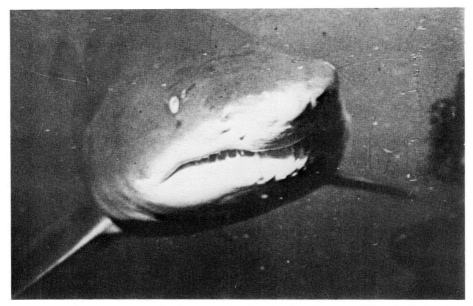

**Figure 24.1** Shark: photograph taken seconds before leaving the water. (Photo by P. Lane)

fatality per year, from millions of bathers at risk. Rescue and first aid groups also have ulterior motives in sometimes exaggerating the risk of shark attack.

Shark attack remains a genuine, but unlikely, danger to seafaring people. Although rare, the attack is often terrifying in intensity, and the degree of mutilation produced has a strong emotive effect on civilized people.

## Data on shark attacks

There has been very little factual research on shark attacks. This is, perhaps, related to the understandable difficulty of experimenting with these animals. Basically, our information comes from two sources: detailed data collection from specific case histories, as illustrated by the pioneering work of Coppleson, and the interpretation of computerized statistical data, as obtained from the 'shark attack' file. Neither source is comprehensive, and neither is adequate by itself. The detailed case histories demonstrate the range of possibilities, whereas the statistical information indicates probable behaviour. The difficulty in obtaining accurate details of any specific shark attack is readily understandable when considering the suddenness of the accident and the emotional involvement of the participants.

The problem in assessing the statistical information is that much of the data was insufficient and unreliable. Application of the statistical figures to an open-water situation is not warranted. Nevertheless, a great deal of interesting information is available from the statistics.

Shark attacks are more frequent when there are more people at risk (i.e. during warm weather and on weekends and holidays). Attacks are also more likely at the shark's natural feeding times, at dusk, near deep channels, in turbid waters in estuaries and where animal products are dumped.

## Anatomy

Of the 350 species of sharks, only 30 have been implicated in attacks on people. Sharks allegedly have a low intelligence, but this has not interfered with their ability to survive far longer than humans in the evolutionary time scale. They are well equipped to locate prey and others of their own species, conduct seasonal migrations and identify specific localities. They react to multiple stimuli, with the sense of smell being a principal means of locating prey. They can detect some substances in minute quantities, e.g. blood in less than one part per million. Although their visual acuity for differentiating form or colour may not be very selective, their ability to discriminate movements and minor contrast variations in low illumination conditions is extremely efficient.

They have an ability to detect low frequency vibrations (e.g. the flapping of an injured fish). Their hearing is especially sensitive to low-frequency sounds and they have an extraordinary faculty for directional localization of this sound. Their taste is not very well developed, but preferences for some foodstuffs have been suggested. The lateral line is a multisensory system commencing at the head and passing along the body. This system receives a variety of information, including vibrations of low frequency, temperature, salinity, pressure and minute electrical fields such as those produced by other fish or humans in the vicinity.

It seems that the feeding response is related more to the presence of specific stimuli than to the nutritional requirements of the animal. The presence of chemical stimuli, such as those released from freshly killed animals, can cause considerable attraction to sharks and may result in the so-called 'feeding frenzy'. It has often been noted that sharks may swim together in an orderly and smooth manner, but when abnormal vibrations are set up (e.g. by one of the animals being shot or hooked), then the abnormal activity of that animal may trigger feeding responses in the others, and this may progressively increase into a feeding frenzy.

## Attack patterns

There are several different types of attack. These may be identified by the behaviour of the animals and the subsequent nature of the injury. Four of these types represent different degrees of a feeding attack, and the fifth represents a territorial intrusion.

1.  Sharks in a feeding pattern tend to circle the victim, gradually increasing their swimming speed. As the circles begin to tighten, the sharks may commence a criss-cross pattern (i.e. going across the circle). At this stage, they may produce injury by **contact**, when they bump or brush against the prey. The shark's abrasive skin can cause extensive injuries and it is thought that the informa-

tion obtained by the animal at this time may influence the likelihood of progression of the feeding pattern.

2.  The **shark bite** is usually performed with the animal in a horizontal or slightly upward direction, with the head swung backward and the upper teeth, therefore, projecting in a forward direction. This results in a great increase in the mouth size and a display of the razor sharp teeth. The physical force involved is of considerable magnitude. The attack is often enough to eject the victim well clear of the water. The bite force is up to 7 tons per square inch, with some species. Once the animal has a grip on the prey, if the feeding pattern continues, the mouthful will usually be either torn out sideways or the area will be totally severed.

3.  If other sharks are in the vicinity, they may respond reflexly to the stimuli created by the attack and commence a feeding pattern behaviour called a **feeding frenzy**. In this instance the sharks are likely to attack both the original prey and the predator or any other moving object. During this feeding frenzy, cannibalism has been observed, and the subsequent carnage can be extensive.

4.  A variant, often used by the great white shark when attacking a larger animal which could possibly inflict damage on the shark, is the **'bite and spit'** behaviour. The bite and spit behaviour is seen not only against seals and sea lions, but also against other prey which may have a similar silhouette on the surface – such as surfboard riders, surface swimmers etc. The shark may make one sudden dash, taking one bite and then releasing the prey, which then bleeds to death. Once the prey has stopped moving, the shark can then continue the feeding pattern in relative safety.

5.  The fifth type of attack is termed **'agonistic'** and is that of an animal which is having its territorial rights infringed on by an intruder – either a swimmer or a diver. This is quite unlike the feeding pattern. The shark tends to swim in a far more awkward manner, exaggerating a lateral motion with its head, arching the spine and angling its pectoral fins downward. In this position, it appears to be more rigid and awkward in its movements than the feeding animal. It has been compared, both in appearance and motivation,

to a cornered animal, adopting a defensive and snapping position. If the intruder diver vacates the area, confrontation will be avoided and an attack prevented.

## Clinical features (see Plate 7)

The lesions produced by shark bite are usually readily identifiable. The rim of the bite will usually have a crescentic shape, delineating the animal's jaw line. There will be separate incisions from each tooth along the line, with occasional fragments of the teeth in the wound. Identification of the shark species is possible from these teeth. There may be crushing injuries to the tissues, and variable amounts of the victim may be torn away. Haemorrhage is usually very severe, in excess of that noted in motor vehicle accidents – probably due to ragged laceration of vessels preventing control by vasoconstriction.

A great variety of damage is noted in different attacks. In some cases, merely the brushing and abrasive lesions of the skin may be present. In others, the teeth marks may still be evident, encircling either the victim's body or even his neck – when the shark has had an appreciable amount of the victim within his mouth, but has still not proceeded with the bite. In most cases, there is a single bite, but occasionally several attacks and bites are made on the one victim. When the latter does occur, adjacent people are rarely attacked. Amputations and extensive body wounds are common. In those victims not killed immediately, the major problem is massive haemorrhage and shock.

## Treatment

In most cases, the most valuable first aid is to protect the patient from further attack and reduce or stop haemorrhage. The rescuer is rarely injured, because the shark tends to concentrate on the original victim. Once the patient is removed from the shark and prevented from drowning, attention should be paid to the prevention of further blood loss. This should be achieved by any means available, e.g. pressure on the site of bleeding or proximal to this site, tourniquets or pressure

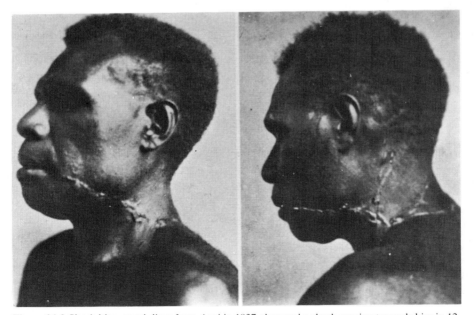

**Figure 24.2** Shark bite: pearl diver Iona Asai in 1937 observed a shark coming towards him in 12 feet of water. The shark enclosed Asai's head within its jaws and Asai claims to have felt for and squeezed the shark's eyes – causing it to release him. Asai was pulled on board the boat, bleeding profusely, before he lost consciousness. Two rows of teeth cuts were sutured in hospital (requiring about 200 stitches) and 3 weeks later the tooth of a tiger shark was removed from a neck abscess. Iona had been injured in a shark attack off Cairns 19 years earlier, and is therefore one of the few men to have survived two separate shark attacks

bandages, tying of blood vessels etc. Use should be made of any material available. The mortality rate is such that there need be no apprehension regarding either the use of tourniquets or the contamination of wounds.

The patient should be lying down with his legs elevated. He should be covered only lightly with clothing or a towel and reassured as much as possible. Medical treatment is best commenced prior to transfer of the patient to the hospital. Infusion of blood, plasma or other intravenous replacement fluid should be given top priority until the state of shock has been adequately controlled. This can be ascertained by the clinical state of the patient, his pulse rate, blood pressure, central venous pressure etc. The use of morphine intravenously is likely to give considerable benefit, despite its mild respiratory depressant effect. Recording and assessing the vital signs then becomes an integral part of the management; they should be monitored throughout the transfer of the patient to the hospital.

At all stages, the first aid resuscitation takes priority over the need for hospitalization. Transport to hospital should be performed in as gentle and orderly a manner as possible. Excess activity aggravates the shock state in these patients. Case reports abound with statements that the victims died in transit. They could more accurately state that the victims died because they were transported.

After stabilizing the clinical state, the patient is transferred by the least traumatic means available. The surgical procedures are not significantly different from those used for a motor vehicle accident case. The areas are swabbed, and bacteriological culture and sensitivities are subsequently obtained. X-rays should be performed, both to show bone damage and also to detect foreign bodies. Under anaesthesia, surgical excision of the obviously necrotic material is required. The surgical techniques should otherwise be of a conservative type, especially if the blood supply is still intact. Tendon suture should not be attempted, unless the wound is very clear. Skin grafting is performed early, whenever possible, to preserve nerves, tendons, vessels, joints and even muscles.

Broad-spectrum antibiotics are indicated, and it should be remembered that the bacteriological contamination is sometimes extensive, both with marine and terrestrial organisms. *Clostridium tetanus* and *Clostridium perfringens (welchii)* have both been isolated from shark wounds, although the contamination almost certainly would have occurred after the initial injury.

## Prevention

Prevention of shark attack depends on the marine locality being considered. The following procedures will be relevant in different situations.

### *Heavily populated beaches*

The most effective method of reducing the incidence of shark attack is by enclosures or meshing. Total bay enclosures are effective in sheltered areas, if consistent surveillance is carried out to ensure the integrity of the net. Areas exposed to adverse weather or surf are best protected by meshing.

Meshing involves the occasional use of a heavy gauge net, which is submerged from a buoy to the seaward side of the breaking waves for 24 hours and then retrieved. The shark tends to swim into it. The net wraps around the animal and interferes with its gill function. As the shark is unable to retreat, it will struggle and attempt to push itself forward through the mesh. This results in the shark being further immobilized and, thus, produces death by suffocation. The net, together with the shark, is brought on board a special vessel, where accurate records are kept of the type, number and size of the 'catch'. Most of the sharks are dead by the time the mesh is retrieved, and the others are killed at the time of the retrieval.

Using this technique, the shark population in any one area is decimated. The experience found on the relatively heavily shark-populated beaches of Australia and South Africa is similar. Shark attacks could still occur despite meshing. Nevertheless, the results are dramatic. Not only does the shark population decrease, shark sightings also decrease, and the shark attacks are virtually eliminated. The local population develops much more confidence in the safety of their surfing area, and increased tourism will often compensate for the cost of the shark meshing.

## Alternative techniques

Other techniques, such as bubble curtains, sound and ultrasonic waves, electric repellents etc., do not have the same excellent record as the enclosure or meshing techniques. Many methods of repelling sharks will, given different conditions and different-sized animals, result in an alerting or an attraction response in the very animals that they are meant to deter. Such is certainly the case with some electrical and explosive devices.

## Survival situation

The crashing of a plane or the noises associated with a ship sinking, may attract sharks to that area. Thus, the survivors of such accidents may become the victim of shark attack. The most effective way to prevent this is to use life rafts and have the survivors move into them as quickly as possible. As an alternative, the Johnson Shark Screen is very effective. The Shark Screen is a bag of thin, tough plastic with a collar consisting of three inflatable rings. The survivor partially inflates one of the rings, by mouth, and then gets into the bag. He fills it with water by dipping the edge so that it becomes full, presenting to any shark as a large, solid-looking black object. The other rings can be inflated at leisure. The bag retains fluids and excreta which may stimulate shark attack. It also attenuates the bioelectric and galvanic fields produced by the survivors.

The 'Shark Chaser' is of value only to the manufacturer. It consists of a dye and 20% copper acetate and was meant to work by the black dye confusing the shark's visual localization, while the copper acetate was thought to be similar to a deterrent chemical, produced in decaying shark tissues. The Shark Chaser does not work. Another chemical, produced by the Peacock or Moses sole, is being investigated at present.

## Swimmers

Swimmers are advised not to urinate in the water or swim with abrasions or bleeding wounds. They are also advised to move gently and not thrash around on the surface. They should stay with a group, or at least with a buddy. This is cynically claimed to reduce the chance of shark attack by 50%, but, in fact, it probably reduces it far more. Swimmers are also advised not to swim in water with low visibility, near drop-offs or deep channels or during late afternoon or night, when sharks tend to be involved in feeding.

## Divers

The incidence of shark attacks on scuba divers appears to be increasing and now comprises one-third of all shark attacks. Wet suits offer no protection and may well increase the likelihood of shark attack, despite popular hopes to the contrary. Divers are advised in the same way as swimmers, but with added precautions. Underwater explosives tend to attract sharks. Shark attacks are more likely with increased depth and can be provoked by playing with or killing sharks. If diving in shark-infested waters, the use of a shark billy (a stout rod with a metal spike) can be effective in pushing the animals away. Powerheads, carbon dioxide darts and the drogue dart (this has a small parachute attached which disrupts the shark's orientation and swimming efficiency) are all specialized pieces of equipment which may be appropriate in certain diving situations.

Divers are also advised not to catch fish or abalone or tether them near their body, as this may attract sharks. If sharks are encountered, it is best to descend to the seabed or to the protection of rocks, a cliff face or some other obstacle so as to interfere with the normal feeding attack pattern described earlier. If the diver recognizes an agonistic attack pattern from the shark, he should vacate the area, swimming backward.

Chain mail (stainless steel) suits discourage sharks from continuing an attack, but incur buoyancy problems for divers and swimmers which usually outweigh the risks of shark attack. Experiments are being conducted on the use of Kevlar incorporated into wet suits, as a shark-bite-resistant material.

It is sometimes claimed that women should not dive or swim while menstruating. There is no evidence to support the belief that decomposing blood will attract sharks; in fact, the experimental and statistical evidence is in the opposite direction.

## Crocodiles, alligators and caimans

### General

Crocodiles cause as many human fatalities as sharks, in the areas where both are found. This was not always so, but while there is a diminishing number of shark attacks due to meshing, there is an increased crocodile attack frequency because the animals have recently been protected and allowed to grow longer and larger. There is also an increase of tourism into remote crocodile territories. They become more aggressive during the breeding times, the young being hatched from eggs and protected by both parents.

All crocodilians are carnivorous. They range in size from 1 to 10 metres long, and the larger specimens are the ones potentially dangerous to humans. The largest grow up to a ton in weight. They are often believed to compete with fishermen, damaging nets, and may prey on both domestic animals and humans.

The species considered as man eaters are the salt-water crocodile and the Nile crocodile, which grow to 8 metres, and the American crocodile and American alligator, which grow to 3.5 metres. South American caimans are of the same family as alligators and grow up to 5.5 metres, but are usually much smaller. Even the Indian mugger crocodile may attack humans if provoked while nesting.

Alligators are slower moving, and generally less dangerous to humans. Crocodiles have narrower snouts than alligators, and the fourth tooth in each side of the lower jaw is usually visible when the mouth is closed.

Salt-water crocodiles may be found in fresh water. They may have swum inland from an estuary or travelled many kilometres overland. Fresh-water crocodiles are also found in lakes and rivers that have no connection with the sea, and in some countries they may be both large and dangerous. Crocodiles are important predators in the food chain, eating water beetles, water spiders, dragon flies etc. in their earlier life, and reptiles, amphibians, crustaceans, molluscs and fish as they become older. If humans or other animals intrude into their territory, the crocodile sometimes give warning by exhaling loudly or even growling at the intruder.

For reptiles, they have very complex brains and are intelligent enough to stalk a human, strong enough to destroy a water buffalo and gentle enough to release its own young from the eggs – with its teeth. It even carries the newly hatched babies in its massive jaws.

Crocodiles tear their food from the carcass, twisting and turning in the water to achieve this. They then swallow it whole. Once an attack pattern has begun, the crocodile will attack repeatedly until the prey is captured, and it may follow the victim from the water if necessary. If the animal captures large prey, it may hide the carcass under water, entangled in submerged trees or under ledges, until it is ready to resume feeding.

The animal often lies along the banks of rivers, with only the nostrils protruding above water to breathe. The prey, especially land animals such as horses, cattle, giraffe, rhinoceros, kangaroo and wallaby, come to the river bank to drink and may be suddenly grabbed in the immensely strong jaws of the crocodile, and twisted off its feet. This movement will sometimes break the neck of the victim. Once the prey is in the water, it is more vulnerable to panic and drowning. Although this is the classic attack pattern, crocodiles can move fast on land and in water, and recent attacks in Australia have included attacks with the victim free swimming in deep water, on dry land and in a canoe.

On land the attacks are more common at night when the animal stalks for food. They can move surprisingly fast – faster than most humans – issue a hissing sound and sometimes attack by sweeping the victim with its powerful tail.

The first aid, medical treatment and investigations are the same as for shark attack. Occasionally, a tooth fragment will be found by X-ray of the wound.

## Other biting marine animals

Little space has been allocated to the other marine animals that are said to bite because it is difficult to find more than one or two cases throughout the world literature of a verified fatal bite on a human.

### Barracuda

Barracuda have occasionally been known to attack. They are sometimes attracted by bright-coloured objects and lights, if diving is performed at night.

## Grouper

There have been reported cases of a grouper attacking a human. As a general rule, these heavyweight bulldogs of the sea have built up a reputation for friendliness more than forcefulness. They are, however, feared in some areas, e.g. the pearl-diving beds between New Guinea and Australia.

## Killer whale

This is the largest of the dolphin family. It acquired its name from its tendency to travel in packs, feeding on other marine creatures such as seals, larger whales etc. Although Scott's journal of his exploration of the Antarctic is often quoted as having an authoritative description of a killer whale attack on a human, perusal of the journal does not lend support to the fable.

## Eel

Many eel attacks have been reported. Moray eels can grow up to 3 m in length and up to 30 cm in diameter. They will rarely attack without provocation, and the attack is usually precipitated by an intrusion into their domain, or after they have been injured or caught on lines or spear guns. Divers who feed the eels inadvertently encourage them to be more adventurous and less fearful, thus increasing the attack potential – for food. Certainly, once they do attack, they are likely to be difficult to dislodge and may even resume the attack once they are dislodged. The wound is likely to be badly lacerated and heavily infected. The medical and surgical treatments conform to those normally used with other damaged and infected tissues.

# Sea snake

## General

These air-breathing reptiles, numbering some 50 species, usually restrict themselves to tropical or temperate zones, being more frequent in the Indo-Pacific area. Sea snakes can be subdivided into two major types according to their feeding habits. The bottom feeders have the capability of diving to considerable depths, over 100 metres to locate and devour their prey (eels, fish etc.). The laticauda, or banded sea snakes, are characteristic of this type. They inhabit coastal and relatively

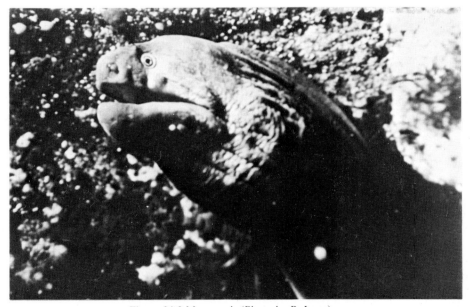

**Figure 24.3** Moray eel. (Photo by P. Lane)

shallow waters, often breed and lay their eggs onshore, in crevices or caves, and are capable of existing for long times out of water.

The second group is the pelagic 'blue water' type, exemplified by the yellow bellied sea snake, *Pelamis platurus*. This is a surface feeder that drifts with the warm tides. Mating takes place at sea and the snake is viviparous. It may be found in packs, far out to sea, but if it is washed up on to beaches or land it is unable to survive. This snake does not tolerate extremes of temperature, and is rarely found when the average sea temperature drops below 20°C. The lethal limit for the snake's body temperature is 33–36°C and high temperatures are avoided by the snake diving into the cool waters away from the surface, when it is travelling in tropical regions. It is for this reason that they are more frequently found on the surface during rain or on cloudy days.

The sea snake is an efficient swimmer. It is capable of remaining submerged for 2 hours. They are inquisitive, and are sometimes aggressive, especially if handled or trodden on. They appear to be attracted by fast moving objects, e.g. divers who are being towed by a boat and, under these circumstances, they can congregate and become troublesome. They are also caught in trawling nets, especially in the Tropics. Land snakes may also take to the water, sometimes causing difficulty with identification. The identification of sea snake is confirmed by the observation of a paddle-shaped tail. No land snake has this flattened tail.

Sea snake venom is 2–10 times as toxic as that of the cobra, but they tend to deliver less of it, and only about one-quarter of those bitten by sea snakes ever show signs of poisoning. It appears that there is some reluctance to inject venom even when they do bite. Nevertheless, the venom that can be injected by one fresh adult sea snake of certain species is enough to kill three men. In most species, the apparatus for delivering the venom is poorly developed even though the mouth can open widely, whereas in a few others the mouth is small and the snake has difficulty in obtaining a wide enough bite to pierce the clothing or any other protective layer that the diver may wear. Sea snake venom is a heat-stable, non-enzymatic protein, which appears to block neuromuscular transmission by acting on the postsynaptic membrane and may affect the motor nerve terminals. It has a specific action in blocking the effects of acetylcholine. Autopsy findings include patchy and selective necrosis of skeletal muscles, and renal tubular damage if the illness lasts longer than 48 hours.

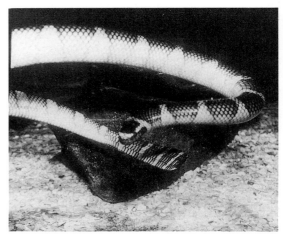

**Figure 24.4** Sea snake: note the flattened, paddle-shaped tail

## Clinical features

An initial puncture at the time of biting is usually noted. Fang and teeth marks may vary from 1 to 20, but usually there are 4 and the teeth may remain in the wound. After a latent period without symptoms, from 10 minutes to several hours, generalized features will develop in approximately one-quarter of the cases.

Mild symptoms include a psychological reaction such as euphoria, anxiety, restlessness etc. The tongue may feel thick. Thirst, dry throat, nausea and vomiting occasionally develop. Generalized stiffness and aching may then supervene. If weakness does progress into paralysis, then it is usually either of the ascending Guillain–Barré type, with the legs being involved an hour or so before the trunk, then the arms and neck. The other manifestation of paralysis is one which extends centrally from the area of the bite, e.g. from the bite on the hand to the forearm, arm, other arm, body and legs. Usually the proximal muscle groups are the most affected and trismus and ptosis are characteristic. Muscular twitchings, writhings and spasms may be seen and the patient may develop difficulty with speech and swallowing as the paralysis extends to the bulbar areas. Facial and ocular palsies then develop. Respiratory distress, due to involvement of the diaphragm, may result in dyspnoea, cyanosis and finally death in a small number of the cases affected. Cardiac failure convulsions and coma may be seen terminally.

Myoglobinuria may develop. When this is seen, the other possible effects of myonecrosis must be considered, namely an acute renal failure, with electrolyte and potassium changes and uraemia, and an aggravation of the muscular paralysis and weakness. This myonecrotic syndrome with renal failure usually supervenes on the other muscular paralysis and may thus prolong and aggravate this state.

When recovery occurs it is usually rapid and complete.

## First aid

The current treatment is the use of pressure bandage (applying a wide strap using about the same tension that would be used for a sprained ankle, first wrapped around the area of the bite, and then proximal and distal to it) together with immobilization. This is thought to reduce both venous and lymphatic drainage to the area. Under these conditions it is possible slowly to transport the patient to medical treatment.

It was originally taught that a venous ligature above the site, together with removal of the surface venom, was indicated. This is thought to reduce both venous and lymphatic drainage of the area, but is now superseded by the pressure bandage/immobilization.

Reassurance is needed and exertion is to be avoided. The limb is immobilized as should the patient. If possible, the snake (dead, to avoid further problems) should be retained for identification because, although it may be harmless, the treatment certainly is not.

In the event of respiratory paralysis, mouth-to-mouth respiration may be required.

## Medical treatment

Once the patient is transported to adequate medical facilities, and the clinicians have been able to review the therapy indicated, the pressure bandage may be removed. Once this happens the envenomation will have its effect on the patient, and preferably the treatment, including the antivenom regime, must be instituted.

Apart from the above first aid procedures, full cardiopulmonary resuscitation may be required. Fluid and electrolyte balance must be corrected. Acute renal failure is usually obvious from the oliguria, raised serum creatinine and electrolyte changes. A high serum potassium is particularly dangerous and treatment by haemodialysis is then required. This may result in a dramatic improvement in the muscular paralysis and the general clinical condition. The acute renal tubular necrosis and the myonecrosis are considered temporary, if life can be maintained.

Treatment may be necessary for the cardiovascular shock and convulsions, and often respiration requires assistance or even complete control. Sea snake antivenom from the Commonwealth Serum Laboratories (CSL) (Australia) can be used cautiously in serious cases. It contains 1000 units per ampoule. Care must be taken to administer it strictly in accordance with the directions in the brochure. The antivenom can be dangerous to patients who are allergic. Emergency precautions for anaphylactic shock are required. The sea snake antivenom is composed of two antivenoms, and each has a very specific action. Unfortunately, although it does counter the most common sea snake venoms, there are others that are not covered. If it is necessary to use land snake antivenom, then probably the Tiger snake type is to be preferred. Polyvalent land snake antivenom can also be used, although the value has yet to be determined.

Patients with sea snake bite should be hospitalized for 24 hours, because of the delay in symptoms developing. Sedatives may be required, and it is reasonable to administer diazepam as required. This will assist in sedating the patient, without interfering significantly with respiration. Preparation for treatment of anaphylactic shock should be available.

## Prevention

This is usually achieved by not handling sea snakes. It is suggested that the feet be shuffled when walking along a muddy sea bed, and that protective clothing be worn when under water. The wet suit is usually sufficient, and if collecting sea snakes it is wise to use a special sea snake tong.

# Fish stings

Many fish have spines and a venom apparatus, usually for protection and occasionally for incapacitating their prey. Spines may be concealed, only becoming obvious when in use (e.g. stonefish), or highlighted as an apparent warning to predators (e.g. butterfly cod or firefish).

Some fish envenomations have resulted in death, especially by the stonefish and stingray. These will be described separately. Others, such as the infamous scorpion and firefish (family Scorpaenidae), catfish (family Plotsidae and Ariidae), stargazers (family Uranoscopidae), have also been responsible for occasional deaths in humans. As a general rule, fish that have been damaged – such as those in fishing nets – cause less problems clinically, probably because some of the envenomation system may have been previously used. Those wounds that bleed profusely are also less likely to have intense symptoms. Some spines are inexplicably not associated with venom sacs.

Other fish may produce injury by the knife-like spines which may or may not be related to envenomation, e.g. old wife (family Enoplosidae), surgeon and unicorn fish (family Acanthuridae), ratfish (family Chimaeridae).

## General

Identification of the species of fish responsible is not always possible. Fortunately, there is often not a great variety in the symptomatology.

### Clinical features

If venom is injected, the first symptom is usually a local pain which increases in intensity over the next few minutes. It may become excruciating, but usually lessens after a few hours ('with the change of the tide' – an old mariner's attempt at reassurance). The puncture wound is anaesthetic, and the surrounding area hypersensitive. Pain and tenderness in the regional lymph glands may extend even more centrally.

Locally, the appearance is that of one or more puncture wounds, with an inflamed and sometimes cyanotic zone around this. The surrounding area becomes pale and swollen, with pitting oedema.

Generalized symptoms are sometimes severe. The patient is often very distressed by the degree of pain, which is disproportionate to the clinical signs. This distress can merge into a delirious state. Malaise, nausea, vomiting and sweating may be associated with a mild temperature elevation and a leucocytosis. Occasionally, a cardiovascular shock state may supervene and cause death. Respiratory distress may develop in severe cases.

### First aid

The patient should be laid down and reassured. The affected area should be rested in an elevated position. Arrangements can then be made to immerse the wound in hot (up to 45°C) water for 30–90 minutes – or until the pain no longer recurs. The wound should be washed and cleaned. As well as the wound, some normal skin must also be immersed in the hot water to ensure that there is no scalding produced. The injured skin may well be hypoaesthetic, and not give adequate warning of this danger.

Fishermen often make a small incision across the wound and parallel to the long axis of the limb, to encourage mild bleeding and relieve pain if other methods are not available.

### Medical treatment

This includes first aid, as above. Local anaesthetic, e.g. 5–10 mg lignocaine 2%, without adrenaline (epinephrine), if injected through the puncture wound, will give considerable relief. Local or regional anaesthetic blocks may also be of value.

Symptomatic treatment may be needed for generalized symptoms of cardiogenic shock or respiratory depression. Sytemic analgesics or opiates are rarely needed; however, they may be of value in severe cases.

Exploration and cleansing of the wound, with removal of any broken spines or their integuments, is best followed by the application of local antibiotic such as neomycin or bacitracin. Tetanus prophylaxis may be indicated if there is necrotic tissue or if the wound has been contaminated.

## Stingrays

### General

This vertebrate lies in the sand and the unwary victim may tread on its dorsal surface or dive over it. The stingray swings its tail upward and forward, driving the spine into the limb or body of the victim. An integument over the serrated spine is ruptured. Venom escapes and passes along grooves into the perforated wound. Extraction of the spine results in a laceration due to the serrations and retro-pointed barbs, and may leave spine or sheath within the wound.

The venom is a protein (molecular weight greater than 100 000), heat labile, water soluble, and with an intravenous $LD_{50}$ of 28.0 mg/kg body weight. Low concentrations cause electrocardiographic effects of increased P–R intervals associated with bradycardia. A first-degree atrioventricular block may occur with mild hypotension. Larger doses produce vasoconstriction, second- and third-degree atrioventricular block and signs of cardiac ischaemia. Most cardiac changes are reversible within 24 hours. Some degree of respiratory depression is noted with greater amounts of venom. This is probably secondary to the neurotoxic effect of the venom on the medullary centres. Convulsions may also occur.

Fishermen who handle these fish in nets are less seriously affected as the integumentary sheath is probably already damaged.

### Clinical features

#### Local

Pain is usually immediate and is the predominant symptom, increasing over 1–2 hours and easing after 6–10, but may persist for some days. Aggravation of pain within days may be due to secondary infection. The pain may be constant, pulsating or stabbing. Bleeding may be profuse, and may relieve the pain. A mucoid secretion may follow. Integument from the spine may be visible in the wound, which may gape and extend for a few centimetres in length. The area is swollen and pale, with a bluish rim, centimetres in width, spreading around the wound after an hour or two. Local necrosis, ulceration and/or secondary infection are common and, if unchecked, may cause incapacity for many months. Osteomyelitis in the underlying bone has been reported.

#### General

The following manifestations have been noted: anorexia, nausea, vomiting, diarrhoea, frequent micturition and salivation. There is extension of pain to the area of lymphatic drainage. Muscular cramp, tremor and tonic paralysis may occur in the affected limb, or be more generalized. Syncope, palpitations, hypotension, cardiac irregularities (conduction abnormalities, blocks) and ischaemia are possible. Respiratory depression may occur, with difficulty in breathing, cough and pain on inspiration. Other features include nocturnal pyrexia with copious sweating, nervousness, confusion or delirium.

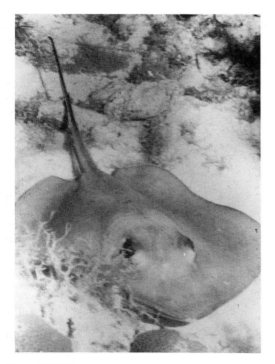

**Figure 24.5** Stingray

Fatalities are possible, especially if the spine perforates the pericardial, peritoneal or pleural cavities. The symptoms may last from hours to many months.

### Treatment

#### First aid

The patient should be laid down, with the affected area in an elevated position. Surface venom is removed by washing or irrigating the area, e.g. with water. If the spine or integument is still present, it should be gently extracted. Bleeding may need to be encouraged by a temporary ligature or, as some people propose, a small incision – if bleeding has not occurred naturally.

The area is immersed in hot water, up to 45°C, until pain has stopped, i.e. usually in 30–90 minutes. Adjacent unaffected skin should also be immersed to prevent scalding. Following pain relief, the limb should be immobilized in an elevated position and covered with a clean dressing. The patient's state may subsequently become far more serious than it first appears.

#### Medical treatment

Local anaesthetic without adrenaline (epinephrine), infiltrated into and around the wound, or by regional block, will relieve the pain. Systemic analgesia may be required, e.g. with opiates. Thorough cleansing of the wound, once the local anaesthetic has been effective, is required.

A soft tissue X-ray may demonstrate foreign body or bone injury. The basic physiological signs (TPR, BP, CVP, urine output etc.), serum electrolytes, electroencephalogram and electrocardiogram are monitored as indicated. Broad-spectrum antibiotics, e.g. tetracycline 250 mg four times a day and local application of neomycin, are used at an early stage. Symptomatic treatment is given for the clinical features present. Tetanus prophylaxis may be indicated.

#### Prevention

Divers are advised to shuffle the feet when walking in the water. This gives the ray time to remove itself – which it cannot do with a foot on its dorsum. While wearing rubber boots decreases the severity of the sting, the spine will penetrate most protective material. Care is needed when handling fishing nets.

### Stonefish

#### General

This fish grows to about 30 cm in length. It lies dormant in shallow waters, buried in sand, mud, coral or rocks, and is practically indistinguishable from the surroundings. The 13 dorsal spines, capable of piercing a sandshoe, are covered by loose skin or integument. When pressure is applied over them, two venom glands discharge along ducts on each spine, into the penetrating wound. The fish may live for many hours out of the water.

The venom is an unstable protein, with a pH of 6.0 and a molecular weight of 150 000. It produces an intense vasoconstriction, and therefore tends to localize itself. It is destroyed by heat (2 minutes at 50°C) alkalis and acids (pH greater than 9 or less than 4), potassium permanganate and Congo red. The toxin is a myotoxin which acts on skeletal, involuntary and cardiac muscles, blocking conduction in these tissues. This results in a muscular paralysis, respiratory depression, peripheral vasodilatation, shock and cardiac arrest. It is also capable of producing cardiac dysrhythmias.

Each spine has 5–10 mg venom associated with it, and is said to be neutralized by 1 ml antivenom from the Australian Commonwealth Serum Laboratories. Occasionally, a stonefish spine may have no venom associated with it. It is thought that the venom is regenerated very slowly, if at all.

#### Clinical features

Whether the local or generalized symptoms predominate seems to depend on many factors, such as the geographical locality, the number of spines involved, protective covering, previous sting, first aid treatment etc.

#### Local

Immediate pain is noted. This will increase in severity over the ensuing 10 minutes or more.

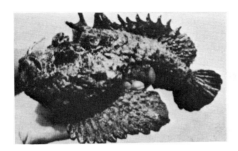

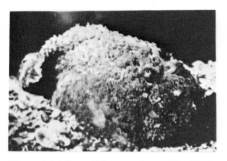

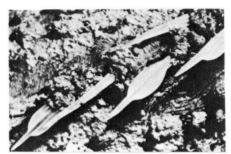

**Figure 24.6** Stonefish: top: cleaned for filming – specimen length 25 cm. Lower left: au naturel. Lower right: spines with venom sacs

The pain, which is excruciating in severity, may be sufficient in some to cause unconsciousness, and thus drowning. Ischaemia of the area is followed by cyanosis which is probably due to local dirculatory stasis. The area becomes swollen and oedematous, often hot, with numbness in the centre and extreme tenderness around the periphery. The oedema and swelling may become quite gross, extending up the limb. Paralysis of the adjacent muscles is said to immobilize the limb, as may pain.

The pain is likely to spread proximally to the regional lymph glands, e.g. axilla or groin. Both the pain and the other signs of inflammation may last for many days. Necrosis and ulceration can persist for many months.

### General

Signs of mild cardiovascular collapse are not uncommon. Pallor, sweating, hypotension and syncope on standing may be present. Respiratory failure may be due to haemorrhagic pulmonary oedema, depression of the respiratory centre, cardiac failure and/or paralysis of the respiratory musculature. Bradycardia, cardiac dysrhythmias and arrest are also possible.

Malaise, exhaustion, fever and shivering may progress to delirium, incoordination, generalized paralysis, convulsions and death. Convalescence may take many months, and may be characterized by periods of malaise and nausea.

---

*FIRST AID TREATMENT OF FISH STING (venom injected by spine):*
- *Lay patient down with affected limb elevated*
- *Wash surface venom away and gently remove spine or integument if present*
- *Immersion in hot water (up to 45°C) will reduce severity of pain*
- *Injection of local anaesthetic without adrenaline into and around the wound*

---

### Treatment

#### First aid

Rescue the patient from the water. Immobilize him and keep the affected limb in an elevated position. Immerse the limb in hot water (up to 45°C) for 30 minutes. This may produce rapid relief, especially if given early. Adjacent unaffected skin should also be immersed to ensure that scalding does not occur. The local application of a weak solution of potassium permanganate may relieve pain. Reassurance is necessary. In cases of loss of consciousness, apply external cardiac massage and mouth-to-mouth respiration as indicated. Resuscitation may be required for many hours.

### Medical treatment

This depends on the site and severity of the symptoms.

### Local

Local anaesthetic agent without adrenaline, infiltrated into and around the wound, is the treatment of choice, especially if administered early. The wound should be thoroughly cleansed, after the local anaesthetic has been effective. It may also remove the pain in the regional lymphatic area. A repeat injection will probably be needed.

Local injection into the site with either hyoscine *N*-butylbromide (Buscopan) or emetine hydrochloride (pH 3.4) is a conventional and effective remedy which gives relief if injected within the first 15 minutes. Emetine may be given in a dose of 25 mg in 0.5 ml.

Elevate the limb to reduce pain and swelling and apply local antibiotics to prevent secondary infection.

### General

Stonefish antivenom may be administered with 1 ml neutralizing 10 mg venom (i.e. the venom from one spine). Initially, 2 ml antivenom is given intramuscularly, although in severe cases the intravenous route can be used. Further doses can be given if required, but it should never be given to people with horse serum allergy. It should be stored between 0°C and 5°C but not frozen, and protected from light. It should be used immediately on opening.

Systemic analgesics and opiates are seldom indicated or useful, although intravenous opiates are sometimes used. Tetanus prophylaxis is sometimes recommended. Systemic antibiotics may be used because secondary infection is likely. Débridement should be considered if there is significant tissue damage and necrosis, or if foreign material could be left in the wound.

Appropriate resuscitation techniques may have to be applied. These include external cardiac massage and defibrillation and endotracheal intubation with controlled ventilation. Monitoring procedures may need to include records of clinical state (pulse, respiration), BP, CVP, pulse oximetry, electrocardiogram, lung function tests, arterial gases and pH. Clinical complications of bulbar paralysis should be treated as they arise.

### Prevention

Wear thick-soled shoes when in danger areas. Be particularly careful on coral reefs and while entering or leaving boats. A stonefish sting is said to confer some degree of immunity for future episodes.

## Coelenterates

### General

This phylum of 9000 species contains jellyfish, sea anemones, fire coral, stinging hydroids etc. It constitutes one of the lowest orders of the animal kingdom, and has members which are grossly dissimilar in general appearance and mobility.

The common factor among the coelenterates is the development of nematocysts or stinging capsules. These capsules are of two types: one which adheres to the animal's prey, either by sticky mucus or by a coiled spring, and the other which acts as a needle, penetrating the prey and discharging venom into it. This may be as long as 0.5 mm. The triggering mechanism which is responsible for the discharge of the nematocyst is thought to be initiated by many factors, e.g. the absorption of water into the nematocyst capsule causing it to swell, trauma etc.

The function of the nematocysts is to incapacitate and retain prey, which is then used as food by the coelenterate. The nematocysts of different types of coelenterate may be identifiable, and therefore of value in the differential diagnosis of marine stings. There may also be a characteristic pattern of nematocyst stings, depending on their aggregation on the tentacle of the coelenterate, and on the morphology of the tentacles. Thus the **Portuguese man-o-'war** usually produces a single long strap with small blisters along it, whereas the **mauve stinger** has short red lines, with the **chironex** having multiple long red lines, often with the tentacle adherent due to a thick sticky substance, when the patient is first seen. **Stinging hydroids** and **fire coral**, being non-mobile, sting only when touched by the diver.

**Clinical** factors may vary from a mild itch locally to severe systemic reactions. The local symptoms vary from a prickly or stinging sensation developing immediately on contact, to a burning or throbbing pain. The intensity increases over 10 minutes or so, and the erythema may develop papules, vesicles or even pustules and necrotic ulcers in severe cases. The pain may spread centrally, with lymphadenopathy, and may be associated with abdominal pain and chest pain.

Generalized symptoms include fever, increased secretions, gastrointestinal disorders, cardiovascular failure, respiratory distress and signs of a toxic – confusional state.

The intensity of both local and generalized manifestations of coelenterate stinging may vary according to: the species involved, (the chironex is often lethal, whereas the blubber jellyfish can often be handled with impunity);

the extent of the area involved; the body weight of the subject, being more severe in children than in adults; the thickness of the skin in contact; and individual idiosyncrasies such as allergic reactions, pre-existing cardio-respiratory disease etc. As the most dangerous coelenterate is the chironex, this is dealt with in detail.

The **Portuguese man-o'-war** or bluebottle (*Physalia*) sting is one of the most common problems encountered by bathers. The first aid treatments have been based on the use of empirical and fashionable treatments, such as vinegar, dehydrating agents (alcohols) or denaturing agents (acetic acid, ammonia, papaine in meat tenderizers) to reduce the discharge of further nematocysts. Some of these have aggravated the symptoms. Current treatments include the use of anti-burn preparations, cold packs, and the application of local anaesthetic ointments and steroids to reduce symptoms of pain or itch, respectively.

The reason that most coelenterates do not injure humans is that the nematocyst is incapable of penetrating the depth of skin necessary to cause symptoms. Variations of this mode of injury occur in four instances.

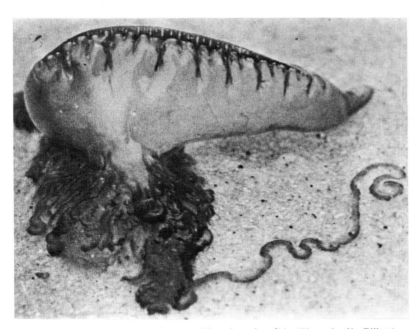

**Figure 24.7** Portugese man-'o-war (*Physalia physalis*). (Photo by K. Gillett)

### Direct entry

Coral cuts are often experienced in the Tropics, and in these cases there is a laceration of the skin, which allows nematocysts to discharge directly into the wound tissues. This is supplemented by a foreign body reaction to the nematocysts, coral pieces and organisms. Pacific islanders spread coelenterates over spears.

### Nudibranchs

These, especially the **glaucus**, ingest certain coelenterates and utilize these nematocysts for their own aggressive purposes. This means that humans who come in contact with these nudibranchs may then sustain an injury having a distribution which corresponds to the area of contact with the nudibranch.

### Ingestion and inhalation

Allergy and anaphylaxis may develop from contact, inhalation or ingestion, Some are poisonous to eat.

### Irukandji

Some jellyfish produce a minimal sting, but inject a toxin that causes severe generalized muscular spasms, especially affecting the large muscle masses of the spine and abdomen up to 2 hours later. Because of the latent period, the relationship may not be realized and diagnostic problems arise. Although the Irukandji have only been described in the tropical and subtropical parts of the southern Indo-Pacific, many jellyfish stings may have a muscular spasm/pain component to their injury – as may many other marine animals.

## Chironex (box jellyfish, sea wasp)

### General

These cubomedusae are restricted to the warm waters of the Indo-Pacific region. Fatalities are more numerous in the waters off northern Australia.

This is said to be the most venomous marine animal known. It is especially dangerous to children and patients with cardiorespiratory

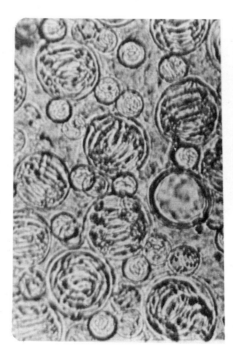

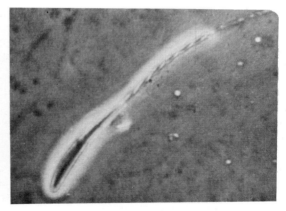

**Figure 24.8** Nematocysts: left: both discharged and undischarged nematocysts of *Physalia* (Portuguese man-'o-war). Right: discharging nematocyst of *Chironex fleckeri* (sea wasp). (Photo by K. Gillett)

disorders (asthmatics and coronary artery disease). Its box-shaped body can measure 20 cm along each side and has up to 15 tentacles measuring up to 3 metres in length on each of its four pedalia. The animal is usually small at the beginning of the 'hot' season, and increases in size and toxicity as it matures during the season. It is especially common after bad weather and on cloudy days, when it moves into more shallow water. It is almost invisible in its natural habitat, being pale blue and transparent. It tends to avoid noise, e.g. speed boats, and turbulence, e.g. the surf – but this should not be relied upon. It is claimed to reach several knots, but it often drifts with the wind and tide when near the surface.

The severity of the sting increases with the size of the animal, the extent of contact with the victim and the delicacy of the victim's skin. Deaths have occurred with as little contact as 6–7 metres of tentacle. Adjacent swimmers may also be affected to a variable degree. The tentacles tend to adhere with a sticky jelly-like substance. They can usually be removed by bystanders, due to the protection afforded by the thick skin on the palmar aspect of their hands. This protection is not always complete, and stinging can occur even through surgical gloves.

## Toxin

The venom is made up of at least two fractions, one with a molecular weight of approximately 75 000 and one of 150 000. The lethal, dermatonecrotic and haemolytic fractions are specific antigens, and cross-immunity probably does not develop to other species. The effects on the cardiovascular system are an initial rise in arterial pressure which is followed by hypotensive/hypertensive oscillations. This is probably due to interference with vasomotor reflex feedback systems. The hypotensive states are related to bradycardia, cardiac irregularities (especially delay in atrioventricular conduction) and apnoea, and these oscillate with hypertensive states. The cardiovascular effects are due to cardiotoxicity, baroceptor stimulation and/or brain-stem depression. Ventricular fibrillation or asystole will precede cerebral death.

## Clinical features

The patient usually screams as a result of the excruciating pain, occurring immediately on contact, and increasing in intensity, often coming in waves. He then claws at the adherent tentacles (whitish strings surrounded by a transparent jelly). He may become confused, act irrationally or lose consciousness, and may drown because of this.

> *Chironex stings are excruciatingly painful and potentially fatal.*

### Local

Multiple interlacing whiplash lines – red, purple or brown – 0.5 cm wide, develop within seconds. The markings are in a 'beaded' or 'ladder' pattern, and are quite characteristic. These acute changes will last for some hours. They are also described as transverse weals. If death occurs, the skin markings fade. If the patient survives, the red, swollen skin may develop large weals and, after 7–10 days, necrosis and ulceration develops over the area of contact. The skin lesions may take many months to heal if deep ulceration occurs. Itching may also be troublesome and recurrent. Pigmentation and scarring at the site of these lesions may be permanent.

### General

Excruciating pain dominates the clinical picture, while impairment of consciousness may lead to coma and death. The pain diminishes in 4–12 hours. Amnesia occurs for most of the incident following the sting. If death occurs, it usually does so within the first 10 minutes; survival is likely after the first hour.

Cardiovascular effects dominate the generalized manifestations. The patient may develop cardiac shock, appearing cold and clammy with a rapid pulse, disturbance of consciousness, hypotension, tachycardia and a raised venous pressure. It is also possible that the cardiac state may oscillate within minutes from episodes of hypertension, tachycardia, rapid respirations and normal venous pressure to hypotension, bradycardia, apnoea and elevated venous pressure. The oscillation may give a false impression of improvement just prior to the patient's death.

Respiratory distress, pulmonary congestion and oedema, and cyanosis, may be due to the cardiac effects or to a direct midbrain depression. Paralysis and abdominal pains may occur. Malaise and restlessness may persist, with physical convalescence requiring up to a week. Irritability and difficulty with psychological adjustment may take weeks or months to disappear. Immunity to the sting is said to occur following repeated and recent contacts, although it is likely that the cross-immunity between the species is incomplete or absent.

---

*TREATMENT OF CHIRONEX STING*
- *Rescue patient from water*
- *Apply vinegar in copious quantities*
- *Mouth-to-mouth respiration and external cardiac massage as required*
- *Box jellyfish antivenom, if available*
- *Application of local anaesthetic ointment*
- *Cardiopulmonary resuscitation techniques*
- *Intravenous opiates or general anaesthesia*
- *Steroids?*

---

## Treatment

### First aid

Prevent drowning. Apply copious quantities of vinegar to reduce the likelihood of discharge of the nematocysts. This may be repeated. Remove the tentacles and undischarged nematocysts. Do this gently but quickly, pulling in one direction only. Rough handling and rubbing will cause further nematocysts to discharge. Some experienced fishermen use a razor blade to pare the tentacles off the exposed skin. Local remedies, such as lemon or lime juice, have yet to be evaluated.

If vinegar is not available other materials may be of value but there is much conflict over which substances may aggravate the condition.

Mouth-to-mouth artificial respiration is required if the patient has stopped breathing. External cardiac massage is needed if no pulse is detectable. This must always be considered when the patient is shocked or losing consciousness and must be combined with mouth-to-mouth respiration. The resuscitation (mouth-to-mouth respiration and external cardiac massage) should be continued and reapplied whenever there is any deterioration in the patient's condition. Do not assume, because there is initial improvement, that he or she will not relapse.

### Medical

Local applications include lignocaine or other local anaesthetic ointment. This may assist even after the first few minutes, during which time the traditional vinegar is believed to be of prophylactic value. Analgesics include morphine 15 mg or pethidine (Demerol) 100 mg, intravenously in divided doses. This may also protect against shock.

Hydrocortisone 100 mg may be administered intravenously every 2 hours if needed. Local steroid preparations are valuable for treating local manifestations such as swelling, pain and itching etc. Intermittent positive pressure respiration, possibly with oxygen, replaces mouth-to-mouth artificial respiration, if needed. This will require constant attention because of the varying degree of respiratory depression. General anaesthesia with endotracheal intubation and controlled ventilation is needed if analgesia cannot otherwise be obtained.

Chlorpromazine 100 mg intramuscularly, or diazepam 10 mg intravenously etc., may be of value after the immediate resuscitation, as they will assist in sedating and tranquillizing the patient without causing significant respiratory depression. Other drugs may be used but are unproven in this clinical disorder. These include noradrenaline (Levophed) or dopamine drips for hypotension, respiratory or cardiac stimulants, verapamil etc. Continuous electrocardiogram monitoring is indicated, as are pulse rate, BP, CVP, respiratory rate, arterial gases, pulse oximetry and pH levels. External cardiac massage and defibrillation is given if required.

Chironex (box jellyfish) antivenom has been developed by the Australian Commonwealth Serum Laboratories (CSL), and is derived from the serum of hyperimmunized sheep. It is of value against both the local and general manifestations. Local steroid ointment may relieve the severe itching which may follow the acute skin lesion.

### Prevention

This includes the wearing of adequate protective clothing (overalls, wet suits, body stockings etc.). Restrict swimming or wading to the safe months of the year. Care is especially needed on cloudy days towards the end of the hot season. Dragging a section of a beach with a 2.5 cm mesh has been used, not very successfully, to clear an area for bathing. Development of a CSL toxoid has been abandoned.

## Cone shells

### General

Highly favoured by shell collectors of the Tropics and warm temperate regions, these attractive univalve molluscs have a proboscis extendable from the narrow end, but able to reach most of the shell. Holding the shell even by the 'big end' may not be entirely safe, and may court a sting with a resultant 25% mortality. The cone shell inhabits shallow waters, reefs, ponds and rubble. Its size is usually up to 10 cm. It has a siphon, sometimes ringed with orange, which detects its prey, and may be the only part visible if the cone burrows under the sand. The proboscis, which delivers the coup-de-grâce, carries 1 to 10 radular teeth which penetrate and inject venom into its prey thus immobilizing the victim.

Probably only the fish-eating cones are dangerous to humans, but as these are difficult to distinguish at first sight, discretion on the part of shell collectors is recommended. The venom is composed of two or more substances. One interferes with the neuromuscular activity and elicits a substained muscular contracture; the other abolishes the excitability of muscle fibre and summates with tubocurarine, but is uninfluenced by eserine. The major effect appears to be directly on skeletal muscular activity. Children are particularly vulnerable.

> *Cone shell venom causes skeletal muscle paresis or paralysis, with or without myalgia.*

### Clinical features

#### Local

The initial puncture effects may vary from no pain to excruciating agony and may be aggravated by salt water. It may become inflamed and swollen, sometimes white and ischaemic, with a cyanotic area surrounding it, and it may be numb to touch.

#### General

Numbness and tingling may ascend from the bite to involve the whole body, and especially the mouth and lips. This may take about 10 minutes to develop. Skeletal muscular paralysis may spread from the site of injury, and result in anything from mild weariness to complete flaccid paralysis. Difficulty with swallowing and speech may occur prior to total paralysis. Visual disturbances may include double and blurred vision (paralysis of voluntary muscles and pupillary reactions). These changes may take place within 10–30 minutes of the bite. Respiratory paralysis may dominate the clinical picture. This results in shallow rapid breathing and a cyanotic appearance, proceeding to apnoea, unconsciousness and death. Other cases are said to result in cardiac failure, although this is probably

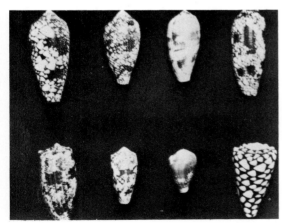

**Figure 24.9** Poisonous cone shells: lengths 5–10 cm

secondary to the respiratory paralysis. The extent of neurotoxic damage is variable. If the patient survives, he is active and mobile within 24 hours. Neurological sequelae and the local reaction may last many weeks.

### Treatment

#### First aid

The following recommendations are made depending on the presence of paralysis.

#### Without paralysis

The limb must be immobilized and a pressure bandage applied to reduce the speed of venom absorption. The patient should be rested and reassured.

#### With paralysis

Mouth-to-mouth respiration may be needed. This may have to be continued for hours, or until medical facilities are reached. This artificial respiration is the major contribution to saving the patient's life. External cardiac massage, as well as mouth-to-mouth respiration, is needed if the patient has neither pulse nor respiration. The patient may be able to hear but not communicate and thus requires reassurance. If he is shocked, ensure he is lying down with his feet elevated.

#### Medical treatment

With respiratory paralysis, administer artificial respiration with intermittent positive pressure adequate to maintain normal arterial gases and pH. Endotracheal intubation prevents aspiration of vomitus and facilitates ventilation and tracheobronchial toilet, when indicated. Routine care and management of the unconscious patient is required. External cardiac massage, defibrillation, vasopressors etc. may be indicated by the clinical state and electrocardiogram. Local anaesthetic can be injected into the wound. Respiratory depressants, respiratory stimulants and drugs used against neuromuscular blockade are not indicated.

### Prevention

The people at risk, e.g. shell collectors, visitors to the reefs, schoolchildren etc., need to be educated about this danger. They should avoid contact with the cone shell. Probably no part of it can be touched with impunity, unless the animal is dead. Despite advice to the contrary, touching the 'big end' is not always safe. If these shells must be collected, it is advisable to use forceps and a tough receptacle.

## Blue ringed octopus

### General

This animal usually weighs from 10 to 100 g and is currently found only in the Australasian and Indo-Pacific region. Its span, with tentacles extended, is from 2 to 20 cm, but usually less than 10 cm. It is found in rock pools, in clumps of cunjevoi and in shells, from the tidal zone to a depth of 10 metres. The colour is yellowish brown with ringed marking on the tentacles and striations on the body. These markings change to a vivid iridescent blue when the animal is feeding, becomes angry, excited, disturbed or hypoxic. The heavier specimens are more dangerous and handling these attractive creatures has resulted in death within a few minutes. Many such incidents have probably escaped detection by the coroner. Autopsy features are non-specific and the bite fades after death.

The toxin ('maculotoxin') is more potent than that of any land animal. Analysis of posterior salivary extracts demonstrates a hyaluronidase and cephalotoxins of low molecular weight (less than 500). The octopus toxin may be identical to tetrodotoxin. The effects are that of a neurotoxin and a neuromuscular blocking agent. It is not curare-like, and is not influenced by neostigmine and atropine, at least during the acute phase. Hypotension may develop.

> *The maculotoxin of the blue ringed octopus is similar to tetrodotoxin from the puffer fish. It is a neurotoxin and a neuromuscular blocker, resulting in painless skeletal muscle paralysis.*

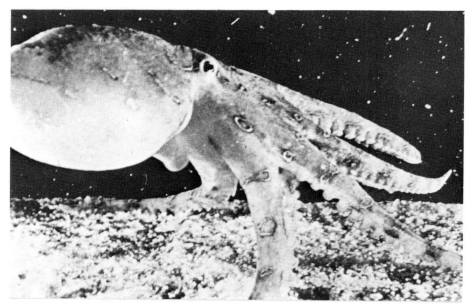

**Figure 24.10** Blue ringed octopus: specimen 12 cm outstretched. (Photo by K. Gillett)

### Clinical features

#### Local

Initially the bite is usually painless, and may thus go unnoticed. A 1-cm circle of blanching becomes oedematous and swollen in 15 minutes. It then becomes haemorrhagic and resembles a blood blister. If the patient survives the next hour, he notices a local stinging sensation for 6 hours. A serous or bloody discharge may occur. Local muscular twitching may persist for some weeks.

#### General

A few minutes after the bite, a rapid, painless paralysis dominates the clinical picture, which progresses in this order: abnormal sensations around mouth, neck and head; nausea and/or vomiting may occur; dyspnoea with rapid, shallow and stertorous respirations leading to apnoea, asphyxia and cyanosis; visual disturbances, involvement of the extraocular eye muscles resulting in double vision, blurred vision and ptosis, whereas intraocular paralysis results in a fixed dilated pupil; difficulty in speech and swallowing, general weakness and incoordination progresses to complete paralysis; the duration of paralysis is between 4 and 12 hours, but the weakness and incoordination may persist for another day. The patient's conscious state is initially normal, even though he may not be able to open his eyes or respond to his environment. The respiratory paralysis (causing hypoxia and hypercapnia) finally results in unconsciousness and then death, often within minutes of the commencement of symptoms, unless resuscitation is continued. Cardiovascular effects of hypotension and bradycardia are noted in severe cases.

There may be a cessation at any stage of the above clinical sequence, i.e. the effects may cease with the local reaction, a partial paralysis, or proceed to a complete paralysis and death. Less severe bites may result in generalized and local muscular contractions, which may continue intermittently for 6 hours or more. This occurs with a subparalytic dose. Other symptoms noted in mild cases include a light-headed feeling, depersonalization, paraesthesia, weakness and exhaustion.

### Treatment

#### First aid

The following recommendations are made before and with paralysis.

### Before paralysis

Immobilization of the limb and application of a pressure bandage will reduce the absorption of venom. Rest the patient, preferably lying on his side in case of vomiting, and do not leave him unattended. Only after hospitalization, where preparations have been made for respiratory support, should the pressure bandage be removed.

### With paralysis

Apply mouth-to-mouth respiration to ensure that the patient does not become cyanotic. Attention must be paid to the clearing of his airway of vomitus, tongue obstruction, dentures etc. If an airway is available, this should be inserted – but it is not essential. Artificial respiration may have to be continued for hours, until the patient reaches hospital. If delay has occurred, then external cardiac massage may also be required. Reassure the patient, who can hear but not communicate, that you understand his condition. Enlist medical aid, but never leave him unattended to obtain this.

### *Medical*

For respiratory paralysis, intubation and artificial respiration with intermittent positive pressure respiration are necessary to maintain normal arterial blood gases. Endotracheal intubation also prevents aspiration of vomitus and facilitates tracheobronchial toilet, when indicated. The usual management of the unconscious patient is required.

Edrophonium (Tensilon) and neostigmine are of no value during the deeply paralysed state. Other central respiratory stimulants have sometimes been used in borderline cases or during the recovery period. Local anaesthetic infiltration to the painful area will give local relief of the delayed pain. For delayed allergic reactions, intravenous hydrocortisone for systemic effects, subcutaneous adrenaline for bronchospasm or oral antihistamines for skin lesions are indicated.

### *Prevention*

Contact with the octopus should be avoided and empty shells should be treated with suspi-

cion. Requests by scientific groups for collection of these specimens should be tempered with caution. A public programme on the dangers of this animal should be directed especially to children, who are attracted by the bright coloration.

## Other marine animal injuries

Only a few of these are mentioned in this text. The sea urchin, electric rays and coral cuts are selected for inclusion because of their interest and frequency in tropical and temperate regions.

### Sea urchin

Of the 6000 species of sea urchins, approximately 80 are thought to be venomous or poisonous to humans. They belong to the phylum Echinodermata, named after the hedgehog (*Echinos*) because of the many-spined appearance. In some, such as *Diadema setosum*, the **long spined** or **black sea urchin**, the damage is mainly done by the breaking off of the sharp brittle spines after they have penetrated the diver's skin. Sometimes the spines have disappeared within a few days, but in other cases they become encrusted and may remain for many months, to emerge at sites distant from the original wound. They are commonly covered by a black pigment, which can then be mistaken for the actual spine during its removal.

Other sea urchins, such as the **crown of thorns,** *Acanthaster planci*, can also cause damage by the spines piercing the skin, but these seem to have a far more inflammatory action, suggestive of a venom. Injuries from the crown of thorns have been more commonly reported since divers attempted to eradicate them from reefs.

The most potent sea urchins are the **Toxopneustidae** which have short thick spines poking through an array of flower-like pedicellariae. Deaths have been reported from this. The venom is thought to be a dialysable acetylcholine-like substance.

### *Treatment*

The long spines tend to break easily, and therefore need to be pulled out, without any bending. A local anaesthetic may be required if surgical extraction is contemplated. Drawing pastes such as magnesium sulphate have been used. Some find relief with the use of heat, and others have removed the spines by the use of a snake-bite suction cap.

A variety of interesting treatments has developed. In Nauru, it is claimed that urinating on the wound immediately after the injury produces excellent results. This presumably relieves the bladder, if not the pain. The use of meat tenderizer owes more to good advertising than to therapeutic efficiency, although it may given benefit in jelly fish stings.

One technique which would be described as barbaric, had it not been for the fact that it seems to work, is to apply extra trauma and movement to the area – to break up the spines within the tissue. It does seem as if, in this case, activity is more beneficial than rest and immobilization. With the latter, the limb tends to swell and become more painful.

Spines may remain in tissues for several months, sometimes causing little disability before emerging through the skin.

Occasionally patients will present having eaten sea urchins. In Tonga they are used as an aphrodisiac; however, the ovaries may be poisonous and produce both gastrointestinal and migraine-like symptoms.

## Electric rays

Electric rays are found in temperate and tropical oceans, as is the other marine fish which produces electric discharge, the stargazer. The rays are commonly encountered by divers, because they are found in relatively shallow depths and submerged in mud or sand.

The electrical discharge varies from 8 to 220 volts, and is passed between the electrically negative ventral side of the ray to the positive dorsal side. The thick electric organs are usually discernible on each side. Activation of an electric discharge is a reflex action, the result of tactile stimulation. The ray can deliver a successive series of discharges, but these are of lessening intensity. There is then a latent period in which the fish regains his electric charge. It is not necessary to have direct contact with the ray.

The electric shock may have a serious effect in disabling an adult temporarily, and presumably could be more hazardous to a child.

Subsequent danger may come from drowning or aspiration. There are usually no local manifestations visible on the affected skin.

Recovery is uneventful, and treatment is not usually required.

## Sponges

These sedentary animals require some defence from mobile predators and they have developed a skeleton of calcareous and silicaceous spicules. They also have a form of toxin which is not well understood. About a dozen sponges have been incriminated as toxic, from the 5000 or so species, and they are mainly in the temperate or tropical zones. Skin lesions have developed from sponges which have been deep frozen or dried for many years.

### *Clinical features*

One group of symptoms relates to the contact dermatitis associated with the areas of sponge contact. After a variable time, between 5 minutes and 2 hours, the dermal irritation is felt. It may be precipitated by wetting or rubbing the area. It may progress over the next day or so and feel as if ground glass has been abraded into the skin. Hyperaesthesia and paraesthesia may be noted. The symptoms can persist for a week or more with inflammatory and painful reactions around the area. The degree of severity is not related to the clinical signs and some patients may be incapacitated by the symptoms without any objective manifestations.

The dermal reaction may appear as an erythema, with or without papule and vesicle development. There is sometimes a desquamation of the skin in the second or third week, but in other cases the skin lesions have recurred over many months.

### *Treatment*

The only adequate treatment is prevention, using gloves when handling sponges and not touching anything that has been in contact with the sponge.

The use of alcohol, lotions or hot water will usually aggravate the condition. Local application of cooling lotion such as Calamine may be of some value, but the treatment with the conventional dermatological preparations has limited success.

## Coral cuts

### General

Corals, because of their sharp edges combined with the awkwardness of humans in the sea environment, often cause lacerations. The sequelae of this may well equal the intensity of the more impressive marine animal injuries. Not only is the coral covered by infected slime, but also pieces of coral or other foreign bodies will often remain in the laceration. It is possible that some of the manifestations, especially initially, are due to the presence of discharging nematocysts. There have also been occasional patients who have been affected by the marine organism *Erysipelothrix*.

Certain vibrios may be present in the marine environment and can cause serious infection. These may be cultured in a saline media if identification is to be made (see Chapter 23).

### Clinical features

A small, often clean-looking laceration is usually on the hand or foot. It causes little inconvenience at the time of injury and may well go unnoticed. A few hours later, there may be a 'smarting' sensation, especially during washing. At that stage, there is a mild inflammatory reaction around the cut. Within the next day or two, the inflammation becomes more widespread with local swelling, discoloration and tenderness. In severe cases there may be abscess formation with chronic ulceration and even osteomyelitis.

After healing, there may be a small numb area of skin with a fibrous nodule beneath it – a keloid reaction to the foreign body (coral).

### Treatment

This involves thorough cleansing of the area, removal of the foreign material and the application of an antibody powder or ointment, e.g. neomycin.

One sequel of coral cuts is sometimes a very unpleasant pruritus which can be troublesome for many weeks. It responds to the use of a local steroid ointment.

# Poisonous marine animals

Food poisoning from ingested marine animals is a serious hazard to many populations who live on or near the sea. This is especially so in tropical or temperate climates where the outbreaks tend to be sporadic and less predictable. Commercially valuable industries have been either curtailed or prohibited because of the serious threat to the consumers of this high-protein, readily available food. In the cold climates, poisoning from marine and polar animals is also of serious import, but it is more predictable and can therefore be avoided.

Diseases which can destroy whole communities, change the fate of military operations, decimate fishing industries, yet still arise sporadically in a previously safe marine environment, are surely worthy of considerable investigation and research. Such has not been the case. This whole subject is sadly neglected, both in medical research and in medical training.

To those physicians who are associated with marine medicine, yachting, diving or travel, or those who conduct their general practice near coastlines, a knowledge of seafood poisoning is essential. It is at least as important to those involved in public health, industrial medicine and the general health of island communities.

Space allows the description of only a few of the more significant fish poisonings. Ciguatera, tetrodotoxin and scombroid poisoning will be dealt with separately because of their commercial implications. Shellfish and crustacean poisoning will be summarized. Only brief mention can be made of barracouta poisoning, hallucinatory fish poisoning, mercury poisoning, other pollutions, seal liver poisoning, shark and ray poisoning, turtle poisoning and many others. One complicating factor is that there may be more than one type of marine poison responsible for the clinical manifestations in the patient.

## Ciguatera poisoning

On a worldwide basis, ciguatera poisoning is the most serious of the marine toxins. It is mainly a disorder of the Tropics and, to a lesser degree, the semitropical and temperate zones. It is mostly found between the 35° latitudes north and south of the equator. The fish cannot be identified as poisonous by their external appearance. They tend to be reef fish, and they may ingest *Gambierdiscus toxicus* which is thought to be the originator of the toxin, or they may acquire it from eating other fish. The toxin is harmless to the fish themselves, but it tends to accumulate as it is passed to the more active carnivorous predators. It is for this reason that the larger fish tend to be more toxic than the smaller ones.

Local knowledge regarding areas in which the fish are poisonous should be seriously considered in all cases. Unfortunately, it is not entirely reliable, as the areas themselves may be constantly changing. Poisoning is also more likely to develop when reefs have been interfered with by natural damage such as hurricanes or artificial damage such as constructions, atomic blasting etc., helping proliferation of *Gambierdiscus toxicus*.

A variety of techniques has been promulgated by folklore to predict which fish will be safe to eat. Observations which are totally irrelevant, despite parochial beliefs, include:

- The presence of worms in the fish.
- Whether ants or flies refuse it.
- Whether a silver coin will turn black.
- Whether grated coconut will turn green if cooked with the fish.

Perhaps the safest method is to feed a small amount of the fish to a kitten, which is highly sensitive to most fish poisons. If the animal is still alive and unaffected a few hours later, then the fish is probably safe to eat. A traditional variant to this, is the rather pragmatic system of feeding the older members of the family first; if they are unaffected, the remainder of the fish is used to feed the children and the more productive members of the society.*

In a survival situation, the advice is as follows: do not eat the viscera of the fish (e.g. liver, gonads, intestines etc.). Avoid the exceptionally large reef predators and those species often implicated in ciguatera poisoning. These include barracuda, grouper, snapper, sea bass, surgeon fish, parrot fish, wrasses, jacks and many others. Moray eels are particularly virulent. Boiling the fish many times and discarding the water after each boiling may sometimes be helpful. As an alternative to this last technique, the fish may be sliced and continually soaked in water which should be changed every 30 minutes or so. Eat only small quantities.

### Clinical features

Symptoms usually develop 2–12 hours after ingestion of the food. More severe cases tend to occur earlier.

Generalized non-specific symptoms may develop, including weakness and dull aches in the limbs and head. These muscle pains may progress to a more severe weakness, with or without cramps. The pains differentiate this disorder from tetrodotoxin poisoning. Paraesthesiae and numbness are noted around the mouth and sometimes in the peripheries. Gastrointestinal problems, including anorexia, nausea, vomiting and diarrhoea, may last for a few days. Severe neurological disturbances may develop and include delirium, cranial nerve involvement, incoordination and ataxia, with occasional extrapyramidal disorders, convulsions, coma and even death. Death is likely to be due to respiratory failure, although in severe cases there is evidence of hypotension, cardiac dysrhythmias and other cardiovascular problems.

Skin lesions are very characteristic and include erythema, pruritus or a burning sensation – sometimes with vesicular formation. They may be very severe for a few days, but then usually subside. Hair and nail loss may supervene. In the severely affected cases, these skin lesions may be troublesome for many weeks. In females, the vagina and urethra may also be affected, sometimes very severely, causing symptoms of cystitis or dyspareunia. Less commonly, males may notice pain during ejaculations.

The death rate from different series varies from 0.1% to 10%. In severe outbreaks, the presentation of the disease can be acute and widespread. In most Indo-Pacific regions, the disease tends to be sporadic and mild. In these cases the main symptoms can clear within 1 or 2 days, although residual weakness and paraesthesia, together with a reversal of temperature perception, may persist for long periods. Severe cases may take many months or up to a

---

* The senior author takes exception to this deplorable practice.

year for full recovery. Exacerbations can be precipitated by alcohol, nicotinic acid and other vasoactive drugs. The production of an erythematous area associated with a burning sensation following intake of alcohol is pathognomonic of this disorder. The illness can also recur following stress or the ingestion of certain fish. Immunity does not develop and subsequent poisonings may be even more severe.

### Treatment

Treatment includes the removal of unabsorbed material by induction of vomiting or gastric lavage in patients who do not have respiratory depression. Rest and observation in a hospital are required until the patient has recovered.

With respiratory paralysis, respiration must be assisted. Once medical assistance is obtained, exhaled air resuscitation (as a first aid measure) is replaced by endotracheal intubation with assisted respiration.

The medical treatment is basically symptomatic; however, there have been many different pharmacological remedies proposed. None has been consistently demonstrated to be effective. A recent treatment is the use of intravenous mannitol, especially if given early. Twenty per cent mannitol 250 ml intravenously in a 6-hour period with maximum of 1 g/kg given over 30 minutes, together with a 5% dextrose infusion, has produced some good results.

Drugs which have been suggested and which seem to do no harm include steroids, e.g. hydrocortisone 100–200 mg, 6-hourly i.v. during the first 3 days, and calcium gluconate 10% i.v. to relieve the neuromuscular or neurological features and perhaps increase muscle tone. Atropine, edrophonium, neostigmine, pralidoxime etc. have all been used at different times, possibly with some effect. Vitamin treatments have been employed in the Pacific Islands. Nicotinic acid preparations have also been recommended, but these sometimes aggravate the clinical manifestations. As a general rule, pharmacological treatment does not have nearly the effectiveness of general medical care. Symptomatic treatment, while not using vasoactive drugs, seems most valuable. Diazepam can be given safely, and severe cases may require the assistance of a neurologist or an organically oriented psychiatrist for pharmacological advice. A tricyclic antidepressant may be of benefit if given in small dosages, e.g. amitriptyline 25–50 mg at night.

## Tetrodotoxin poisoning

### General

Of all that are in the waters you may eat these: whatever has fins and scales you may eat. And whatever does not have fins and scales you shall not eat; it is unclean for you.

Deuteronomy 14:9,10.

Tetrodotoxin poisoning follows the ingestion of puffer fish, ocean sunfish or porcupine fish. The name puffer comes from the ability of the fish to inflate itself by taking in large quantities of air or water. The scales have been modified to form protective plates or spikes. They are recognized as poisonous throughout the world, although they are more common in the tropical and temperate regions. The toxin is concentrated mainly in the ovaries, liver and intestines. Lesser amounts occur in the skin but the body musculature is usually free of poison. The toxicity is related to the reproductive cycle.

With two exceptions, these fish are usually considered inedible. The first exception is the uninformed consumer. Examples range from Captain James Cook (who, on September 7, 1774, sampled this fish in New Caledonia with near fatal results) to the poor of southern California and Florida looking for a cheap meal. The other exception is the Asiatic gourmet consuming 'Fugu'. After a prolonged apprenticeship, specially licensed chefs in Japan are allowed to prepare this fish, receiving considerable kudos by retaining enough of the toxin to produce a numbing effect in the mouth – but not enough to cause tetrodotoxin poisoning. Nevertheless, accidents do happen, and the death rate from Fugu poisoning reaches approximately 50 cases per year.

The toxin interferes with neuromuscular transmission in motor and sensory nerves and in the sympathetic nervous system by interfering with sodium transfer. It also has a direct depressant effect on medullary centres, skeletal muscles (reducing excitability), intracardiac conduction and myocardial contractility. Hypotension may be due to either the effects on the preganglionic cholinergic fibres or the direct effect on the heart. Respiratory depression precedes cardiovascular depression.

### Clinical features

The onset and severity of symptoms vary greatly according to the amount of toxin ingested. Usually within the first hour, the patient will notice muscular weakness and other effects of blockage of the motor and sensory systems. This may progress to total skeletal paralysis, including respiratory paralysis.

Paraesthesia around the mouth may also extend to the extremities, or it may become generalized. Autonomic effects include salivation, sweating, chest pain and headache. Gastrointestinal symptoms of nausea, vomiting, diarrhoea etc. may develop, and there is sometimes a decrease in temperature, pulse rate and blood pressure.

A coagulation disturbance, which is an occasional complication, may lead to systemic bleeding or desquamation from haemorrhagic bullae.

The neurological involvement may commence as muscular twitching and incoordination and may proceed to a complete skeletal muscular paralysis. Bulbar paralysis may produce interference with speech and swallowing. The pupils, after initially being constricted, may become fixed and dilated. The clinical picture is, therefore, one of a generalized paralysis with the patient maintaining a fully conscious state while oxygenation is maintained. This is important in the treatment, because the patient is able to hear and appreciate the statements made by people around him.

The death rate from this disorder is approximately 60%. It is usually due to respiratory paralysis and occurs within 24 hours of ingestion. It is a reflection of incorrect diagnosis or inadequate resuscitation techniques, in most cases.

### Treatment

Before the patient shows signs of paralysis or weakness, the use of an emetic or gastric lavage may be of value in removing poisonous material. Lavage may also be employed if controlled respiration has required the insertion of an endotracheal tube, which will prevent aspiration of stomach contents.

After weakness has become apparent, the treatment is entirely symptomatic, i.e. maintenance of an adequate respiratory state, monitoring of vital signs, measurement of arterial blood gas and biochemical profile. The patient may require mechanical ventilation for up to 24 hours, prior to regaining muscular control. Because of the likelihood of consciousness being retained in the absence of skeletal or respiratory movement, the periodic administration of a minor tranquillizer such as diazepam seems prudent. Continuous explanation and reassurance should be given, even though the patient cannot respond physically to these.

Various pharmacological treatments have been proposed, including intravenous calcium gluconate 10%, anticholinesterases, respiratory stimulants, steroids etc. There is no firm evidence that they are of value.

General nursing care, with special attention to pressure areas, eye and mouth toilets etc., is axiomatic in these paralysed and debilitated patients.

### Prevention

'Scaleless' fish should not be eaten unless they are known to be harmless. If one is forced to eat Fugu in Japan, it should be purchased from a first-class restaurant with a licensed cook. All the viscera and skin must be removed. In a survival situation, these fish should be eviscerated and only the musculature should be consumed. The meat should be cut or torn into small bits and soaked in water for at least 4 hours. The fish should be kneaded during this time and the water changed at frequent intervals. The toxin is partly water soluble, therefore this soaking may help to remove it. Do not eat more than is required to maintain life. Feeding of the fish to test animals has been suggested.

## Scombroid poisoning

### General

This disorder is possible wherever mackerel-like fish, tuna, bonito or albacore are caught and eaten without adequate care or preparation. It has also occurred in epidemics due to contaminated canned tuna. The fish, which are normally safe to eat, become poisonous when handled incorrectly. If left for several hours at room temperature or in the sun, the histidine in their muscular tissues is changed by bacterial action into saurine, a histamine-like substance. The bacteria implicated include *Proteus morganii, Clostridium, Salmonella, Escherichia* spp. etc. Laboratory verification of contaminated fish is obtained by demonstrating a histamine content in excess of 100 mg/100 g fish muscle.

### Clinical features

The fish may have a characteristic 'peppery' taste. After $\frac{1}{2}$–1 hour, other symptoms characteristic of histamine toxicity develop. Gastrointestinal symptoms associated with headache, palpitations and tachycardia with hypotension, are followed by a typical 'allergic' syndrome. The latter may involve the skin with an erythematous or urticarial reaction, the respiratory system with bronchospasm or the cardiovascular system in the form of anaphylactic shock.

### Treatment

The first aid treatment includes the removal of unabsorbed material by vomiting or gastric lavage if the patient is not too severely distressed. Treatment involves the customary techniques for handling dermatological, respiratory or cardiovascular manifestations of allergy.

### Prevention

Prevention is possible by correct care, storage and preparation of the fish. Prompt refrigeration and not leaving the fish exposed to the sun or room temperature has reduced the incidence of this disease. It is believed that pallor of the gills, or an odour or staleness, may indicate that saurine may be present in the fish.

## Shellfish and crustacean poisoning

Shellfish include oysters, clams, mussels, cockles etc.; crustaceans include lobsters, crayfish, prawns, crabs, yabbies etc. Four different types of poisoning may develop from ingestion of these animals.

### Gastrointestinal type

This is the most common type, and it develops many hours after ingestion of the contaminated shellfish. Viruses, marine vibrios, *Escherichia coli*, and other bacteria and organisms have been implicated. Manifestations last about 36 hours and are treated according to general medical principles.

### Allergic type

The allergic type of reaction appears to be a typical hypersensitivity reaction to a protein in the shellfish. It is likely that the victim has previously been exposed to the same or similar protein to which he has developed an antibody reaction. Symptoms develop after the second and subsequent exposures and are aggravated by exercise, heat and emotion. There may be a history of allergy to other foreign proteins, e.g. hay fever, antitoxins, horse serum etc. The clinical features are dermatological, respiratory and/or cardiovascular in type and may, therefore, mimic scombroid poisoning. Antihistamines, sympathomimetic drugs and steroids tend to be used in the three manifestations, respectively.

### Hepatic disease

There appears to be a hepatotoxin especially concentrated in molluscs and perhaps related to the presence of a toxic dinoflagellate or vibrio. This may result in severe hepatocellular disease with the clinical picture of acute yellow atrophy. Viral infection, causing infectious hepatitis, has also been reported.

### Paralytic shellfish poisoning

This disorder (PSP) is due to the ingestion of a neurotoxin in shellfish called saxitoxin. The poison is associated with the 'red tide' or 'water bloom' – a discoloration of the sea due to masses of dinoflagellates. It accumulates and is concentrated by shellfish which filter the organisms from the contaminated water. It usually occurs in epidemics, with all consumers of the shellfish being affected. One plankton protozoa implicated is the species *Gonyaulax catanella*. The major effect of PSP is respiratory paralysis due to a peripheral action (probably by blocking conduction in the motor nerves) and a direct effect on skeletal muscles.

The clinical effects and treatment are similar in many ways to tetrodotoxin poisoning.

## Recommended reading

BALDRIDGE, D. (1975). *Shark Attack*. Available from author, Box 15216, Sarasota, Fla 33579, USA.

EDMONDS, C. (1989). *Dangerous Marine Creatures*. Sydney: Reed.

HALSTEAD, B. *Poisonous and Venomous Marine Animals of the World* (Vols 1–3). Washington DC: US Government Printing Office.

SUTHERLAND, S.K. (1983). *Australian Animal Toxins*. Melbourne: Oxford University Press.

# 25

# Underwater explosions

## Introduction

Although most of our information on this topic has been acquired from naval research work, it is still relevant to some civilian divers. Explosives are used in salvage, mining and dredging operations, as well as in war-like activities which involve divers and shipwreck survivors. During World War II there were many deaths of divers and swimmers following air, surface ship or submarine attack. One report claimed that mortality from the underwater blast injuries could approach 80%.

For an explosion with the same energy and at the same distance, an underwater blast is more dangerous than an air blast. This is because in air the blast dissipates more rapidly and tends to be reflected at the body surface; in water the blast wave travels through the body and causes internal injuries.

## Physics of blast waves

Some understanding of underwater explosions is of assistance in understanding its clinical manifestations. An explosion is a very fast chemical reaction. The process propagates through the explosive at 2–9 km/s. The products of the chemical reaction are heat and combustion products such as carbon dioxide. A bubble of gas is produced in the water. The gas in the bubble may be at a pressure of 50 000 atmospheres and temperature of 3000°C. The bubble rapidly expands in a spherical form, displacing water. This rapid expansion generates the first pressure wave as the pressure in the gas bubble is transferred into the water, producing a pressure pulse that is transmitted through the water. It is sometimes called the **short pulse** or **primary pulse**. The initial pressure change of the wave is steep, rising to the peak pressure within a few microseconds. The pressure in the bubble falls as it expands and the gas cools. The fall of pressure at the end of the explosion reflects the end of the expansion of the gases and takes milliseconds.

The momentum of the water which has been displaced by the bubble enlarges the bubble past its equilibrium volume and a series of volume swings can be initiated. The volume oscillations of the gas bubble cause a series of pressure waves.

Near the point of detonation, the velocity of the first pressure wave is great, and is related to the speed that the explosive detonates. Some explosives produce high pressures for a short period, others, with a slower reaction rate, produce less intense pressure waves that have a longer duration.

At a point some distance from the detonation, the velocity of the pressure waves slows to that of sound – about 1.5 km/s. From then on, the pressure waves follow the laws of sound in water. The energy of the waves decreases with distance and they are reflected and absorbed in a similar fashion to sound waves.

In water the pressure pulse is not absorbed as rapidly as in air. In air the gas surrounding the explosion is compressed and so absorbs energy from the explosion. In water, which is far less compressible, there is little absorption. The pressure pulse is transmitted with greater intensity over a longer range. Thus the lethal range of an explosion is normally far greater than the same mass of explosive in air.

An example of the increased damage an explosion can cause in water can be demonstrated by a simple experiment. A small charge of chosen size is detonated in an empty, open drum and does not dent it. The drum is then filled with water. When another charge of the same size is detonated in the drum, it ruptures.

> *A pressure wave is transmitted over a greater range in water than in air.*

As mentioned above, the expanding gas bubble in the water pushes the water away from the centre of the explosion. Due to the momentum of the moving water, the bubble expands past its equilibrium volume, so it contracts, again with a momentum that carries it past its equilibrium volume. In this manner a series of **secondary pulses** may be generated by the bubble.

The energy in a typical blast is distributed in the following proportions: the initial pressure wave has approximately one-quarter of the energy, subsequent waves total one-quarter and the other manifestations, such as heat and turbulence, comprise the remaining half. In an explosion most of the damage is achieved by the initial pressure wave.

Other waves may result from an explosion. If the initial waves reach the sea bottom they may be reflected and/or absorbed. The proportions depend on the nature of the sea bed. If it is hard, there is little absorption and much reflection. The angle of incidence, i.e. the angle at which the waves strike the sea bed, will be equal to the angle of reflection. The **reflected wave** coming from the sea bed may combine with the other waves, causing increased damage. If the sea bed is distant from the point of detonation, this effect is negligible.

At the water surface the reflected wave is a negative pressure pulse rather than a positive pulse. As a result of this, a diver may experience a less intense pressure wave if he is close to the surface. The negative reflected pulse tends to cancel the positive direct path pulse.

At the surface a series of events may modify the pressure waves. Above a certain intensity the surface of the water will be broken or shredded, and thrown up into a **dome**, termed 'the dome effect'. This dissipates a small part of the pressure wave, and the remainder is reflected back into the water. Other disturbances which may be observed on the surface following the dome phenomenon include the slick and plume. The **slick** is a rapidly expanding ring of darkened water due to the advancing of the pressure waves. The **plume** is the last manifestation of the explosion and is the result of gas reaching and breaking the surface of the water. Although the plume may be spectacular, it does little damage.

The surface phenomenon varies with the size and depth of the explosion. Beyond a certain depth or with a small explosion, the dome may not form, as there may be insufficient energy to shred the water. The slick tends to be retained to a greater depth, being dependent only on the presence of the pulse wave.

Thermal layers may also reflect the pressure waves from the explosion as may other objects such as large ships. The size of the charge, depth of detonation and distance from target will have an influence on the potential damage by the initial and subsequent pressure waves.

## Charge size, distance and the risk of injury

The risk of injury or death will be dependent on several variables: the size of the charge, the victim's distance from it and the nature of the bottom. American sources give the relationship below for estimating the effect of a TNT charge. Other explosives behave differently; the longer pulse from a slower detonating explosion can cause more damage than the same pressure from a more rapidly detonating explosive.

$$P \text{ (lb/in}^2) = \frac{13\,000 \times \text{charge size (lb)}^{\frac{1}{3}}}{\text{Distance from charge (feet)}}$$

where $P$ = pressure.

Pressures over 2000 lb/in² will cause death, pressures of over 500 lb/in² are likely to cause death or serious injury. Pressures in the range 50–500 lb/in² are likely to cause injury, but those less than 50 lb/in² are unlikely to cause any harm.

## Mechanism of blast injury

In air explosions, the main cause of damage is from the fragments from the charge container, shrapnel and foreign bodies drawn into the explosive wave, as well as the pressure wave. In the water these particles are retarded by the medium. Also, with air explosions much of the pressure wave is reflected at the body surface, because this is an interface between media of different densities, any blast effect probably acting through the mouth, nose and ears.

Intestinal injury as a result of blast damage rarely occurs in explosions in air.

In water, the blast wave passes through the body as it is of a similar consistency to water. The individual molecules are displaced very little except in areas capable of compression, i.e. gas spaces. Damage is mainly at the air–water interfaces within the body. The gas in the gas-filled cavities is almost instantaneously compressed as the pressure wave passes. The walls of these spaces are torn as the wave passes.

Damage can be expected in the lung, air-filled viscera in the abdomen, sinus cavities and the ear. In the lungs, the damage is not due to pressure transmitted via the upper airways, but is the result of transmission of the wave directly through the thoracic wall. The pressure wave reaches the gas–tissue interface at the respiratory mucosa and it is there that the tissues are 'shredded' or torn apart.

> *Injury from underwater blast occurs mainly at gas–tissue interfaces, as in barotrauma.*

## Animal experiments

The effects of underwater blast on animals have been studied. The respiratory and gastro-intestinal tracts were the most significantly affected. Pathological examinations revealed injury to the lungs and gas-filled abdominal viscera. Central nervous system lesions have also been observed.

The respiratory damage included pulmonary haemorrhage, usually at the bases, bronchi and trachea, acute vesicular and interstitial emphysema, pneumothorax and haemothorax. Intestinal injury consisted mainly of subserous and submucosal haemorrhage and perforation of the gas-filled viscera. Renal and hepatic systems were not affected, with no evidence of gall-bladder or urinary bladder damage. If both the thorax and abdomen were immersed the lungs would be consistently more affected than the intestines. If only the abdomen were immersed, then this would be most affected, with bleeding via the rectum.

The above results show the importance of the air–water interface in damage from an underwater blast. Wolf (1970) cites experiments to confirm this phenomenon. If three loops of bowel are prepared and occluded, collapsing one, filling another with saline and filling a third with air, only the air-containing loop sustained injury.

There is some contention regarding the cause of death in animals exposed to underwater explosions. In most cases early deaths are probably due to pulmonary lesions. These animals usually had a low arterial oxygen saturation, correctable by 100% oxygen inhalation, with a respiratory acidosis and carbon dioxide retention. Some early deaths may be due to central nervous system involvement. Petechial haemorrhage and oedema have been noted in the brain. These might be caused by a rapid increase in the venous pressure, following compression of the chest and abdominal venous reservoirs by the pressure wave. With this transmission of pressure into the cerebral venous system, small blood vessels may rupture. Another postulate is that pressurizing the air in the alveoli, or rupture of alveoli, may result in the production of air emboli. Air has been demonstrated in the cerebrovascular system of animals who were in the upright position during the blast.

> Brain damage is thought to be caused by a rapid rise in venous pressure following compression of the chest and abdomen by the pressure wave.

Late deaths result from the complications of respiratory, abdominal and neurological injuries. These include bronchopneumonia, peritonitis, coma and its sequelae.

## Clinical features

Information on the clinical features of underwater explosions in humans is mainly derived from case reports. Most of the physical parameters such as distance from the blast, intensity etc. are not known, and thus clinical correlation with the physical parameters is not possible. Autopsies are usually complicated by the effects of drowning and immersion.

A recent paper by Huller and Bazini (1970) gives a good outline of the literature on the subject and describes 32 casualties from an Israeli destroyer. While they were in the water they were exposed to blast from an exploding missile. Nineteen had both pulmonary and abdominal injuries. Five had only abdominal injuries and eight had only pulmonary injuries. It is not possible to determine if there was any physical reason for this distribution of symptoms.

**Table 25.1 Pulmonary symptoms and radiological findings**

| Pulmonary symptoms (27 patients) | Percentage |
| --- | --- |
| Haemoptysis | 56 |
| Dyspnoea | 41 |
| Abnormal auscultatory findings | 41 |
| Chest pain | 22 |
| Cyanosis | 19 |

| Radiological findings | Percentage |
| --- | --- |
| Mild to severe infiltrates | 100 |
| Pneumomediastinum | 22 |
| Haemothorax | 19 |
| Interstitial emphysema | 11 |
| Pneumatocele | 11 |
| Pneumothorax | 4 |

From Huller and Bazini (1970).

Twenty-four laparotomies were performed: 22 had tears of the bowel, 11 had subserosal bleeding in other parts of the bowel. In one case the perforations were only found at a second operation and in one case there was also a lacerated liver. One had an isolated rupture of the spleen, but this may have been due to an incident before the patient entered the water.

An unexpected finding was that four cases had ECG changes consistent with myocardial injury. Three cases died within 8 hours of operation from cardiorespiratory failure. One lasted 48 hours before dying from peritonitis and sepsis.

In other reports neurological involvement has been described. Abnormalities of consciousness, varying from a mild delirium to coma, have been reported. The patients may suffer severe headaches and there may be evidence of an upper motor neuron lesion.

There may also be interference with the spinal cord and the autonomic nervous system. It is possible that the paralytic ileus, which is quite common in this disorder, is at least partly due to a neuronal reflex phenomenon. Subdural haematomas have been reported. Pain has been reported in the testes and legs as well as the abdomen and chest.

## Management

Blast injuries cause severe body trauma. The patient must be admitted to hospital for observation, even though he may not appear seriously affected in the early stages. There are often no external signs of injury, such as bruising or lacerations, despite the internal damage. Exposure to altitude may aggravate or precipitate respiratory difficulties. Gastrointestinal perforations should also be considered before evacuating by air.

> *The patient may not appear to be seriously injured in the early stages and there may be no external signs of injury.*

The patient should have no oral intake and be maintained on intravenous fluids and gastric suction until the full extent of the damage has been assessed. The appropriate studies to ascertain the degree of lung or abdominal injury should be performed. When there are signs of peritonitis, such as rebound tenderness, rigidity or decreased bowel sounds, a decision has to be made regarding the possibility of surgical intervention and repair. Unfortunately, these signs may be due to the haemorrhagic lesions throughout the bowel, affecting the peritoneal cavity, and do not necessarily indicate a perforation. Before surgical exploration is performed, there should be a reasonable presumption of gastrointestinal perforation. Bleeding from the rectum is common, and is not itself an indication for surgery.

Bowel perforations presenting within the first 2 days are usually ragged, requiring resection and anastomosis. Later perforations normally develop from haematomas. They are generally clean-cut and may be oversewn.

> *Management is similar to that of severe body trauma from other causes.*

Treatment of the respiratory damage is based on general medical principles. Care must be taken in the use of positive pressure ventilation, although the administration of 100% oxygen is needed if there is significant hypoxaemia. It may also be of benefit in cases with signs of cerebral or cardiac air embolism.

Antibiotics and tranquillizers may be indicated, but care must be taken to avoid respiratory depression and the making of symptoms. Intravenous fluids and transfusions should be decided on the clinical state of the patient, serial haematological and biochemical studies.

If the signs of peritonitis continue despite the above regime, then surgery is probably needed. A perforated viscus may be present in the absence of radiological signs.

Hyperbaric oxygen therapy has been proposed to reduce cerebral oedema, eliminate cerebral bubbles and improve tissue oxygenation. Except in sophisticated hyperbaric units, it is likely to delay and complicate the cardiopulmonary support and gastrointestinal surgery.

## Prevention

The obvious measure is to avoid diving in areas where explosions are possible. If this is unavoidable, the diver should wear protective clothing. This may be a dry suit which gives the most protection. An air-containing vest gives some protection, because they reflect a great deal of the pressure pulse at the first water–air interface and absorb some of the remainder. If it is possible for the diver to reach the surface and float face up, the effect of the pressure wave will be decreased. If he is near the surface, the pressure wave may be attenuated by reflected waves.

> *Elevation of the chest and abdomen out of the water reduces the severity of blast injury.*

Lifting the chest and abdomen out of the water will lessen the effect of the blast. This is especially so if the swimmer can lie on some piece of debris or solid support. Facing away from the explosion is said to give some protection.

# Recommended reading and references

HULLER, T. and BAZINI, Y. (1970). Blast injuries of the chest and abdomen. *Archives of Surgery* **100**, 24–30.

MILLER, J.W. (Ed.) (1979). US *NOAA Diving Manual*. US Department of Commerce.

SHILLING, C.W., WERTS, M.F. and SCHANDELMEIER, N.R. (Eds) (1976). *The Underwater Handbook, A Guide to Physiology and Performance for the Engineer*. New York: Plenum.

WOLF, N.M. (1970). *Underwater Blast Injury: A Review of the Literature*. US Navy Submarine Research Laboratory Report Number 646.

# 26

# Sudden (cardiac) death syndromes

It is not the delicate, neurotic person who is prone to angina, but the robust, the vigorous in mind and body, the keen ambitious man, the indicator of whose engine is always set 'full speed ahead'.

William Osler

## Introduction

There is little doubt that the immediate cause of many scuba fatalities is either myocardial infarction or a serious cardiac dysrhythmia. This is increasing in frequency, possibly due to the increasing age of the diving population.

It would be too easy to dismiss the 12% (or up to 21%) of deaths in scuba divers as just cardiac disease. Unfortunately, such an over-simplification, although appropriate for the death certificate, does not give a full understanding of the dynamic progress of events. It belittles the complexities and inter-relationships between the diver, his equipment and the environment.

Diving induces a series of stresses which may interfere with cardiac function, affecting the conducting system, coronary blood supply or efficient muscular contraction. Environmental factors result in a reduction of blood volume, either tachycardia or bradycardia, hypertension and an increased work of the heart.

Dysrhythmias, including various degrees of heart block, ventricular tachycardia and fibrillation, further reduce the efficiency of the heart's ability to supply an adequate blood flow, in the face of the heavy physiological demands imposed by the environment.

Exceeding the coronary arteries' ability to supply the myocardium with oxygen may result in coronary insufficiency and myocardial ischaemia, causing myocardinal infarction. Although this is possible with normal coronary arteries, it is much more likely when the diver has reached an age at which coronary pathology has developed. This pathology may have been otherwise undetected, in the absence of this excessive stress.

The following summary is based on the investigations into sudden death in scuba diving by Eldridge (1979). A substantial number of middle-aged males suddenly and inexplicably lost consciousness and died while scuba diving in cold water. The behaviour of the victims, the ineffectiveness of resuscitation and the timing of the brain damage and death suggest a cardiac dysrhythmia as the underlying cause. Most of the victims had either previous cardiovascular symptoms such as hypertension or dysrhythmia and/or showed significant coronary artery stenosis or pathology at autopsy. Her report concluded with a plea for physicians conducting diving medical examinations to be aware that minor cardiac irregularities may preface major problems to people diving in cold water.

After detailed assessment of the case histories, the following observations were made. The victim often appeared calm just before his final collapse. Some were unusually tired or resting, having previously exerted themselves, or were being towed at the time – suggesting some degree of exhaustion. Some acted as if they did not feel well before their final collapse. Some complained of difficulty in breathing only a few seconds before the collapse, others under water signalled that they needed to buddy breathe, but rejected the offered regulator. Explanations for the dyspnoea include psychogenic hyperventilation and pulmonary oedema – the latter being demonstrated at autopsy. Currently, this is one of the newly developing diseases of diving medicine. The hypotheses used to explain it are often based on anecdotes or conjectural data. Some victims lost consciousness without giving any signal to their buddy; others requested help in a calm manner.

Most of the autopsies revealed a stenosis of at least 50% of a coronary artery. Some showed a 100% blockage and others had evidence of infarction. Victims who did not have substantial arteriosclerosis often had pre-existing hypertension. Pulmonary oedema, to a degree frequently associated with left ventricular failure, was seen in some of the cases. A few had medical records of cardiac symptoms such as dysrhythmias and one had had coronary bypass surgery.

Case report analyses suggested that the diagnosis of drowning was over-emphasized, it being a consequence of the environment in which the disorder occurred, rather than an aetiological factor. It is very likely that these cases of sudden death are similar to others associated with swimming and cold water immersion. It is probable that they are related to other sudden death syndromes in sports such as in squash, athletics etc., although in these particular environments there is much more opportunity to desist and obtain relief from physical stress, and for subsequent resuscitation, than in the water.

The data were supported by the research of McDonough and his colleagues showing strikingly higher frequencies of dysrhythmias when scuba diving. These included both supraventricular and ventricular premature contractions and dysrhythmias. Breath-holding and facial immersion produced other dysrhythmias, and was considered to identify susceptible individuals.

Autonomic nerve control of the heart, either by overactivity or imbalance, is thought to be responsible for most of the dysrhythmias of diving. Many of the diving activities involve an increase in sympathetic tone on the heart. Others induce parasympathetic effects.

The likelihood of provoking a cardiac incident is related to the number and severity of **trigger factors**. Some of these are:

1. Exercise.
2. Personality and psychological factors.
3. Cold.
4. Reflexes associated with diving.
5. Hyperbaric conditions.
6. Immersion and aspiration.
7. Electrolyte and pH changes.
8. Drugs.
9. Pre-existing cardiac disease.

# Cardiac stress factors

## Exercise

Perhaps the most famous example of death due to exercise is that incorrectly attributed to the famous athlete Pheidippides (490 BC). A young Greek soldier ran from the battlefield of Marathon to the city of Athens, delivering news of victory over the Persians, and then dropped dead. The feat is commemorated by the present-day marathon which is an athletic event of 26 miles' distance.

The increased parasympathetic (vagal) tone associated with fitness training may make the fit individual more susceptible to a variety of atrial dysrhythmias. Alternatively, fatigue is more likely in unfit individuals and has been shown to be a dangerous factor in those susceptible to dysrhythmias.

Increased cardiac output and heart rate do not produce blood pressure elevation on land, due to vasodilatation in the muscles and the skin. The latter is inhibited when the skin is exposed to cold water. The inclination to perform heavy work with elevated oxygen consumption is enhanced in the sea because of the more pleasant conditions. The diver rarely feels overheated and uncomfortable.

Vigorous exercise does not usually prevent, and may even intensify, the conventional diving bradycardia.

The metabolic acidosis and hypercapnia associated with extreme exercise, and the cardiorespiratory effects of diving which hinder carbon dioxide elimination, will aggravate any tendency to cardiac dysrhythmia. Myocardial hypoxia, a complication of inadequate cardiac output, will complicate this condition and both will predispose to myocardial ischaemia and sudden death.

Both clinically and on exercise provocation in the laboratory, dysrhythmias are often observed 5–10 minutes after the maximal effort, and are therefore more likely at the end of a dive.

## Personality and psychological factors

Although still contentious, it is likely that personality influences cardiac disease.

The **type A personality**, aged 35–55, still carries the same characteristics which resulted in his life successes as a younger man. He is a strong, controlled individual committed to achievement in both sporting and occupational activities, oriented to determination, courage and self-esteem. He exhibits 'time urgency', a busy man competing against both time and people. There is a tendency to hypertension. He is vigorous, physically fit and somewhat of an extravert, or at least appears to be so. Life is a challenge.

As a result of these personality characteristics, he may continue to practise and excel at physically demanding sports, such as squash, spear fishing etc., and take pride in his ability to equal or surpass his younger rivals in physical prowess. In a psychological context, he continues to prove his manhood through competitive activities. He differs from a type B personality who is easy going, does one thing at a time, feels satisfied and competent in his position, normotensive and has a lower incidence of heart disease.

Unfortunately, although the spirit is willing, hypertension increases and the coronary arteries become less patent as the years progress. Because this type A personality will subject himself to extreme levels of stress and not 'give in', he is likely to precipitate coronary insufficiency earlier, and in a more hazardous environment, than his less exciting contemporaries.

It is traditional to think of the type A personality as being aggressively male. With changes in social attitudes, female liberation has increased the potential for women to be trapped into this competitive and aggressive work and sport ethic.

**Anxiety** and the sympathetic response may have a deleterious effect on cardiac function, especially if there is already cardiac pathology. This is appreciated by physicians, and is well typified by the demise of John Hunter – the eminent pathologist and surgeon who inoculated himself with syphilis, believing it to be gonorrhoea, while performing research for his treatise on venereal disease. When confronting a particularly disturbing managerial committee of the hospital, he clutched his heart, stated 'Gentlemen, you have killed me' and slumped over the table dead.

If the diver believes that there is a threat to him, whether real or not, there will be an autonomic stress response. During this anxiety state a massive sympathetic discharge is present, with blood pressure reaching very high levels and causing excessive strain on the heart. Heart rates of up to 180 per minute can be produced and will reduce cardiac output, diminishing coronary blood flow proportionately.

The sympathetic autonomic response to stress can result in dysrhythmias, myocardial ischaemia and even sudden death in the presence of underlying cardiovascular disease.

Another form of psychic stress is the **vagal response** which produces exactly the opposite effects from the above, i.e. hypotension and bradycardia to the stage of cardiac standstill. This is analogous to the fainting or syncopal episodes of people who respond with an extremely exaggerated reaction to stress, e.g. fainting at the sight of blood, or on receipt of tragic news. The vagal response is a parasympathetic one, and could combine with other parasympathetic influences to cause an inappropriate cardiac inhibition in the aquatic environment, with unconsciousness leading to drowning. One such influence is the diving reflex, which is precipitated by exposure to cold, such as with cold water on the face.

## Cold

Any patient with angina pectoris will bear witness to the deleterious effects of cold in aggravating his condition. In the case reports on exercise stress precipitating cardiac death during scuba diving, a common factor was the association with cold water. Cold can produce a variety of cardiac insults, with various types of responses (see Chapter 22).

During cold water immersion, there is usually an increase in the sympathetic activity, as indicated by a rise in circulating noradrenaline, concurrent with or just preceding the release of adrenaline from the adrenal glands. The sympathetic activity will be responsible for the increase in heart rate, systolic blood pressure and ventilation. The deleterious effect on cardiac efficiency may be very significant. An increase in the diastolic blood pressure is also possible, but not invariable. It may be overridden by the adrenaline effect which at physiological levels causes a drop in the diastolic pressure. The sympathetic response is observed to be greater in subjects who are physically unfit and who have not adapted to cold water exposure.

Sudden death from a parasympathetic reflex can be associated with a vagal arrest of heart action, following inhalation of water into the nasopharynx and on the glottis. There is also thought to be a reflex following cutaneous stimulation from cold, producing coronary spasm or sudden death in people who are immersed in very cold water. Another cutaneous reflex induces considerable hyperventilation, sufficient to reduce carbon dioxide tension in the arterial blood, to levels which have been associated with the ventricular fibrillation in both animals and human beings.

In general, the degree of the 'diving reflex' bradycardia is greater with lower water temperatures. With the development of hypothermia, the myocardium becomes hyperexcitable, and is susceptible to episodes of ventricular extrasystoles, tachycardia and fibrillation. This becomes more frequent in the late stages and during rewarming.

Peripheral vasoconstriction will result in central pooling of the blood, with diuresis, and associated fluid and electrolyte loss.

## Reflexes associated with diving
### Diving reflex

In diving mammals, the diving reflex is accompanied by intense peripheral and visceral vasoconstriction (except in the heart and brain) and a dramatic reduction in cardiac output. This combination of effects results in a maintenance of normal arterial blood pressure, a reduction of heat loss and a conservation of oxygen, with a shunting of blood to the vital organs, the heart and brain.

In humans, the diving reflex is more rudimentary and undeveloped. Although there is a diving bradycardia, it is often complicated by the development of idioventricular foci producing ectopic beats. ECG abnormalities are frequent during or after the dive. T-wave inversion, premature ventricular excitation and atrial fibrillation, together with other irregularities and dysrhythmias, are common. They reflect inhibition of vagal rhythms and interference with atrioventricular conduction. Hong et al. showed an incidence of cardiac dysrhythmias in the Korean Ama women divers, increasing from 43% in summer (water tempe-

27°C) to 72% in winter (water temperature 10°C).

The drop in cardiac output noted in the diving mammals is seen to only a slight degree in humans. The intense vasoconstriction of the peripheral vessels resulting when a person is immersed in cold water is not compensated for by a proportional drop in cardiac output, and therefore there is a significant rise in arterial blood pressure.

The diving reflex may well have some protective value in the drowning situation. It has been used in the treatment of paroxysmal atrial tachycardia. Nevertheless, it is possible that it may contribute to the otherwise inexplicable diving deaths.

### Carotid sinus syndrome

This disorder is frequently observed, although often not recognized as such, by divers whose wet suit or close-fitting dry suit applies pressure to the carotid bifurcation. The neck constriction is especially noted with wet suit tops which are pulled over the head. Bradycardia and hypotension are produced reflexly resulting in a sensation of fainting, dizziness or even convulsions.

The extent of the relationship of the carotid sinus syndrome to sudden deaths in scuba divers is not yet clarified. Certainly, the cardiovascular effects are dramatic and the disorder is not uncommon among divers who wear tight-fitting 'pullover' wet suits. It also increases in frequency and severity with advancing age. Occasionally divers in great distress will be seen pulling the neck of the wet suit away from the throat, and sometimes this is done prior to the loss of consciousness. The carotid sinus reflex was incriminated in only one of 100 well-documented deaths in the ANZ series, but in others there were complaints of dyspnoea and tight-fitting wet suits, which could well be related to this syndrome.

### Other cardiac reflexes

A variety of other reflexes influence dysrhythmias, some having the afferent stimuli from skin or mucosal areas (e.g. the pharynx) and others associated with breath-holding, Valsalva manoeuvres and exercise. A French electrocardiographic study into experienced breath-hold divers, reaching a maximum of 15 metres in 28°C water during repeated diving, showed the expected bradycardia but also dysrhythmias in six of the ten. The atrial dysrhythmias were frequently multiple, and the ventricular dysrhythmias were often bigeminal.

### Hyperbaric exposure

Pacemaker automaticity, conduction and repolarization are all affected by hyperbaric exposure.

Experiments on subjects with prolonged exposure to hyperbaric air, between 2 and 132 feet (0.6–39.6 m) of equivalent sea water depth, in a dry chamber, verified that the hyperbaric air caused an increase in parasympathetic tone of sufficient magnitude to induce cardiac dysrhythmias. Hyperoxia is one cause of this, and nitrogen has been incriminated as a cause of beta blockade. Associated with the reduction in heart rate and the increase in Q–T interval in the ECG, asymptomatic supraventricular dysrhythmias (generally atrioventricular nodal escape rhythms) were seen in 10% of the subjects.

### Immersion and aspiration

An immediate reflex from immersion causes a sudden and temporary increase in cardiac output and stroke volume, each by up to 100%, before stabilizing at a lower level.

Immersion counters the effect of gravity and expedites fluid transport from the tissues and vessels of the limbs, increasing the cardiac return, the central blood volume, the work load on the heart and the possibility of coronary insufficiency. It may also subsequently lead to water and electrolyte loss from the body, and then an increased susceptibility to syncopal episodes. 'Negative pressure' breathing – a result of immersing the body but breathing through a snorkel, from the atmosphere – also increases the diuretic effect of immersion.

Aspiration of sea water produces some immediate reflex changes, and and also some delayed effects on pulmonary gas exchange – often with a significant drop in arterial oxygen and variable responses in arterial carbon-dioxide levels (see Chapter 21).

## Electrolyte and pH changes

Many of the effects noted above will influence the cardiac contractility and efficiency. The influence of exercise on both pH and metabolic biochemical changes has been mentioned. The production of hypocapnia following cold water stimulation and hyperventilation, diuresis and changes of blood volume from the effects of immersion, and the effects of salt water aspiration, will all ultimately act towards altering the internal composition. These effects will be aggravated when superimposed on pathological changes of age and disease.

Acidosis, produced by the effects of exertion, breathing against a resistance (regulator and increased gas density) and carbon dioxide accumulation, reduces the ventricular fibrillation threshold and depresses myocardial contractility. Underwater exertion, while breathing through scuba regulators, has been shown to produce end-tidal carbon dioxide levels of above 70 mmHg.

The interrelationships of many of the above factors may lead to either cardiac dysrhythmias or myocardial ischaemia. The dysrhythmia is made more likely by the occurrence of sympathetic and parasympathetic stimuli separately or combined, when there is a potentiation that is more than merely a summation of effects. The ischaemia may be due to diminished cardiac output, coronary occlusion or spasm, and increased metabolic demands of the myocardium.

## Drugs (see also Chapter 31)

Certain drugs are likely to increase the possibility of cardiac events during diving. They include the following:

- Alcohol.
- Nicotine – cigarette smoking.
- Caffeine – coffee
- Sympathomimetics – stimulants such as nasal decongestants and asthma medications.
- Beta-blockers – antihypertensive drugs.
- Calcium channel blockers – antihypertensive drugs.
- Cocaine – social and metabolic stimulation.

Many of the antihypertensive drugs cause an interference in autonomic regulatory control of the heart rhythms, reduced exercise tolerance, exertional syncope, syncope when climbing from the water and increased restriction of the airways (especially from beta-blockers).

As demonstrated with quinidine and its derivatives, antidysrhythmic drugs can become prodysrhythmic, under certain circumstances. These effects have recently been explained. They may affect the original dysrhythmia by increasing its incidence, its frequency or its haemodynamic consequences. They may also induce new dysrhythmias due to their effect on re-entrant circuits, or torsades de pointes due to marked QT prolongation. They may produce more bradycardia and increased ectopic beats, triggering the induction of spontaneous clinical re-entrant dysrhythmias.

This has been observed with beta-blockers. The calcium channel blockers and the beta-blockers have some characteristics in common. They both induce a bradycardia, aggravating the reflex and the metabolic effects mentioned above. A ventricular rhythm breakthrough is then possible. In both cases the ventricular dysrhythmias are more likely if the diver has coincidental or occult coronary artery disease or conductive abnormalities. There is inadequate clinical experience with use of the anticholinesterase inhibitors by divers to draw conclusions.

Cocaine is already infamous for its ability to cause ventricular dysrhythmias and sudden death, even in young fit athletes.

## Pre-existing cardiac disease

In younger divers, the presence of myocarditis (often associated with generalized infections) or hypertrophic cardiomyopathy may predispose to the sudden death syndrome. Many conduction abnormalities and other cardiac diseases are likewise a source of concern if there is any increased likelihood of dysrhythmias or ischaemia.

With increased age, there is a development of pathology which produces myocardial infarction and cardiac dysrhythmias.

The rise in heart rate is an integral part of the cardiovascular response to exercise. However, in the transition from rest to exercise, older individuals do not adapt as well, having a less adequate increase in both heart rate and cardiac output. Occasionally tachy-cardia may be excessive and result in a decrease in efficiency by interfering with venous return and thereby reducing cardiac output.

Some divers continue diving despite them having known cardiac disease, and these patients are likely to have increased risk of the sudden death syndrome. This results from both the disease entity being aggravated by the dive and drugs being taken. Following myocardial infarction, the likelihood of dysrhythmias is increased. Underwater swimming has been shown to increase extrasystoles in these patients. Also, the awareness of angina is rare under water, compared to an equivalent land exercise with similar ST depression.

The increased freqency of infarction and dysrhythmias, following coronary bypass surgery, is observed even on land.

The investigations in questionable cases include maximal stress electrocardiography, 24-hour Holter monitoring, and echocardiography.

For assessment of cardiac fitness for diving see Chapter 35.

## Breath-hold diving

The dysrhythmias identified with breath-hold diving are mainly those of alterations in respiratory patterns, submersion, exercise and cold exposure. Many of these may have implications for scuba diving.

Dysrhythmias are found even in common respiratory manoeuvres, such as deep inspiration, prolonged inspiration, breath-holding and release of breath-holding. The effects of breathing against resistances, skip breathing and the change of respiratory patterns which occur with snorkel and scuba diving are presumably related, but have yet to be investigated.

Submersion increases the central blood volume, and elevates arterial pressure and stroke volume.

The exercise of swimming fast under water for 50 metres produces a heart rate of about 55 beats per minute. This requires an oxygen consumption of five to ten times the resting level, and would have caused a rate of about 180 beats per minute on land!

The bradycardia of breath-hold diving is greatest when exercise is combined with cold water exposure. There are a dozen reports of the bradycardia being 20 beats per minute or less, with some at 10 or less.

## Unconsciousness

It has been postulated that transitory dysrhythmias, such as paroxysmal atrial tachycardia and reflex bradycardia, may induce unconsciousness while diving, without necessarily resulting in death. Environmental and physiological stresses may precipitate these abnormalities. The clinical significance and relevance of this observation to diving accidents awaits clarification.

**Syncopal episodes**, with the diver losing consciousness as he moves from the gravity-reduced environment of the ocean, often occur as he climbs the diving ladder or stands up in the boat. Unconsciousness (see Chapter 32) may be related to a variety of causes, such as:

- Peripheral venous pooling in the legs.
- Dehydration from the osmotic diuresis of immersion.
- Dehydration from hyperthermia.
- Vasodilatation from hypercapnia.
- Carbon monoxide toxicity.
- Oxygen off-effect, with rebreathing equipment.
- Hypoxia from any cause.
- Decompression sickness.
- Cerebral arterial gas embolism.
- Hypotensive drugs.
- Cardiac disease.
- Marine venoms.

## Pulmonary oedema

Immersion is known to increase the venous return (preload) to the heart and cold increases both this and the work of the heart (afterload) by vasoconstriction. The combination of immersion and cold exposure might therefore be expected to precipitate heart failure in those with impaired cardiac function.

Those cases with overt cardiac disease, especially with ischaemic heart disease, left heart failure from any cause or dysrhythmias as described above, would not be unexpected candidates for pulmonary oedema.

Diving diseases, discussed elsewhere in this text, including aspiration or drowning, pulmonary barotrauma, severe decompression sickness and some marine animal toxins, may also cause pulmonary oedema.

What is less expected is the observation of cardiac decompensation producing pulmonary oedema, without evidence of cardiac disease or other diving cause. In the series by Wilmshurst et al. (1989) of 11 such patients, 9 demonstrated a pathological vasoconstriction and 9 showed signs of cardiac decompensation when stimulated by cold. Follow-up many years later showed the development of hypertension in 7, Raynaud's phenomenon in 1 and atrial fibrillation in 1. There were no cardiovascular events and/or deaths. The case histories showed a relationship between the episode of pulmonary oedema and exposure to cold.

Another cause of pulmonary symptomatology, perhaps with pulmonary oedema, includes the occasional case of cold urticaria. This is a generalized disorder and can cause dyspnoea from the inhalation of cold air, because of the adiabatic expansion of gas from the scuba cylinder through the regulator.

## Acknowledgements

With acknowledgements to Professor A.A. Bove, Temple University, Philadelphia and Dr H.H. Rasmussen, Cardiology Department, Royal North Shore Hospital, Sydney for their comments and assistance in reviewing this chapter.

## Recommended reading

BACHRACH, A.J. and EGSTROM, G.H. (1987). *Stress and Performance in Diving*. San Pedro, CA: Best.

BONNEAU, A., FRIEMEL, F. and LAPIERRE, D. (1989). Electrocardiographic aspects of skin diving. *European Journal of Applied Physiology* **58**, 487–493.

BOVE, A.A. (1979). *Weekly Update on Hyperbaric and Undersea Medicine*. New Jersey, Biomedia Inc.

BOVE, A.A. (1990). In: *Diving Medicine*, edited by A. A. Bove and W.B. Davis. Philadelphia: Saunders.

ECKENHOFF, R.G. and KNIGHT, D.R. (1984). Cardiac arrhythmias and heart rate changes in prolonged hyperbaric air exposures. *Undersea Biomedical Research* **11**, 335–367.

EDMONDS, C. and WALKER, D. (1989). Scuba diving fatalities in Australia and New Zealand. The human factor. *SPUMS Journal* **19**(3), 94–104.

ELDRIDGE, L. (1979). Sudden death syndromes. *Proceedings of the Undersea Medical Society Meeting*, Miami, June, 1979.

FLETCHER, P.J. (1990). Antiarrhythmic or proarrhythmic: Editorial. *Australian Prescriber* **13** (1), 2–4.

LUNDGREN, C.E.G. and FERRIGNO, M. (Eds) (1987). *The Physiology of Breathhold Diving*. Washington: Undersea and Hyperbaric Medical Society.

McDONOUGH, J.R., BARUTT, B.S. and SAFFRON, R.N. (1987). Cardiac arrhythmias as a precursor to drowning accidents. In: *The Physiology of Breathhold Diving*, edited by C.E.G. Lundgren and M. Ferrigno. Washington: Undersea and Hyperbaric Medical Society.

MURRAY, W.B. (1986). Problems of the cardiovascular system in relation to diving. In *Diving and Submarine Medicine*, Chap. 20, edited by L. Terblanché. South African Navy, Simons Town.

PENTEL, P.R. and SALERNO, D.M. (1990). Cardiac drug toxicity *Medical Journal of Australia* **152**, 88–94.

ROSS, D.L. COOPER M.J., CHEE, C.K. et al. (1990). Proarrhythmic effects of antiarrhythmic drugs. *Medical Journal of Australia* **153**, 37–47.

SEM-JACOBSEN, C.W. and STYRI, O.B. (1970). EKG arrhythmias monitored from free swimming scuba divers. Proceedings: *Journale Internationale Hyperbarie et Physiologie Subaquatique*. Marseilles 8–11 June.

STRAUSS, M.B. (1973). *The Physician in Sports Medicine*, vol. 1, no. 1. New York: McGraw-Hill.

WILMSHURST, P.D., CROWTER, A., NURI, M. et al (1989). Cold induced pulmonary oedema in scuba divers and swimmers and subsequent development of hypertension. *The Lancet* **i** , 62–65.

YU-CHONG, L. (1990). Physiological limitations of humans as breathhold divers. In: *Man In The Sea*, vol. 2. chap. 2. San Pedro: Best.

# 27

# The ear and diving

## Introduction

An explanation is needed for the inclusion of a chapter on specialized clinical medicine in a diving medical text. Ear problems are the most common of all occupational diseases of diving, and so the diving physician should have a working knowledge of otology, both clinical and investigatory. It is not always possible to obtain specialist assistance at an early stage in the assessment of a diving accident, i.e. at the time when therapeutic decisions need to be made.

The ideal combination is, of course, a diving physician and an otologist who both have an understanding of the other's speciality and who work together. It is for the diving physician that this chapter is included.

## Pathophysiology

### External ear

#### Anatomy

The external ear comprises the pinna and the external ear canal, which captures sound waves and directs them to the middle ear – separated from the external ear by the ear drum or tympanic membrane.

The external ear canal is approximately 3 cm long; the outer third is surrounded by cartilage and the inner two-thirds by bone. It is lined by stratified squamous epithelium which tends to migrate outwards carrying casts of dead epithelial cells, foreign bodies such as dust and cerumen.

**Cerumen** or wax forms in the outer one-third of the canal. At body temperature, the wax has bacteriostatic fatty acids and produces a hydro-phobic lining which prevents the epithelium from being wetted, becoming soggy and there-by creating a culture medium for infections of the external canal – **otitis externa**. The pH of the external canal lining is usually slightly acidic, which also works as a bacteriostatic factor.

Interference with the function of the external canal can be produced by removal of the cerumen, either by **syringing of the ear**, long periods of **immersion**, or by **traumatic gouging** of the canal with cotton buds, finger nails, hair pins etc. The presence of cerumen or wax should not be an indication for external ear toilet or syringing. On the contrary, it is likely to increase the subsequent otitis externa if this is performed before diving. The normal protective mechanisms against organisms invading the external ear are presumably disrupted following disturbance of the cerumen layer by even the most careful ear toilet. The paediatricians' maxim to 'not put anything in your ear, smaller than your elbow', has much to commend it. By immersion, divers can lose most of the cerumen from their ears and it is very rare to see a subject, who is in frequent, diving practice, who has any significant amount of cerumen blockage, unless he wears a hood which prevents the entry of water.

During a diving medical seminar at Tahiti, a heated discussion ensued on the value of ear syringing to remove cerumen. Of the 44 divers present only 3 were required by a Club Mediter-anee physician to have cerumen removed from their ears, even though in none of these cases was the external ear obstructed. Otitis externa developed in four ears during the subsequent week, one bilateral and two unilateral, and these were in the three subjects who had their ears syringed. It demonstrated statistically what most of us knew clinically.

Avid swimmers and surfers will recognize their predisposition to otitis externa ('swim-mer's ear'). It becomes an occupational hazard in many cases and especially when the water is warm and the environment humid, e.g. in the Tropics ('tropical ear'). Many use prophylactic acetic acid or oil ear drops, both of which are of considerable value. The environmental heat and humidity within some saturation or hyper-baric complexes may also predispose to otitis externa, which has been the cause of suffering and the termination of major hyperbaric projects.

Those unfortunate patients with seborrhoeic dermatitis, often presenting as dandruff, may have episodes of external ear itchiness. If they respond to this by scratching the ear, they gouge out furrows of wax and excoriate the skin – breaking the two protective linings. Otitis externa often develops within hours. If they refrain from inflicting this trauma, and especially if they treat the inflammation and itch by the use of a non-water-based, anti-inflammatory steroid ointment (e.g. fluo-cortolone), then this unpleasant sequence of events does not eventuate.

Another reaction to aquatic irritation in the external ear canals is the development of **exostoses** – usually in three sites. Being oste-omas, they are very hard white masses and are tightly covered by epithelium. Sometimes they grow to such a size that they may occlude the external canal and cause a conductive deaf-ness. Under these conditions they may require removal by an otological surgeon. Less exten-sive lesions can still produce problems by blocking the drainage of cerumen, debris and water – predisposing to otitis externa. Conver-sely, the otitis externa may complete the par-tial occlusion of the canal, produced by the exostoses.

## Middle ear

The **tympanic membrane**, separating the external and middle ears, is a thin but tough and flexible conical membrane. It mirrors the pathology of both the external and the middle ear.

The middle ear is a gas-containing cavity separated from the external ear by the tympan-ic membrane, and the inner ear by the round window and oval window. Between the tympan-ic membrane and the oval window, three small bones are linked together – the ossicular chain, comprising the malleus, incus and stapes. They transmit the sound wave pressure on the ear drum to the fluid-filled inner ear.

The promontory and handle of the malleus can be seen impinging on the tympanic membrane. The incus is the middle bone and it articulates with the stapes, which in turn is attached by a strong fibrous band to the oval window. An inward movement of the oval window is transmitted through the inner-ear hydraulic system and reflected by a similar but opposite movement of the round window, outwards into the middle ear.

The middle-ear cleft extends into the mastoid air cells and the eustachian tube, and includes the middle-ear cavity. It is lined with mucosa which constantly absorbs oxygen from the enclosed space, thereby giving the middle ear a negative pressure (0–20 mmH$_2$O) relative to the environment. This is usually brought back to environmental pressure by the opening of the eustachian tube. This tube is 3.5–4.0 cm long and is directed downwards, forwards and medially from the middle ear to the nasopharynx. It is lined by respiratory epithelium and is subject to all the allergies, irritants and infections of this system.

The purpose of the eustachian tube is to maintain equal pressures across the tympanic membrane – between the middle ear and the environment. At the potential nasopharyngeal opening, the pressure is at environmental or ambient levels, whereas the middle-ear opening of the eustachian tube is at middle-ear pressure. If there is a continual blockage of the eustachian tube, the middle ear cannot be aerated regularly and therefore a significant negative pressure develops at a rate of 50 mmH$_2$O per hour, as oxygen is being absorbed from this cavity. This results in a retracted tympanic membrane and/or an effusion, both of which will partly reduce the negative pressure.

The eustachian tube usually opens once a minute while awake and every 5 minutes when asleep. Swallowing and yawning will commonly open this tube and allow replenishment of the gas to the middle ear from the nasopharynx, without any active or artificial overpressurization.

The eustachian tube may be opened actively by increasing the pressure in the nasopharynx by 50–250 mmH$_2$O in excess of the pressure in the middle ear. This commonly opens the eustachian tube and gas passes from the nasopharynx into the middle ear, alleviating the middle-ear negative pressure produced when the diver descends. If equalization of the pressures is not achieved during descent, by the time a gradient of 400–1200 mmH$_2$O is reached, this pressure may produce a locking effect on the valve-like cushions of the eustachian tube, preventing active or passive equalization of the pressures.

If the pressure in the middle ear for any reason exceeds that in the nasopharynx by 100–200 mmH$_2$O then the eustachian tube usually opens passively and gas passes from the middle ear into the nasopharynx. This mechanism is applicable when the diver ascends towards the surface.

It must be noted that the pressures above refer to pressure differences between the spaces mentioned. These should not be directly extrapolated to water depths, as there is considerable tissue movement and distortion which reduces some of the effects of ascent and descent. Thus a diver with a very mobile tympanic membrane, and a small volume middle-ear cleft, would be able to tolerate a much greater descent without experiencing any change in his middle-ear pressures. In practice it is found that, if the eustachian tubes are not open, the diver may experience some subjective sensation at a depth of 250 mmH$_2$O (1 foot or 0.3 m). Discomfort or pain may be noted when as shallow as 2 metres; this is also the depth at which the 'locking effect' may develop and the tympanic membrane may rupture at a depth varying between 2 and 10 metres.

Abnormalities of eustachian tube function in divers or other groups exposed to variations in pressure result in middle-ear barotrauma and indirectly in inner-ear barotrauma, with mucosal and membrane haemorrhage and ruptures. These clinical entities are dealt with under barotrauma (Chapter 10) and in the differential diagnosis of deafness and disorientation (Chapter 28).

## Inner ear

The inner ear is composed of the cochlea, a snail-like structure which is responsible for hearing, and the vestibular system responsible for the orientation of the animal in space, i.e. the sensation of acceleration, equilibrium, balance and positioning (Figure 27.1 and see Figure 10.4).

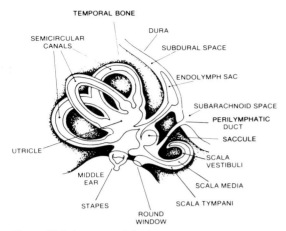

Figure 27.1 Anatomy of the inner ear

## Sound and hearing

The hearing part of the inner ear, the cochlea, is composed of three adjoining tubes or scalae:

1. The scala vestibuli (or inner tube) connected to the middle ear by the oval window membrane and the footplate of the stapes. It contains perilymph, which is similar in composition to extracellular fluid.
2. The scala tympani (or outer tube) – connected to the middle ear via the thin and fragile, but flexible, round window membrane. This also contains perilymph, which is continuous with that of the vestibuli. The vestibuli and the tympani communicate at the apex, the helicotrema.
3. The scala media (or middle tube) – lies between the other two channels, demarcated from the scala vestibuli by a fragile Reissner's or vestibular membrane. This separates the fluid of the two tubes but is so thin that it does not impede the pressure waves passing between them. Between the media and the tympani, there is the much thicker basilar membrane, which does impede sound waves and which supports the 25 000 reed-like basilar fibres, which are connected to the sound receptors called hair cells. Each sound frequency causes a vibration at a different sector of the basilar membrane. Near the oval and round windows the basilar fibres are short and rigid, and are sensitive to high frequency sounds, whereas further up the cochlea they become

longer and more flexible and respond to low frequency sounds. The fluid within the media is endolymph, similar in composition to intracellular find.

The integrity of the above membranes, together with the different composition and electrical potential of the inner ear fluids, are required for normal hearing.

Sound is caused by the vibration of an object in a compressible media, at frequencies between 20 and 20 000 cycles per second (20–20 000 hertz). It is transmitted to the ear by pressure waves in air or water. The external ear directs the sound waves to the tympanic membrane. This vibrates with the fluctuations of sound pressure and transmits these vibrations through the ossicular chain of the middle ear to the oval window, and thence to the cochlear fluid of the inner ear.

The tympanic membrane has a surface area 17–22 times that of the oval window. When a sound wave moves the tympanic membrane, there is a deflection of the oval window and a transmission of this pressure wave in the cochlear fluid, distorting the basilar membrane and triggering off the nerve impulses from the hair cells – thereby converting pressure waves into electrical impulses which are then passed to the brain via the eighth (auditory) nerve, where it is identified and interpreted as sound stimuli. The pressure wave disperses itself by distending the round window into the middle ear. Once the sound stops, the tympanic membrane no longer vibrates, the ossicular chain then moves to its resting position, the oval window, which is bound to the stapes by a thick fibrous band, resumes its neutral position, the cochlear fluid moves back to its normal position and the round window no longer distends into the middle ear.

The hair cells of the cochlea may also be stimulated by vibration of the bones of the skull. Sounds which cause this vibration and which are heard in this manner are transmitted by bone conduction. This method of hearing is less sensitive than the air condition pathway, but it is of importance for hearing under water. It is the pathway by which people with middle-ear damage hear.

Symptoms of cochlear impairment include tinnitus, dysacusis and hearing loss.

## Spatial orientation

The balance organ of the inner ear is called the vestibular apparatus and is made up of three loops termed the 'semicircular canals', positioned at right angles to each other, together with the utricle and the saccule. The membranous semicircular canals and the utricle are fluid-filled cavities with sensory end-organs able to detect movement of this fluid. They are responsible for supplying information to the central nervous system about acceleration and deceleration of the head through space. The end-organ in the utricle is responsible for supplying information about the position of the head in space and is influenced by gravity.

The vestibular system can only be understood as a very dynamic one with constant input from all areas at all times. The vestibular end-organs fire electrical discharges even in the resting state. If there is an increase in the stimuli in one area, then there must be a corresponding decrease in a complementary area on the other side, otherwise conflicting messages are received by the brain and are interpreted incorrectly. These impulses, giving information regarding position and movement in space, are transmitted to the brain by the vestibular part of the eighth cranial nerve.

The membranous labyrinth is somewhat like an inflated inner tube of an automobile tyre, and contains endolymph continuous with that of the scala media. Around the membranous labyrinth there is perilymph, which is continuous with the perilymph of the scala vestibuli and scala tympani, and is also connected to the cerebrospinal fluid by the perilymphatic or cochlear duct.

Vestibular damage may lead to symptoms of disorientation and imbalance, vertigo and associated vagal complaints such as nausea, vomiting, syncope etc. Nystagmus, the ocular movement with a quick and slow component, is an objective manifestation of vertigo. It, like vertigo, can be suppressed by other sensory input, cortical inhibition, drugs etc.

Vestibular injury may be irritating (increasing discharges) or, more commonly, destructive. If the vestibular system is damaged irreparably, the clinical features may diminish over the subsequent weeks or months, as the brain accommodates the inequality by suppressing responses from the undamaged side. Nevertheless, the damage can still be demonstrated by provocative tests (e.g. caloric electronystagmograms – ENGs) or movements (sudden head turning).

## Clinical otoscopy

Visual inspection of the external ear canal and tympanic membrane is one of the more valuable clinical examinations to be made on diving candidates. Otological disorders such as cholesteatoma may be diagnosed or there may be a condition, such as otitis externa, which is aggravated by diving, or a perforated tympanic membrane which makes diving unsafe. An external ear blockage predisposes to otological diving problems, and aural barotraumas are identifiable diving diseases. As well as identifying these clinical disorders, a major value of otoscopy is the verification of a successful middle-ear autoinflation (see page 121).

The tympanic membrane is viewed while the candidate attempts to inflate the middle ear by active manoeuvres (very commonly one ear remains consistently easier to autoinflate than the other). Physicians who have experience in diving medicine will spend considerable time ensuring that diving candidates understand the techniques and sensations experienced during middle-ear autoinflation. Inadequate middle-ear autoinflation is responsible for the most common and preventable of diving accidents – middle-ear barotrauma of descent.

In one Australian series, the tympanic membrane was viewed initially in 87% of cases, with 84% being mobile during the autoinflation. In the remaining 13%, 12% claimed subjective autoinflation. The otoscopic view was obstructed by cerumen in 9%, an unusual canal alignment or structure in 3% and extoses in 1%.

## Hearing assessments

### Clinical

The symptom of deafness is perhaps one of the most common encountered in diving medicine. In most cases, the complaint of deafness is not supported by conventional audiometric testing. The diver often refers to a feeling of 'fullness' or 'blockage' within the middle ear. This is probably a sensation associated with congestion and swelling of the tympanic membrane and mucosal lining of the middle-ear cavity. It is most commonly related to the middle-ear barotrauma of descent, which is described elsewhere, and normally resolves within a week.

Objective **hearing loss** may be of four types

1. **Conductive** due to problems of the conductive apparatus (external ear, tympanic membrane, ossicles, middle ear).
2. **Sensorineural** – when the problem lies in the cochlea or the auditory nerve.
3. **Central** – due to lesions of the auditory pathways in the brain, central to the cochlear nuclei.
4. **Mixed** – various combinations of the above. Usually it indicates a combination of conductive and sensorineural hearing loss.

The type of hearing loss can be inferred from the **patient's speech**. Soft but articulate speech associated with a moderately severe hearing loss is suggestive of conductive deafness. Loud clear speech suggests an acquired bilateral sensorineural hearing loss. Slurred, hesitant, inarticulate and inaccurate speech is more compatible with central lesions.

Impaired speech discrimination by the patient may be obvious during the interview. The otological examination may include the **tuning fork tests**. The Rinne test becomes abnormal when the fork is heard louder by bone conduction (fork held on the mastoid bone) than by air conduction (tuning fork placed over the auditory meatus). This indicates a 'conductive' deafness. A Bárány noise box may 'mask' the other ear during the tests, which may extend between 64- and 4096-Hz forks. The Weber test is performed with a 256- or 512-Hz fork. It is placed on the vertex of the skull and the subject indicates in which ear he hears the fork. He will hear it in the affected ear with conductive deafness, the unaffected ear with sensorineural deafness or both ears in mixed or bilateral deafness. Schwarbach's test is performed by comparing the patient's and the examiner's ability to hear the tuning fork tests by bone conduction.

## Hearing tests

In remote environments, use has to be made of even more primitive techniques. The ticking or alarms from a wrist watch, has a reliable sound intensity and frequency of considerable value. The frequencies are commonly about 4000–6000 Hz and this is the area that is less noticeable to the diver than the usual voice frequencies of 250–2000 Hz. Comparison is made between the diver's two ears and the examiner's. The finding that the watch can be heard only in one ear, or that the hearing acuity for the watch ticking is below that of the examiners, suggests that pure-tone audiometry is a very much needed next step. For divers who have subjective sensations of 'dullness', the hearing of the watch gives some reassurance to the examiner that a gross sensorineural loss is unlikely.

> *As a rough general indicator, for use in remote or isolated areas, an approximation of the diving accident victim's hearing can be made by:*
>
> - *Speech*
> - *Associated symptoms (tinnitus, vertigo etc.)*
> - *Hearing tests with watch and whispered speech*
> - *'Tuning fork' tests – Rinne, Weber and Schwarbach*

## Pure-tone audiometry

This measures the ability to hear pure tones in octaves between 125 and 8000 Hz (cycles per second). The hearing loss in each frequency is measured in decibels – a logarithmic scale which means that a loss of 10 decibels represents a ten-fold change in intensity of the noise, 20 decibels a 100-fold, 30 decibels a 1000-fold etc. Testing is carried out initially for air conduction, but, if this is significantly impaired, then bone conduction should be measured. With sensorineural deafness, the impairment is the same for both air and bone conduction.

If bone conduction is adequate and normal, then it infers that the cochlea is picking up sound waves transmitted via the bone, and therefore the sensorineural component of the hearing is normal. If there is a considerable discrepancy, with the air conduction being poor but the bone conduction normal, then this suggests that there is a 'conductive' deafness, i.e. involving the external or middle ear.

A very quiet area, usually a sound-proof audiogram booth, is necessary for reliable testing. With a severe unilateral deafness, sound levels of 40–60 dB can be heard by cross-hearing and therefore masking is needed in that ear while the damaged one is being tested above this level. As a general rule, conductive deafness tends to be first noted in the lower frequencies (250–2000 Hz), whereas the sensorineural damage is first noted somewhere in the range 4000–8000 Hz. If there is serious and significant nerve damage, then all frequencies will be involved.

More elaborate audiology, utilizing such devices and techniques as recruitment, brainstem and Békésy audiometry, short increment sensitivity index (SISI) and pure-tone decay are used by otologists – but are of little interest to the diving physician. Speech discrimination testing is probably of considerable value, especially in the more sophisticated diving medical establishments.

Perhaps the most valuable of all ear function tests is the comparison of repeated pure-tone audiograms. If these measurements are made prior to the diver commencing his hyperbaric experiences, and routinely carried out during his diving career, then any discrepancies can be readily detected.

It should also be performed immediately if there is any subjective complaint of hearing loss, or evidence of inner-ear disorder such as tinnitus, vestibular symptoms etc. Once evidence of sensorineural impairment is found, then repeated serial audiometry should be performed to ensure that deterioration does not supervene and that therapeutic measures are having their desired effect.

## Tympanometry

Indirect assessments of the function of the middle-ear cavity and the eustachian tube are obtained from most of the otological investigations. Techniques to measure directly the middle-ear pressures and movements have recently been made available to clinicians – although for some reason diving physicians have been slow to appreciate the value of these developments. Perhaps the explanation for this reluctance lies in an understanding of the history and the difficulty in applying the tympanometry techniques in non-specialized laboratories and in non-expert hands. If so, there is no reason to continue this reluctance since the development of the impedance or acoustic audiometer.

The tympanometer or acoustic impedance meter (impedance audiometer, admittance audiometer) is now clinically available. It is designed to facilitate the quick, objective testing of middle-ear function, measuring the mobility of the middle-ear system (usually called compliance), the pressure within the middle-ear cavity and the variation in middle-ear mobility reacting to variations of pressure from −300 to +300 mmH$_2$O applied in the external ear. It can also react to an autoinflation of the middle ear through the eustachian tube – and herein lies its specific value to the diving clinician.

A graph produced on an $xy$ plotter is termed a 'tympanogram', with the peak height on the $y$ axis showing the degree of compliance and the position on the $x$ axis showing the middle-ear pressure. Both of these may be of considerable interest to the diving physician, as it is possible to change the middle-ear pressure with either the Valsalva or the Toynbee manoeuvre (or others referred to in Chapter 10 and Figure 27.3).

The middle-ear pressures, recorded as the position of the tympanogram peak on the $x$ axis, changes with different diving environments and accidents. There is a decrease of middle-ear pressure when 100% oxygen is breathed, or alternatively the increase in

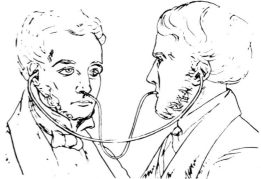

**Figure 27.2** Toynbee (on right) blowing air into eustachian tube catheter and listening for the movement of the patient's tympanic membrane on the same side

middle-ear pressure when helium/oxygen (Heliox) is breathed. In the first case, nitrogen is lost and oxygen is absorbed very rapidly from the middle ear, and this is one of the causes of serous otitis media with oxygen-breathing divers. The increase in middle-ear pressure while breathing Heliox is due to the rapid movement of helium as compared to nitrogen and therefore the helium moves into the middle ear faster than the nitrogen moves out. This results in at least a temporary increase in middle-ear pressure. As the oxygen percentage is increased and the helium reduced, there is a cancelling of the above effects.

Pathological conditions which may cause a positive pressure peak are: acute otitis media in the very early stages, middle-ear barotrauma of descent (after subsequent ascent), following haemorrhage and exudation in the middle ear, and during overpressure from middle-ear barotrauma of ascent (Figure 27.4).

A negative pressure peak may develop with middle-ear barotrauma of descent (ear squeeze), while still at depth. Negative pressure peaks are related to poor eustachian tube function and associated absorption of gas from the middle-ear cavity. This may result in effusion and, if the middle ear contains a significant amount of fluid, the pressure peak may disappear and the tympanogram becomes flat.

Middle-ear barotrauma of descent, which produces congestion and swelling within the middle ear, will produce a decreased peak within the tympanogram, demonstrating a drop in compliance. This rises as the structures and lining of the middle ear return to normal.

With perforation of the tympanic membrane, no pressure gradient can exist between each side, and therefore there is no peak. This information is used clinically to show the patency of grommets (ventilation tubes) inserted into the tympanic membrane, but may also be of value to demonstrate perforated tympanic membranes which cannot be seen otoscopically.

Tympanograms, with increased amplitude or notches, may be due to an ear-drum abnormality as well as ossicular discontinuity. The examples of increased amplitude or notching of the tympanogram may be seen with healed perforations and a W-shaped pattern is commonly

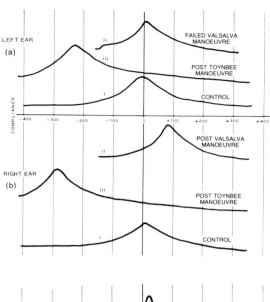

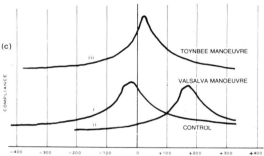

**Figure 27.3** 'Diving' tympanogram: the tympanometry demonstration of the effect of Valsalva and Toynbee manoeuvres on middle-ear pressures. (a) Left ear: (i) normal control tympanogram, passing from $-400$ mmH$_2$O on the left to $+300$ mmH$_2$O on the right (note: opposite to the conventional technique). (ii) Valsalva manoeuvre attempted at the neutral position (peak of control tympanogram) and a repeat tympanogram from $-100$ mmH$_2$O to $+300$ mmH$_2$O shows no substantial movement of the peak, i.e. middle-ear pressures were not influenced by the procedure. Valsalva manoeuvre failed! (iii) Toynbee manoeuvre performed at $+300$ mmH$_2$O, with the subsequent tympanogram showing a 225 mmH$_2$O negative pressure being produced in the middle ear. Toynbee manoeuvre successful. (b) Right ear: (i) normal control tympanogram; (ii) Valsalva manoeuvre produced a 80 mmH$_2$O positive pressure in the middle ear; (iii) Toynbee manoeuvre at $+300$ mmH$_2$O produced a 280 mmH$_2$O negative pressure to the middle ear. Toynbee manoeuvre successful. Note: for patient tolerance, the technique has been modified to extend between pressures $-300$ and $+300$ mmH$_2$O. (c) Diving tympanogram: performed as above. This tympanogram demonstrates an increase in middle-ear pressure from $-25$ mmH$_2$O (normal) to $+175$ mmH$_2$O with Valsalva manoeuvre and then a partially successful Toynbee manoeuvre – reducing the middle-ear pressure to $+25$ mmH$_2$O.

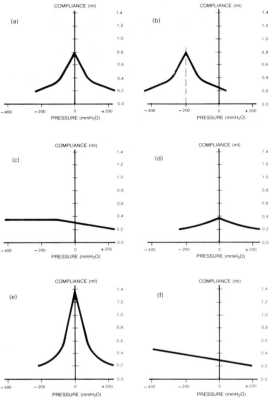

**Figure 27.4** Diagrammatic tympanogram responses: (a) normal; (b) negative middle-ear pressure, e.g. eustachian tube obstruction; (c) fluid-filled, middle-ear cavity, e.g. haemorrhage from severe middle-ear barotrauma; (d) reduced compliance, e.g. otosclerosis or mucosal congestion in the middle ear from barotrauma; (e) increased compliance seen with disarticulation of the ossicles, scarred or very mobile tympanic membranes; (f) perforated tympanic membrane

observed. Ossicular chain discontinuity may produce deep and multiple notches.

The presence of a respiratory wave in the tympanogram suggests a continuously open eustachian tube, an occasional sequela of middle-ear barotrauma, especially with overforceful Valsalva manoeuvres.

A way of verifying inner-ear fistula, which is currently under investigation, integrates an impedance audiometer and an electronystagmogram (ENG) with both horizontal and vertical leads. The induction of nystagmus during the external-ear pressure change may give some support to the diagnosis, but should only be performed if facilities exist for immediate inner-ear surgery – if the procedure

enlarges the fistula. This application remains only a research tool at this stage and is not recommended for general usage.

### Edmonds' diving tympanogram (see Figure 27.3)

For eustachian tube assessments on divers, a tympanogram is performed, with the pressure in the external ear passing from −300 to +300 mmH$_2$O and this is used as a control. The pressure in the external ear is then moved to zero and a Valsalva manoeuvre is performed by the subject. A tympanogram is then repeated moving from −100 to +300 mmH$_2$O and if the Valsalva manoeuvre has been successful this will demonstrate a significant movement of the peak, illustrating the increase in the middle-ear pressure due to the Valsalva manoeuvre forcing more gas into this cavity. At the completion of this second tympanogram, at +300 mmH$_2$O, the subject is then asked to perform the Toynbee manoeuvre and the third tympanogram is recorded, passing from +300 mmH$_2$O to −300 mmH$_2$O. If the Toynbee manoeuvre is successful, then the peak of the tympanogram will have returned towards the control or even beyond it to demonstrate a more negative middle-ear pressure.

This allows an objective way of measuring the effects of autoinflation and deflation on the middle ear during simulated conditions of descent and ascent. This technique is somewhat different to the conventional one. The modification is carried out to ensure that inadvertent opening of the eustachian tube – and consequent release of post-Valsalva pressure – is not produced by the excess external-ear pressure induced during the traditional procedure.

It can be seen from the above that the impedance audiometer is a valuable instrument for use in both the clinical and research aspects of diving medicine.

## Disorientation under water

### Introduction

The diver needs an accurate appreciation of his orientation, depth and distance from boat or shore, to enable him to return safely. With the advent of free and scuba diving without an attachment to the surface, the importance of **spatial orientation** under water has increased.

Under terrestrial conditions, spatial orientation depends mainly on information from three systems: visual, proprioceptive and vestibular. The visual system usually dominates the other two, unless there is abnormal sensory input, or gross damage or stimulation of the other systems.

Even under good diving conditions, it is likely that there will be a severe interference to the diver's visual cues, and they are lost in adverse circumstances such as in murky water or at night. Proprioceptive information is seriously distorted or reduced by the loss of gravity cues. Under diving conditions of neutral buoyancy, much of the gravity-induced proprioceptive input is lost and either insufficient or inaccurate information may be available for the diver to perceive his relative position under water. An extraordinary significance may then be placed on vestibular responses – greatly in excess of that customary on land. This is aggravated if the vestibular stimulation is increased, as is likely to happen in the aquatic dysbaric environment.

If vertigo occurs to such a degree that the diver cannot compensate, or if it is associated with vomiting, visual disturbances or unconsciousness, then his safety will be seriously impaired.

> *Awareness of body position in space involves integration of visual, proprioceptive and vestibular input information.*

With experience, certain clues to spatial orientation are available to the diver. He will realize that his exhaust bubbles, which can often be felt on the skin, are moving towards the surface. In certain positions his inhalation or exhalation may be expedited, especially with the use of twin hose regulators and rebreathing equipment requiring a counterlung. Inhalation is easier if the counterlung is below the diver in the water. If the counterlung and relief valve are above the diver then it is easier to exhale.

Heavy objects with negative buoyancy, e.g. weight belts, pressure gauge, knife etc., still obey gravity and press or fall downwards. Buoyancy compensators pull upwards. Gas spaces within the body can be felt to expand during ascent and contract during descent; this may be noted in the diver's lungs, middle ear or face mask. When the diver is immobile his legs will tend to sink and his chest to rise – fins which are negatively buoyant accentuate this tendency. These clues are of immense value to the alert, experienced and composed diver, but are ignored by the trainee or during a panic situation.

> *Diving reduces visual and proprioceptive input thus placing greater reliance on the vestibular system.*

The most likely cause of disorientation under water is the reduction of sensory input. With greatly impaired vision and reduced proprioception in an unfamiliar environment, disorientation is more likely. Also, in contrast to the situation on land, there is an added dimension of vertical movement. This becomes important when the diver has lost sight of the sea bed, and is distant from the surface. Other sensory inputs are also modified, e.g. the speed of sound is increased, making localization and discrimination much more difficult.

This lack of orientation is independent of the vestibular system, and occurs under predictable environmental conditions, e.g. at night, diving in murky water, diving without a companion, buddy line, surface line or boat contact, or diving far from the surface, sea bed or other marine objects. Under these conditions the diver may become disoriented and also develop symptoms of an agoraphobic reaction (see Chapter 29), a sensation of depersonalization, derealization or isolation, associated with anxiety which may extend to panic. Frequently, the diver overcomes this by visual fixation on objects that are associated with him, such as a companion diver, a buddy or surface line, a compass etc. The syndrome can be prevented by avoiding the conditions mentioned above, and may be corrected by swimming to the surface, the seabed or along ledges.

**Psychological** factors are believed to play a considerable part in disorientation. Neuroticism, and its associated anxiety state, may result in neglect of many of the orientation clues that have been learnt, and may interfere with an appreciation of the significance of these.

Disorientation, as an early manifestation of a toxic–confusional state, is a characteristic feature of breathing **abnormal gas pressures**, e.g. carbon dioxide toxicity, hypocapnia, oxygen toxicity, hypoxia, nitrogen narcosis, high-pressure neurological syndrome, carbon monoxide toxicity etc. These toxicities are mentioned elsewhere, and are verified by an appraisal of the diving profile, and examination of the breathing gas mixtures. Disorientation in these states, although it may be of extreme importance as an early symptom, is usually overshadowed by the subsequent events – unconsciousness or drowning.

In other diving accidents, there may also be a prodromal sensation of disorientation, but this becomes obliterated with the impairment of cerebral function. Such instances are seen with pulmonary barotrauma, decompression sickness, syncope of ascent etc.

## Vestibular disease

When the disorientation of the diver is due to a disorder of the vestibular system, it is commonly a transient and mild effect resulting from the unequal stimulation of the two labyrinths (caused by pressure changes, caloric changes etc). Under these conditions, the disorder may persist for as long as the unequal stimuli remain, or perhaps a few minutes longer. During this period, however, accidents may be produced either directly from the effects of vertigo, disorientation, nausea or vomiting, or because of the dive profile.

Other peripheral vestibular disorders may be more severe and longer lasting, e.g. for weeks until central compensatory mechanisms suppress the unequal vestibular responses. This may be seen in the decompression sickness associated with deep and helium diving and the more common effects of labyrinthine window fistulae, from middle-ear barotrauma. Under these conditions, the clinical effects may be catastrophic and endanger even the habitat or

saturation diver – let alone the free swimming, recreational scuba diver.

Central neurological disease, which interferes with vestibular and cerebellar connections, may produce very long lasting signs – but these are less common than the peripheral manifestation of vestibular disease in divers.

Once vestibular disease has developed, then a full otological investigation is indicated – both of middle-ear and inner-ear function, both auditory and vestibular.

Symptomatically, the diagnosis of peripheral vestibular disease may be indicated by a typical rotatory vertigo. More often in diving accidents it is less clear, and problems such as 'dizziness' and 'confusion' are described.

In true vestibular disease there is a nystagmus demonstrable at the time of the abnormal sensation – either during the causal incident or during its simulation in water and/or under hyperbaric conditions.

In diving accidents, the vertigo due to barotrauma may have a rotatory component, whereas that due to caloric (water irrigation) stimuli produces a pure horizontal or lateral nystagmus.

## Vestibular testing

Spontaneous nystagmus is an important sign of vestibular disorder. Positional vestibular testing refers to the effects of certain head, neck and eye positions in producing abnormal vestibular responses in some patients.

The Hallpike caloric tests were the traditional tests used to demonstrate the activity of the vestibular system stimulated by water at temperature of 30°C and 44°C, i.e. 7°C above and below body temperature, with the subject lying supine and his head elevated to 30 degrees. The temperature change causes convection currents in the horizontal or lateral semicircular canal and this stimulates the vestibular system. The response to hot and cold water on both sides is compared and conclusions are drawn as to whether there is unequal function of the two vestibular systems to identical stimuli and whether there is preponderance of responses to either side. The first suggests a peripheral lesion and the second a more central one.

In the event of no response from one side, greater stimuli may be given, e.g. iced water calorics (more practical than the standard calorics under most operational hyperbaric conditions) or even drug provocation such as intravenous methylamphetamine. With peripheral vestibular lesions, the eye movements are sometimes best observed by having the subject close his eyes and perform distracting exercises such as mental arithmetic. The eyes can then be seen rolling with fast and slow components, beneath the closed lids. These primitive techniques of assessing vestibular function in the field are rarely needed nowadays. Vestibular function assessment has been revolutionized by the addition of the ENG to detect spontaneous nystagmus and the effects of both positional and caloric provocation.

## Electronystagmogram

When there is an imbalance in the neural activity from the vestibular systems on each side, involuntary eye movements develop and are termed 'nystagmus'. This is the physical sign that corresponds to the sensation of vertigo; however, the exact relationship depends on the method of measuring the nystagmus.

If it is measured clinically, i.e. by observation or by the use of Frenzel glasses, then it is a crude sign and is associated with many false positive and negative results. If it is measured by electronystagmography, then it is not only a quantitative measure of the ocular movement, but it is also a sensitive measurement of vestibular dysfunction. The ENG is also far more sensitive than the clinical sensation of vertigo, and therefore depicts subclinical levels of vestibular disease. It may demonstrate asymmetry long after the symptoms have disappeared.

The electrical recordings are not dissimilar to those of an electroencephalogram, but the electrodes are positioned lateral to the outer canthus of each eye so that the movement of the eye causes a deflection on the recording paper. The reason this is produced is that the retina has a negative charge when compared to the cornea, and as the eyes move so does the electrical field, and this movement is recorded by the two electrodes.

In clinical practice, the conventional ENG is a graphic record of vestibular function made during positional tests and also during caloric stimulation – the Hallpike tests referred to above. Thus the horizontal electrodes are commonly used. In diving there is sometimes a rotatory nystagmus. Therefore, in diving research it is recommended that the tracings record both the horizontal movement and the vertical, i.e. as well as electrodes placed near the outer canthus of the eyes, there are also electrodes placed above and below one eye.

By the use of this very valuable and objective test (electronystagmography), vestibular dysfunction can be demonstrated and quantified. The duration of the nystagmus can be observed, reviewed and measured and the degree of nystagmus can be quantified by different parameters (rate, height and deflection of the slow and fast components). The vestibular responses can be stimulated in a provocative but selective manner by the use of the Hallpike caloric test, positional tests and even changing pressures – by altering the subject's ambient pressure in recompression and decompression chambers, or by the use of an impedance audiometer, referred to previously.

The use of this equipment has revolutionized our approach to vertigo and its relationship to diving, and has allowed us to clarify and verify clinical impressions, often demonstrating significant pathophysiology in cases which may otherwise have been classified as functional. It has an application as an electrodiagnostic procedure in recompression chambers, with the electrode leads under pressure and the equipment outside the chamber to assist in diagnosis and to monitor the effects of therapeutic agents such as recompression and gas mixture alterations.

ENGs may be used to differentiate end-organ (vestibular) disease from central (brain) causes of vertigo and dizziness. The ENG of peripheral vestibular end-organ disease produces a spontaneous nystagmus greater than 7 degree/s, due to a reduction in the tonic discharge from the affected vestibule. The nystagmus (fast phase) is thus towards the side of increased vestibular activity. It is strongest when the subject looks to the same side as the fast phase. It is suppressed by visual fixation (more than 40%) and augmented by eye closing and mental concentration (e.g. calculations).

## Acknowledgements

We would like to make acknowledgement to Professor J. Farmer, Duke University Medical Centre, USA, who has constructively criticized many of our reports on this subject, and whom the senior author has constantly referred to for guidance in this field. Similar acknowledgement is made to Dr John Tonkin, Sydney, and Dr Peter Freeman, Melbourne.

## Recommended reading

EDMONDS, C. (1971). Vertigo in divers. *Royal Australian Navy SUM Report* 1–71.

EDMONDS, C., FREEMAN, P., TONKIN, J., THOMAS, R. and

BLACKWOOD, F. (1973). *Otological Aspects of Diving.* Sydney: Australia Medical Publishing.

EDMONDS, C., PENNEFATHER, J. and BLACKWOOD, F. (1980). Manometric audiometry for the evaluation of Eustachian tube function. Royal Australian Navy, RANSUM Research Project Report 3/80.

ELNER, A., INGELSTEDT, S. and IVARSSON, A. (1971). A method
for studies of the middle ear mechanics. *Acta Oto-Laryngologica* **72**, 191.

GERSDORFF, M.C. (1977). Tubal-impedance-manometry. *Archives of Oto-Rhino-Laryngology* **217**, 319–407.

HOLMQUIST, J. (1976). In: *Acoustic Impedance and Admittance*, edited by A.S. Feldman and L.A. Wilber. Baltimore: William's & Wilkins.

INGELSTEDT, S., INVARSSON, A. and JONSON, B. (1967). Mechanics of the human middle ear. *Acta Oto-Laryngologica Supplementum* 228.

RIU, R., HOTTES, L., GIULLERMA, R., BADRES, R. and LEDEN, R. (1969). La trompe d'eustache dans la plongee. *Rev. Physiol. Subaquatique Med. Hyperbare* **1**, 194–198.

TJERNSTRÖM, O. (1973). On alternobaric vertigo – experimental studies. *Forsvarsmedicin* **9**, 410–415.

# 28

# Hearing loss and vertigo

## Hearing loss

### Introduction

The symptom of deafness is perhaps one of the most common encountered in diving medicine. In most cases, the complaint of deafness is not supported by conventional audiometric testing. The diver often refers to a feeling of 'fullness' or 'blockage' within the middle ear. This is probably the sensation associated with congestion and swelling of the tympanic membrane and mucosal lining of the middle-ear cavity. It is most commonly related to the middle-ear barotrauma of descent, which is described elsewhere (Chapter 10), and normally resolves within a week.

> *Dullness of hearing, dampening of sound, deafness and 'fullness' or 'blockage' within the ear are common symptoms reported by divers. The most common cause is middle-ear barotrauma of descent.*

Any hearing loss is confirmed by audiometric testing (see Chapter 27). This can be achieved by comparison of the diver's post-incident audiograms with the one which should have been performed prior the diver undergoing diver training, or previous annual audiograms if he is an experienced diver. For a more definitive assessment, air and bone conduction should be measured in the audiogram performed after the accident. A classification of the types of hearing loss can be made, based on whether it is predominantly conductive or sensorineural.

# Hearing loss in diving – aetiological classification

1. Conductive:
   (a) external ear obstruction
       (i) cerumen
       (ii) otitis externa
       (iii) exostoses
   (b) tympanic membrane perforation
       (i) middle-ear barotrauma of descent
       (ii) forceful autoinflation
       (iii) shock wave
   (c) middle-ear disease
       (i) middle-ear barotrauma of descent
       (ii) otitis media
       (iii) forceful autoinflation
       (iv) increased gas density in middle ear
       (v) ossicular disruptions
2. Sensorineural:
   (a) noise induced
   (b) decompression sickness
   (c) inner-ear barotrauma
3. Others: dysacusis

# Conductive deafness

## External-ear obstruction

This is not uncommon in divers. It is easily diagnosed both on history and on otoscopic examination. It is also a cause of vertigo induced by unequal caloric stimuli, i.e. the result of cold water entering one external ear more readily than the other. The causes are as follows.

## Cerumen plug

Conductive deafness may result from the movement of cerumen in the external ear, due to gas space alterations with diving. Water will cause swelling of the desquamated tissue and cerumen, possibly obstructing an external canal which was already partly blocked.

## Otitis externa

Infection is aggravated by immersion of the ear in water

## Exostoses

Exostoses may be single or multiple. Although rarely causing complete obstruction of the external canal by themselves, obstruction may result in the presence of cerumen or otitis externa.

## Tympanic membrane perforation

This is a not uncommon complication of diving. There is usually a well-defined reason, which is discussed later. The patient may complain of a hissing sensation or a feeling of air flowing through the tympanic membrane, especially when he autoinflates the middle ear, producing transient vertigo. There may be a hearing loss, mainly conductive, but usually of only 5–15 dB. The lower frequencies may be most affected. This hearing loss is rectified when the tympanic membrane is almost closed, and this may take a few days with small perforations, or weeks with larger perforations. Clinical management includes keeping the ear dry. Divers must be advised not to aggravate this disorder by exposing their middle ears to further pressure changes, e.g. by flying, diving, nose-blowing or autoinflation. Prophylactic antibiotics may be indicated. In some cases the diver may become aware of the perforation only at a later date, e.g. when returning from a diving expedition.

The causes of perforation of the tympanic membrane during diving include the following:

### Middle-ear barotrauma of descent

If the diver is unable to autoinflate the middle ear during descent, the tympanic membrane may rupture inwards. In some cases the perforation occurs at a shallow depth (e.g. 2–4 metres), in which case there is little else to observe on otoscopic examination other than the oval or crescent-shaped perforation just posterior to the handle of the malleus. In those cases who experience more characteristic symptoms of middle-ear barotrauma of descent, and continue on to greater depths (e.g. 5–10 metres) without equalizing the middle-ear pressures, there may be signs of gross haemorrhage within the tympanic membrane, as well as perforation.

### Forceful autoinflation

The Valsalva manoeuvre may cause perforation of the tympanic membrane, especially if this has been damaged previously, e.g. by middle-ear barotrauma, otitis externa, old perforations etc.

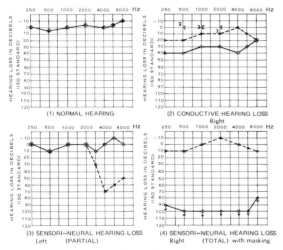

**Figure 28.1** Examples of typical audiograms

### Shock wave

This may be due to underwater explosion or the pressure wave from another diver's fin. These cases often develop vertigo and there are usually no signs of middle-ear barotrauma of descent on otoscopic examination.

### Middle-ear disease

Many divers complain of hearing loss, which is also described as a dullness of hearing, a dampening of blurring of sound. It may be noticed after diving, and in many cases is related to less severe grades of middle-ear barotrauma of descent. Pure-tone audiometry,

from 250 to 8000 cycles/s (Hz), usually reveals only slight difference between the affected and the unaffected ear, or between the pre- and post-incident audiograms.

Middle-ear diseases associated with diving are as follows.

### Middle-ear barotrauma of descent ('ear squeeze')

Despite complaints related to hearing most cases have no significant pure-tone loss (see page 116). In some cases, especially those with a severe middle-ear barotrauma of descent, there is an appreciable conductive loss. These cases presumably have impairment of sound conduction due to either haemotympanum, fluid in the middle ear dampening conduction by the ossicular chain, or temporary damage to the ossicles by subluxation or trauma.

In those cases in which it is associated with the symptoms or signs of aural barotrauma, dullness of hearing is likely to last between 1 and 2 weeks, and then resolve. It is sometimes associated with a sensation of bubbling in the middle ear and, in these cases, it is likely to be due to the middle ear being congested and swollen, or even having free fluid within it.

Treatment is not usually required but, in the presence of nasal congestion, systematic (oral) decongestants may have some value in re-establishing patency and drainage of the eustachian tube.

### Otitis media

The hearing loss, in those cases in which the infection remains strictly an otitis media without extension, is of the conductive type. Infection may follow contamination of the middle ear with nasopharyngeal organisms, introduced with autoinflation. It may progress because of the culture media of blood and effusion, caused by middle-ear barotrauma of descent. The patient usually presents with pain which has developed within 6–24 hours of a dive. The prognosis and treatment are based on general medical principles (see page 310).

### Forceful autoinflation of the middle ear

This is associated with middle-ear barotrauma of descent, and may be an indirect cause of some of the damage noted with this disorder. The Valsalva manoeuvre is often necessary in an attempt to overcome the difficulty in equalizing pressures within the middle ear, but when excess force is required to achieve this, the pressure is then transmitted into the inner and middle ear, aggravating pre-existing damage and producing damage in its own right. The damage may be to either the tympanic membrane, the ossicles, the oval window, the cochlea or the round window. The last three may result in a sensorineural deafness. Dysacusis may also develop (see page 379).

### Increased gas density

With exposure to increased pressure and increased depth, more gas molecules must pass into the middle ear to ensure that its volume remains constant. In this condition the gas is more dense – causing a depth-related, reversible hearing loss, due to increased impedance of the middle-ear transformer. This explains the impairment of hearing noted in recompression chamber experiments and helmet diving. The use of helium, which will reverse this trend to increased gas density in the middle ear, unfortunately changes the middle-ear resonant frequency, thereby also interfering with normal hearing. Under water, bone conduction is the major hearing mechanism.

### Ossicular disruption

This may follow middle-ear barotrauma and may cause a mixed hearing loss. It is more easily detected by the use of the impedance audiogram (see page 369).

---

*Hearing loss in diving may be either conductive or sensorineural, the latter being more serious, the former more common.*

---

## Sensorineural deafness

It has become obvious that pure-tone audiograms must be performed on all divers prior to exposing them to hyperbaric conditions. Without these pre-incident audiograms an assessment of hearing damage would be most difficult, especially as it predominantly involves the asymptomatic high frequencies in mild or early cases. In mild sensorineural deafness, unlike the conductive deafness that interferes with speech frequencies, the diver may not be aware of the deafness.

### Noise-induced deafness

Extreme noise exposure may result in either temporary or permanent threshold shifts which present as a sensorineural deafness. The sensorineural deafness is usually bilateral and partial.

A temporary threshold shift may occur whenever subjects are exposed to loud noises, e.g. in a compression chamber, in diving helmets, near compressors etc. The hearing loss is confined almost entirely to frequencies higher than the frequency of the offending noise, the greatest shift being for tones about half an octave above the exposure tone, but all of the higher frequencies may be more or less affected. Hearing for lower tones remains almost unaffected. Exposure to a 1000-Hz signal at 120 dB (the threshold of discomfort) for half an hour usually causes a temporary threshold shift of about 35 dB over the upper half of the speech range. These changes are normally reversible, but the frequencies which are least likely to recover are those between 3000 and 6000 Hz. This band seems to represent a vulnerable area in the sense organs of hearing, and in this range the recovery is slower.

---

*Frequencies between 3000 and 6000 Hz are particularly sensitive to noise-induced deafness.*

---

Repeated exposure to loud noise may cause a permanent threshold shift in which the multiple threshold shifts summate, especially if there is little time between the exposures. Prolonged and repeated exposure to noise is especially likely to occur in attendants who work in association with compressors and compression chambers. Under these conditions it would be expected that the noise-induced deafness would be bilateral.

Many reports of sensorineural deafness associated with diving have been complicated by other environmental factors to which divers are exposed, and noise is the most important of these.

Hearing impairment is also thought to be aggravated by noise, even though this may not have been the original cause. This is particularly so in cases of pre-existing sensorineural deafness, and therefore is to be considered whenever divers develop this type of deafness. Divers, at least in the armed services, are often trained in gunnery and explosives – both predispose to sensorineural deafness.

### Decompression sickness

See page 170.

### Inner-ear barotrauma

See page 124.

# Dysacusis

This word, which has been used to denote 'faulty' hearing, does not include hearing loss, but the terms are not mutually exclusive – both may exist from the one cause. In diving medicine the most common types of dysacusis are painful hearing and echo hearing.

Dysacusis, presenting as **painful hearing**, may follow injury to the inner ear from noise damage, secondary to middle-ear barotrauma, or due to successful but excessive Valsalva manoeuvres. There may be an associated hearing loss, either temporary or permanent. The pain, which is usually associated with loud noise, may persist for a variable time.

Any excessive noise may produce pain, especially sound levels of 120 dB or greater. This is possible in either helmet diving or in compression chambers. It has been known to damage the vestibular part of the inner ear and to produce the **Tullio phenomenon** (vertigo and nystagmus associated with excessive noise stimulation).

A dysacusis effect from a **patulous eustachian tube** may present as an echo, excessive awareness of the patient's respiration or his own speech (causing him to speak softly), or the reverberation of sounds such as his footsteps. The eustachian tube may be over-stretched and made 'patulous' by the excessive pressure employed with the Valsalva manoeuvre. Other medical causes should be excluded.

The clinical otoscopic sign of tympanic membrane movement during respiration is considered pathognomonic of a patulous eustachian tube in the general population. This is not necessarily so among divers, many of whom are quite capable of opening the eustachian tube at will and during normal breathing.

The symptoms may be relieved or abolished by reclining or lowering the head between the legs – thus increasing venous and lymphatic congestion in the soft tissue of the eustachian tube. They are also temporarily relieved by sniffing, or by the nasal congestion associated with upper respiratory tract infections.

The disorder may be transitory, or last for many months. Treatment is not usually indicated and those procedures which have been employed in otological practice – such as paraffin or Teflon paste injections around the eustachian cushions – may not be appreciated by divers who need adequately patent eustachian tubes to resume their diving activities.

# Vertigo

## Introduction

The most dramatic and demonstrable cause of disorientation underwater is that due to vertigo. The perennial problem of differentiating vertigo from other disturbances of equilibrium, such as dizziness, giddiness, unsteadiness, faintness, lightheadedness, swaying etc., is nowhere more prominent than in the early diving literature. In this chapter, the term 'vertigo' is reserved for those conditions in which there is an hallucination of movement, resulting in either the impression that objects are moving in a certain direction (objective vertigo), or in which the patient is moving in a certain direction (subjective vertigo). Because vertigo is associated with nystagmus, and this can be demonstrated in an objective manner, an attempt has been made to differentiate the specific causes of vertigo from those of disorientation in general. It must be appreciated that there is a strong correlation between these two symptoms (see Chapter 27).

Vertigo is likely to be a more serious symptom in breath-hold diving than with scuba, when there is adequate air supply and orientation cues, such as direction of bubbles, can be thought out with more time available.

Investigations of cases of vertigo in diving should involve:

- Physical examination.
- Pure-tone audiometry.
- Electronystagmography – with positional and sometimes caloric or dysbaric provocation.

## Vertigo in diving – aetiological classification

### Due to unequal vestibular stimulation

1. Caloric
   (a) unilateral external auditory canal obstruction
       (i) cerumen
       (ii) otitis externa
       (iii) miscellaneous
   (b) tympanic membrane perforation
       (i) shock wave
       (ii) middle-ear barotrauma of descent
       (iii) forceful autoinflation
2. Barotrauma
   (a) external-ear barotrauma
   (b) middle-ear barotrauma of descent
   (c) middle-ear barotrauma of ascent
   (d) forceful autoinflation
   (e) inner-ear -barotrauma
       (i) fistula of the inner-ear windows
       (ii) other causes
3. Decompression sickness
4. Miscellaneous: Tullio phenomenon

### Due to unequal vestibular responses

1. Caloric
2. Barotrauma
3. Gas toxicity
4. Sensory deprivation

## Vertigo due to unequal vestibular stimulation

Exposure to both hyperbaric and diving environments results in stimuli to both vestibular end-organs. Under most diving conditions, the stimulus on each side will be equal, but in certain situations this is not so, especially when there is a pathological process involving one external or middle ear. Under these conditions the dominant stimulus effect on one side may well produce vertigo.

### Caloric

When the diver immerses himself in water there is normally an equal flow of cold water into both external auditory canals. This stimulation is therefore symmetrical, and thus no vertigo is expected – nor does it occur in the vast majority of dives. If the stimulus is disproportionately great on one side, vertigo would be expected – with an intensity and duration related to this inequality.

In the production of vertigo by means of a unilateral caloric stimulation, or a bilateral stimulation with unilateral dominance, the spatial orientation of the subject is very relevant. In an experimental situation, caloric stimulus will produce the most intense vertigo and nystagmus when the subject is placed in a position either lying supine with his head elevated at 30 degrees, or lying prone with his head depressed at an angle of 30 degrees. In both these positions the horizontal semicircular canal becomes vertical. This has been repeatedly demonstrated in the supine position during the conventional Hallpike caloric tests, but a more usual position for subjects involved in diving is the prone position. This is more common when the diver is underweighted, i.e. with slight positive buoyancy, or when his fins are positively buoyant – he automatically assumes the prone, head-down position in which vertigo is experienced most intensely and nystagmus demonstrated most vividly. Resumption of an upright posture terminates the vertigo.

Vertigo may result when there is unilateral obstruction to water flow into the external canal, when the tympanic membrane perforates, or where there is bilateral and equal caloric stimulation with unequal vestibular responses (see later).

### Unilateral external auditory canal obstruction

Free flow of cold water into only one external auditory canal can induce vertigo. None of the

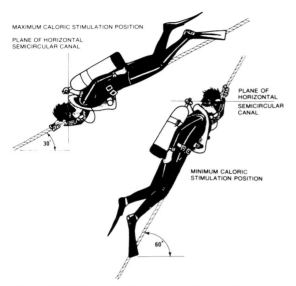

**Figure 28.2** Caloric stimulation related to spatial orientation

foreign body, ear plug, air bubble etc. may allow water to flow into one ear and produce this effect.

### Cerumen

Those who spend much time under water, without hoods, quickly lose any cerumen accumulation they may have had. Those who commence formal diving courses have an otoscopic examination to ensure patency of the external ear canal and to observe tympanic membrane movement during autoinflation. An occlusive cerumen plug, uncommon in this selected population, is now known to be of aetiological import in cases of vertigo, because it obstructs the free flow of water into one external ear.

cases has shown any permanent vestibular effects, and the only effect on audiometry is that due to the canal obstruction, i.e. a remedial conduction deafness. Two common causes observed are cerumen and otitis externa, although others such as exostosis,

### *Otitis externa*

Patients with otitis externa should not dive, but sometimes they do. This cause of vertigo has not often been reported. The swelling and congestion of one external auditory canal may greatly restrict water entry, resulting in asymmetrical caloric stimuli and vertigo.

---

## CASE REPORT 28.1

This diver had no difficulty in autoinflating his ears during a descent to 10 metres. While swimming along a horizontal underwater line, he felt as if he were rotating to one side around the line. As the line was on the sea bed, he knew that his sensation was abnormal, and he decided to surface. The vertigo, which lasted for some 10–20 seconds, did not trouble him during the ascent and he had no further difficulty.

On clinical examination there was no abnormality other than the presence of a large plug of hard cerumen noted in the left ear. Prior to removal of the plug it was decided to carry out ENG with caloric testing, to ascertain whether sufficient water was likely to pass this obstruction. The positional electronystagmogram was normal, but the caloric test demonstrated a false picture of a total left canal paresis. The cerumen was removed, and no evidence of external- or middle-ear barotrauma was noted. It was postulated that the cerumen plug was large enough to obstruct the free flow of water, but not complete enough to prevent some water from equalizing the changing pressures within the external ear. The caloric stimulus was therefore much greater in the unobstructed ear, producing transient vertigo. No further incidents occurred after the plug was removed.

*Diagnosis:* vertigo from a unilateral caloric stimulus, due to unilateral auditory canal obstruction by a cerumen plug.

## Tympanic membrane perforation

This is a dramatic cause of transient, but often disabling, vertigo. It is well recognized by most doctors dealing dealing with diving accidents, and by divers. It has a characteristic symptomatology. First, there is a loud noise associated with a sensation of cold water rushing into the middle ear. Vertigo follows almost immediately and usually lasts for less than a minute. It is believed that the inrush of cold water to the middle ear through the ruptured tympanic membrane is the cause of the transient vertigo, and that this small amount of cold water rapidly warms to body temperature, removing the caloric stimulus. On surfacing, the diver often has blood-stained fluid running from the external auditory canal, probably expelled when the gases which have remained in the middle ear expand during ascent, and force the blood out through the perforation.

There may be no vertiginous symptoms in those less common cases in which the tympanic membrane ruptures without entry of water into the middle-ear cavity. Entry of water into the middle ear may be prevented if either this space is occupied by blood or the perforation occurs during ascent. These patients usually notice the hissing of gas through the perforation with ascent or autoinflation. Occasionally they present with vertigo, noted while driving their motor vehicles after the dive. Whether this is due to head movements aggravating positional vertigo, air currents replacing water in producing caloric stimulation or eddy current movements of the tympanic membrane and ossicles is unknown.

On otoscopic examination, the perforation is often circular and seen either at the site of previous pathology or posterior to the lower half of the handle of the malleus. With pure-tone audiometry, it is often possible to detect a 5–15 dB loss in the affected ear. This is of the conductive type, especially affecting lower tones, and usually returns to normal within a week or two, i.e. when the perforation has almost closed. Caloric tests are contra-indicated. As neither the vertigo nor the hearing loss is permanent in the vast majority of these cases, it is believed that the inner ear is not seriously damaged. If prolonged or progressive inner-ear changes are noted, second-ary inner-ear barotrauma should be considered as an associated abnormality.

When perforation is suspected but cannot be visualized, impedance audiometry is useful to confirm, or more often to refute, the diagnosis.

It is customary to advise patients with tympanic membrane perforation against diving, flying or middle-ear autoinflation for at least a month. The ear should be kept dry and no ear drops are indicated. Some advise the use of systemic decongestants, but this is not usually required. Prophylactic antibiotics are administered, as contaminated water frequently has entered the middle-ear cavity. The tympanic membrane often appears healed within a week or two, but it remains susceptible to a recurrence if diving is then resumed within the next 2 or 3 months.

There are three major predisposing causes of tympanic membrane perforation leading to vertigo whilst diving: a shock wave, middle-ear barotrauma of descent and autoinflation of the middle ear.

### Shock wave

This is a disorder easily diagnosed on history, and is said to have been common when Navy divers were routinely subjected to underwater explosions, especially when they faced at right angles to the source of the explosion (see Chapter 25). The blast wave may damage any tissue which is capable of distortion, and especially if it is associated with a compressible gas-containing cavity. The tympanic membrane is such a tissue, although whether the shock wave moves easily into the external auditory canal to reach the membrane, or whether it receives significant interference by deflection waves, is a matter of individual fortune. In these days of sport diving the most common underwater shock wave causing perforation of the tympanic membrane and vertigo is due to being 'finned'. When a diver swims past another diver, considerable pressure waves are generated from the fin (or flipper) movements. If fins are used near another diver's ear, perforation of the tympanic membrane is possible. Manometric testing within a short distance of the fin action commonly employed by divers showed that pressures varied rapidly from + 30 to − 10 cmH$_2$O. The shock wave, which is a water wave, is probably also responsible for the entry of water into the middle ear following the perforation. Most cases reported have no permanent vestibular or hearing sequelae, although these could occur in more severe cases with inner-ear barotrauma.

### Middle-ear barotrauma of descent ('ear squeeze') (see page 116)

This is due to the inability to autoinflate the middle-ear cavity, and to equalize its pressure with the increasing ambient water and body pressure during descent. The diver is almost always aware of this inequality and its origin. Under. these conditions, most divers experience considerable discomfort, preventing further descent in the water, and sustain haemorrhage within the middle-ear mucosa, in the tympanic membrane, above and along the handle of the malleus. It is commonly inferred that perforation is the ultimate damage from not equalizing the pressure in the middle-ear cavity, and follows the extreme degrees of haemorrhage described in gradings of middle-ear barotrauma of descent. Despite this, many tympanic membrane perforations due to diving are not associated with these gross haemorrhages in the tympanic membrane. It is possible that perforation competes with middle-ear haemorrhage as a pressure-equalizing process – the former demonstrating tympanic membrane fragility and the latter demonstrating vascular capillary fragility.

### Autoinflation of the middle ear ('clearing the ear')

In some cases the tympanic membrane is perforated during the performance of autoinflation by the Valsalva manoeuvre, presumably following the transmission of pressure from the nasopharynx, through the eustachian tube into the middle ear, and then bulging the tympanic membrane outwards, resulting in rupture. In these cases there is more likely to be vertigo if water then enters the perforated tympanic membrane, into the middle ear. This would be particularly likely if the diver continues his descent.

### Barotrauma

In relation to vertigo there are five clinically important types of barotrauma. They are all dependent upon the changing of volume with pressure, in accordance with Boyle's law. They comprise:

1. External-ear barotrauma of descent ('reversed ear').
2. Middle-ear barotrauma of descent ('ear squeeze').
3. Middle-ear barotrauma of ascent (alternobaric vertigo).
4. Forceful autoinflation of middle ear.
5. Inner-ear barotrauma.

It appears that vertigo due to barotrauma is more likely when the diver is upright (vertical) than when he is horizontal or in the position needed for caloric stimulation. Attempts to reproduce vertigo due to barotrauma, in a recompression chamber with electronystagmogram monitoring verify this clinical observation.

This spatial orientation infers involvement of the utricular/saccular divisions. The unequal pressure gradients may themselves produce vestibular irregularities or they may, especially when associated with forceful autoinflation, result in a fistula of the round window, producing a much more permanent effect. This is described later.

### External ear barotrauma of descent ('reversed ear')

This is due to an obstruction preventing water from replacing the contracting air space in the external auditory canal during the diver's descent. It is commonly due to the incorrect use of hoods which cover the ear, or ear plugs. Cerumen has also been incriminated. Although most cases have minimal discomfort, occasionally the middle or inner ear is involved. Other symptoms of this disorder are mild, but examination of the external canal reveals haemorrhage and vesicle formation, with the tympanic membrane free of haemorrhages or perforations.

### Middle-ear barotrauma of descent ('ear squeeze')

If the diver fails to equalize the pressures in the middle-ear cavities during descent, haemorrhages occur in the middle ear and vertigo can result. In some of these cases, this transitory vertigo occurs during or soon after the descent and there may be an associated mild transient conductive deafness. In other cases the vertigo appears to be more serious and persistent, and related to inner-ear barotrauma. In these cases there may be an associated sensorineural deafness.

Case report 28.2 demonstrated, in an objective manner, that vertigo and nystagmus can be precipitated with the middle-ear pressure changes during descent.

Case report 28.3 demonstrated that middle-ear barotrauma of descent can initiate vertigo and nystagmus, that this manifestation may continue and that the condition need not be merely transitory.

---

### CASE REPORT 28.2

The patient, a certified diver, frequently developed dizziness during descent. She commonly experienced difficulty in equalizing the middle-ear spaces and frequently resorted to nasal decongestants. There were no symptoms suggestive of disorientation during ascent, and usually the sensation of dizziness reduced as she remained at a constant depth.

On examination, there was no conventional evidence of any abnormality in ear functions; she had normal pure-tone audiograms and normal electronystagmograms to positional and bithermal caloric stimuli.

Dysbaric electronystagmograms (as described by Edmonds et al., 1973) were performed with the diver in the sitting upright position with the eyes closed and positioned centrally. ENG monitoring was continued while the patient was subjected to changes in pressure. The compression was at the rate of 9 m/min to a depth of 18 metres. The patient was then kept at the depth of 18 m for 2 min and ascended at the same rate. Minor problems were encountered with middle-ear equalization during descent, but did not require cessation or delay of this descent.

The ENG results verified the subject's observation of vertigo associated with compression, which was relieved by maintenance of pressure and absent during decompression (Figure 28.3). The nystagmus 'saw tooth' pattern is obvious during and immediately after descent.

---

### CASE REPORT 28.3

This subject also had normal hearing and vestibular function demonstrated before having difficulty in equalizing both middle-ear pressures during a recompression chamber descent. Because of the inability to achieve this middle-ear equalization, the compression was terminated at 4.5 m. At that time the ENG monitoring (performed in conjunction with another experimental aim) demonstrated severe nystagmus associated with the subjective complaint of vertigo. The diver was in the supine position. Vertigo was stated to persist for many minutes after the initial middle-ear injury, and nystagmus was demonstrated to persist in a progressively decreasing degree, for appropriately 12 minutes (see ENG). The nystagmus 'saw tooth' pattern is maximal between 3.0 and 4.5 metres during descent, is less at 5 minutes and almost gone at 12 minutes.

DIVE VELOCITY: 9.0 m/min.

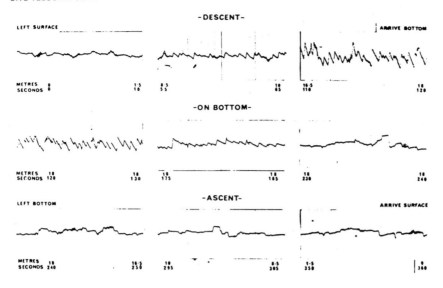

**Figure 28.3** Case 28.2

DIVE VELOCITY: 9.0 m/min.

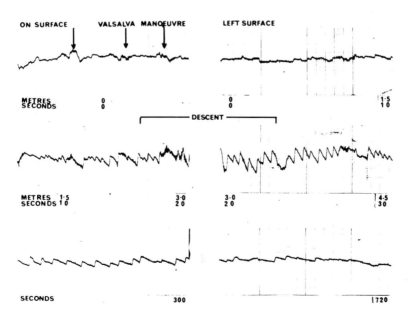

**Figure 28.4** Case 28.3

Because there is no evidence of either abnormal cochlear or vestibular function prior to the dives referred to above, there is no reason to believe that the vestibular response is due to an underlying vestibular inequality. In both cases there is a history of inability in equalizing the middle-ear spaces, and it is presumed that the inequality of middle-ear pressure is the cause for both the transitory and the persistent abnormal vestibular response. The transitory response could be the result of unequal physiological stimuli, i.e. unequal middle-ear pressures; the persistent nystagmus may be related to more persistent barotraumatic pathology in the vestibule. These descriptions are thus similar in concept, although opposite in direction, to the alternobaric vertigo described by Lundgren (1965) and confirmed independently by Edmonds (1973) and Tjernström (1973). The nystagmus responses described in this and previous reports are abolished or inhibited by eye opening, supporting the peripheral nature of the disorder.

Dysbaric electronystagmograms supplement formal vestibular function tests in aviators and divers, and may be needed to demonstrate vestibular pathology.

### Middle-ear barotrauma of ascent ('alternobaric vertigo')

The unequal release of gas from the middle-ear cavities, especially during the initial stages of ascent, results in a pressure difference between the two middle ears, and unequal stimuli to the vestibular systems. The nystagmus is towards the side of the block, with the diver's spinning sensation towards that ear with the higher middle-ear pressure (Chapter 27).

During this ascent the diver may develop a mild vertigo, often rectified by further ascent which may open the less patent eustachian tube. When this does occur, the pressures are then both equalized with the ambient pressure, and the stimulus to vertigo ceases. Also, subsequent opening of the tube seems easier. Other cases may reach the surface while still having an asymmetry of pressure within the middle-ear cavities, or the residual effects of previous asymmetries, and they will experience vertigo following the ascent.

The vestibular system is sensitive to pressure changes in the middle ear. Vertigo is produced probably by a pressure difference of 60 cmH$_2$O or more between the middle ears.

Most cases of middle-ear barotrauma of ascent are mild, i.e. the eustachian tube finally opens and thus prevents further aural damage. The equalization is usually accompanied by an escape of gas bubbles down the eustachian tube, and is felt by the diver. Such is not always the case and there have been instances of inner-ear damage, and of progressive pain during ascent, which may result in perforation of the tympanic membrane. The appearance of the tympanic membrane in cases of middle-ear barotrauma of ascent is quite unlike that of middle-ear barotrauma of descent, with virtually no haemorrhage around the handle of the malleus.

### Forceful autoinflation ('clearing the ears')

Some subjects can produce vertigo merely by performing autoinflation, and it may be presumed that the middle ears are ventilated unequally, because of unequal eustachian tube patency. Another proposed mechanism is an abnormally mobile stapes.

### Inner-ear barotrauma (see page 124)

Cochlear trauma, haemorrhage, inner-ear membrane rupture and/or fistula of the round or oval window, with or without air entry into the perilymph, are serious complications of barotrauma and forceful autoinflation of the middle ear.

If a fistula of the round or oval window results, it can be observed surgically as a leakage of perilymph into the middle ear and can be repaired. It is not known how long surgery can be delayed and yet still be of value. In the cases which initially, predominantly or solely involve vestibular function, the symptoms may progressively diminish as adaptation occurs. In others, vertigo may persist or recur while the fistula persists or recurs. Even though the symptoms may diminish, the lesion may progress to complete destruction – with certain sequelae. Unless this lesion is corrected the patient will never be able to dive or fly safely, and may continue to have occasional vertigo, aggravated by sudden head movement, which is then a hazard in all occupations that involve balance, exposure to heights or driving. Associated cochlear damage is also present in most cases.

Unfortunately, some of the causes of inner-ear barotrauma do not lend themselves to reconstructive surgery. In some, the vestibular lesion is minor, and may only be detected by ENG. Such cases do not suffer permanent vestibular complications.

### Decompression sickness ('bends')
(see page 170)

Although vertigo has often been reported among air scuba divers with this condition, there is considerable doubt about the validity of the diagnosis when, as in many of the cases reported, there are no other manifestations of the disease. It is likely that many of the permanent vestibular damage cases originally reported as decompression sickness were really due to inner-ear barotrauma. The delay of onset of symptoms is not necessarily a diagnostic feature favouring decompression sickness, as it is not uncommon in cases of inner-ear barotrauma resulting in a fistula of the round window. Vertigo may occur without any loss of hearing in both diseases.

Even allowing for the misdiagnoses, there are still some cases which presented with hearing loss and/or vertigo, probably due to decompression sickness. This is especially so with deep diving, using helium as a breathing gas. In these cases, it is necessary to institute recompression therapy to prevent permanent inner-ear damage.

The consequences of vertigo, such as near drowning, vomiting, dehydration, electrolyte disturbances and distress, are more important in a patient who is already seriously ill with decompression sickness. There are also long-term sequelae. With vestibular damage, there is a likelihood that the diver may not be able to continue with his occupation, and that he may be restricted from other occupations, such as flying or driving vehicles. If incorrectly diagnosed during decompression (e.g. if the symptoms are attributed to seasickness), then further decompression may result in more damage to the vestibular apparatus.

Recompression therapy, if promptly instituted, should result in cure. Objective tests of vestibular function can and should be performed under hyperbaric conditions, when doubt exists regarding clinical management. These investigations include ENG and iced-water caloric tests, and are valuable in differential diagnosis, prognosis and response to treatment.

### Miscellaneous conditions

Motion sickness is a complication of certain diving operations, e.g. on the diving boat, while decompressing on a platform or rope under water, or surface swimming. Certain specific medical causes of vertigo are also occupational complications of diving. Migraine (page 406) is a typical example – and it is recommended that patients with this disorder should limit their diving. Otitis media can also be classified both as an occupational disease of divers and as a cause of vertigo.

#### *Tullio phenomenon*

The observation by Tullio early this century that sound can stimulate the vestibular system has received much attention from the 1930s onwards. Vertigo may be experienced, and nystagmus identified, when subjects are exposed to pure tones ranging from 200 to 2500 Hz at intensities from 120 to 160 dB. Dizziness, nausea and disturbances of postural equilibrium have been correlated with sound stimulation at intensities and frequencies lower than these.

In diving, the Tullio phenomenon is seen particularly with compression chambers that do not have muffling systems over the air inlets and in which there is excessive enthusiasm to 'flush-through' the chamber with the compressed gas – producing very loud noises. It may also be observed in helmet divers, divers near sonar domes, caisson workers and aircraft personnel.

### Vertigo due to unequal vestibular responses

This group includes subjects who, under almost any conditions other than flying or diving, would be considered 'normal'. In these people, vertigo may be the end-result of unequal vestibular responses to equal stimuli, i.e. one vestibular apparatus being more sensitive than the other.

## CASE REPORT 28.4

A 35-year-old male was subjected to a recompression chamber dive to 9 metres (30 feet). There were no problems with middle-ear equalization during descent, and the procedure was a routine one carried out every few months. While in the outer lock, and before equalizing the chambers, the subject used the intercom phone system, with the earpiece next to his right ear. The chamber pressures were equalized and the subject moved from the outer to the inner lock. A 'flush-through' was then performed. This procedure involves the replacement of a large quantity of compressed air in the chamber, exchanging the chamber air and removing carbon dioxide. In this particular case, it was performed by a chamber operator under training and an excessive zeal was used in opening the inlet and outer valves, producing a great deal of noise. After approximately 20 seconds, the noise of the 'flush-through' was so intense that 'it knocked me off balance'. There was no actual change of pressure during this period and therefore no need to perform Valsalva manoeuvres or middle-ear equalization. The diver felt severely giddy and disoriented, and was unable to stand. His right ear was nearer the inflow of the gas and, when he attempted to use this ear to communicate through the telephone intercom, he was unable to hear the voice of the surface attendant. He was able to use his left ear for this. He noted that he was falling to the left when he finally got out of the chamber, and was feeling off balance through most of that day. He claimed that he was far more sensitive to noise, even though his audiograms had not changed. Impedance audiometry revealed a tympanic membrane far more mobile on the right side than on the left. Electronystagmograms demonstrated nystagmus on the vertical tracing in the positional test, even though the caloric tests appeared normal.

Clinical examination of the ear, nose and throat was normal, without any evidence of patulous eustachian tubes. The tympanic membranes were easily moved with middle-ear autoinflation, and there was no evidence of middle-ear barotrauma.

*Diagnosis:* Tullio phenomenon, presenting with vertigo and dysacusis.

---

Even small differences in the vestibular response of each side may produce some demonstrable dysfunction when exposed to the multiple stimuli encountered with diving or hyperbaric environments. The fact that, with caloric tests, asymmetry cannot be demonstrated in most patients probably highlights the relative crudity of this investigation. As electronystagmography becomes precise, and with more accurate and controlled stimuli, marginal asymmetry of vestibular function may be demonstrated.

### Caloric stimulation

A very common syndrome of vertigo induced by diving seems explicable only by postulating a greater caloric response from one vestibular apparatus than from the other. There is usually no abnormality evident on otoscopic examination, or on the formal testing of hearing or vestibular function. There is no reason to postulate barotrauma, sensory deprivation, decompression sickness, inert gas narcosis etc. There remains the possibility that the vertigo is due to unequal vestibular responses, but even this must remain conjecture without more comprehensive vestibular function assessments than are currently available. The caloric aetiology is consistent with the usual position of the diver, i.e. prone with head slightly lowered, when he develops this vertigo, as has been described previously. It is most commonly experienced by divers who have descended without any difficulty in equalizing pressures in the middle-ear cavities, and have reached a level at which they then perform a horizontal swim. The vertigo normally comes on approximately 5–10 minutes after the commencement of the dive, and tends to recur when the diver attempts similar dives under similar conditions within the next few weeks. These cases, have previously been given the nondescript term 'idiopathic vertigo of divers'.

The belief that this particular syndrome is due to unequal vestibular response to caloric stimulation is supported by: the time delay prior to vertigo being produced, unlike vertigo from barotrauma; the spatial orientation of the diver during the swim, suggestive of caloric-induced vertigo; and the tendency for this to recur during similar dives and without any otoscopic abnormalities present, refuting the likelihood of unequal stimulation.

Other cases, who have demonstrable pathology of one inner ear, and thus unequal vestibular responses, are easier to comprehend.

## Barotrauma

Vertigo induced by unequal pressure stimulation (barotrauma) of the vestibular apparatus has been described. The middle-ear spaces are likely to contract during descent and expand during ascent in the water. Even though the eustachian tubes may be patent and equal, ensuring symmetrical pressure changes in the middle-ear cavities, vertigo may result if one vestibular apparatus is relatively hypofunctional. Under these conditions, the vertigo occurs during or immediately following the changes of pressure, i.e. descent and ascent.

In some cases a damaged vestibular apparatus on one side may have been the result of a previous diving accident, whereas in other cases non-diving aetiologies may be postulated. An example of the latter is the inner-ear damage which occurs due to gunfire, especially when this is unilateral.

Vertigo from barotrauma is more severe when the diver is in the upright position than in the almost horizontal 'caloric' position.

## Gas toxicity

This field has been almost unexplored by otophysiologists. The difficulty of differentiating vertigo from such terms as dizziness, lightheadedness and disorientation makes any review of the diving literature almost valueless in this context. Each of the conditions described below will seriously interfere with cerebral function and thus a subjective assessment of vertigo is particularly difficult, and an objective measurement becomes imperative. Due to the interference in cerebral function, each of these conditions may result in serious disorientation whether or not vertigo is noted or nystagmus demonstrated.

### Inert gas narcosis (nitrogen narcosis)

As divers descend beyond 30 metres while breathing air, they become progressively sedated and narcotic from the influence of nitrogen. Dizziness has been described by many divers under these conditions, but there is considerable doubt as to whether this proceeds to true vertigo. If this dizziness does represent a true vertigo in some cases, then like other symptoms of nitrogen narcosis, it should be quickly corrected by reducing the nitrogen pressures, i.e. with ascent. However, nystagmus does seem to be accentuated by exposure to high nitrogen pressures, supporting the possibility of nitrogen narcosis as an accessory aetiological factor, in conjunction with the other stimuli to which subjects are exposed during diving (dysbaric and caloric).

### High-pressure neurological syndrome

Vertigo, nausea and tremor are some of the symptoms reported with this syndrome. Nystagmus and vertigo are not now believed to be characteristic features of this. The effects are probably either in the subcortical or reticular activating system, and are aggravated by too rapid a compression, and are relieved within a few hours of reaching depth.

### Oxygen toxicity

Vertigo is a documented symptom of this disorder when it affects the neurological system, i.e. when the oxygen partial pressure is 2 ATA or greater. Vertigo may be a warning symptom. It is also precipitated during the reduction from high oxygen pressures, i.e. an 'oxygen off effect', as well as following oxygen convulsions. These situations are only likely when divers use oxygen or rebreathing equipment, when the safe limits for oxygen pressures or durations are exceeded. Nausea or vomiting are also associated with somewhat lower oxygen pressures (1–2 ATA) but whether these are related to vertigo is unknown at this stage.

### Carbon dioxide toxicity

Disorientation is a characteristic feature of this toxicity, but vertigo is far less definite. It has been reported in association with vomiting by submariners who have become acclimatized to breathing high carbon dioxide pressures and then revert to breathing air or oxygen. This is known as the 'carbon dioxide off effect'. A similar state occurs clinically in divers using rebreathing equipment with partially ineffective carbon dioxide absorbent systems, when they stop their high carbon dioxide exposure, e.g. if they rest after an energetic swim.

### Other gases

The effect of hypoxia, hypocapnia, carbon monoxide poisoning etc. may well include vertigo, as this is a possible symptom with any factor which disturbs the state of consciousness. In these cases the effects are analogous to drug effects.

### Sensory deprivation

Sensory deprivation, especially when it involves those senses involved in spatial orientation, is likely to aggravate vertigo and to produce disorientation. Abnormalities of vestibular or cochlear function would not be expected in most of these cases. Many of the clinical case reports are characterized by complaints of poor visibility. The reduction of incoming stimuli is particularly disturbing to novice and amateur divers, as when diving in murky waters or at night, when visual cues may be totally lost. It is possible that sensory deprivation will serve to decrease the threshold for vertigo and nystagmus. This belief receives support from the techniques aimed at reducing extraneous stimuli, which are utilized during vestibular testing in otological laboratories. The effect of sensory deprivation in the production of disorientation is unquestioned.

> *Despite the multitude of causes of disorientation under water, as described above, the most common is inadequate sensory input experienced by the novice diver.*

## Recommended reading and references

APPAIX, A., DEMARD, E., BONNAUD, G. and JACQUIN, M. (1973). Otorhinolaryngology, diving and hyperbaric medicine. *Journal Français d' Otorhinolaryngologie* **22**, 559–593.

AXELSSON, A., MILLER, J. and SILVERMAN, M. (1979). Anatomical effects of sudden middle ear pressure changes. *Annals of Otology* **88**, 368–376.

DEMARD, F. (1973). Les accidents labyrinthiques aigus au cours de la plongée sous-marine. *Forsvarsmedicin* **9**, 416–422

EDMONDS, C. (1973). Round window rupture in diving. *Forsvarsmedicin* **9**, 404–405.

EDMONDS, C. and BLACKWOOD, R. (1975). Disorientation with middle ear barotrauma of descent. *Undersea Biomedical Research* **2**, 311–314.

EDMONDS, C., FREEMAN, P., THOMAS, R., TONKIN, J., and BLACKWOOD, F.A. (1973). *Otological Aspects of Diving*. NSW. Australia: Australian Medical Publishing Co.

FARMER, J.C. (1981). *Otolaryngology and Diving in Hyperbaric and Undersea Medicine*. San Antonio: Medical Seminars Inc.

FARMER, J.C. (1990). Ear and sinus problems in diving. *Diving Medicine*, edited by A.A. Bove and J.C. Davis. Philadelphia: W.B. Saunders.

FARMER, J.C., THOMAS, W.G., YOUNGBLOOD, D.G. and BENNETT, P.B. (1976). Inner ear decompression sickness. *The Laryngoscope* **86**, 1315–1327.

FIELDS, J.A. (1988). Skin diving. *Archives of Otolaryngology* **68**, 531

KENNEDY, R.S. (1972). *A bibliography of the role of the vestibular apparatus under water and pressure*. USN MRI M4306-03. 5000BAK9. Report No. 1

LUNDGREN, G.E.C. (1965). Alternobaric vertigo – a diving hazard. *British Medical Journal* 1, 511.

McCORMICK, J.G., HOLLAND, W., HOLLEMAN, I. and BRAUER, R. (1974). Consideration of the pathophysiology and histopathology of deafness associated with decompression sickness and absence of middle ear barotrauma. *Proceedings of UMS Annual Scientific Meeting, Undersea Biomedical Research* vol. 1, no. 1

MOLVAER, O.I. (1980). Acute hearing loss following diving. *South Pacific Underwater Medical Society Journal*, April, pp. 3–12.

MOLVAER, O.I. and ALBREKTSEN, G. (1988). Alternobaric vertigo in professional divers. *Undersea Biomedical Research* **15**, 271–282.

MOLVAER, O.I. and ALBREKTSEN, G. (1990). Hearing deterioration in professional divers: An epidemiological survey. *Undersea Biomedical Research* **17**, 231–246.

MONEY, K.E., BUCKINGHAM, I.P., CALDER, I.M., et al. (1985). Damage to the middle ear and the inner ear in underwater divers. *Undersea Biomedical Research* **12**, 77–84.

NISHIOKA, I., and YANAGIHARA, N. (1986). Role of air bubbles in the perilymph as a cause of sudden deafness. *The American Journal of Otology* **3**, 430–438.

PARKER, D.E., RESCHKE, M.F. and TUBBS, R.L. (1973). Effects of sound on the vestibular system. *Agard Conference*, No. 128, NATO Publication.

PULEC, J.G. and HAHN, F.W. (1970). The abnormally patulous Eustachian tube. *Otological Clinics of North America*, February.

TERRY, L. and DENNISON, W.L. (1966). Vertigo amongst divers. *Special Report 66-2*. U.S. Navy Submarine Medical Centre, Groton, Conn.

TJERNSTRÖM, O. (1973). Alternobaric vertigo. Proceedings of the First European Undersea Biomedical Symposium, Stockholm, *Forsvarsmedicin* **9**, 410–415.

VOROSMARTI, J. and BRADLEY, M.E. (1970). Alternobaric vertigo in military divers. *Military Medicine* **135**, 182–185.

YANAGITA, N., MIYAKE, H., SAKAKIBARA, K., SAKAKIBARA, B. and TAKAHASHI H. (1973). Sudden deafness and hyperbaric oxygen therapy – clinical reports of 25 patients. *Fifth International Hyperbaric Conference*, 389–401.

# 29

# Psychological and neuropsychological disturbances

PSYCHOLOGICAL DISTURBANCES
    Anxiety states: claustrophobia, agoraphobia
    Panic
    Hysteria: Munchausen's syndrome
    Illusions
    Organic psychological responses

PSYCHOSES
    Schizophrenia, affective disorders, suicide

NEUROPSYCHOLOGICAL
IMPAIRMENT – DEMENTIA
    Aetiology
    Diving folklore
    Circumstantial evidence
    Dementia and diving surveys
    Australian 'excessive diver' surveys
    Discussion

RECOMMENDED READING AND
REFERENCES

## Psychological disturbances

### Psychological traits of divers

There have been few studies of the relationship between personality structure and diving (page 55). It is known that successful divers are characterized by an average or below-average neuroticism level. Psychometric tests show that intelligence is positively correlated with successful diving, as are emotional stability and self-sufficiency. The psychological mechanism of denial, in which the subject refuses consciously to acknowledge the hazards, is thought to have some adaptive value under some diving conditions. This allows divers to continue to work despite stress which would be disruptive to many 'normals'.

Some psychological disturbances experienced during diving are well known, but poorly documented. They are as follows.

### Anxiety states

In susceptible people, the normal anxiety induced by the undersea environment may be complicated by an over-awareness of the potential but definite danger, with a resultant increase in anxiety. A vicious circle results. The diver may then develop an actual **phobia** to being under water.

Some candidates develop this prior to ever attempting a diving course and realize that they would be apprehensive in this particular environment, but other motivating factors may temporarily override this fear.

In other cases, there is a history of traumatic exposure to water (such as a near-drowning incident) which initiates the phobic state.

There are isolated cases of genuine **claustrophobia**, preventing either the immersion of the subject in water, or entry into a confined recompression chamber. This syndrome is not often seen in its full form, and may only present during times of diminished visibility (murky water, night diving etc.) or prolonged exposure.

The **agoraphobic reaction** is also termed the **'blue orb'** or **'blue dome syndrome'**. It develops progressively as the diver becomes more aware of his isolation and his lack of contact with people or objects. It may be aggravated by nitrogen narcosis, at depth. The diver is usually diving alone, without physical or visual contact to either diving craft or sea bed. The fear is one of isolation in the vastness and depth of the water. He becomes apprehensive, and may note palpitations, increased rate of breathing and epigastric sensations. These symptoms of anxiety are interpreted as being indicative of 'something wrong', and thus result in more anxiety. If reassurance, in the form of a companion diver or visual orientation with familiar objects, is not available, then the diver may panic and ascend rapidly. Drowning, decompression sickness or pulmonary barotrauma are possible complications. If the diver regains physical or visual contact with the sea bed, the diving boat or a companion diver, the symptoms usually abate. Divers who develop the illness repetitively may take the obvious precautions of buddy diving, or may undergo typical desensitization therapy with great benefits.

All phobic anxiety states can be treated by desensitization or deconditioning techniques. They are prevented by avoiding the environmental circumstances which predispose them, and also by diving with a team or companion. The use of sedatives is to be discouraged, but diazepam may be indicated during the deconditioning process.

### Acute overreactive anxiety state (panic)

Due to some misfortune, the diver panics and is likely to behave irrationally. This may result in ascent to the surface without taking adequate precautions, frantic search for alternative air supplies, lack of concern for other personnel etc. This is more likely in those divers with a normal or above-normal neuroticism (trait anxiety) level.

It is also more likely when the diver attempts tasks beyond his capability, when there is an aggravation by environmental hazards or when inadequate safety precautions and back-up facilities exist. Inadequate physical fitness and exhaustion will predispose to panic. (See Chapter 5 for a detailed account of this important subject.)

---

### CASE REPORT 29.1

AR, a 21-year-old diver with limited open water experience, was testing out his new equipment. After anchoring his boat over a reef, he dived into clear water, without tidal currents. He made no use of any safety precautions such as float, surface line, buddy compass, contents or depth gauges. The water was known to be 70 metres deep off the edge of the reef although the diver depth was probably no deeper than 15 metres. Approximately 10 minutes after commencing the dive, AR noted a queasy feeling in his stomach, together with a sensation of fear. His breathing became deep and he started to panic with an overwhelming desire to return to the safety of his boat. He ascended to the surface, observed his boat and started to swim back to it. His anxiety remained until he saw the reef coming into his visual range, 5 metres below him. Once back on board he felt quite well.

*Diagnosis:* agoraphobic reaction.

## Hysteria

This may be the basis of some false claims related to diving. A number of cases have presented with a diving history and clinical symptomatology suggestive of a diving disorder, usually decompression sickness. The patient may move from one hyperbaric unit to another, for repetitive treatments – presumably either as an attention-seeking device or for the warmth and support that such a therapeutic unit may engender. These cases are the aquatic equivalent of the surgical **Munchausen's syndrome**. There is an analogous syndrome recorded in caisson workers.

## Illusions

Sensory deprivation, especially in the form of impaired visibility, is likely to aggravate the tendency to misinterpret stimuli. Anxiety associated with this environment results in heightened suggestibility, e.g. terror on sighting unexpected objects, mistaking another diver for a shark etc.

## Organic psychological responses

The psychological response of any subject to an abnormal physiological state is likely to be related to both the personality structure and

---

### CASE REPORT 29.2

During a flight from a northern, New South Wales, coastal town to Sydney, Miss PH, aged 30, developed episodes of breathlessness, unconsciousness with cyanosis, followed by a convulsive state. Between episodes she explained to the stewardess that she had been diving to 50 metres for approximately 35 minutes, 2 hours prior to the flight. There was a past history of a laminectomy.

On examination at a Sydney hospital she complained of pain on deep inspiration and a slight ache in the right knee exacerbated by movement. Over the next few hours she had three grand mal convulsions with associated epistaxis and the development of periorbital petechiae. The pain over the right knee had become worse and there was an overlying area of diminished sensation. A diagnosis of decompression sickness was made and treatment arranged at a nearby recompression chamber.

Prior to recompression she was conscious, rational and gave a history of the above dive in some detail. She complained of pain in the right knee and in the chest on deep inspiration. Apart from the area of diminished sensation over the right knee and decreased knee and ankle reflexes, no other neurological signs were detected. She was placed in the recompression chamber and pressurized to 18 metres on 100% oxygen initially and she improved symptomatically. During the subsequent decompression she had three grand mal epileptic convulsions. Upon recovery she complained of worsening of her knee and chest symptoms. She was therefore pressurized to 50 metres, where she again showed improvement, but again subsequently deteriorated. Following a series of epileptiform seizures, she became unresponsive to vocal and painful stimuli for some time. Some hours later, consciousness returned and she complained of severe abdominal, chest, right hip and right knee pain.

At this stage investigations by telephone revealed that she had not, in fact, been diving. She had a long psychiatric history of hysterical symptoms, genuine epilepsy and a recent interest in a 'skin diver' article on decompression sickness. Because of the long duration of exposure to pressure of both the patient and the attendants, subsequent decompression proceeded at a slow rate. The chamber reached the 'surface' after approximately 48 hours.

*Provisional diagnosis:* an aquatic Munchausen's syndrome.

the environment. Such diving situations include variations in inert gas pressure, carbon dioxide and oxygen tensions, hypothermia etc. Variations in the type and intensity of the reaction may range from the psychoneurotic to the organic cerebral syndromes.

The presence of cerebral involvement, with decompression sickness or arterial gas embolism, produces both psychological responses and sometimes organic psychiatric syndromes such as toxic–confusional states and symptomatic depressions which may last for months after all physical signs have gone.

If symptomatic depression remains after the course of hyperbaric therapy has been completed, the diver may have a modification of personality, with anxiety, emotional lability, difficulty in coping, delayed insomnia (waking up in the early hours) and even suicide ideas. Small doses of tricyclic antidepressants, such as amitriptyline 25–75 mg nightly, may have a beneficial result in a week of two. Otherwise an organically oriented psychiatrist may be required.

A common mistake made by hyperbaric clinicians is to interpret the behavioural abnormalities of an acute organic brain syndrome – as happens with both cerebral arterial gas embolism and decompression sickness – with hysterical and psychopathic diagnoses. Thus the obstreperous diver, with an illogical reluctance to enter the recompression chamber, is the very patient who may need it. The best assessors of apparent behaviour disorder are the diver's colleagues and family. They will recognize the behaviour as atypical, and thus indicate that it may be based on recent brain disease.

## Psychoses

Although psychosis should automatically preclude a candidate from diving training, certain diseases may result in pathological delusions related to diving, a misuse of the diving environment or false claims related to diving.

The incidence of psychiatric morbidity in divers is approximately twice as great as that in a comparable non-diving population – although there is a normal distribution pattern of the various psychiatric disorders. However, psychiatric disease is much less protracted among divers, and they return to their occupation quicker than the controls.

**Schizophrenia** may result in a diver developing primary delusions centred on his diving activity, e.g. a paranoia towards sharks resulting in a personal vendetta being waged against them. The development of a complex delusion system regarding international undersea control, radioactivity, diving inventions etc. has also been observed.

**Affective disorders**, such as a cyclic, manic–depressive psychosis, may be dangerous along both psychological axes. The grandiosity and self-assurance in a hypomanic state are as potentially dangerous as the suicidal inclinations during depression.

**Suicide** – although not well recognized, it is possible that this is not a rare event among those who have access to the sea. With the more widespread attraction to this sport among a greater range of personalities, the incidence must increase. The aetiology of suicide is not different to that of general medicine, but the means may differ considerably.

Swimming into the oceanic horizon has a certain Hollywood appeal, and has been used by some prosaic souls. One diver completed the suicide formalities by documenting his intent to free ascent while breath-holding, and succeeded in bursting his lungs. Others use more mundane methods despite the exotic environment (see Case report 29.3).

## Neuropsychological impairment – dementia

The neurological insults from diving may be many and varied, and may summate. There are often neurological signs of cerebral or cerebellar disorder. The judgement of such a patient, especially if he is in a powerful administrative position, may result in damage to other divers. The anecdotal observations of dementia in middle-aged professional divers, who do not adhere to established safety regulations and decompression procedures, are contentious and deserve investigation.

### Aetiology

The possible causes of intellectual impairment from compressed-air diving include neurological decompression sickness, air embolism

---

## CASE REPORT 29.3

FR refilled his scuba cylinder from the local diver shop, and hired a boat and diver to take him on a dive. He quietly read a science fiction book on the way out. He then entered the water, surfaced very soon and asked the boatman to hand him a bag he had bought. He was found the next morning by the water police still wearing his scuba equipment and with a 0.22 calibre bullet through his brain.

---

from pulmonary barotrauma, carbon monoxide toxicity and hypoxia. The ill-defined and unquantified damage from other gas toxicities may involve carbon dioxide, nitrogen, oxygen and contaminants. Repeated neuropsychological effects of immersion, such as dehydration and hypothermia, as well as subclinical decompression sickness (silent bubbles), are uncertain aetiological factors.

### Diving folklore

In a symposium in Norway in 1983, there was apparent acceptance of the neuropsychological complications of diving with compressed air at shallow depths, even though no consensus was reached regarding the long-term neuropsychological complications of deeper diving.

The anecdotal or folklore belief developed among many occupational diving groups that a dementia (diver's dumbness or the 'punch drunk' syndrome) was produced by prolonged compressed-air diving. This presumption was supported by media reports of brain damage in divers during the 1980s.

In the United Kingdom, clinical observations from the Royal Navy and pilot studies from the University of Lancaster have been widely quoted, and have probably heightened the concern about this topic by suggesting that it may have a basis in fact.

In a report on abalone divers in Australia, it was stated that 30% of the divers suffered chronic ear damage, 20% had dysbaric osteonecrosis and 10% had brain damage, but no supporting evidence was submitted.

### Circumstantial evidence

A number of diverse reports all seem to support the association of compressed-air div-

ing and neuropsychological damage. Clinical decompression sickness cases among recreational divers from Hawaii, Australia and Israel, during the last decade, showed an increased proportion of neurological manifestations, compared to the joint bends from the earlier navy studies.

In Sweden, abnormal EEGs were noted in 3.5% of free ascent trainees, suggesting the presence of cerebral arterial gas emboli.

Kwaitowski (1979) investigated 150 professional Polish divers and found abnormal EEGs in 43%, compared to 10% in the normal population.

Extrapolation from the animal models suggests a clinical value from EEGs and evoked cortical potentials in divers, at least in the acute stages of decompression sickness.

An investigation by Gorman et al. (1987) on civilian divers who had been treated for decompression sickness by the Royal Australian Navy, demonstrated a large number of neurological, EEG and psychometric abnormalities during the following 1–2 weeks. This was so even with divers who had no obvious clinical neurological component to their decompression sickness. These manifestations seemed to disappear with time.

Recently, imaging techniques have been used to demonstrate cerebral damage and perfusion abnormalities, after appropriate treatment has been instituted. This confirmed the presence of both anticipated and unexpected lesions (see page 168).

Calder (1983) demonstrated neuropathology findings at autopsy, which were more extensive than would have been anticipated from the mild or treated decompression sickness to which subjects had been coincidentally exposed. There was, however, more spinal than cerebral damage.

## Dementia and diving surveys

Reports from the 1950s and 1970s claimed that divers who suffered severe neurological decompression sickness were likely to sustain permanent brain dysfunction. These reports are widely cited as demonstrating the relationship between neurological decompression sickness and disruption of intellectual functioning. They are also quoted as evidence of diving, as such, as a cause of dementia. There are good reasons, however, for treating the findings of these reports with caution.

In 1959, **Rozsahegyi**, in Hungary, examined 100 subjects between 2.5 and 5 years after neurological decompression sickness, and concluded that over a half had some form of psychological disorder. Three-quarters of these had neurological findings on clinical examination. He noted that quiet men would frequently become irritable and uncontrolled after the injury, and that pathological drunkenness and alcohol intolerance were frequent.

He also observed an association between neurological and EEG abnormalities with psychiatric disturbance, leading him to postulate that these consequences were organic as opposed to psychogenic in nature. Rozsahegyi concluded that a chronic, progressive encephalomyelopathy resulted from repeated decompressions.

Although these observations were of value in prompting later research on the relationship between the neurological sequelae of decompression sickness and intellectual functioning, they do not constitute firm evidence for an association between the two. Rozsahegyi's paper reported his clinical conclusions, rather more than details or investigative data. There was no control group, no psychometric testing and considerable doubt about the contamination of diagnostic categories, because many of the patients suffered from inner-ear and possibly other barotraumatic lesions.

Between 1975 and 1977, three **Texas studies** (based on the same subjects) reported neurological and psychological problems in a small number of divers who experienced decompression sickness affecting the nervous system.

They also reported a correlation between neurological features and psychological impairment on a range of neuropsychological tests.

Unfortunately, there are some difficulties in evaluating the reports. The patients studied were probably not a representative group because 'litigation was pending in most cases', and it could be argued that such a situation could influence the neurological symptomatology, 'soft' neurological signs and motivation during psychological testing.

No attempt was made to control for the time lapse since the injury, in that patients were examined some time between 1 day and 2 years after the incident. Tests performed shortly after a neurological injury will, in many cases, overestimate the amount of damage that will remain in the future. It is important to report the time interval and, if necessary, control for it in the statistical analysis.

The way in which the control group was obtained also raises doubts about the validity of the conclusions regarding impaired performance in neuropsychological tests. Apparently the groups were determined by performance on the very tests that were then used to compare them. Under such circumstances, it is not surprising that the two groups differed on the test results. The error is analogous to dividing patients into groups of tall and short, and then using statistical tests to show that one group is taller than the other. Other divers were excluded from the comparison 'with equivocal neuropsychological findings', thereby maximizing the difference between the groups.

**Norwegian** reports claimed neuropsychological damage after 'near miss' diving accidents. They compared 9 divers who had accidents to 15 non-accident divers and an age-controlled reference group. The findings of the Texans, i.e. impaired intelligence among diving accident victims as assessed by the Wechsler Adult Intelligence Scale (WAIS), were not replicated. However, they did report that 8 of the 9 diving accident victims developed a syndrome in which there appeared to be a change in cognitive functioning; most reported impaired memory capacity as the main problem. In addition, difficulty in concentration, irritability, alcoholism and aphasia were noted. The interval between accident and neuropsychological testing was not reported.

The control group – divers who did not have a diving accident – differed from the accident group in a number of ways. They had a higher mean IQ (111) and were younger on average (26 years) than the accident group (mean IQ of 106 and mean age of 36 years). In this study, the effects of age and IQ on test performance operated in the same direction as the obtained results. Some account should have been made for these effects of age and IQ, using an analysis of co-variance.

There is also considerable difficulty in determining exactly which accidents were being investigated. In their accident table, the cause in three cases was listed as 'carbon dioxide'. The problems did not seem to be related to decompression sickness. There were a number of references to hypoxia, and in the remainder of the nine cases the suspected accident was listed as 'emboli'.

The authors stated that EEGs were performed and brain-stem auditory evoked potentials were taken; however, the results were not reported in the paper. They stated that a longitudinal study had been instigated, but no reference to this was made in subsequent symposia. This is unfortunate because the results, even if negative, would have been of interest.

### Australian 'excessive diver' surveys

In 1985, an opportunity became available to investigate a very special group of divers. The Australian abalone divers were interesting because of their extremely provocative diving procedures, the high prevalence of conventional occupational diseases of diving and the alleged presence of a punch drunk syndrome. It was presumed that, if this excessive diving group showed no evidence of intellectual impairment, the disorder would be an unlikely or uncommon complication in more conventional air diving groups. Conversely, if damage was present, its specific nature would be more obvious in this group.

After an initial pilot survey, which indicated that there may be such a problem, special interest researchers were asked to investigate the larger population of these excessive divers – using their own specialized psychological, neurological and electrophysiological tests. The purpose was to employ objective investigations, standardized and extensively used on the Australian population, to indicate the existence or otherwise of brain damage.

This excessive diving population of 152 divers had, on average:

1. been diving over 16 years;
2. spent 12 years in professional abalone diving;
3. spent over 5 hours per day on compressed air (Hookah) for 105 days each year;
4. reached just over 50 feet (15.25 m) on a typical day.
5. claimed to have been 'bent' over four times, but probably did not recognize the less dramatic types of decompression sickness.

Routinely, 58% of the excessive divers employed a dive profile that required some time for decompression, but which was omitted. Sixty-nine instances of decompression sickness were diagnosed and treated by recompression therapy in a recompression chamber. Of these, at least 39 seemed neurological in nature.

Because of the contradictory findings between the Texan and Norwegian studies on the WAIS, this approach was repeated by Edmonds and Coulton (1986) on a much larger ($n=67$), 'excessive' diving population.

A multiple regression analysis was made against all diving co-variants and the 10 subtext scores (verbal IQ, performance IQ, total IQ) and deterioration index ('dementia score'), corrected for age. Apart from very minor and unimportant associations, the analysis showed no relationship between the type of diving and these measurements of intellectual functioning. Nor was there an abnormal profile or scatter in the divers' results, which would have supported brain damage. This investigation indicated that if neuropsychological changes were present, they would be of a more subtle nature than those detected by such multiple aptitude batteries.

Neurobehavioural researchers, who specialized in detection of minor abnormalities among occupational groups exposed to chemicals, heavy metals and toxins, also examined a group of excessive divers. Williamson et al. (1987, 1989) reported two studies, one looking at whether divers differed from carefully selected controls in their performance in a variety of tests and the second looking at the relationship between the test performances and the indices of diving exposure.

In the first study, they found that the divers did as well or better than the controls on some tests (reaction time, some memory and motor tests) and worse than controls on others (visual and short-term memory and some psycho-motor learning skills). However, the way in which divers chose to complete their tests differed from the controls, in that they were more likely to take risks and substitute speed for accuracy. This sort of difference in behaviour must be taken into account when interpreting neuropsychological assessments in other surveys.

The second study focused on neuropsychological functioning and a number of diving-related variables, but the associations found were weak. What it did demonstrate was that the deficit in neurobehavioural tests was shown in those divers who consistently exposed themselves to gross decompression omissions and decompression sickness.

Another subgroup of 48 excessive divers was subjected to the more conventional psychometric tests by Andrews et al. (1986). This study compared excessive divers to non-diving fishermen controls living in the same locality. They found that the differences were small, and the divers' scores were within normal limits for the general population.

A valuable approach in the Andrews' survey was the comparison of the 'abnormal low' performance members from both the divers and control groups, and they found no evidence for a subset of divers with abnormal scores. The authors concluded that 'there was no evidence for the accumulation of subclinical insults leading to a dementing process'.

Hjorth et al. (1986) performed double-blind assessments on EEGs and carried out multiple evoked cortical potentials on 20 excessive divers. Apart from a couple of minor abnormalities in the EEGs, no significant findings were made. Visual evoked cortical potentials and upper and lower limb somatosensory evoked cortical potentials were all normal.

## Discussion

Brain damage can supervene if there is an obvious cerebral injury (severe hypoxia, carbon monoxide toxicity, cerebral embolism or cerebral decompression sickness). Otological, visual, spinal and peripheral neuropathies from decompression sickness, oxygen toxicity and other diving may affect neurobehavioural function.

Earlier studies, although contributing to the concept of neurological decompression sickness causing permanent neuropsychological damage, had serious limitations in their diagnostic categories, statistical analysis and use of control groups.

There was some relationship between excessive decompression stress (decompression sickness and grossly omitted decompression) and some short-term memory decrement in the Williamson et al. Australian series, supporting the observations that decompression sickness may induce some changes consistent with organic brain damage.

The adverse effect of decompression sickness and its treatment on the anxiety and self-esteem of the diver, together with attitudes of both peer and therapist groups, may well have psychological effects. The post-traumatic stress syndrome is a possible sequel to all diving, and non-diving, accidents. These effects, together with the physiological influences of sleep deprivation, hyperbaric therapy, drug administration and non-cerebral manifestations of decompression sickness, may well complicate the interpretation of psychometric tests performed soon after the incident.

In the Australian excessive diver cross-sectional survey, tests of neuropsychological impairment were performed to ascertain whether excessive diving, as such, is associated with changes in intellectual functioning in this population. Even in these excessive divers, there was no evidence of a diving-related dementia. There was no evidence that diving, per se, causes any mental impairment.

There is ample evidence that acute and temporary neurological insults are experienced by compressed-air divers. These were not commonly translated into hard evidence of permanent brain damage or dementia. If such a deterioration does occur, it is likely to be either minor or rare in compressed-air diving.

The investigations into the neuropsychological effects of deep and helium diving bear a definite similarity to the earlier amateurish psychometric approaches applied to the compressed-air diving. The added long-term effects of the high-pressure neurological syndrome have yet to be adequately defined, qualitatively and quantitatively.

# References and recommended reading

ANDREWS, G., HOLT, P., EDMONDS, C. et al. (1986). Does non-clinical decompression stress lead to brain damage in abalone divers? *Medical Journal of Australia* **144**, 399–401.

CALDER, I.M. (1983). The long-term neurological consequences of deep diving. In: *EUBS and NPD Workshop*, Stavanger, Norway.

EDMONDS, C. and COULTON, T. (1986). Multiple aptitude assessments on abalone divers. In: *The Abalone Diver*, edited by C. Edmonds. Morwell, Victoria: National Safety Council of Australia.

EDMONDS, C. and HAYWARD, L. (1987). Intellectual impairment with diving. A review. *Ninth International Symposium on Underwater and Hyperbaric Physiology*. Bethesda, MD: Undersea and Hyperbaric Medical Society.

GORMAN, D., BERAN, R., EDMONDS, C. et al. (1987). The neurological sequelae of decompression sickness. A preliminary report. *Ninth International Symposium on Underwater and Hyperbaric Physiology*. Bethesda MD: Undersea and Hyperbaric Medical Society.

HJORTH, R., VIGNAENDRA, V. and EDMONDS, C. (1986). Electroencephalographic and evoked cortical potential assessments in divers. In: *The Abalone Diver*, edited by C. Edmonds. Morwell, Victoria: National Safety Council of Australia.

INGVAR, D.H., ADOLFSON, J. and LINDEMARK, C.O. (1973). Cerebral air embolism during training of submarine personnel in free escape: an electroencephalographic study. *Aerospace Medicine* **44**, 628–653.

KELLY, P.J. and PETERS, B.H. (1975). The neurological manifestations of decompression accidents. In: *International Symposium on Man in the Sea*, edited by S.K. Hong, pp. 227–232. Bethesda, MD: Undersea Medical Society.

KWAITOWSKI, S.R. (1979). Analysis of the E.E.G. records among divers. *Bulletin of the Institute of Maritime and Tropical Medicine*, **30**, 131–135.

LEVIN, H.S. (1975). Neuropsychological sequelae of diving accidents. In: *International Symposium on Man in the Sea*, edited by S.K. Hong, pp. 233–241. Bethesda, MD: Undersea Medical Society.

PETERS, B.H., LEVIN, H.S. and KELLY, P.J. (1977). Neurologic and psychologic manifestations of decompression illness in divers. *Neurology* **27**, 125–127.

ROZSAHEGYI, I. (1959). Late consequences of the neurological forms of decompression sickness. *British Journal of Industrial Medicine* **16**, 311–317.

SYMPOSIUM PROCEEDINGS (1983). The long-term neurological consequences of deep diving. *EUBS and NPD Workshop*, Stavanger, Norway.

VAERNES, R.J. and EIDSVIK, S. (1982). Central nervous dysfunction after near miss accidents in diving. *Aviation Space and Environmental Medicine* **53**, 803–807.

WILLIAMSON, A. and CLARKE, B. (1986). Relationships between neurobehavioural factors and diving exposure. In: *The Abalone Diver*, edited by C. Edmonds. Morwell, Victoria: National Safety Council of Australia.

WILLIAMSON, A., EDMONDS, C. and CLARKE, B. (1987). The neurobehavioural effects of professional abalone diving. *British Journal of Industrial Medicine* **44**, 459–466.

WILLIAMSON, A., CLARKE, B. and EDMONDS, C. (1989). The influence of diving variables on perceptual and cognitive functions in professional shallow-water divers. *Environmental Research* **50**, 93–102.

# Other disorders

## Introduction

This chapter includes many less known or less appreciated disorders which have not been well defined. With future editions, some of these topics will warrant their own chapters.

## Carotid sinus syndrome

Pressure may be exerted over the carotid sinus by tight-fitting wet suits, especially when they are of the 'pullover' variety without zippers. Most divers will be aware of the unpleasant sensation while wearing these, and will cut the neckline to release the pressure before other symptoms supervene. In some cases, the sensation of confusion and disorientation may have a demonstrable nystagmus associated with it. Such cases may be verified by electronystagmography (ENG). Other mechanisms may be needed to explain some of these cases.

Others may experience a sensation of fainting and have the bradycardia and hypotension which result from pressure on the carotid sinus. This may contribute to the 'sudden death syndrome' (see page 358).

In all these cases it is necessary to reduce the pressure around the neck, by removing or cutting the wet suit.

# Caustic cocktail

This only occurs when rebreathing equipment is used. It is variously termed 'proto cocktail' when Protosorb is the carbon dioxide absorbent used, and 'soda cocktail' when Sodasorb is used.

Exogenous or endogenous water, when mixed with carbon dioxide absorbent, will produce an alkaline solution which may not remain in the absorbent canister. If it travels into the breathing tubing, it may be taken into the mouth and inhaled or swallowed. A severe inflammation, possibly with mucosal ulceration, can result. The extent of these injuries is related to the amount, concentration and distribution of the 'cocktail'.

Traditionally, treatment involves rinsing of the mouth with vinegar or other acidic mixture to neutralize the alkaline cocktail. This therapy may itself be very painful because of the mucosal damage. Probably, a rapid irrigation of the area with fresh or sea water will expedite the removal of the irritant material, and reduce the symptoms and subsequent damage. Respiratory and gastric involvement is treated according to general medical principles.

# Cold urticaria

This is a predominantly localized response to cold – whether it be cold water, ice, wind or volatile fluids. It is usually noticed on the exposed skin, but may also affect mucosa in the respiratory system (by breathing cold air) or in the mouth and gastrointestinal tract (by swallowing cold drinks). The symptoms may thus vary from skin rash, punctate erythema or urticaria, to nasal congestion, swelling of the lips and mouth, cough and dyspnoea, dysphagia and abdominal cramps.

It can often be replicated by placing the hand and forearm in iced water for 5 minutes and observing the development of the skin manifestations over the next 5–10 minutes. Occasionally it can be reproduced by an ice cube (see Plate 8).

Generalized symptoms and signs may develop, probably due to histamine release, and produce headache, flushing, hypertension, syncope and increased gastric secretion. In a highly sensitized patient, swimming in cold water may precipitate cardiovascular collapse and death.

Investigations may reveal cold precipitated plasma proteins, such as cryoglobulin, cold agglutinin, cryofibrinogen etc. Other allergic responses may also be present.

The stimulus to tissue damage and mast cell histamine release is the rate of decrease of temperature, more than the absolute temperature. The symptoms tend to develop after the return to normal temperatures. The syndrome may develop spontaneously or after some illness or injury (one case followed a jelly fish sting).

The response to systematic antihistamines and topical steroids is usually poor (although oral cyproheptadine has been used with benefit). Desensitization by gradually increasing the severity of the stimulus from warm acceptable showers to cold water swimming (under competent supervision) has worked in some cases. The disease tends to clear over some months or years, but may recur. It is sometimes familial.

# Dental disorders

**Barotrauma** (see page 129) affecting the teeth, sinuses with pain referred to the teeth and subcutaneous emphysema (also submucous) from dental procedures has already been mentioned.

**Dental electrolysis** may be experienced by divers who do electric welding. They notice a metallic taste in the mouth adjacent to amalgam fillings. The electrical field set up by the equipment causes the metal in the filling to be released, producing both the metallic taste and the premature destruction of the fillings.

**Dental plates** must be secure and not easily displaced either during buddy breathing, vomiting, resuscitation or otherwise. A candidate who exhales his plate while performing lung function tests is just as likely to inhale it while diving. Deaths have been caused by a loose dental plate.

# Hyperthermia

The sea is commonly a heat-extracting environment because of its high conductivity and spec-

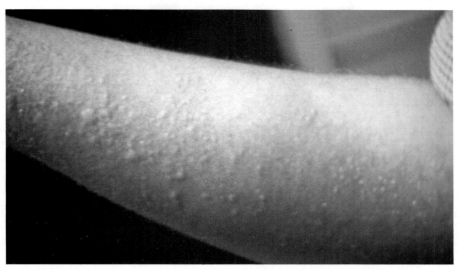

**Plate 8**  Cold urticaria: histamine skin reaction developing 5–10 minutes after exposure to cold water. Mucosal surfaces were affected by drinking cold liquids. Diving had to be suspended for 6 months. (See Chapter 30)

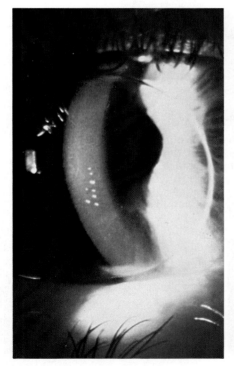

**Plate 9**  Bubbles developing between the hard contact lens and the cornea; developed during decompression

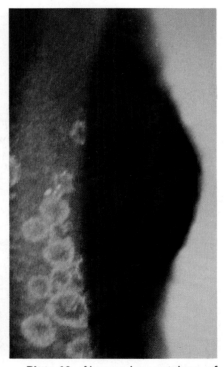

**Plate 10**  Nummular patches of corneal epithelial oedema, where the bubbles injure the cornea. (See Chapter 30.) (Photos in Plates 9 and 10 courtesy of Drs Mark E. Bradley and David Simon)

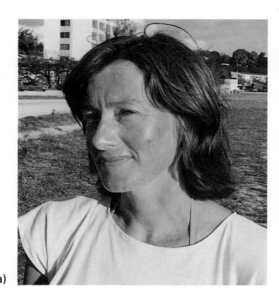

(a)

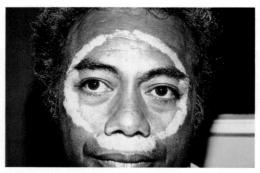

(b)

**Plate 11** Mask burn: (a) inflammation around the mask/skin contact. Mild and lasting only a few hours, this disorder leaves the conjunctiva unaffected. Compare Plate 2, showing mask barotrauma. (Courtesy of Mrs R. Lowry.) (b) Using a full face mask, this islander experienced a severe reaction to the mask, with blistering, scarring and depigmentation. (Courtesy of Dr C. W. Williams)

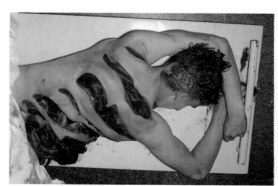

**Plate 12** Parallel lacerations from propellor injury. (Courtesy of Dr W. Brighton – in Plueckhahn, V.D. (1991) *Ethics, Legal Medicine and Forensic Medicine,* 2nd edn)

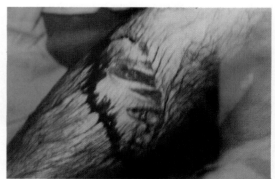

**Plate 13** Triangular teeth marks of shark bite. (Courtesy of Dr C. Barnes)

ific heat, and low temperature. Despite this, hyperthermia has claimed the lives of some divers. It may develop in three ways.

Thermal protection suits, which effectively insulate the diver from low water temperatures, also help to retain the diver's own heat output. Both wet suits and dry suits, worn before or after immersion, may produce hyperthermia and heat stroke in temperate climates. When these divers also wear their suits at tropical diving resorts, or perform exercise, the danger is increased. The suit may still be worn for mechanical protection, without realizing its thermal disadvantages. Armoured diving suits, such as the 1 atmosphere 'Jim', may predispose to hyperthermia because of inadequate ventilation.

Actively produced hyperthermia may result from wearing hot water or other heated suits, or by breathing heated gases of high thermal conductivity, such as helium. In deep diving operations, this gas may need to be heated to reduce respiratory heat loss, but the operating range is small and it is easy to overstep the margins. A further complication is the heat produced by compression of the chamber gas to simulate descent.

Divers with hyperthermia may lose consciousness from postural hypotension when, in their vasodilated state, they are exposed to the effect of gravity – as they emerge from the water onto the dive boat or into the diving bell.

Hyperthermia is a recognized complication of the treatment of hypothermia, by hot water immersion or by active core rewarming.

The prevention is by avoiding the above circumstances. Treatment includes removal of the cause, applying cooling techniques, rehydration and electrolyte replacement.

# Musculoskeletal problems

The musculoskeletal problems of decompression sickness (Chapter 12), dysbaric osteonecrosis (Chapter 14) and Irukandji stings (see page 334) have been described previously.

## Compression (hyperbaric) arthralgia

With the advent of deep and helium diving, a syndrome of joint noises and sensations was recorded. The noises were described as crack-ing, creaking or popping, and the sensations varied from discomfort, to a dry and gritty feeling, to frank pain precipitated by movement.

The symptoms can appear as early in compression as 30 metres, but are more common at depths exceeding 100 metres. They are aggravated by a fast compression, but improve as the exposure at depth continues. The divers show considerable individual susceptibility, and it is more likely to be noted in compression chambers than in water, when fast movements are limited and little mechanical load is placed on the joints.

The current explanation of this disorder involves a gas-induced osmosis interfering with joint lubrication and producing cavitation. As the subject is compressed, a relative imbalance is present between the concentration of inert gas in the blood and that in the synovial fluid, and articular cartilage, and causes a water shift from the joint to the higher osmolarity blood. As equilibration of inert gas develops with a continuation of this exposure to pressure, the original fluid volumes should become re-established.

## Cramp

Divers seem particularly prone to muscle spasms, resulting in temporary pain and disability, which may have disproportionately severe complications under water. It usually develops in muscles that are exposed to atypical exertion, e.g. physically unfit divers, the use of new fins etc. Although the most common sites are the calf of the leg and the sole of the foot, other muscle masses may be affected. These include the thighs (especially hamstrings), upper limbs, abdomen etc. Diagnosis is made by observation and palpation of the tight muscle mass. Any damage to the neuromuscular system will predispose to muscle cramp.

The immediate treatment consists of a slow, passive extension of the cramped muscle, and then a return to safety. Prevention includes the maintenance of an adequate standard of physical fitness, constant diving exercise and practice, the fitting of comfortable equipment and fins, avoidance of dehydration and sweating, good nutrition and adequate thermal protection.

## Decompression sickness

The musculoskeletal ('bends') pains of decompression sickness have already been dealt with in Chapter 12. Such symptoms are thought to be due to tissue distortion from bubbles, and are relieved rapidly (within minutes) during hyperbaric exposure and less rapidly (hours) by inhalation of 100% oxygen.

There are many less obvious and less well-defined musculoskeletal or arthralgic symptoms which may follow decompression sickness and which are possibly attributable to subsequent tissue damage (in tendons, muscles etc.) or even to early injury within the bones – which may or may not progress to dysbaric osteonecrosis. Such symptoms may improve somewhat with non-steroidal anti-inflammatory drugs, such as paracetamol, ibuprofen or piroxicam. A technetium bone scan may be of value in excluding early and progressive osteonecrosis pathology. The symptoms usually diminish and gradually disappear over weeks or months.

## Lumbosacral lesions

Prolonged underwater swimming, in an abnormal hyperextended spinal position – such as is employed by shell fisherman scanning the seabed – can aggravate lumbosacral pathology. The positioning of the heavy weight belt around the waist may make this worse. Many divers so affected have replaced the weight belt with a much wider weight-containing corset. For cervical spine lesions see page 406.

## Temporomandibular joint dysfunction

In the early stages of diving training, a novice may experience apprehension with regard to the air supply. Consequently, he is likely to clamp his teeth hard onto the mouth piece to such a degree that considerable temporomandibular joint stress is caused with a resultant arthritis. Pain and tenderness are felt just anterior to the ear. Alternative or associated symptoms include trismus, restriction of the ability to open the mouth widely, 'clicking' of the joint and occasionally tinnitus and vertigo. The syndrome is readily relieved by education of the diver and encouraging him to relax.

Recurrent problems of temporomandibular arthritis and subluxation of this joint are also likely to be aggravated by diving. Apart from the above cause, which is unlikely in experienced divers, there are other stresses placed on the temporomandibular joint which are not normally experienced in non-divers. These include the use of mouth pieces not individually fashioned to the diver's oral and dental configuration, prolonged exposure to a chilling environment, and finally the use of equipment which tends to pull vertically or to one side of the diver's mouth. Most mouth pieces require the diver to hold his mouth open with the mandible protruded, tugging on the mouth piece – an abnormal position. The symptoms are similar to those described above, but in the chronic cases, radiological evidence will demonstrate the extent of joint damage and dysfunction. The remedy is to avoid the provoking situations, i.e. use well-fitting mouth pieces or an oronasal mask, ensure there is no strain on the demand valve or its hose, and wear a well-fitting hood to avoid cold.

## Tank carriers' lateral epicondylitis

The aquatic equivalent of 'tennis elbow' is due to the strain on the extensor tendon attached to the lateral condyle, from carrying heavy tanks.

# Neurological problems

Many neurological problems have already been dealt with. They include: CAGE (see Chapter 9), neurological DCS (see Chapter 12), nitrogen narcosis (see Chapter 15), the HPNS (see Chapter 16) and neuropsychological disorders (see Chapter 29).

Others include: headaches in diving, brachial plexus lesions, scuba diver's thigh, epilepsy, and other neuralgias and nerve lesions.

## Headache

This is a common symptom in diving medicine, but is not usually well documented. The following causes are not all inclusive, and the clinical details of each type of headache are to be found either in the appropriate sections of this book, or in general medical texts. The differential diagnosis will depend on a detailed clinical and diving history, a physical examination and laboratory investigation.

### Anxiety (tension)

The psychological reaction, induced in susceptible novice divers exposed to a stressful underwater environment, may produce a typical
tension headache.

### Sinus barotrauma (page 128)

Pain occurs during the diver's change of depth
– caused by the volume changes on the sinus
gas spaces. Barotrauma of descent affecting
the frontal sinus is the most common. It is
often relieved by ascent. Ethmoidal sinus pain
is referred to the intraorbital area and maxillary sinus pain may be referred to the teeth.
Sphenoidal sinus pain may be referred to the
parieto-occipital area.

### Sinus pathology

Mucocele or other **sinus pathology** can be
produced by diving. Rupture of the cells in the
ethmoidal sinus air cells can cause a sudden
and explosive headache and result in a small
haematoma or bruising below the glabella, at
the root of the nose, following sinus barotrauma. A similar explosive headache can
develop, often during ascent and following
middle-ear barotrauma, with rupture of the
mastoid air cells causing a generalized pain,
localizing later to the mastoid region. Pneumocephalus can follow the sinus ruptures (see
Figure 10.11). CT skull scans demonstrate
these lesions with precision.

### Infections (Chapter 23)

In the mastoid cavities or sinuses infections
usually cause pain 4–24 hours after the dive
and are commonly associated with a pre-
existing upper respiratory tract infection and/
or barotrauma. Other generalized infections,
including *Naegleria* spp., are related to marine
exposure.

### Cold

In some susceptible subjects, exposure to cold
water may induce a throbbing pain particularly
over the frontal area, but sometimes also
including the occipital area. It is probably
analogous to the head pain experienced by

some people when eating cold food, such as ice
cream. The onset may be rapid after cold water
contact, or it may progressively increase in
intensity with the duration of exposure. It
usually remains for some minutes after the
diver has left the water. Whether this is a
migraine variant, a neurocirculatory reflex or
merely due to an increase in muscular tone is
not known. Prevention is by the use of a
protective hood to ensure warmth.

### Salt water aspiration

Headache following aspiration of sea water
usually follows a latent period of 30 minutes or
more, is usually associated with myalgia and is
aggravated by exercise and cold.

### Mask tension

Inexperienced divers tend to adjust the face
mask straps far too tightly and this may result
in a headache not dissimilar to that of a tight
hat, misfitting spectacle frames etc. due to
direct local pressure effects. It is related to the
duration of the dive, and clears in an hour or
so. A similar disorder, called 'swim goggle'
headache, may be related to migraine.

### Gas toxicity

Specific gas toxicities may sometimes cause a
characteristic headache. The carbon dioxide-
induced headache usually develops with a gradually increasing carbon dioxide tension, or
follows a reduction in a sharply rising carbon
dioxide tension, i.e. a carbon dioxide 'off
effect'. The carbon dioxide-induced headache
is throbbing in nature, lasts a few hours and is
not relieved by analgesics or anti-migraine
preparations. Headaches have also been
described with oxygen toxicity, carbon monoxide toxicity and other gas contaminations.

### Decompression sickness (see Chapter 12) and pulmonary barotrauma (see Chapter 9)

Headache is an ominous symptom in both
neurological decompression sickness and air
embolism from pulmonary barotrauma. It is
associated with intracerebral bubbles and/or
raised intracranial pressure. Usually it arises
within minutes of ascent, and is thus suggestive

of bubbles of intravascular origin. Other neurological manifestations and a disturbance of conscious state are often associated. The headache is likely to persist for a week or more, but is rapidly relieved by recompression therapy. Its recurrence is indicative of a deterioration in the patient's neurological state and is also amenable to recompression or oxygen therapy.

### Migraine

Traditionally migraine sufferers have been advised not to take up diving. Attacks are rarely induced by the diving environment, but may be of greatly increased severity when they do develop. The precipitation of the migraine attack may be due to any of the other headache-producing stimuli discussed in this section, e.g. cold, anxiety, oxygen or carbon dioxide tensions, intravascular bubbles etc.

Once a migraine attack has commenced during diving activities, the patient is at considerable risk from the following: disturbance in neurological function, i.e. interference of consciousness, perception and motor activity; vertigo; psychological complications; and vomiting. A number of subjects have had their first migraine episode under water – although there is usually a positive family history to aid in diagnosis. This may lead to diagnostic confusion with cerebral decompression sickness and/or air embolism. Then the oxygen therapy tables pose therapeutic problems.

Prevention is best achieved by either not diving, or avoiding the specific provoking stimulus, e.g. use of a wet suit hood if cold is the precipitant, or limit of diving exposures to shallow no-decompression diving with generous safety margins. Safety techniques such as buddy diving techniques are also very important for those migraine subjects who insist on diving.

### Neuromuscular pain

Headaches produced by the environment or by locomotor stress may produce severe pains which are difficult to assess and diagnose. Many such patients give consistent accounts of headaches being induced by diving, and sometimes only by scuba diving, but with none of the specific features mentioned above. Some may be psychogenic or tension headaches, whereas others seem more vascular in nature.

One specific type, due to minor degrees of cervical spondylosis, aggravated by excessive provocation, may be confirmed by cervical spine X-rays. In these there may be loss of lordotic curvature, narrowing of intervertebral spaces and osteophytosis in the lateral views. Many divers who develop this disorder are in the older age bracket or have a history of head and neck trauma. They often swim under water with flexion of the lower cervical spine (to avoid the tank) and their upper cervical spine hyperextended (to view where they are going). This produces C1, C2 and C3 compression and distortion of the cervicocranial relationships – an unnatural posture aggravating underlying disease, which may otherwise be asymptomatic.

The headache is usually occipital and may persist for many hours after the dive. The area is often tender on palpation. Persistent occipital neuralgia can have a similar aetiology. Occasionally the pain is referred to the top and front of the head, possibly due to fibres of the trigeminal nerve passing down the cervical cord and being affected by damage to the upper cervical vertebrae.

### Others

Many other obvious reasons may be incriminated in the aetiology of headache in divers. These include such diverse factors as alcohol overindulgence, head injury usually sustained during ascent, glare from the sun, drugs such as vasodilators and calcium channel blockers, computing the US Navy repetitive dive tables etc.

### Brachial plexus injury

This disorder is related to the use of standard diving equipment, when the weight of the helmet is taken directly on the supraclavicular region. This may be from mishandling the helmet or by having inadequate or incorrectly placed padding over the area between the neck and shoulder. It is more likely to be caused out of the water, when the weight factor is greatest. The standby diver is thus more prone to this disorder. The middle and lower cervical nerves are more likely to be involved, i.e. the

> *Some causes of headache in diving:*
> 1. *Anxiety*
> 2. *Sinus barotrauma, sinusitis and other pathology*
> 3. *Cold exposure*
> 4. *Salt water aspiration*
> 5. *Tight face mask straps*
> 6. *Carbon dioxide and carbon monoxide toxicity*
> 7. *Decompression sickness*
> 8. *Pulmonary barotrauma*
> 9. *Migraine*
> 10. *Cervical spondylosis*
> 11. *Drugs*

fifth to seventh, and this may be either temporary or permanent. The minor cases present with paraesthesia and numbness of the lateral aspect of the arm, forearm, thumb and adjacent fingers. Severe cases result in both motor and sensory damage over the affected nerve distribution. Rigid shoulder harnesses of scuba can also produce this.

## Epilepsy

Epilepsy is a total contraindication to diving, but not infrequently the first epileptic convulsion develops under water. In some cases the cause may be obvious, such as oxygen toxicity (see Chapter 18), cerebral arterial gas embolism (see Chapter 9) or neurological decompression sickness (see Chapter 12).

A variety of medical causes also could be responsible, including previous idiopathic epilepsy, hypoglycaemia, cerebrovascular accidents, cerebral trauma or tumours etc. These are the easier cases to diagnose and the management extends beyond the diving situation. The dilemma is the case without an established cause, and this is the most frequent situation in recreational diving. It appears as if diving lowers the seizure threshold in general. It is commonly seen in oxygen convulsions, where 'dry' exposures may be much longer than in-water durations, using high oxygen mixtures or rebreathing equipment.

Perhaps the reasons in non-specific convulsions are multifactorial and include:

- Sensory deprivation.
- Hyperventilation from positive pressure demand valves.
- Nitrogen narcosis (sedation).
- Acidosis from carbon dioxide retention.
- Anxiety.
- Misdiagnosis of hypoxic and carbon dioxide convulsions.

The first four of these conditions have been used in general medicine to provoke convulsions.

Management of an epileptic attack under water poses unsolvable problems. The confusional state during the aura may cause unpredictable behaviour. The fear of pulmonary barotrauma during ascent, at least in the tonic phase, has to be weighed against the likelihood of drowning during the clonic and post-ictal phase, when the diver is unconscious. It is our experience that the diver is best served by risking an ascent in a face-down position, until the surface is reached. This is certainly so once the clonic phase has begun.

Subsequent management includes the exclusion of other causes, appropriate investigations, exclusion from diving and the warning that subsequent episodes may occur on land, even years later.

## Scuba diver's thigh (meralgia paraesthetica)

The lateral femoral cutaneous nerve is vulnerable to compression neuropathy by pregnancy, tight trousers, pelvic tilt, harnesses and low positioned weight belts. It results in a numbness over the upper thigh, anteriorly and laterally. It usually clears up in a few months.

## Neuralgias and other nerve lesions

Chronic and sometimes severe pain, referable to either nerves, nerve roots or plexus, may follow neurological decompression sickness (see page 172), when myelin sheaths may be damaged. Spinal cord lesions may also be responsible for some of these cases.

Oxygen toxicity may produce a variably persistent bilateral peripheral neuropathy, as may many of the fish poisons and marine toxins.

Involvement of the trigeminal and facial nerves may follow sinus or middle-ear barotraumas (see page 135).

# Ocular disorders

## 'Bubble eyes'

Some divers complain of gas bubbling from the inner canthus of the eye. The cause is an excessively patent nasolacrimal duct. This structure frequently has an imperfect valve, formed by the mucous membrane in the nasal cavity. The normal passage of tears from the eye and down the duct is not impeded. Unfortunately, the passage of air up the duct may be expedited when the diver increases nasopharyngeal pressure, such as during the Valsalva manoeuvre. It can be demonstrated by viewing the air bubbling out of the lacrimal canals during this manoeuvre. There is a possibility of spreading organisms from the nasopharynx and causing conjunctivitis.

## Ocular damage from corneal lens

Recent work on the use of contact lenses during diving has demonstrated that the soft corneal microlens is permeable to gas and nutrients. They are therefore safe, except for the likelihood of being lost during such diving techniques as face mask removal, followed by opening the eyes under water.

Ophthalmologists claim that soft lenses shrink when exposed to fresh water, and may cling to the cornea and be temporarily difficult to remove. If exposed to sea water they swell and can float out of the eye. Within the mask this should not cause a problem. The fresh water organism *Acanthamoeba*, which can cause severe infections, corneal ulcerations and blindness, should not be a problem in sea water or inside face masks.

The smaller, hard contact lenses are also not very secure in that they cover less of the cornea. Some are less permeable and have the potential of causing problems during decompression (see Plate 9).

Underneath the hard lenses, small bubbles develop during decompression, in the precorneal tear film. They coalesce and expand during decompression and may damage the corneal tissue. Divers may be aware of a sensation of discomfort in the eyes, the appearance of haloes radiating spokes when looking at lights, and also a decreased visual acuity. In mild cases the symptoms last only a few hours.

The symptoms may be prevented by the use of a small 0.4-mm hole made near the centre of the hard lens, and this is then termed a 'fenestrated hard lens'. The hole serves as a channel through which the small amounts of tear fluid can pass, carrying the gas with it.

These problems are likely to occur especially in deeper or longer dives, or in hyperbaric chambers. The problem of loss of a lens during any diving operations makes these visual aids unacceptable for many professional divers. The increased likelihood of eye infections and the difficulty with eye toilet and lens disinfection procedures, as well as the blurred vision that sometimes accompanies the lens usage, makes them an unnecessary and often unacceptable hazard in remote areas and oil rigs.

## Ocular fundus – lesions in divers

The ocular lesions of hyperoxia are described elsewhere (see page 254).

Recently, retinal fluorescein angiography has shown that the retinal capillary density at the fovea was low, and microaneurysm and small areas of capillary non-perfusion were seen, more often in divers than in non-divers (see page 177). The prevalence of the fundus abnormality is related to the length of diving exposure. The changes were consistent with the obstruction of the retinal and choroidal circulations. This obstruction could be due either to intravascular bubbles, formed during decompression, or to altered behaviour of blood constituents and blood vessels in hyperbaric conditions.

These lesions did not appear to have any influence on visual acuity, and there was an increased prevalence of such lesions in divers who had had decompression sickness; this was significantly higher than in divers of equivalent experience but without a history of decompression sickness. Nevertheless, even if the divers with decompression sickness were excluded, this did not abolish the correlation between diving experience and pigment epithelial changes. The statistics refer specifically to pigment epithelial changes.

The defects in the retinal pigment epithelium are indistinguishable from those documented in eyes following choroidal ischaemia.

It is possible, but there is no actual evidence, that these abnormalities may cause problems in later life. It is also necessary that these observations be verified by other workers, prior to preventive advice or action being taken.

### Swimmers' eyes

Keratitis may cause blurred vision and 'rainbow' or 'halo' effects because of the corneal irritation from exposure to suspended particles and hypertonic saline (sea water), chlorine, ammonia and hypotonic water (swimming pools and fresh water). This is less likely with mask-wearing divers than with swimmers, but it is not uncommon when divers use chemical preparations to clean and demist the mask's glass face plate.

### Trauma

Damage to the eyes can result from face mask implosion, from inadequately strengthened glass during descent or from confronting a released anchor as the diver swims down the chain. Dramatic injuries have been due to spear guns (see page 413).

It has been demonstrated that divers with radial keratotomy (usually used for surgical treatment of myopia) may have a weakened cornea and be more susceptible to trauma – with rupture along the lines of the incision. Barotrauma effects in the face mask with descent, causing rupture of the eyeball, are a possibility. For this reason, such patients are usually advised not to dive with the usual (half) face masks. Alternatives may include: gas-filled contact lenses, face masks with openings to the water, and full face masks connected to the air supply (Visionaire, Auer).

### Others

Refer to **Oxygen toxicity** (page 254), **Infections** (page 313) **Decompression sickness** (page 172), **Facial barotrauma** (page 132) and **Mask burn** (page 411). See Chapter 35 regarding medical selection for diving.

## Seasickness (motion sickness)

Almost everybody is susceptible to motion sickness. In general the population can be divided roughly into one-third who are highly susceptible, one-third who react only under rough conditions and one-third who become sick only under extreme conditions. Although anyone with a normally functioning vestibular system is susceptible, there are some patients who are totally deaf and have unresponsive vestibular systems, and who are immune.

In diving there are two major situations predisposing to seasickness. The first is on the boat going towards the dive site, and the second is while the diver is actually in the water, particularly if he is attached to the boat, e.g. on a shot line or during decompression. Most divers swimming under water are less susceptible to seasickness than while on board. It is for this reason that many divers hurry to enter the water, following exposure to adverse sea conditions en route to the dive site. Problems develop because of divers being inadequately prepared and equipped due to haste or the debilitating and demoralizing effects of seasickness.

Usually the first sign of seasickness is pallor, although this occasionally may be preceded by a flushed appearance. It may be followed by yawning, restlessness and a cold sweat, often noticeable on the forehead and upper lip. Malaise, nausea and vomiting may progress to prostration, dehydration, electrolyte and acid–base imbalance. During this progression, there is often a waxing and waning of symptoms especially prior to the actual development of vomiting.

Tolerance does develop to a particular group of circumstances, and a subject may become totally immune under specific conditions. If, however, there is a change in the intensity or nature of the motion, then the individual is again susceptible. Continuous exposure to constant conditions will usually produce tolerance within 2–3 days. This can also develop to repeated shorter exposures. There is a central nervous system habituation, to such a degree that when the motion is stopped, the subject may then experience 'sea legs' in which stationary objects appear to be rocking at the frequency of the original ship exposure, after the subjects disembark.

There is considerable variation in susceptibility to seasickness. With increasing age individuals tend to become more resistant and females are said to be more susceptible – but this is probably due to a lack of experience with the situations which produce seasickness. Overindulgence in food and alcohol prior to exposure, and especially the night before, predisposes to motion sickness. It probably has a direct effect on accentuating vestibular responses. The position on board the vessel can also be important, with least stimuli if the patient is placed amidships, using the horizon as a visual reference at sea and with the head braced in a fixed position. Any attempt to read will aggravate the motion sickness. Psychological factors do play a part, especially with the seasickness that develops prior to boarding the vessel. Once one person becomes seasick, there is a rapid increase in frequency among the others.

### Anti-seasickness drugs

These drugs work in both preventing and to a lesser degree relieving seasickness. Hyoscine (scopolamine) has been found to be the drug of choice for short exposures, under 4 hours, and severe motion. The antihistamines are more effective for longer exposures (6–12 hours) in moderate conditions. Repeated doses during long exposures are necessary. Probably dexamphetamine is effective when used alone, but is extremely effective when in combination with hyoscine.

Motion sickness is due to a mismatch or conflict of sensory neural information. Normally, the vestibular stimuli are consistent with the visual and proprioceptive stimuli, all informing the brain of the position of the body – even when it is in motion. When the environment starts moving as well, the information becomes conflicting. The motion sickness occurs at the onset and cessation of sensory rearrangements, when input of vision, vestibular and proprioception is at variance with the stored patterns of recent stimulus information.

It is mainly a central nervous system reaction to vestibular impulses transmitted to the vestibular nuclei in the 'old' areas of the cerebellum and the brain-stem reticular system. In these areas, neurons are responsive to acetylcholine and noradrenaline and thus some of the effects can be reduced with drugs which influence these neurotransmitters. The acetylcholine neurons appear to be responsible for increasing activity from vestibular stimulation, building

up to activate the vomiting centre. Hyoscine has strong nervous system anticholinergic effects and it is possible that the antihistamines have a similar anticholinergic effect, rather than through any effect on histamine. Neurons responding to noradrenaline produce a stabilizing influence which resists the development of motion sickness.

### Drug treatment

If seriously ill or if vomiting has commenced, the pylorus will be constricted and oral drugs may not reach their site of absorption. The drugs must be administered parenterally. Promethazine 12.5–50 mg is effective.

### Prevention

For **sailing**, acclimatization will develop if progressively increasing periods are spent at sea. Otherwise, it usually takes 2–5 days to accommodate to the new conditions. Cinnarazine has a large cult following among yachtsmen, but is probably more effective in treating vertigo than motion sickness.

The sources of vestibular and proprioceptive stimulation should be reduced to a minimum. This usually means either lying down or being as still as possible. Unnecessary head movements are avoided. In small craft, staying along the centre line of the boat towards the stern incurs the least complex motion. Conflicting visual stimulation is reduced by keeping the eyes closed, or focusing on the horizon.

Inhibition of the conflicting stimuli can be achieved by mental activity (e.g. watching distant videos), but reading requires visual convergence, which will increase conflicting visual stimuli and aggravate seasickness.

By far the most effective preparation is hyoscine 0.3–0.5 mg with dexamphetamine 5–10 mg, as used by the Luftwaffe in World War II. Unfortunately hyoscine, except for the transdermal form (Transderm, Scop), cannot be taken for a period in excess of 12 hours because of its central nervous system effects. Dexamphetamine being a potent stimulant is best avoided. Thus, this most effective combined preparation for seasickness is incompatible with safe diving.

The combination of promethazine and ephedrine is very effective, and more easily available than other anticholinergic/sympathomimetic mixtures. The sedation produced by the promethazine is partly countered by the ephedrine, whereas the anti-motion sickness effects are synergistic.

- For short trips of 4–6 hours, cyclizine 50 mg is effective taken 1 hour beforehand.
- For medium duration of 6–12 hours, meclozine 25 mg is effective, taken 2 hours beforehand.
- For long durations 1–3+ days, transdermal hyoscine is applied 6 hours beforehand.
- For extra protection, promethazine 25 mg may be taken at night before and during the trip.
- Reduction of sedation can be achieved by caffeine (coffee) or ephedrine.
- For **diving** both the therapeutic procedures and the diving depths need modification.
- For early morning dives, promethazine 25 mg taken the night before will still have anti-seasickness effects even after the sedation has worn off. Cyclizine 25 mg may be used, if necessary, 1 hour before departure.
- For later dives, meclozine 25 mg is taken 8 hours beforehand. Cyclizine 25 mg may be used, if necessary, 1 hour before departure.
- In each of these cases the drugs must be tried beforehand to ensure there are no untoward reactions. There should be no undue sedation immediately prior to the dive and the dive must be shallower than 18 metres (60 feet) to avoid significant narcosis dangers.
- In diving the numerous side effects of hyoscine, including reduced respiratory secretions, dry mouth, blurred vision, psychotic episodes and drowsiness, make it unacceptable.

# Skin reactions to equipment

A plethora of dermatological disorders may be found in diving medicine. Some of these, e.g. decompression sickness, barotrauma etc., can be found in other chapters. There are, however, a small group of illnesses which are apparently skin reactions to materials used in the equipment, or may be related to the direct effect of the equipment, without any specific diving medical illness. A few such disorders are described below, but many others are possible.

**Contact dermatitis** (mask, mouth-piece and fin burn)

Rubber may often have included in its composition an antioxidant or accelerator, mercaptobenzothiazole, and others. The chemical acts as an irritant and, because of the minor insult to the skin, may then sensitize the diver to further contact. The diver may then note an irritation with inflammation around the contact area. A similar disorder is seen among some surgeons who wear rubber gloves. The three manifestations in diving are the following.

### Mask burn

This varies from a red imprint of the mask skirt to a more generalized inflammation with vesicles, exudate, crusting etc. (Plate 11). It may take weeks before the mask can be worn again, and will recur if a similar type of mask is used. To overcome this, silicone rubber masks are made from Dow Corning medical grade silicone.

The treatment is either by soothing lotion, such as Calamine, or more effectively by the

**Table 30.1 Anti-seasickness drugs**

| Drugs | Dose (mg) | Duration (hours) | Condition |
|---|---|---|---|
| Hyoscine + dexamphetamine | 0.3–0.6 + 5–10 | 6 | Severe |
| Promethazine + ephedrine | 25 + 25 | 12 | Severe |
| Hyoscine | 0.3–0.6 | 4 | Severe |
| Promethazine | 25 | 12 | Severe |
| Dimenhydrinate | 50 | 6 | Moderate |
| Cyclizine | 50 | 4 | Mild |
| Meclozine | 50 | 6 | Mild |

use of a steroid preparation, applied regularly until relief is obtained.

### Mouthpiece burn

This may present as a burning sensation on the lips especially associated with hot drinks, fruit juices or spicy material. There may be an inflammation and vesiculation of the lips, tongue and pharynx.

A similar product to that described above, using silicone to replace the rubber mouth piece, may be obtained. For treatment hydrocortisone linguets may be effective.

### Fin or flipper burn

This is a very similar reaction to these described above, but may be mistaken for more common infections of the feet, and has been mistreated as a fungal disease. The disease will of course continue while the fins or flippers are being used, and will not respond to fungicides. Wearing protective footwear, of a non-rubber nature, under the fins, will prevent recurrence. The treatment is as described above for mask burn.

### Angioneurotic oedema (dermatographia)

The effect of localized pressure on one part of the skin producing a histamine response has been well recorded in other texts. This is occasionally seen among divers when the ridges or seams of the wet suit push onto the skin. Under these conditions there are often stripes on the skin, with either erythema and/or oedema along these lines. It can be reproduced by firm local pressure.

The disorder can be confused with an allergy response to the resins and adhesives used in joining the seams.

It can be prevented by either wearing wet suits which do not have such internal seams or, alternatively, using undergarments which protect the skin from the localized pressure of the seams.

### Allergic reactions

Unlike the above two complaints, there are rarely cases of allergy to either the wet suit material, the dyes used in it or the adhesives used in its manufacture. Where this is the case there is a rash over the incriminated area.

### Nappy rash (diaper rash)

The micturition that follows immersion, exposure to cold and emotional stress may be performed during a normal dive. The urine usually has little effect, as it is diluted with water and gradually washed away with the pumping action of the diver's movements in the suit. Unfortunately, if there is excess ammonia present, the diver may react with the equivalent of a nappy rash of children. Sometimes the divers are unaware of the aetiology, and there is some embarrassment when this diagnosis is imparted to them.

### Fin ulcers

Erosion by the hard edge of the fin, on the dorsum of the foot, may cause an ulcer. It is likely with new or ill-fitting fins, and may be prevented by wearing booties as protection. Secondary infection by both marine and terrestrial organisms is common, and is aided by softening and maceration of the skin due to immersion.

The inflammation, which develops within a few hours of the trauma, may then prevent the subsequent use of fins, and endanger the diving operation. A prolonged period out of the water, and the administration of local antibiotics, may be required to achieve healing. The prompt use of these, such as neomycin, within an hour or two of the injury and the subsequent wearing of booties with fins, may avoid this situation. Chronic ulcers are mainly a problem in the Tropics.

## Trauma

Because divers use motorized **boats** as tenders, and because they use the same environment as other motor boats, speedboats etc., there is always a risk of boating injuries, such as lacerations from **propellers**. The risk is enhanced by the problem the diver has in locating boats by either vision or hearing. Although the boats are readily heard under water, the sound waves are more rapid, making directional assessment by binaural discrimination very difficult.

Usually, by the time the diver sees a boat coming over him it is too late to take evasive action. All diving tenders should have guards over the propellors to reduce the hazard, and divers should employ floats with diving flags if they dive in boating waterways.

The lacerations inflicted by propellers tend to be parallel and linear along one aspect of the body or limb (Plate 12) – unlike the concentric crescents on opposite sides, as seen in shark attack. The treatment is along the same general lines as shark attack (Plate 13).

Head injury from ascending under the boat and hitting the hull is not uncommon (thus the advised technique of holding the hand above the head during ascent), and also from injury as the diver swims alongside the hull (explaining the reason for holding an arm between the diver and the boat in that situation).

Other causes of trauma are numerous. **Weights** and **scuba cylinders** take their toll of broken toes and metatarsals, subungual haematoma etc.

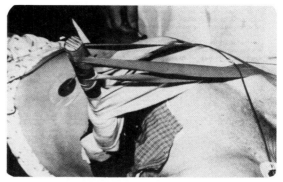

**Figure 30.2** Speargun injury: this spearfisherman stumbled on the way to the water, and caught a 180 lb amphibian – himself. The five spear prongs penetrated the pleura and pericardium on the left side. The 2-metre spear caused excessive leverage and pain when the victim laughed or breathed, and so the first aid team wisely cut the shaft 20 cm from its tip. Cardiothoracic surgical intervention was successful. *Note:* more divers are killed or injured each year by spearguns than by sharks in Australian waters.

**Spear guns** account for as much morbidity and death as sharks in Australia (Figures 30.1 and 30.2). Power heads, carbon dioxide darts and other underwater weapons cause a variety of injuries.

**Dam outlets** and underwater siphons can trap divers, then plug the outlet with the diver's body – which then is exposed to the full pressure gradient from the weight of water above him. This causes massive and grotesque injuries and death.

Others forms of environmental trauma are described in Chapter 7.

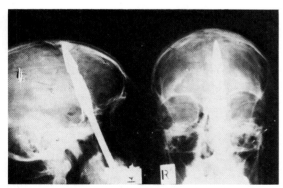

**Figure 30.1** Speargun injury: this 40-year-old male presented to a casualty department fully conscious and cooperative, with a 1-metre spear penetrating from underneath his chin to the coronal suture of his skull. The injury included a large palatal wound, penetration of the ethmoidal sinus and the sphenoidal region, severed left optic nerve and damage to the mesial cortex of the left frontal lobe. Craniotomy was performed and the cut spear was extracted through the craniotomy wound. Subsequent oronasal reconstructive surgery left the victim only with impaired vision and smell on the left side, and a functional left leucotomy – a contented customer and a happy diver?

# Recommended reading

LAURENCE, D.R. and BENNETT, P.N. (1987). *Clinical Pharmacology*, 6th edn. Edinburgh: Churchill Livingstone.

REASON, J.T., and BRAND, J.J. (1975). *Motion Sickness*. New York: Academic Press.

WOOD, C.D. (1979). Antimotion sickness and antiemetic drugs. *Current Therapeutics (Australia)* 155–168.

# 31

# Drugs and diving

## Introduction

A drug is defined as 'any substance, synthetic or extracted from plant or animal tissue . . . which is used as a medicament to prevent or cure disease' (*Butterworths Medical Dictionary*). A drug may also be considered as any agent, which, when introduced into the body, produces a biochemical or physiological change. In this sense, oxygen, nitrogen and carbon dioxide under increased partial pressures may be considered as drugs and, as such, are important in considering interactions with agents more conventionally regarded as drugs.

The modern community has come to rely on drugs to overcome illness and cope with life, and the diving population is probably little different. Many divers do take drugs either routinely or intermittently, despite the limited information of the effects of drugs under diving conditions.

In the **hyperbaric** context, drugs should be considered in terms of their principal therapeutic effects, their possible side effects in the underwater environment and their interaction with hyperbaria. The most important areas of concern in diving are the effects on the central nervous system and autonomic nervous system. Many studies have concentrated on the neurobehavioural effects of drugs under pressure, but other effects such as production of cardiac arrythmias or aggravation of oxygen toxicity may be equally important.

There is a paucity of information on the effects drugs have on human physiological or psychological performance in the **aquatic** hyperbaric environment. Conversely, there is information on the effect of certain drugs on animals under extreme hyperbaric conditions. This research is often designed as much to elucidate mechanisms of drug action and biochemical functions as to define the safe uses of drugs under pressure. There are relatively few research data at conventional scuba depths.

Two widely different examples of the interaction of drug and pressure variables to produce altered responses are: the pressure reversal of some general anaesthetic agents (see Chapter 15) and severe pulmonary toxicity caused by bleomycin and raised partial pressures of oxygen.

> *Drug–diving interactions are unpredictable.*

Other aquatic environmental influences, such as cold, sensory deprivation, spatial disorientation, reduced vision, reduced sound localization, vertigo and weightlessness, may also profoundly alter the behavioural effects of certain drugs. Another largely unresearched area is the effect that drugs may have on the uptake and elimination of inert gas, thereby altering the propensity to decompression sickness. For example, dehydration has been associated with increased decompression sickness. Certain drugs, such as alcohol, diuretics etc. may induce dehydration thus increasing the likelihood of decompression sickness.

The significance in diving of certain side effects may not be immediately apparent. For example, aspirin has a profound effect on platelet function, causing an increased bleeding tendency. This effect may be crucial in, say, inner-ear barotrauma or severe decompression sickness, where its effect may be disastrous. Aspirin may also cause increased airway resistance in some individuals. It is therefore important that all the effects of a drug be considered.

Side effects of many drugs which may be important in the underwater environment include:

- *Nervous system:* headache, dizziness, acute psychosis, tinnitus, tremor, extrapyramidal syndromes, paraesthesiae, peripheral neuropathy.
- *Cardiovascular system:* tachycardia, bradycardia, arrhythmias, hypotension (postural), chest pain, oedema.
- *Blood:* anaemia, thrombocytopenia, neutropenia, disturbances of coagulation.
- *Alimentary system:* nausea, vomiting, abdominal cramps, heartburn, diarrhoea, altered liver function, liver failure.
- *Renal:* renal failure, electrolyte disturbances, disturbances of micturition.

- *Musculoskeletal:* myalgia, arthralgia, fatigue.
- *Skin and mucosa:* pruritus, rash, angioneurotic oedema, photosensitivity.
- *Eye:* glaucoma, photophobia, blurred vision, scintillation.

The mechanism may be an exaggerated normal effect, a toxic reaction, hypersensitivity (idiosyncrasy) or true allergy.

There are two possible attitudes to the use of drugs and diving. One is that some drugs will counteract minor problems such as eustachian tube dysfunction, seasickness etc., and that these drugs will make diving safer. The other view is that the diver should not be under the influence of drugs and any possible side effects. The latter concept would require divers to stop taking some drugs many weeks prior to the dive, and the more conservative physicians would include such drugs as alcohol, nicotine and caffeine in their recommendations.

As discussed in Chapter 35, a history of drug ingestion may give important clues as to the presence of otherwise undetected organic or psychological disorders.

> *As in pregnancy, the safe use of many drugs in diving has not been established.*

## Drugs under pressure

Even if the effect of a drug at 1 ATA is well understood, it may be very different at hyperbaric pressures. Physiological influences, such as the increased hydrostatic pressure, varying pressures of oxygen and nitrogen or other diluent gases, may alter drug activity. Carbon dioxide retention may develop at depth due to the function of the diving equipment, perhaps augmented by the increased gas density and work of breathing at depth. For example, the addition of some degree of nitrogen narcosis or elevated carbon dioxide may combine with a central nervous system depressant drug (such as alcohol, antihistamines or opiates) to produce an unexpectedly severe impairment of mental function or even unconsciousness.

Animal experiments have been carried out on a number of drugs, usually at very great pressures. Such information, whilst valuable in elucidating mechanisms of drug action and pressure interaction, is of limited value in the normal current diving range of pressures. Information in this area comes from a limited number of human and animal studies of the effects of drugs and pressure on behavioural and other physiological functions.

There is very little information about alteration of therapeutic effects or side effects of drugs under hyperbaria. As with nitrogen narcosis and oxygen toxicity, the effects may be quite different in a dry chamber than in the open water at equal pressure.

Some information comes from anecdotal reports of the use of drugs in hyperbaric or saturation diving operations. The fact that drugs have occasionally been used safely in such situations does not mean that they can be regarded as safe for diving.

Walsh and Burch (1979) have studied the behavioural effects of some commonly used drugs at air pressures of 1.8 ATA, 3.6 ATA and 5.4 ATA. They found that, at pressure, all drugs studied impaired learning (i.e. cognitive functioning). Of the drugs, diphenhydramine had the most effect, caffeine and dimenhydrinate (Dramamine) varied widely with individual susceptibility, and aspirin and acetaminophen had less effect.

Illustrating the difficulty in interpreting animal experiments, the same authors found that, in rats, 5–10 times 'normal' doses at pressures of 3, 5 and 7 ATA were required to show performance decrements with diphenhydramine and pseudoephedrine, but with dimenhydrinate no effect was seen.

Amphetamines (in animals) exacerbate the behavioural effects of hyperbaric air (not ameliorate as expected). Hyperbaric air and amphetamines combine to produce behavioural changes not seen with either alone. Conversely, hyperbaric nitrogen can decrease the incidence of convulsions initiated by amphetamines.

Pressure and cold both increase the barbiturate sleep time in mice.

A clear synergistic relationship between alcohol (2 ml/kg) and pressure (air at 4 and 6 ATA) in humans, in the processing of visual information, has been demonstrated.

Pharmacological studies (including $LD_{50}$) in animals have not shown important changes at pressure equivalents of 200 metres sea water with morphine, pentobarbitone (pentobarbital), lignocaine, ethanol or digoxin.

There are isolated anecdotal reports of therapeutic drugs producing unexpected effects on divers at pressure. The effects are usually on judgement, behaviour or level of consciousness and involve: paracetamol (32 ATA), dextropropoxyphene (4 ATA), hyoscine (scopolamine), oxymetazoline spray (5 ATA) and phenylbutazone.

---

*The combination of drugs and pressure may produce:*

- *No change*
- *Antagonism*
- *Summation or potentiation*
- *Unpredictable effect*

---

Drugs may be associated with diving in four ways:

1. The prevention of disorders produced by the diving environment.
2. The treatment of dysbaric induced diseases.
3. The treatment of concurrent diseases, either acute or chronic.
4. The consumption of drugs for 'recreational' or social purposes.

# Drug prophylaxis and therapy of diving disorders

### Barotrauma

Divers seek drug therapy to allow them to enter the water when they might otherwise be unfit. The most common use of drugs is to prevent barotrauma of the middle ear or sinuses. Both topical and systemic vasoconstrictors are employed to shrink nasopharyngeal mucosa to allow pressure equalization through sinus ostia or eustachian tubes.

Some state that the widespread use of these drugs testifies to their safety. Problems accompany this usage. Too often the drugs are used to overcome incorrect diving techniques, upper respiratory tract infections or allergies. Diving clinicians are aware of the problem of rebound congestion leading to either barotrauma of ascent or descent problems later in the dive with topical vasoconstrictors.

Pseudophedrine is used alone or as a common component of systemic preparations. Side effects may include tachycardia, palpitations, hypertension, anxiety, tremor, vertigo, headache, insomnia, drowsiness and rarely hallucinations. Some individuals show a marked intolerance.

One diver suffered severe vertigo and unconsciousness in a dive to 136 feet after having used an excessive amount of oxymetazoline spray prior to the dive.

### Oxygen toxicity, nitrogen narcosis

Drugs have been sought to prevent or reduce the effects of raised partial pressures of these gases, but they remain in the research field and are of no practical value to the diver (see Chapters 15 and 18). No drug has been shown to overcome nitrogen narcosis in humans.

Diazepam has been used to prevent or treat the convulsions of oxygen toxicity. The role of gamma-aminobutyric acid (GABA) analogues, superoxide dismutase, catalase, ergot derivatives and magnesium sulphate is under investigation. The use of drugs to prevent toxicity in lungs or brain may allow the development of toxicity in other organs.

### High-pressure neurological syndrome (HPNS)

The addition of nitrogen or hydrogen to helium–oxygen to reduce the onset and severity of this syndrome is an interesting example of the interaction of pressure and a 'drug' (see Chapter 16). Drugs which potentiate transmission at GABA synapses, such as the anticonvulsant sodium valproate and flurazepam, protect against HPNS in small mammals.

### Decompression sickness (DCS)

#### Prophylaxis

Researchers have considered the use of drugs to try to prevent or minimize this disease. Drugs which inhibit platelet adhesiveness have been shown to reduce morbidity and mortality from DCS in animals.

Post-decompression thrombocytopenia is well known in humans. Aspirin has been advocated as a drug that might prevent DCS by inhibiting platelet aggregation induced by intravascular bubbles. Possible disastrous haemorrhagic effects in, say, the inner ear or barotrauma or spinal DCS preclude its clinical use.

A number of other drugs have been suggested because of a possible influence on the blood–bubble interface. Heparin, superoxide dismutase and catalase did not prevent or ameliorate decompression sickness in dogs subjected to provocative dives. Alternatively, drugs might be used to reduce the release of tissue injury mediators from cells.

Drugs, such as isoprenaline (isoproterenol), which enhance cardiac output and cause general vasodilatation have been shown to shorten time to desaturate slower tissues in rats.

#### Therapy

Drugs as an adjunct to the treatment of DCS are discussed in Chapter 13. Until recently, low-molecular-weight dextran and steroids (dexamethasone, methylprednisolone) were used. Other drugs such as tranquillizers or anticonvulsants may be employed to treat symptoms rather than the underlying pathological process.

Aminophylline, given for bronchospasm in divers with decompression sickness, may lead to trapped air emboli moving out of the pulmonary into the systemic circulation with disastrous consequences.

## Drug therapy of coincident illness

Quite apart from the unknown effect of many therapeutic drugs in the aquatic and/or hyperbaric environment, it is often the condition for which these drugs are taken that renders diving unwise (see Chapter 35). For example, the use of a tetracycline antibiotic might be acceptable for chronic acne but not for bronchitis. A thiazide diuretic may be acceptable for mild hypertension but not for congestive cardiac failure.

Even if the medical condition for which the drugs are taken, and the possible interaction

---

**CASE REPORT 31.1**

DS, a 20-year-old man, dived to a depth of between 45 metres and 50 metres with companions, all of whom were deliberately under the influence of large oral doses of barbiturates, taken while on the way out to the dive site by boat. After an undetermined period under water, the patient lost consciousness at depth and was taken rapidly to the surface by his companion. On returning to shore, he was driven to his companions' flat, where he remained unconscious, presumably sleeping off the drugs. On regaining semi-consciousness 48 hours later, he found that both legs were partially paralysed and that he had paraesthesiae below the knees and in the palm of his left hand. He was dizzy and ataxic. He presented to hospital 60 hours after diving. A diagnosis of spinal decompression sickness was made with possible cerebral involvement from air embolism, although no firm evidence of pulmonary barotrauma was found.

Immediate management was by intravenous infusion of fluids, high doses of steroids with hyperbaric oxygen (USN Table 6). He improved rapidly with recompression.

(Courtesy of Dr I.P. Unsworth)

---

with pressure, are ignored many drugs may themselves produce unwarranted risks. This is reflected in the denial of flying or driving licences to people who require certain therapeutic drugs. Much more stringent considerations apply to the use of drugs in the subaquatic environment.

The mode of administration of drugs is relevant in certain situations. For example, drugs given in depot form may lead to localized scarring and be a nidus for bubble development. Certain implantable infusion pumps, especially those with a rigid casing, are designed to operate under positive internal pressure to deliver the drug and to prevent leakage of body fluids back into the pump. If the external pressure exceeds this, then not only is the drug not delivered, but body fluids will leak into the pump. Upon decompression, the increased pressure in the pump may suddenly dispense the contents into the tissues or blood with potentially disastrous consequences.

Some drugs or classes of drugs which might be encountered in the diving population with possible associated risks in diving are discussed.

**Beta-adrenergic blockers**, often prescribed for hypertension, cause an inadequate heart rate response to exercise, and reduce exercise tolerance – an effect which may be critical in an emergency situation. They may also cause bronchoconstriction.

**Topical beta blockade** for control of glaucoma may be absorbed systemically and cause bronchospasm, bradycardia, arrhythmias or hypotension, and decreased stress response. Newer agents such as betaxolol are more specific and cause fewer cardiorespiratory effects than, for example, timolol drops. Candidates using one of these specific eye drops should have no underlying cardiac disease and no abnormalities on cardiorespiratory assessment (e.g. stress ECG, Holter monitoring, and respiratory function testing – see page 457).

**Anti-arrhythmics** may themselves, under certain circumstances, provoke arrhythmias.

**Diuretics** may cause dehydration, or electrolyte loss, especially in a tropical environmental.

**Peripheral vasodilators** may produce orthostatic hypotension, not under the water but at the moment of exit, due to loss of hydrostatic support.

**'ACE'** (angiotensin-converting enzyme) inhibitors are known to produce a dry cough which may be dangerous or diagnostically confusing in the diving/hyperbaric environment.

**Psychoactive** drugs, including sedatives and tranquillizers, produce varying degrees of drowsiness. The recipients are advised to avoid activities such as driving a car or operating machinery, where decreased alertness may be dangerous.

**Phenothiazines** may produce extrapyramidal syndromes and some of these used for nausea or motion sickness such as prochlorperazine may produce oculogyric crises.

**Tricyclic antidepressants** are known to cause cardiac arrhythmias and under conditions of increased sympathetic stimulation this effect may be exacerbated.

**Antihistamines** – this class of drugs is mainly used for their anti-allergy effects (urticaria, hayfever, allergic rhinitis, anticholinergic effects, drying effect with the 'common cold') or as anti-emetics (e.g. motion sickness). The main side effect important in diving is sedation. Newer agents such as terfenadine, a specific $H_1$-receptor blocker, do not appear to cross the blood–brain barrier significantly so drowsiness is not as much of a problem. Its use is anti-allergy, not anti-emetic.

**Antibiotics** are probably safe for the diver provided there are no side effects. In the diving context photosensitivity, especially to tetracyclines, may be relevant. Many also cause nausea and vomiting.

**Antimalarials** may be prescribed for divers visiting tropical areas. Divers and their medical advisers should be aware of the side effects of any antimalarials prescribed. Most antimalarial chemoprophylactic regimes must be commenced 1–2 weeks prior to departure. This allows time for blood levels to reach a steady state. It also allows adverse reactions to occur, so that medications can be altered before departure. Apart from idiosyncratic adverse reactions, a major worry among the widely prescribed antimalarials now relates to mefloquine (Lariam). Common side effects include vertigo, visual disturbances and difficulty with coordination. As the drug has a half-life of approximately 3 weeks, these effects can take some time to subside if they occur. Severe neurological symptoms have been reported 2–3 weeks after a single dose. Mefloquine can also cause bradycardia, an effect potentiated by concurrent administration of beta blockers. Safer alternatives for divers would include doxycycline, chloroquine, pyrimethamine (Maloprim), proguanil.

**Analgesics** should not be required by the diver although they may be requested in the decompression chamber. The problems of aspirin have been discussed. Paracetamol is usually safe. Stronger analgesics decrease mental performance and may combine with inert gas narcosis to produce a marked degree of central nervous system depression as well as complicating the therapeutic assessment of pressure effects.

**Anticholinergics**, used as antispasmodics for the gastrointestinal and urinary systems, cause dry mouth, blurred vision, photophobia and tachycardia. Decreased sweating may lead to heart stroke in the Tropics.

**Insulin** and **oral hypoglycaemics** may cause severe hypoglycaemia with altered consciousness and convulsions.

**Thyroxine** may cause tachycardia, arrhythmias, tremor, excitability and headache. Oxygen toxicity is enhanced.

**Steroids** may produce a wide variety of adverse reactions such as: fluid and sodium retention and potassium loss, perforation or haemorrhage of peptic ulceration, avascular necrosis of femoral or humeral head (see also Chapter 14), thromboembolism, increased susceptibility to hyperbaric oxygen toxicity and infection.

**Oral contraceptives**, because of their tendency to cause hypercoagulability of the blood, were postulated to cause increased decompression sickness. This is probably not significant with the modern, low-dose agents. Some women experience migraine, nausea and increased mucosal congestion.

**Bronchodilators** should not be taken by divers because, very clearly, the indication for their use precludes diving. Nevertheless, some physicians have advocated their use prior to diving. This is to be condemned. **Theophylline** and derivatives may produce cardiac arrhythmias and central nervous system **adrenergic** drugs, even beta-2 selective drugs, taken orally or more usually as inhaled aerosols, may precipitate cardiac stimulant effect. Aerosols, while producing marked improvement or prevention of symptoms, may still leave small regional microscopic areas of lung unaffected leading to localized air trapping.

Histamine **$H_2$-receptor blockers**, such as **cimetidine**, used for peptic ulceration, may produce central nervous system effects such as drowsiness and headache. **Ranitidine** is said to have a lower incidence of such side effects.

## Anaesthesia under pressure

Anaesthesia may be required for operative procedures during decompression and saturation dives. The use of regional or intravenous anaesthesia is usually preferred to gaseous anaesthesia. Theoretically, **nitrogen** could be anaesthetic, but very great depths/pressures and a long period of decompression would be required.

**Nitrous oxide** would require a partial pressure of greater than 800 mmHg for surgical anaesthesia. This pressure exposure is associated with signs of increased sympathetic activity such as tachycardia, hypertension and mydriasis. Clonus and opisthotonus may develop. A stable physiological state is difficult to maintain. Its use is also precluded by its high lipid solubility and tissue uptake as well as counterdiffusion problems (see page 149) increasing the risk of subsequent decompression sickness.

**Halothane** and **enflurane** have been used to about 4 ATA pressure. They have the pharmacological advantage of reducing the cerebral vasoconstriction of hyperbaric oxygen. There is little dose–response information at very great pressures, especially regarding organ toxicity if higher doses are required to overcome pressure reversal effects.

**Neuromuscular blocking drugs** are unaltered in effect at low (hyperbaric oxygen therapy) pressures, although they mask an oxygen convulsion.

**Regional anaesthetic** techniques (with care not to introduce gas) have theoretical support and major procedures may be carried out. The minor effects of pressure-reversal are not relevant considering the doses applied to nerves, but effects on toxicity and pharmacokinetics due to altered effects on blood flow and tissue binding may be. Surface doses of **lignocaine** have been used up to 6 ATA.

**Ketamine**, in combination with a benzodiazepine to prevent psychological phenomena, is a useful anaesthetic and shows the least pressure-reversal effect of intravenous agents and studied.

**Opiates** appear to have similar effects under some saturation diving conditions as at the surface, but respiratory depression would be a possibility in hyperbaric air (due to narcotic effect of nitrogen) or at very great depth (due to increased gas density and increased work of breathing).

**Emergency drugs** should not be withheld because of uncertainty about their effects in a hyperbaric environment.

## Recreational drugs

These drugs, which may be either legal or illegal under various national legislations, may be consumed regularly or spasmodically for social, peer pressure or mood-altering qualities. They include: tobacco, alcohol, marijuana, sedatives/tranquillizers, hallucinogenics, cocaine and opiates (heroin, morphine, pethidine etc.) These drugs may be taken singly or in combination. A Los Angeles coroner reported that 20% of diving deaths in southern California were associated with the use of drugs.

### Tobacco

The acute effects of nicotine include increased blood pressure and heart rate, and coronary vasoconstriction. The inhalation of tobacco smoke containing nicotine and tar causes increased bronchospasm, depressed cilial activity and increased mucus production in bronchial mucosa. This may lead to intrapulmonary air trapping and increased pulmonary infection. There is therefore an increased possibility of ascent pulmonary barotrauma.

Carboxyhaemoglobin (COHb) levels in smokers range from 5% to 9%. Significant psychomotor effects from exposure to this level of carbon monoxide have been reported.

Many studies of smoking on physical fitness training show detrimental effects. Increased heart rate and decreased stroke volume are the opposite of the changes with aerobic training. Oxygen debt accumulation after exercise is greater among smokers.

Long-term use may lead to chronic bronchitis and emphysema with decreased exercise tolerance and eventually marked hypoxaemia. It may also lead to coronary artery disease (angina, myocardial infarction), peripheral vascular disease, oral and lung cancer. Reduced blood volume and decreased haematocrit also develop with long exposure to increased carboxyhaemoglobin.

Nasopharyngeal mucosal congestion may predispose to sinus and middle-ear baro-trauma.

## Alcohol

The acute effects of alcohol are well known, with its depressant effects on central nervous system functioning. Alcohol is associated with up to 80% of drowning episodes in adult males. Some aspects relevant to diving will be discussed.

The harmful effect on intellectual function, judgement and coordination is well known. The addition of hyperbaric air (nitrogen narcosis) has a synergistic action in impairing mental performance.

Alcohol consumption is associated with an increased risk of vomiting.

Peripheral vasodilatation increases heat loss and may lead to hypothermia.

Acute alcoholic intoxication causes a dose-dependent impairment of left ventricular emptying at rest, probably acting directly on the myocardium.

Alcohol is a diuretic and the post-alcoholic-indulgence 'hangover' may be in part attributable to dehydration which may, in turn, increases the risk of decompression sickness.

The long-term over-use of alcohol is associated with damage to the liver, brain and heart as well as an increased risk of a number of other diseases.

## Marijuana

Cannabis intoxication alters perception of the environment and impairs cognitive and psychomotor performance. The 'mind-expanding' experience produces a sensation of heightened awareness even for things that are not physically present. There may be feelings of euphoria, indifference, anxiety or even para-noia. Subjects may experience fears or 'hang-ups' of which they were not previously aware.

An acute toxic psychosis can develop with 'flashbacks', depersonalization and derealiza-tion.

Physiological effects include conjunctival injection, tachycardia, increased oxygen consumption and heat loss with decreased shiver-ing threshold. Hypothermia may develop.

Regular use is associated with suppression of the immune system and respiratory disease. Heavy smoking can produce respiratory irritation and isolated uvulitis.

## Caffeine

Caffeine is present in coffee and a variety of cola drinks. Moderate coffee drinking is not proven to be associated with increased risk of coronary heart disease and is probably safe in most healthy persons. However, acute consumption does produce a small increase in blood pressure and may induce cardiac arrhythmias or even lethal ventricular ectopic activity in certain susceptible individuals.

Caffeine withdrawal symptoms include headache and fatigue. Less often anxiety, nausea, vomiting and impaired psychomotor performance are seen.

## Cocaine

The most marked pharmacological effect of this useful topical local anaesthetic and vaso-constrictor drug is intense sympathetic stimulation both centrally and peripherally.

Symptoms include changes in activity, mood, respiration and body temperature, blood pressure and cardiac rhythm. Morbidity and mortality are mainly associated with its cardiac toxicity producing myocardial infarction in young people and sudden cardiac arrhythmias. Sudden cardiac death syndrome in athletes taking cocaine is well known. Cerebrovascular accidents, pneumomediastin-um, rhabdomyolsis with renal failure and intestinal ischaemia have also been reported.

Cocaine smoking has been reported to produce severe reactive airway disease.

Withdrawal symptoms are marked by severe depression.

## Opiates

This class of drugs covers heroin and its derivatives, including morphine, papaveratum and synthetic opiates such as pethidine, fentanyl, dextromoramide, dextropropoxyphene etc.

Although the analgesic effects of morphine have been shown to be little affected at pressure, the behavioural effects of these drugs with hyperbaric air have not been widely investigated.

High doses of these drugs can produce respiratory depression, whilst lesser doses can produce alterations of mood and impair psychomotor performance. These effects may be altered in an unpredictable way by immersion and hyperbaria.

The development of novel methods of self-administration of illicit substances has increased the incidence of pulmonary complications. This may be due to the route of administration, the presence of contaminating foreign material or microbiological pathogens, or altered host immune response.

## Summary

More research is required into the effects of drugs in diving. There are many variables which make assessment difficult. The action of a drug may depend to a large degree on the physiological and psychological characteristics of the individual at that time. The drug effects may also vary with the environmental conditions, and all these factors may change from time to time. Some people are particularly sensitive to certain side effects, and may thus tolerate only very small doses. Others may be allergic to the drug so that it is not safe in any dose.

It is not possible to discuss all of the drugs that may be either prescribed or self-administered by the diver. Examples of therapeutic drugs which may prejudice diver safety include: sedatives, tranquillizers, antidepressants, antihistamines, hypoglycaemics, steroids, antiarrhythmics and other drugs affecting the central nervous system, the autonomic nervous system and the heart.

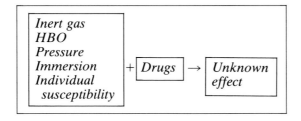

## Recommended reading and references

HEFFER, J.E., HARLEY, R.A. and SCHABEL, S.I. (1990). Pulmonary reactions from illicit substance abuse. *Clinical Chest Medicine* **11**, 151–162.

JENNINGS, R.D., JONES, W., ADOLFSON, J., GOLDBERG, L. and HESSER, C.M. (1977). Changes in man's standing steadiness in the presence of alcohol and hyperbaric air. *Undersea Biomedical Research* **4**, A16.

JOHNSON, B.A. (1990). Psychopharmacological effects of cannabis. *British Journal of Hospital Medicine* **43**, 114–122.

KENDING, J.J. (1979). Interactions between hyperbaric pressure and drugs on excitable cells (nerve and muscle). In: *Proceedings of the Twenty-first Undersea Medical Society Workshop*, edited by J.M. Walsh. Undersea Medical Society, Bethesda, MA.

LOPER, K.A. (1989). Clinical toxicology of cocaine. *Medical Toxicology and Adverse Drug Experience* **4**(3), 174–185.

PHILIP, R.B. (1979). Drugs and diving. In: *Proceedings of the Twenty-first Undersea Medical Society Workshop*, edited by J.M. Walsh. Undersea Medical Society, Bethesda, MA.

RUSSELL, G.B., SNIDER, M.T. and LOUMIS, J.L. (1990). Hyperbaric nitrous oxide as a sole anesthetic agent in humans. *Anesthesia and Analgesia* **70**, 289–295.

THOMAS, J.R. and WALSH, J.M. (1978). Behavioral evaluation of pharmacological agents in hyperbaric air and helium–oxygen. In: *Proceedings of the Sixth Symposium on Underwater Physiology*, edited by C.W. Shilling and M.B. Beckett. Bethesda, MD: Federation of American Societies for Experimental Biology.

WALSH, J.M. (1976). Drugs and diving. In: *Diving Medicine*, edited by R.H. Strauss. New York: Grune & Stratton.

WALSH, J.M. (Ed.) (1979). Interaction of drugs in the hyperbaric environment. In: *Proceedings of the Twenty-First Undersea Medical Society Workshop*. Undersea Medical Society, Bethesda, MA.

WALSH, J.M. and BURCH, L.S. (1979). The acute effects of commonly used drugs on human performance in hyperbaric air. *Undersea Biomedical Research* **6** (suppl.), 49.

# 32

# Unconsciousness

## Introduction

Normal brain function depends on a steady supply of oxygen and glucose to the brain. Impairment of cerebral circulation and/or a fall in blood oxygen or glucose will rapidly cause unconsciousness. Cerebral function may also be altered by toxic effects of gases, drugs and metabolites.

Unconsciousness in a diver, during or after a dive, can result from many causes and should be treated as an emergency. Some of the causes require prompt action beyond simple first aid. Attempts should always be made to elucidate the specific factors leading to the unconsciousness.

Drowning is the most likely result of unconsciousness in the water. It may be the final common pathway of a number of interactive situations related to environment, equipment technique or physiology. Many accidents in the water are fatal, not because of the pathology, but because there is no one to rescue the unconscious victim. In the water, unconsciousness from whatever cause may result in loss of

a respirable medium and aspiration of water. This secondary effect may be the fatal one and may obscure the original cause of the 'blackout'.

This chapter deals with the various causes of unconsciousness by relating them to the type of diving equipment used, and indicates the likelihood of a given cause in a given situation. Repeated reference to Table 32.1 is recommended in the consideration of such cases. More detailed discussion of the diagnosis and management of the specific diseases peculiar to diving will be found in the appropriate chapters.

## Causes

### Causes confined to breath-hold diving

#### Hypoxia

*Hyperventilation*

The most common sequence of events leading to unconsciousness and possible drowning in a breath-hold dive is as follows; the diver is

TABLE 32.1 *CAUSES OF UNCONSCIOUSNESS IN DIVERS*

| | Category |
|---|---|
| *Hypoxia* due to prolonged breath-hold enhanced by<br> – prior hyperventilation<br> – deep dive | Confined to breath-hold diving |
| *Hypocapnia* due to hyperventilation | Any type of diving |
| Near *drowning* due to underwater entrapment, faulty equipment or technique | Any type of diving |
| *Cold exposure*<br> – acute leading to cardiac arrhythmias<br> – prolonged leading to hypothermia | Any type of diving |
| *Pulmonary barotrauma of descent (thoracic squeeze)* | Any type of diving |
| *Marine animal injuries* | Any type of diving |
| *Vomiting and aspiration* | Any type of diving |
| *Decompression sickness* | Any type of diving |
| *Sudden death syndrome* | Any type of diving |
| *Miscellaneous medical conditions* | Any type of diving |
| *Syncope due to loss of hydrostatic support* | Any type of diving |
| *Trauma* | Any type of diving |
| *Pulmonary barotrauma of ascent* | Confined to compressed-gas diving |
| *Syncope of ascent* | Confined to compressed-gas diving |
| *Inert gas narcosis* | Confined to compressed-gas diving |
| *Carbon monoxide toxicity* | Confined to compressed-gas diving |
| *Oxygen toxicity* | Usually confined to rebreathing equipment or gas mixture diving |
| *Carbon dioxide toxicity* | Usually confined to rebreathing equipment or gas mixture diving |
| *Hypoxia* due to faulty equipment or technique | Usually confined to rebreathing equipment or gas mixture diving |

Bracket labels (left side, bottom to top): Rebreathing equipment; Open circuit breathing equipment; Breath-hold diving

NOTE: The above list is not meant to signify either incidence or relative importance.

intent on achieving some goal, such as increasing the distance or depth that he can swim under water, or seeing how long he can stay submerged. Prior to entering the water, he overbreathes (hyperventilation) for a variable amount of time producing hypocapnia. The underwater endeavour is then commenced and eventually he loses consciousness, aspirates water and drowns. If the victim is fortunate enough to be rescued, he will not recall the latter stages of the swim because there is no warning of hypoxic sensations, or of impending blackout. This is the most common cause of drowning in experienced swimmers in a pool, often at a depth in which they could have stood up, and is due to hypoxia. It is also thought to be the cause of death in experienced breath-hold spearfishermen. The changes in blood oxygen and carbon dioxide are discussed in Chapters 3 and 17.

> *Hyperventilation prior to breath-hold diving is a dangerous practice because of the sequence of hypoxia, unconsciousness and drowning.*

### Deep breath-hold dive

Breath-holding time can also be prolonged by deep diving without prior hyperventilation. In this case the increased partial pressure of oxygen in the diver's lungs prevents hypoxia until ascent. Thus the blackout frequently occurs near the surface.

## Causes possible in all types of diving

### Hypocapnia due to hyperventilation

Unconsciousness due to this cause is a theoretical possibility before breath-hold diving and during compressed-air diving. It would rapidly correct itself. It is not clear whether hypocapnia contributes to accidents.

Hyperventilation can produce dizziness and altered consciousness. The threshold for syncope is reduced. The postulated mechanism involves cerebral vasoconstriction and reduced cerebral blood flow. It is observed in an anxiety or panic situation and has been suggested as a cause of unconsciousness in divers.

It is an uncommon event because:

1. The resistance of the breathing apparatus and the increased gas density at depth combine to increase the work of breathing.
2. Oxygen is also breathed at higher than normal pressures. This depresses the respiratory response to carbon dioxide. It also interferes with the transport of carbon dioxide in the blood and thus tends to increase tissue carbon dioxide tension.
3. With closed or semi-closed rebreathing apparatus, the resistance and dead space are greater and thus the degree of hypocapnia would be less.

It is concluded that, if hyperventilation does cause unconsciousness during diving, it is only likely with helmets or open circuit scuba at shallow depths.

### Drowning

**Underwater entrapment** is a common cause of drowning even in the experienced diver. Snags include seaweed (especially kelp), rock ledges and caves, wrecks, rope and lines. Accidents resulting from **equipment failure** are not nearly as common as those due to **poor judgement** or **faulty technique**. **Aspiration** is possible when using diving equipment either due to malfunction (purge valves ineffective, damaged diaphragm etc.) or incorrectly performed techniques (buddy breathing, towed search, free ascents etc.)

Near drowning due to **loss of the demand valve** or **exhaustion of the air supply** is more likely in the beginner, but can occur in the experienced diver. Factors contributing to such accidents include inadequate training in safe diving practices, being over-weighted, failure to release weight belts or inflate buoyancy vests in an emergency situation. **Panic** (see Chapter 5) is a potent cause of impaired judgement producing a disaster where an alternative course of action may have avoided it.

### Cold

Sudden exposure to cold water may cause reflex inhalation. In some people cold water in the pharynx may stimulate the vagus nerve causing reflex sinus bradycardia or even asystole. Such exposure is also known to shorten the breath-hold time (see Chapter 22).

A prolonged exposure to cold sufficient to lower the core temperature to less than 30°C will cause unconsciousness, and the possibility of ventricular fibrillation. A fall in core temperature to 33–35°C may lead to an insidious onset of confusion and decreased mental and physical function. In this hypothermic state the diver is likely to drown.

### Pulmonary barotrauma of descent (thoracic squeeze)

This is likely only in the breath-hold diver whose descent involves a pressure change ratio greater than that between his initial lung volume, or total lung capacity with maximum inspiration, and his residual volume (see Chapter 3).

In the scuba diver, thoracic squeeze is unlikely except when the diver is grossly over-weighted and sinks rapidly or first loses consciousness from some other cause and then sinks. In both situations, loss of the air supply before the descent makes the diagnosis more tenable.

The diver supplied with gas from the surface is at greater risk. Thoracic squeeze is possible if the rate of increase of gas pressure does not keep pace with the rate of descent or if the gas pressure fails (e.g. severed gas line) in equipment not protected by a 'non-return' valve.

### Marine animal injuries

Unconsciousness may result from the bite of the sea snake or blue ringed octopus, the sting from coelenterates such as *Chironex* the sea wasp, or the injection of toxin via the spines of stonefish or stingray (see Chapter 24). The casual snorkeller is just as likely a victim as the experienced scuba diver, perhaps even more so because of his ignorance of these dangers.

Accurate diagnosis depends on awareness, knowledge of geographical distribution of dangerous marine animals, the clinical features and, most important, identification of the animal.

### Vomiting and aspiration

Nausea and vomiting under water may result from seasickness, aspiration and swallowing of sea water, unequal vestibular caloric stimulation (e.g. perforated tympanic membrane) and middle- or inner-ear disorders. Causes unrelated to diving itself include over-indulgence in food or alcohol, gastroenteritis etc.

Aspiration of vomitus from the mouth piece is a possibility in the inexperienced diver. Vomitus ejected into a demand valve may interfere with its function, or may damage the absorbent activity in rebreathing sets. If the diver removes his mouth piece to vomit, he may then aspirate sea water during the subsequent reflex inhalation. In severe cases, unconsciousness may result from respiratory obstruction and resultant hypoxia.

### Decompression sickness

This is extremely unlikely in breath-hold divers although DCS has been described in native pearl divers (**Taravana**) and submarine escape training instructors who have a very short surface interval between deep breath-hold dives.

Unconsciousness during, or immediately after, compressed-air diving is occasionally due to cerebral decompression sickness. A typical dive profile is a deep dive on compressed air to greater than 40 metres, with or without prescribed decompression stops. Differential diagnosis from cerebral arterial gas embolism resulting from pulmonary barotrauma of ascent may be difficult, but immediate treatment is similar.

Severe decompression sickness involving the cardiorespiratory system may also lead to unconsciousness due to hypotension (shock) and/or hypoxia.

### Miscellaneous medical conditions

The diver is as prone to the onset of sudden incapacitating illness as the equally fit, or unfit, land athlete. Diagnoses such as myocardial infarction, cardiac arrhythmia, syncope, cerebrovascular accident, diabetes with hypoglycaemia or hyperglycaemia, epilepsy etc. should be considered. The metabolic disturbances of renal failure, liver failure or adrenal failure can affect cerebral function, but would be most improbable in the diver!

**Drugs**, either 'legal' or 'illegal', may depress central nervous system function, enhance carbon dioxide retention (e.g. opiates), affect cardiac performance (e.g. some antihypertensives) or alter blood sugar (insulin or oral hypoglycaemic agents). This is discussed more in Chapters 31 and 35.

## Trauma

A diver could be rendered unconscious by a blow to the head or chest. Underwater explosion is discussed in Chapter 25.

---

*Diagnosis of cause of unconsciousness in a diver:*
- *Type of equipment and breathing gases*
- *Depth/duration, of this and other recent dives*
- *Environmental factors*
- *Clinical signs*

---

## Causes usually confined to compressed-gas diving

### Pulmonary barotrauma of ascent

**Cerebral arterial gas embolism (CAGE)** (see Chapter 9) must be the first diagnosis to be excluded in the diver who surfaces and rapidly becomes unconscious. It is only likely in a diver who has been breathing compressed gas. It cannot be dismissed merely because the diver was seen to exhale or breathe normally during ascent, due to possibility of localized airway obstruction. Although there need not be any evidence of pulmonary damage, the presence of cough or haemoptysis will aid in diagnosis, and clinical evidence of mediastinal emphysema is very supportive of the CAGE association.

Tension **pneumothorax** may conceivably cause unconsciousness due to hypoxia or cardiovascular disturbance.

---

*Unconsciousness developing in a scuba diver immediately after surfacing is presumed due to CAGE, until proven otherwise.*

---

## Syncope

Altered consciousness or syncope may be due to partial breath-holding during ascent. This disorder, called **syncope of ascent**, is thought to be due to the expansion of intrathoracic gas interfering with venous return and thus reducing cardiac output. Unless it proceeds to pulmonary barotrauma or drowning, it is rapidly self-correcting with the resumption of normal respiration.

Syncope due to **postural hypotension** may develop as the diver leaves the water due to loss of hydrostatic circulatory support. This is more likely in the dehydrated or peripherally vasodilated diver, from whatever cause.

## Inert gas narcosis

In deep dives, unconsciousness may result from the narcotic effects of nitrogen in the compressed air (see Chapter 15). An unconscious diver on the surface is not suffering from nitrogen narcosis, because the narcosis is reversible upon reduction of the environmental pressure. However, irrational behaviour or poor judgement due to narcosis may lead to drowning. Unconsciousness due to narcosis is likely to develop at a depth greater than 90 metres, breathing air, but impaired consciousness is seen from 30 metres onwards.

## Carbon monoxide toxicity

Carbon monoxide toxicity is often put forward as a cause of unconsciousness in scuba divers. It is probably not common, despite its theoretical likelihood. Clinical features are similar to carbon monoxide toxicity from other causes (see Chapter 37). Diagnosis is aided by examining compressor facilities, and is confirmed by estimations of carbon monoxide in the gas supply and the victim's blood.

## Causes more likely with rebreathing or mixed gas diving

### Oxygen toxicity

The diver breathing gas mixtures containing high percentages of oxygen is at risk of central nervous system oxygen toxicity if the partial pressure of oxygen exceeds 1.6 ATA, especially with heavy exercise (see Chapter 18). Closed circuit oxygen sets are particularly dangerous because of the complementary $CO_2$ effects. A diver on 100% $O_2$ must not exceed a depth of 8–10 metres (1.8–2.0 ATA). The most serious manifestations are unconsciousness and generalized convulsions. Recovery is usually within minutes of reducing the pressure of oxygen, but the clinical picture may be confused by subsequent aspiration of sea water or vomitus.

A study by Leitch (1981) to elucidate causes of otherwise unexplained loss of consciousness concluded that air diving deeper than 48 metres was unduly hazardous due to the toxic effects of oxygen. He also postulated that raised carbon dioxide, especially with heavy physical work and even pressure alone, may lower the oxygen toxicity threshold.

### Carbon dioxide toxicity

The most common cause of unconsciousness in divers using rebreathing equipment is a build-up of carbon dioxide. The diver's respiration may be rapid and deep and he may appear flushed and sweaty. A history of the dive, noting prolonged or heavy exertion, and an examination of the equipment and the absorbent material help in diagnosis. Recovery is usually fairly rapid once the equipment is removed and the diver breathes from the atmosphere. A characteristic headache may persist for some hours. Carbon dioxide toxicity may also develop due to inadequate ventilation of an enclosed space such as in a diving helmet or chamber.

The possibility exists that some divers, under conditions of increased gas density at depth and heavy exercise, may retain carbon dioxide. Resultant carbon dioxide toxicity may impair consciousness, exacerbate oxygen toxicity or nitrogen narcosis.

### Hypoxia due to faulty equipment or technique

This may be produced by insufficient oxygen in the inspired gas mixture due to dilution, excess oxygen consumption or incorrect gas mixture for the set flow rate. The manifestations are those of hypoxia from any cause. Provided the hypoxia is rapidly corrected, prompt recovery can be expected.

> *A rapid recovery is to be expected in uncomplicated cases of transient hypoxia, carbon dioxide toxicity, syncope of ascent, oxygen toxicity – after the patient is removed from the offending environment.*

## Contributory factors

Several factors, although not direct causes, may contribute to the development of unconsciousness under water. The **inexperienced** diver is more likely to be involved in such an episode. A vigorous Valsalva manoeuvre may increase the likelihood of syncope due to reduced venous return and hence decreased cardiac output. This is less likely in the water because the hydrostatic support reduces peripheral pooling of blood.

The **overheated** diver (e.g. overheated suit) may develop heat exhaustion with mild confusion, but heat stroke with coma and/or convulsions is unlikely.

The diver exposed to cold may have a higher incidence of equipment (and absorbent) failure, dexterity reduction and cardiac reflexes.

A **fall in plasma glucose** may result from fasting or high physical activity. In the normal individual, the degree of **hypoglycaemia** is not enough to produce symptoms. Alcohol, by inhibiting gluconeogenesis, may contribute to significant hypoglycaemia in the fasted (greater than 12 hours) diver. Chronic alcohol abuse damages liver glycogen storage and hypoglycaemia may develop after a shorter fast.

The role of **psychological factors** in causing unconsciousness has often been postulated. The **anxious** diver may be more prone to cardiac arrythmias related to sympathetic nervous system stimulation.

**Cardiac arrhythmias** (see Chapter 26) have been postulated as a cause of otherwise unexplained collapse or death in the water. Postmortem examinations have either shown no significant pathology or coronary artery disease. These incidents tend to occur towards the end of a dive, suggesting that fatigue and hypothermia might be involved. Acute coronary spasm (Prinzmetal's angina) may precipitate arrhythmias. Bradycardia due to laryngeal stimulation, cold-induced reflexes, or carotid sinus pressure due to a tight-fitting wet suit, may also permit ventricular ectopic breakthrough, leading to arrhythmias.

## 'Shallow water blackout'

**'Shallow water blackout'** was used initially by the British to refer to carbon dioxide toxicity with rebreathing equipment, whereas the Americans recently used it to describe unconsciousness following hyperventilation and breath-hold with free diving. The term has created much diagnostic confusion, in that it suggests that there is some mysterious cause of unconsciousness in divers or that there is always a multifactoral aetiology. Attempts to define specific causes of unconsciousness should always be made. Nomenclature should then follow this specific cause, e.g. syncope of ascent, dilution hypoxia, carbon dioxide build-up, oxygen toxicity etc.

## Management

The first step in management of all cases is the establishment and maintenance of respiration and circulation. The administration of 100% oxygen at 1 ATA will do no harm, even in central nervous system oxygen toxicity, and will be of great benefit in most cases. If respiration is not spontaneous, positive pressure will be required, despite the argument that it may be detrimental in cases of pulmonary barotrauma. External cardiac massage may also be necessary. Divers suspected of CAGE or DCS require rapid recompression as well.

---

*The most common causes of unconsciousness in divers*
1. *Breath-hold – hyperventilation plus prolonged breath-hold leading to hypoxia.*
2. *Compressed air equipment – drowning due to faulty equipment or technique.*
3. *Rebreathing equipment – carbon dioxide toxicity.*

---

Clues to accurate diagnosis of the cause of the unconsciousness may be elicited from the diver's companion or other observers. Helpful information includes: depths and duration of the dive; type of equipment used; whether the incident occurred during descent, on the bottom, while surfacing or on the surface; and description of the sequence of events leading to unconsciousness. Unfortunately, in many instances, much of the above information is not available. Clinical examination of the diver and critical examination of his diving equipment are also important.

Maintenance of adequate circulation and ventilation may be all that is required in cases of near drowning, pulmonary barotrauma of descent and marine animal envenomations.

Cases of carbon dioxide toxicity, oxygen toxicity, nitrogen narcosis and temporary hypoxia from whatever cause, uncomplicated by aspiration of sea water, usually recover rapidly with return to normal atmosphere.

Miscellaneous medical conditions, hypothermia, aspiration of vomitus, trauma etc. are managed along general medical principles.

## Recommended reading and references

BARLOW, H.B. and MACINTOSH, F.C. (1944). *Shallow Water Blackout*. RNPL Report 44/125. Royal Navy.

EDMONDS, C. (1968). *Shallow Water Blackout. School of Underwater Medicine Report 8/68*. Royal Australian Navy.

LANPHIER, E.H. (Ed.) (1980). The unconscious diver: respiratory control and other contributing factors. *The Twenty-fifth Undersea Medical Society Workshop*. Undersea Medical Society.

LEITCH, D.R. (1981). A study of unusual incidents in a well-documented series of dives. *Aviation, Space and Environmental Medicine* **52**, 618–624.

MILES, S. (1957). *Unconsciousness in Underwater Swimmers*. RNPL Report 57/901. Royal Navy.

# 33

# First aid and emergency medical treatment

There is no such thing as an accident.
What we call by name is the effect of
some cause which we do not see.

Voltaire

GENERAL

FIRST AID
  Rescue
  Specific treatment at the site

LOCAL MEDICAL TREATMENT
  Minor diving disorders
  Major diving disorders

POSITIONING AND TRANSPORT

RECOMPRESSION THERAPY
  Water recompression
  Recompression chamber therapy
  Recompression facilities

AVIATION MEDIVAC

DIVING MEDICAL KIT

RECOMMENDED READING

## General

This chapter deals with the immediate treatment of diving accidents. The material is discussed in greater detail elsewhere in this book, but an overview is presented here for easy reference.

Priority should be given to the **prevention** of morbidity and mortality. The diver should be medically fit to dive, have received training for that specific diving environment and utilize reliable and appropriate equipment.

When, despite the above precautions, an accident does occur, then the other divers should be able to identify and treat the symptoms and signs. Their knowledge may be augmented by:

1. Preliminary training in first-aid procedures for diving accidents.
2. At least one comprehensive diving medical textbook available, on site, for reference. It would also be advisable to have a general diving manual available (see Appendix V).
3. Direct contact with diving medical expertise – either by telecommunication or by transporting the patient to such care. In remote areas neither capability may be readily available.

# First aid

No matter how much effort is put into prevention, diving accidents will occur. There are two aspects to first aid, one being the rescue and the other the specific first aid treatment.

## Rescue

In 70% of the diving fatalities reviewed in one series, there was a period in excess of 15 minutes between the accident and the rescue. This is an unacceptable time for any patient to remain under water without functioning breathing equipment. Thus, in many cases, there is a progression from unconsciousness to death, which could have been prevented by the institution of the three basic requirements for rescue, namely:

1. A method of requesting immediate assistance from a companion diver.
2. Assistance in returning to the surface or to a habitable environment.
3. The use of basic life support techniques until professional medical treatment is obtained.

In practice the common methods of achieving the above three requirements are:

1. Immediate contact with a buddy (companion diver) or attendant.
2. A buoyancy vest or direct contact with a diving tender.
3. Mouth-to-mouth respiration and external cardiac massage.

The practice of buddy diving is the single most important factor in rescue. It requires that each diver is responsible for the welfare and safety of both himself and his companion. It infers: a reliable method of communication between the divers, a practised rescue technique, and a basic knowledge of resuscitation.

## Specific treatment at the site

Many injuries sustained by divers require a rapid assessment, diagnosis and management. Others are of such a minor nature that expert medical assistance is not needed, although some form of treatment may be indicated. First aid is usually supplied by the diver's associates and may include the following.

- General resuscitation, including mouth-to-mouth respiration and/or external cardiac massage; cardiopulmonary resuscitation and basic life support are dealt with in Chapter 21.
- Oxygen inhalation for near-drowning, decompression sickness (DCS) or pulmonary barotrauma.
- Management of trauma, including haemostasis and tourniquets for shark attack, propellor injuries etc.
- Warming techniques for hypothermia.
- Methods of reducing marine animal envenomation, including pressure bandages and symptomatic relief.
- The general care and specific treatment of various infections ranging from otitis externa to coral cuts.
- An ability to prevent and treat disorders environmentally associated with diving, e.g. seasickness, sunburn, fish poisoning etc.

It is important that the divers' associates realize their limitations in treating such disorders as decompression sickness, barotrauma and hearing loss.

# Local medical treatment

This is usually an exension of the first aid, with the local physician augmenting the treatments by his knowledge of cardiopulmonary physiology, electrolyte disturbances, surgical techniques, the use of antitoxins, antibiotics, steroids, analgesia and, possibly, anaesthesia.

In many cases the local physician can work as a liaison officer between the divers and diving medicine specialist, especially when recompression therapy is required. The local physician will also be important in integrating the transport and medical evacuation needs, if these are required. The local physician should have available to him direct communication with a specialist in diving medicine, so that the measures described in this chapter can be instituted appropriately.

## Minor diving disorders

These include barotrauma of the upper respiratory tract (otological, sinus, dental etc). They also include infections, trauma, sea sickness, sunburn, marine animal injuries, salt water aspiration etc. Most of these are dealt with elsewhere, and sometimes they are not 'minor' in their effect.

A coral cut, left unattended for a few hours, can develop into a serious and rapidly spreading cellulitis.

Hearing loss or vertigo could be the harbinger of a serious case of inner-ear barotrauma which could deteriorate if exposed to further otological pressure changes (diving, flying, exercise, Valsalva manoeuvres etc.).

Infections of the upper respiratory tract, e.g. otitis media, if inadequately treated, can produce permanent damage. Often they follow barotrauma in the middle ear and sinuses. Antibiotics must sometimes be used without a physician's authority, and they should be chosen because of their wide spectrum and minimal side effects.

Marine animal injuries can have their morbidity reduced by rapid first aid, e.g. the use of vinegar to prevent further nematocyst discharge from box jelly fish, application of heat to fish stings etc. Local anaesthetics may relieve pain when applied superficially on jelly fish injuries, or by subcutaneous injection for fish stings. Pressure bandages and immobilization is recommended for sea snake and blue ring octopus bites, to delay toxicity until the appropriate treatment procedures can be arranged.

Hypothermia, if mild, can be treated by immobilization of the patient, protection from further heat loss and rewarming by either warm baths or sharing a sleeping bag – preferably with a warmhearted friend.

Salt water aspiration is relieved by resting the patient, giving oxygen if needed, and waiting.

## Major diving disorders

Many diving accident victims will deteriorate when they are subjected to transportation or even body movements. A variety of cases will benefit by the use of oxygen. These will be discussed later.

In all serious cases of diving disorder, **cardiopulmonary resuscitation** may have to take priority over the other treatments. It is of little value to allocate priority to transport, if the patient has no cardiac activity, or if he has stopped breathing. With such an obvious qualification, the more specific first aid treatments may be summarized for the various disorders.

In cases of **near drowning** there is little to supplement the cardiopulmonary resuscitation techniques, except for the use of 100% oxygen and immobilization. Victims have survived immersion times of up to an hour without breathing, under water, and still survived without clinical sequelae. Careful documentation, if time permits, may assist the medical team that finally takes over the treatment. Observation for at least 24 hours after the patient has apparently recovered is mandatory as relapses are not uncommon.

Active rewarming techniques may be indicated with hypothermia victims and death must not be presumed below 32°C, even without obvious vital signs.

The first aid treatment of **cerebral arterial gas embolism** (CAGE) comprises the correct positioning of the patient (left lateral/horizontal is the current recommendation), the inhalation of oxygen rather than air, and immobilization as far as practicable. Oxygen may reduce the effects of the air emboli by hastening their resolution.

In other forms of **pulmonary barotrauma**, the positioning will depend on the comfort of the patient, but oxygen will often remove the subcutaneous and mediastinal gas pockets and will even hasten resolution of a pneumothorax, if given continuously over many hours.

If **decompression sickness** is suspected, or diagnosed, then general treatment will include the immobilization of the patient, attention to hydration and the administration of 100% oxygen. In the event of cerebral manifestations, the same body positioning may be used as in CAGE. Careful documentation will assist subsequent assessment and will include the development and timing of the clinical features and vital signs, with specific reference to urine production. If the latter is inadequate, the hydration must be increased. If urine output is absent because of neurological induced retention, then bladder catheterization must be performed. There is no indication for aspirin or steroids.

## Positioning, moving and transport of the patient

In some recent publications, a diagram of the head-down position with the patient lying supine was proposed and was advised for CAGE, DCS or near-drowning. In fact such a position would certainly aggravate many near-drowning cases, as aspiration is almost inevitable, unless a cuffed endotracheal tube was inserted. It would also increase cerebral pathology because of the raised central venous pressure and possibly open a patent foramen ovale to increase paradoxical embolism.

Due to recurrent or redistributed emboli, the horizontal, preferably left lateral, position should be maintained in cases of CAGE. The concept of recurrent embolization has been used to describe the cases that suddenly deteriorate after initial symptoms may have cleared, especially when the patient resumes an erect, standing or sitting, position.

Body movement, both active (muscular) and passive (transport) may aggravate a number of diving illnesses. These include:

1. CAGE – the upright position may promote redistribution of emboli in large arteries, towards the cerebral circulation, and reduce the hydrostatic forces that drive obstructed bubbles through the cerebral circulation.
2. DCS – muscular activity or body movement can precipitate and increase venous gas embolism.
3. Near-drowning – movement redistributes loculated intrapulmonary fluids, and decreases compliance.
4. Hypothermia – movement precipitates cardiac dysrhythmias, possibly by returning a bolus of acidotic blood from hypothermic tissues to the heart.
5. Inner-ear barotrauma – by increasing perilymph pressure or haemorrhage.
6. Marine envenomation – muscular activity negates the pressure bandage effect.
7. Shark attack – transport increases blood loss.

## Recompression therapy

In cases of DCS and pulmonary barotrauma, recompression therapy is usually indicated.

The need for prompt recompression in both CAGE and neurological DCS is universally accepted. If there is less than 5 minutes' delay in treatment of CAGE then, even though 5% may die, the morbidity among the survivors is low. In contrast, if the delay exceeds 5 hours, mortality is 5–10% and at least half the survivors are left with residual problems.

In many circumstances the facilities may not be immediately available for formal recompression therapy. Thus a decision has to be made as to whether the patient is to be recompressed by descent in the water, transported to a recompression chamber or have a recompression chamber transported to him.

### Water recompression

In an attempt to initiate early therapy, many divers have been recompressed in the water. Both mechanical and physiological problems are encountered. Requirements for the diver support include a sufficient supply of compressed air, tolerable weather conditions, a full face mask or helmet to prevent aspiration of water, adequate thermal protection and a constant attendant.

The problems often encountered in water recompression therapy include seasickness, drowning, hypothermia, panic and the aggravation of the illness by subjecting the patient to a further uptake of inert gas in the tissues, compounding the problem on subsequent ascent. In many cases, the regime has to be terminated prematurely because of adverse weather conditions, equipment failure, sharks, physiological and finally psychological difficulties. Even when the treatment does give relief, it often needs to be supplemented with the conventional recompression therapy carried out in a chamber, soon after the patient has left the water.

A much more effective water recompression therapy uses 100% oxygen, at a maximum of 9 metres, and is relatively short in duration. This regime, which has been particularly valuable in remote localities, is described in Chapter 13 and Appendix V. It involves a 30–90 minute stay at 9 metres, and ascent at the rate of 12 minutes per metre. It has the advantage of not aggravating the disease by adding more inert gas, being of short duration, avoiding any problem of nitrogen narcosis, and being suited

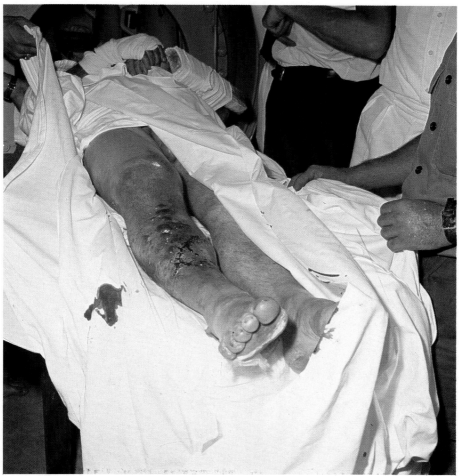

**Plate 14** Gas gangrene: swollen leg with pallor, haemorrhagic bullae and necrosis. Responded to hyperbaric oxygen therapy. (See Chapter 37)

for shallow bays and off wharves, protected from the open sea.

## Recompression chamber therapy

A recompression chamber can almost eliminate mortality from decompression sickness. It also considerably reduces the dangers associated with air embolism. The armed services and national regulating bodies lay down conditions in which a recompression chamber must be available for practising free ascents and for most deep (greater than 30 metres) professional diving operations. The British and Australian regulations require a submersible decompression chamber for dives to a depth greater than 50 metres. Amateur divers have a more casual attitude to safe diving and the treatment is more variable. It depends on the chamber, personnel available and the nature of the diver's ailment.

If CAGE or DCS is diagnosed or suspected, then rapid recompression to 18 metres on oxygen is required. Time should not be wasted, as the diver's life may depend on the speed of compression. After the patient is recompressed, there is time to evaluate the situation; the diagnosis can be confirmed and further treatment instituted. Once the patient is under pressure, and no longer in immediate danger, time is available to read the appropriate chapter or appendix of this or another book or diving manual.

## Recompression facilities

The problem of treatment of the diver in a remote location can be reduced if an efficient transportation and treatment system has been established beforehand. There are three possible strategies:

1. Transporting the diver without compression, breathing 100% oxygen, to the recompression chamber.
2. Keeping the diver on site, breathing 100% oxygen, and bringing a portable recompression chamber to him. Once under pressure his danger may be diminished, but it still remains to treat him in the best chamber available. This portable recompression chamber should have compatible transfer-under-pressure capability with other recompression chambers, for the transfer of both patient and attendants. It may be moved to a more suitable site where the smaller unit can be mated to a major treatment chamber, and the patient transferred.
3. A specialized hyperbaric or water ambulance, available from large, deep sea, oil companies, in certain areas.

The choice of system depends on the seriousness of the injury, the availability and type of recompression chambers, gas supplies, transport, and time and distance relationships. The initial treatment carried out by other divers on site will influence subsequent management. It is important that an experienced authority is responsible for decisions regarding treatment and transportation. This authority is best situated where the major definitive treatment chambers are located. The capability to transfer experienced staff and equipment to remote localities affects the decision of whether to treat on site or to transport.

An ideal system has yet to be designed where divers in all localities can be adequately treated at all times. The following is a suggested scheme for a country where medical knowledge is available in certain centres and where transport is available from most diving localities.

### Major centre

- Large multi-compartment, multi-person recompression chamber with transfer-under-pressure facilities located within a hospital complex.
- Portable (two-person) recompression chamber with gas supplies and compatible transfer-under-pressure capability. These chambers should be at least large enough to accommodate both the patient and an attendant, but should also be capable of transport by air to remote localities.

### Regional centre

- Portable recompression chamber as described above with compatible transfer-under-pressure facilities.

It is important in the above system that all transfer-under-pressure facilities within the one geographical area are compatible. An injured diver can be placed in a portable recompression chamber and treated at the regional centre or transported to the major centre. This system, by enabling rapid recompression of the diver, reduces morbidity. Divers injured at localities remote from the regional or major centre are transported to whichever unit is most appropriate.

# Aviation Medivac

Diving is frequently carried out in localities remote from recompression chambers. Transportation of the patient requiring recompression therapy then becomes a major problem.

The benefit of moving a seriously ill patient to more sophisticated medical facilities must be weighed against the hazards of this procedure. Receiving a diver from an aircraft, in much worse clinical condition than he went in, is a not infrequent experience.

Several problems can develop during aviation medical evacuation.

1. It is possible that the vibration (especially in helicopters) and hypoxia from altitude (especially in fixed wing aircraft) may aggravate the clinical condition.
2. Any exposure to attitude will expand existing bubbles and initiate more bubble formation, thereby increasing damage. This is even observed by patients with DCS in motor vehicles being driven over mountains. There is no 'safe' altitude at which one can fly, once a bubble is present. Whether there is such a safe altitude for asymptomatic divers could be argued, but those with symptoms do not enjoy such a luxury.
3. Often the aircraft can only take one-person chambers. Under these conditions there is an impaired capability of patient care throughout the transfer.
4. Unless there is a formal aviation Medivac facility, such as in the armed forces, more attention and decision-making may be given to transport logistics than patient care.
5. There is often a loss of continuity of treatment and communication during the transport.

Air transport is of most value in **CAGE** and **DCS** if it is carried out with continuous medical support, in the following order:

1. Under hyperbaric conditions (portable recompression chamber) – recommended.
2. With aircraft pressurized to ground level – possible.
3. At altitude pressures – needs careful consideration.

Due to the value of hyperbaric oxygenation in the acute treatment of CAGE and DCS, prompt contact should be made with a recompression facility, to initiate retrieval under hyperbaric conditions.

Most aircraft are pressurized to approximately 2000 metres above sea level (0.8 atmosphere), and ascent will increase the size of the gas bubble and thus the extent of pathology.

If the aircraft cannot be pressurized to 1 atmosphere, then the patient should not be transported at altitude unless there is no other alternative. All these factors must be evaluated before deciding on the best means of transport of the patient or chamber and only after the diver is breathing 100% oxygen (with due precautions against fire and explosions) throughout the whole procedure.

# Diving medical kit

Diving support boats should be equipped for likely accidents. No check list can contain materials needed for all situations, but, as a general guide, the following items should be considered:

- Airways for use in mouth-to-mouth respiration.
- Resuscitator with an oxygen supply and instructions regarding its use and fire risk (in drowning, pulmonary barotrauma, decompression sickness).
- Mechanical suction system, not reliant on scarce oxygen supplies.
- Topical antibiotic or antiseptic for skin injuries.
- Motion sickness tablets.
- Dressings.
- Preparations to prevent and treat cold, sun or wind exposure.

Protection against dangerous marine animals depends upon the fauna of the expected dive site, but may include:

- Tourniquet (sharks, barracuda, eel bite) and ligature or pressure bandages (sea snake, blue ringed octopus and some other venomous animals).
- Local anaesthetic ointment and vinegar for jellyfish.
- Local anaesthetic injection without adrenaline (scorpion fish, stonefish, stingray, catfish).
- Appropriate antivenoms (sea snake, box jelly fish, stonefish).

If DCS is possible, consider:

- Large oxygen cylinder for surface supply to helmet or full-face mask with adaptor to supply surface respirator if needed.
- An underwater recompression unit for remote areas.
- Intravenous infusion system (e.g. physiological saline).
- Urinary catheter.
- Adequate compressor or air bank to support the diving attendants.
- A portable two-person recompression chamber if possible.
- Medical kit required for recompression chamber.

Special circumstances will require supplementation of the above medical kits. In remote localities, diagnostic and therapeutic equipment varying from a thermometer to a thoracotomy set may be appropriate. Ear drops to prevent and/or treat external ear infections are especially necessary in the Tropics. Broad-spectrum antibiotics are also needed. The use of these will depend on the clinical training of the attendants.

A laryngoscope and endotracheal airway may be of use if trained medical assistance is available. It is important that diving support boats have radio communications to obtain expert medical advice on the treatment of difficult or unexpected problems. Frequently, medical or paramedical personnel are available coincidentally.

## Recommended reading

BENNETT, P.B. and MOON, R. (Eds) (1990). *UHMS/NOAA/DAN Workshop on Diver Accident Management*. Duke University.

*British Sub-Aqua Club Diving Manual*. New York: Charles Scribner's Sons.

DICK, A.P.K. MEBANE, G.Y. and JOHNSON, J. (1984). Early oxygen breathing for scuba injuries. Annual Scientific Meeting, Undersea Medical Society.

DUTKA, A.J. (1990). Therapy for dysbaric central nervous system ischaemia. Adjuncts to recompression. *UHMS/NOAA/DAN Workshop on Diver Accident Management*, edited by P.B. Bennett and R. Moon. Duke University.

EDMONDS, C.W. (1990). Diving accident management in remote areas. *UHMS/NOAA/DAN Workshop on Diver Accident Management*, edited by P.B. Bennett and R. Moon. Duke University.

EDMONDS, C. and WALKER, D. (1989). Scuba diving fatalities in Australia and New Zealand. *SPUMS Journal* **19**, 94–104.

GORMAN, D.F. (1989). Decompression sickness and arterial gas emboli. *Sports Medicine* **8**(1), 32–42.

McANIFF, J.J. (1981). *United States Underwater Diving Fatality Statistics/1970–79*. US Department of Commerce, NOAA, Undersea Research Program, Washington DC.

McANIFF, J.J. (1988). *United States Underwater Diving Fatality Statistics/1986–87*. Report number URI-SSR-89-20, University of Rhode Island, National Underwater Accident Data Centre.

*Scuba Safety Report Series Nos 2, 5 and 6*. Department of Ocean Engineering, University of Rhode Island.

*US Navy Diving Manual* (1988). Volume 1, Superintendent of Documents, US Government Printing Office, Washington DC 20420. Revision 2.

# 34

# Investigation of diving fatalities

Full fathom five thy father lies
of his bones are coral made.
Those are pearls that were his eyes:
Nothing of him that doth fade
But doth suffer a sea-change
Into something rich and strange

Shakespeare, *The Tempest*

## Introduction

In the investigation of diving accidents, there are five separate areas which require assessment:

- Personal and past medical history.
- Environmental conditions.
- Dive profile and history.
- Diving equipment.
- Autopsy investigation.

Only the last of these will be discussed in detail in this chapter, the others being more relevant to the investigation by diving authorities, or are discussed in other chapters (Chapters 4, 5, 7 and 8). Details of the specific diving disorders are found in the appropriate chapters.

Once death has been certified, it is important that no further interference occurs with either the body, its clothing or the equipment, except for sealing the equipment and the closure of cylinders and valves, to retain the breathing gas for analysis.

## Personal and past medical history

There are certain personal data that may be relevant in the assessment of the diving accident. First and foremost is the presence of diseases likely to predispose to the diving accident and reference should be made to Chapters 8 and 35. Of recreational divers who died, 25% were not medically fit for diving. Chapter 35 deals with these medical standards.

Other information which may be pertinent is the level of experience of the diver and his companions. Accidents are more likely with the inexperienced diver, and especially during his first 'open water' sea dive.

The history of previous diving accidents should be sought. Many problems experienced by divers in the past are likely to be repeated under similar conditions. These include hypoxia from breath-holding after hyperventilation, panic with hyperventilation, salt water aspiration, alternobaric vertigo, barotrauma and especially pulmonary barotrauma, nitrogen narcosis, syncope of ascent, decompression sickness, oxygen toxicity and carbon dioxide toxicity.

Alcohol and drug history may be very relevant, with both illicit and legal drugs contributing to accidents.

---

***Personal and past medical history***
- *Pre-existing diseases*
- *Past diving experience and training*
- *Any previous diving accidents*
- *Drug and alcohol use*

---

## Environmental conditions

Note should be made of the weather and water conditions prevailing at the time of the accident. Environmental factors contribute to 62% of the deaths. Not only may the diver be exposed to an increased risk of injury during entry to or exit from the water, but also during the dive there may be exceptional stress in the form of impaired visibility, sea sickness, tidal currents, cold etc.

A diver who has to battle a 1-knot current is exerting himself to a significant degree, consuming 2 litres or more of oxygen per minute. It is virtually impossible for an unassisted diver to make headway against a current of 2 knots or more.

The tempertaure of the water will influence hypothermia, manual dexterity, decompression sickness and also the functioning of various pieces of diving equipment. Carbon dioxide absorbents are less effective under cold conditions and, with the temperature approaching freezing point, regulators may cease to function.

Other environmental hazards include exposure to explosives, dangerous marine creatures, inability to surface (e.g. in caves, under ledges, in kelp, wrecks, dam outlets etc.), night diving and others.

---

***Environmental conditions***
- *Wind and weather*
- *Visibility impairment from sediment, 'white water', night diving etc.*
- *Adverse water conditions, waves, rips, currents and 'white water'*
- *Water temperature*
- *Caves, ledges, kelp, fishing nets*
- *Dangerous marine creatures*

---

## Dive profile and history

In the predisposition to decompression sickness, a history of recent dives is of importance. The history may be equally relevant in cases of pulmonary barotrauma, salt water aspiration, hypothermia etc. The log book may indicate the type of diving performed, or accidents suffered. So may witnesses, relatives, dive buddies, dive leaders etc.

In cases of breath-hold diving, the depth and duration are relevant to hypoxia, as is the practice of prior hyperventilation.

With the use of diving equipment, the depth and duration of each dive are relevant to the development of decompression sickness, especially if recommended stoppages have been omitted, or if the dive is in excess of that suggested in the tables, e.g. beyond the 'limiting line' in the Royal Navy tables, or in the extended exposure tables of the US Navy.

The depth is of importance in nitrogen narcosis and its influence on the behaviour of the diver, and also in other gas toxicity disorders, such as carbon dioxide and oxygen.

The speed of ascent, if excessive, can contribute to pulmonary barotrauma, decompression sickness or syncope of ascent. Some recreational divers have been timed to exceed 60 metres per minute in their routine ascents.

Exercise performed during the dive is of considerable importance, especially with rebreathing equipment. With strenuous exercise, the increased oxygen requirement may be in excess of that supplied by the flow rate for the particular gas mixture chosen. With increased oxygen consumption there is also an increased carbon dioxide production, placing an added load on the absorbent system. Thus, the incidence of both hypoxia and carbon dioxide toxicity are increased. Exercise also increases the likelihood of toxicity from high partial pressures of oxygen.

Even with scuba there are problems with increased exercise. First, there is an increased consumption of gas, and this may not be allowed for by the diver who is not wearing or observing a contents gauge to indicate his consumption. Secondly, there is the problem of an increased resistance to breathing with a resultant dyspnoea and physical exhaustion. Panic and fatigue are then common sequelae.

---

*Dive profile and history*
- *Recent dives; log book*
- *Depth/duration*
- *Entry, exit*
- *Speed of descent, ascent and stoppages*
- *Pre-dive exercise, alcohol, drugs or food consumption*
- *Problems – seasickness, stress, exertion, illness etc.*
- *Rescue, first aid and resuscitation attempts*

---

Accidents are likely to involve panic and rapid ascent. Inadequate training will then become manifest. The out-of-air situation, and the measures used to counteract it, are particularly hazards, often resulting in one of the companions making a desperate ascent.

Probably the most neglected information relevant to any accident, and also to the interpretation of the autopsy findings, is that involving the **first aid and resuscitation** methods employed. Such activities as rescue procedures, re-immersion, recompression, intubation and respiratory assistance, cardiac massage, oxygen administration etc. should be recorded in detail, because they influence autopsy findings.

## Diving equipment

It must be ensured that there is minimal or no interference after the accident with any of the diving equipment used by the deceased. Other diving equipment or air supply from the same source, used by other divers, may also be informative when examined by forensic diving experts. Contributions to the accident are often ascertained from the examination of this equipment. The information may vary from such obvious faults as the absence of protective clothing in a diver exposed to cold water, to the analysis for oxygen, carbon dioxide, carbon monoxide, inert gases and their derivatives, hydrocarbons etc. of the remaining contents of gas cylinders. Functioning of the equipment also requires assessment, e.g. demand valve performance and flow rate through the reducer.

The equipment may have been affected by the accident, as can be seen when there is loss or displacement of movable items, damage to protective clothing, diving set or accessories. Gas spaces, such as the face mask, buoyancy vest or counterlung, may be flooded. The lugs of the mouthpiece may be bitten during a convulsion. Vomitus may be present on the equipment or on the mouth piece, and this could either be a cause of the accident or a complication aggravating the situation.

Other observations on the equipment may reflect both on the diver and on the rescue procedure. The absence of specific equipment may be significant, and it must be determined whether this contributed to the incident, was caused by it or the rescue, or was coincidental.

The ease with which the weight belt and other harnesses can be released, or whether this was actually done, is of obvious importance. The protective suit, its thickness and integrity are relevant to both buoyancy and hypothermia. A depth gauge, watch, contents gauge on the gas cylinder, dive profile recorder etc. will be worn by the diver who takes precautions against accidents. A knife is important to overcome entanglements in ropes, kelp etc. The state of inflation of the buoyancy vest, and its ease of operation under similar circumstances, are very relevant to first aid. Similarly, a buddy line or direct contact with the surface support is often necessary for a rapid rescue.

The clothing may be cut off the body at the time of autopsy, but retained for assessment.

---

**Diving equipment**
- *Face mask, snorkel, buoyancy vest, depth gauge, watch, contents gauge on cylinder, buddy line, knife, weights etc – presence, absence or condition*
- *Protective clothing*
- *Functioning demand valve and reducer*
- *Cylinder condition, valve position (number of turns to close)*
- *Correct gas mixture, pressure and flow measurements*
- *Absence of contaminants*
- *Diving profile recorder*
- *Laboratory testing of equipment (regulators, buoyancy compensator, gauges etc.)*
- *In water replica trials*

---

In water, trials of the equipment may be conducted by professional investigators (water police, Navy divers), in cases where the cause of death is not clear. The trial is performed by a professional of approximately the same physical stature as the deceased, using a similar dive profile (if deemed safe to do so) and with appropriate safety procedures. Valuable information regarding problems with equipment is often obtained from these trials.

## Autopsy procedure

This requires specific pathological expertise and diving medical knowledge. Photographs, chest and soft tissue thigh X-rays are taken first. A CT scan of the body, if available, showing the pulmonary and cerebral vessels, can be of value. The presence and distribution of gas in tissues, vessels and body spaces is relevant.

### Site and time of the autopsy

To overcome the generalized and disruptive effects of the liberation of gas from the deceased diver who is brought to the surface, i.e. post-mortem decompression artefact, it is often advantageous to perform the autopsy prior to the decompression (Figures 34.1 and 34.2). This is possible when the death has occurred in a recompression facility, where the pathologist can be transferred to the same pressure, and can perform the autopsy adequately under such conditions. This is only appropriate in saturation diving, where the environment is such as to sustain life for an indefinite time. It is much more difficult under operational diving conditions where the pathologist himself may be exposed to the hazards of nitrogen narcosis and decompression sickness. The former is likely to influence his ability to perform the hyperbaric autopsy and the latter his enthusiasm.

The results of the autopsy must be assessed in relation to the time between the diving accident and the diver's death, and also between the death and the time of autopsy. If there has been a substantial period of time between the accident, injury, drowning or decompression sickness, and the time of death, then many of the pathological changes will have time to be corrected, even though the disease progresses to a fatal termination. Thus, the electrolyte changes of drowning and the gas changes associated with decompression sickness may well be totally corrected. The pathological lesions demonstrated hours or days later may reflect only the previous existence of the disease. A prolonged time between death and autopsy will nullify any electrolyte changes, and putrefaction influences both gas and alcohol production.

The widespread disruptive influence of **'post-mortem decompression artefact'** have already been mentioned. This develops in divers who die under pressure, within minutes and hours after they are brought to the surface, or in divers who retain a nitrogen load and die soon after surfacing.

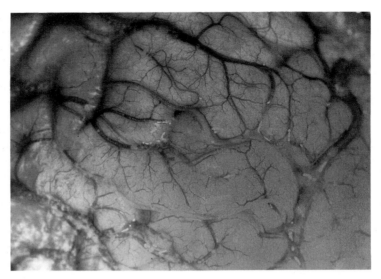

**Figure 34.1** Gas bubbles in the cortical veins of the brain and under the membrane – commonly seen in autopsies carried out on divers. It may be either from dysbaric disease or as a post-mortem artefact

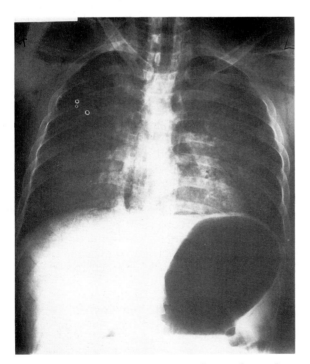

**Figure 34.2** Post-mortem decompression artefact – chest X-ray. There is a lot of gas seen within the heart chambers and the left pulmonary artery, as well as in the major vessels of the neck and the subclavian vessels bilaterally. Subcutaneous emphysema is seen in the chest wall. The gaseous distension of the gastric fundus is well demonstrated. These characteristics are commonly found in divers and caisson workers who die while under pressure and who are then brought to the surface

The results of bacteriological investigations will also be greatly influenced by the above factors. A time delay between the dive and death from encephalitis due to *Naegleria* is expected in divers who have exposed themselves to contaminated fresh water areas. Culture for organisms, such as marine vibrios, should also be performed in hypertonic saline. Unfortunately, many bacteriologically positive results may reflect contamination as opposed to actual aquatic infection. This is so with organisms such as *Clostridium tetani* and *C. perfringens* (*welchii*).

Nematocyst identification on the skin may remain possible for many days, even though the actual lesion may decrease in its florid appearance, not only between the injury and the time of death, but also post mortem. Immunoglobulin titres to coelenterate venoms may take several days to develop. Spines from marine creatures can be demonstrated macroscopically and on histology.

## General

An autopsy on a diver, who has died as a result of a diving accident, should be undertaken by a pathologist who has had experience in these investigations. The presence of a diving physician is an advantage. Otherwise the investigation may be incomplete and misinterpreted.

The deceased is examined prior to cleaning or removal of foreign bodies or clothing. Damage may result from either the cause of the accident, e.g. shark attack, propeller or from the search and recovery, e.g. from a grappling hook or line.

Skin examination may show the duration of exposure (cutis anserine), Tardieu spots of asphyxia, or signs of decompression sickness (see Chapter 12). Trauma to the skin from marine animals may either be caused after death or be instrumental in the death. Small crustaceans and 'sea lice' may cause extensive loss of soft tissues in water, within a day or two of death. If there are marine animal lesions, these are usually easy to diagnose. Shark bites (see plate 13) cause multiple crescentic teeth marks and tearing wounds illustrate the direction of the attack and the size of the animal. Teeth may break in the wound and will assist in identifying the species of shark. Barracuda bites are clean-cut excisions.

Coelenterate injuries may be recognizable by the number and distribution of the whiplike marks, which partly fade after death. An accurate identification of the type of coelenterate or jellyfish is possible by taking a skin scraping for examination of the nematocysts by a marine biologist. Cone shell may leave a tiny harpoon puncture. Blue ringed octopus bite appears as a small angular nick or a single haemorrhagic bleb. The sea snake bite will show two or more fang marks with surrounding teeth impressions. Where an octopus has held a victim, multiple bruising from round sucker pads is seen along this extent of the tentacle contact. Squid and cuttle fish may leave similar circular marks and incisions.

The skin of the fingers may show the effects of immersion, i.e. pale and wrinkled with the so-called 'washerwoman's skin'. There may be lacerations from where the diver has attempted to clutch barnacles, coral etc. Injury inflicted by aquatic animals in the early post-mortem period is especially seen on protuberances – fingers, nose, lips, eyelids etc. – if these are not protected by equipment.

There is often evidence of vomitus, which may be either causative or an important part of the sequence of events. In cases in which sea water has been aspirated there may be white, pink or blood-stained foam in the nose and mouth. Where the patient has been brought to the surface following a significant exposure at depth, there may also be distension of the gas spaces within the body resulting in a distended abdomen, faecal extrusions etc.

External evidence of barotrauma is important in ascertaining the sequence of events. An unconscious diver, or one who has not been able to equalize his physiological or equipment gas spaces during submergence, will have evidence of barotrauma, as described in previous chapters. Thus there should be an examination for evidence of mask or face squeeze with haemorrhage into the conjunctiva, ear squeeze with haemorrhage or perforation of the tympanic membrane, and suit squeeze with long whip-like marks underneath the folds of the protective clothing. Total body squeeze may occur when a standard diving rig is being used. Middle-ear haemorrhage, long considered a sign pathognomonic of drowning, is merely evidence of descent while alive.

Pulmonary barotrauma of ascent may be inferred by evidence of subcutaneous emphysema localized to the supraclavicular and cervical areas. If this finding is generalized over most of the body, then it is more likely to be due to the generalized liberation of gas following death, i.e. 'post-mortem decompression artefact'. This should not be confused with clinical decompression sickness or putrefactive changes. Where the diver has suffered from decompression effects, there is often a reddish or cyanotic distension of the head, arms and upper trunk. The body will therefore have an appearance not unlike that seen in clinical cases of the superior vena cava syndrome.

## Radiology

Prior to any invasive technique, radiology should be performed with under-penetrated films to show evidence of gas within the tissues (easily detected along muscle sheaths in the thigh), mediastinum, pleural cavity and neck, with gas in the great vessels and heart chambers, with fluid levels in the erect chest film. The interpretation of these must include consideration of pulmonary barotrauma, decompression sickness and post-mortem decompression artefact. X-rays may be taken for bone lesions and dysbaric osteonecrosis in the shoulders, hips and knees. In the case of marine animal injuries, there may also be

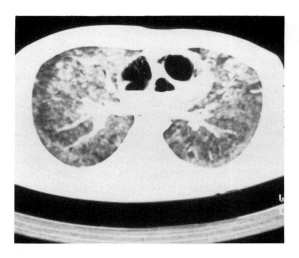

**Figure 34.3** CT scan of the chest. This is an axial CT scan through the heart. On these 'lung settings', diffuse changes are seen throughout both lung fields, particularly anteriorly. The gas within the heart chambers is well visualized

evidence of bone damage and foreign bodies, such as shark teeth, fish spines etc.

Sinus and middle-ear X-rays or CT scan may be performed for completeness, and to demonstrate possible contributing causes of the accident. Upper body (head, neck and thorax) CT scanning is of value in detecting gas in tissues, pleural cavity, mediastinum, cerebral and other vessels or pathology in the paranasal sinuses, middle ears and brain.

### Brain

Gas in the cerebral circulation may be very relevant to the cause of death or may be an artefact. As a cause of death, it results from embolism consequent on pulmonary baro-trauma or antemortem decompression sickness. Gas artefact may occur as a result of post-mortem decompression. Incision of the scalp and removal of the calvarium, or dissection of the neck, may introduce artefactual 'air emboli' into the superficial cerebral veins and venous sinuses, and these are not of diagnostic importance.

The calvarium should be opened at the beginning of the autopsy to obviate these problems. The technical difficulties of opening the skull under water are far outweighed by the advantages. A technique to demonstrate air emboli is of paramount importance in the investigation of diving accidents.

The circle of Willis and its distribution arteries are the areas to be examined meticulously for evidence of the significant air bubbles.

The customary technique is to do the craniotomy and cervical incisions under water, with a constant flushing of the water, avoiding artefactual air being introduced during this or during dissection of the neck. If bubbles are found, they should be photographed in situ, or after clamping the carotid arteries and cutting proximal to the clamp, in order to obtain a better exposure.

Alternatively, the head may be submerged and suspended into a mortuary sink with the body resting on shelving. The scalp is first incised above the water, then reflected under water. The head is again elevated, and the skull cut with a vibrating saw, taking care not to damage the dura. The head is then submerged for a second time, the calvarium dislodged, the dura incised and the brain removed under water. The brain may then be placed directly into a formalin container beneath the water container; formalin and brain then remain when the sink is drained. No air enters the cerebral circulation during the removal of calvarium and brain, and any gas bubbles present when the brain is examined after fixation would have been present at the time of death. Sections of the brain should include the 'watershed' area of the frontal cortex 2.5 cm from the midline.

## Spinal cord

Cord removal may be indicated, and the cord examined after fixation. Antemortem bubble formation may produce microscopic haemorrhages and infarcts, which are most easily recognized in the spinal cord. After fixation, a transverse section of the spinal cord should be taken from each segment and parasagittal longitudinal sections between each transverse section. Air may enter the spinal venous plexus during removal of brain, abdominal and thoracic organs, so that finding gas bubbles in this area in the final stages of the autopsy may not be significant.

## Temporal bones

In diving accidents, in diving pathology, the temporal bone and its associated middle-ear and mastoid air cell cavities are of special importance. Not only will haemorrhage occur in this area, due to barotrauma of descent, but also there are specific disorders related to disorientation which may be instrumental in the diving accident. These include such injuries as tympanic membrane perforation, middle-ear barotrauma of descent and inner-ear disturbances either from haemorrhage or round window rupture. It is thus important to record the appearance of the tympanic membrane or otoscopy, the presence of any fluid within the middle-ear cavity, and finally a histological examination of the temporal bones, ear and

mastoid cavities, performed by a specialist pathologist.

## Cardiothorax

Gas collections should be aspirated, preferably under water or through a water seal. The chest should also be opened beneath water in the bath or a water seal, so that small amounts of gas in the pleural cavities may be detected. Similarly, the pericardium should be opened and gas sought in the pericardial space and visceral pericardial vessels. The heart is removed, and each chamber opened under water. Unless the procedure is carried out under water, large quantities of intracardiac gas can be missed.

If there is doubt about drowning, blood samples should be taken from the vena cava and the pulmonary veins. A routine blood sample should always be taken, either from subclavian vessels or later from a femoral vein.

Mediastinal tissues and the soft tissues of the neck should be examined for interstitial emphysema. The lungs are inflated using compressed air or oxygen and a cuffed endotracheal tube to a pressure of 2.5 kPa (25 cmH$_2$O), producing slight overinflation. With the tube clamped, the lungs are then submerged beneath water, using a coarse metal grill to produce complete submersion. Air leaks are sought from air spaces into the pulmonary veins or from the pleural surfaces. Using an inverted water-filled glass measuring cylinder, some estimate should be made of the volume of air escaping per minute into veins or from pleura. The tube is then removed, the lungs separated, weighed, reinflated at similar pressure with buffered formalin and retained for examination after fixation.

Most of the above procedure can be performed, without the necessity of having the whole body immersed, by immersing only the heart and lungs under water. This is achieved by performing a neck incision extending down the midline from the sternal notch to the midpoint between the xiphisternum and umbilicus, and then to each of the antero-superior iliac spines. The skin and the muscles over the chest and the skin over the abdomen are then widely reflected by undercutting, and the trough between the body and the skin filled with water. The cavities can then be opened, noting the presence of any abnormal gas collection.

The appearance of the lungs may be characteristic for certain diving diseases. In drowning, the lungs are usually heavier than normal, with oedema and haemorrhage in the lung tissue and frothy red sputum in the airways. In fresh water drowning, if sufficient time has elapsed between rescue and death, the lungs may appear 'dry'. Evidence of marine foreign bodies, diatoms etc. should match those of the area where death occurred.

Pulmonary barotrauma may be identified at post mortem by demonstrating air leak from the lungs to pleura, interstitial tissue or blood vessels. These post-mortem findings are interpreted with a knowledge of all the circumstances of the accident so that the event or events leading to the fatality may be fully comprehended.

In pulmonary barotrauma, the voluminous lungs may bulge out to the thoracic cavity, and may have interstitial emphysema, subpleural blebs and mediastinal emphysema. Rupture of alveolar walls may be associated with widespread intra-alveolar haemorrhages. Interstitial emphysema recognized in sections of lung and acute intra-acinar emphysema may be seen in cases of pulmonary barotrauma. Haemorrhage, varying in intensity from lobule to lobule, may also be found when pulmonary barotrauma has occurred.

The pathological cause (e.g. pleural scarring, evidence of chronic asthma) of the barotrauma may also be detected. Acute effects of asthma, although of great importance clinically, will not be evident pathologically within 24 hours. Mucus secretion and eosinophils will usually be present in longer lasting disease, and basement membrane thickening with chronic asthma.

With severe decompression sickness the lungs may be engorged and distended with blood and intravascular gas. These effects are complicated by the addition of disseminated intravascular coagulation.

## Abdomen

Apart from the above observations, it is necessary to inspect the inferior vena cava and descending aorta for gas bubbles, and to examine the gastrointestinal tract for haemorrhages and infarcts, which may be related to either emboli or decompression sickness. In cases of underwater blast, most of the haemorrhages occur between a gas and fluid interface, and the abdomen and gastrointestinal tract are particularly involved. Under these conditions, there are seldom any external signs of violence on the skin or subcutaneous tissue despite severe haemorrhages within the bowel itself.

## Histology

Routine blocks should be taken from the brain, spinal cord, heart and abdominal viscera. After re-inflation and fixation, sections should be taken from the pleural surface of each lung lobe, and sections also across each segmental bronchus, including adjacent lung parenchyma.

Temporal bone studies and those for dysbaric osteonecrosis are specialized investigations and best referred to a specialist pathologist. They may indicate recent or past diving accidents.

Samples should be taken and kept, even if the pathologist does not intend to examine them himself. They will be valuable in future investigations.

## Other laboratory examinations

Urine samples may be tested for drugs and fibrin degradation products (FDPs). Evidence for antemortem intravascular blood coagulation and fibrinolysis may occur when there has been intravascular bubble formation. A blood sample should be examined routinely for alcohol, carbon monoxide and other drugs. Blood from the vena cava and pulmonary veins may be centrifuged, serum separated and examined for haemolysis, and the osmolarity of each sample measured.

It is necessary to test for alcohol and drugs in blood and tissues, as contributors to the diver's death. The alcohol level must be correlated with the postmortem interval to assess the putrefactive neoformation of this substance. Other biochemical investigations which may be relevant include serum electrolytes, performed on both the right and left side of the heart, serum haemoglobin and haptoglobin levels, and especially carboxyhaemoglobin estimation. Various assays may become possible to determine marine animal toxins, with some immunoglobulin analyses already available from specialized laboratories if death has been delayed.

Histological examination of the blood, the tissues and the bone marrow, as well as the material in the respiratory and gastrointestinal tracts, is necessary for the identification of diatroms and aquatic organisms. This information should be compared with similar investigations on a sample of water taken from areas in which the diver could have died.

## Conclusion

There needs to be a close integration of investigations performed by the investigating (police) divers, the diving physician and the pathologist, to obtain data and then to assess it. There is little information on the pathology and autopsy techniques associated with diving accidents.

In most countries, there are no analogous diving units to those which investigate aircraft accidents. Thus the usual practice is for the investigation of the diving accident to be performed by a police inspector moderately ignorant in the technical aspects of diving equipment, a local clinician who has no training in diving medicine and a pathologist who is overworked and not amenable to varying his standardized and venerable techniques. The result is often a mistaken diagnosis of either decompression sickness, air embolism or drowning, without an explanation of the causative sequence of events.

There is thus a loss of valuable information and a failure to learn from the mistakes of the past.

> *Adequate investigation that will result in useful information requires close cooperation between the divers, the diving physician, the police and the pathologist.*

## Acknowledgements

Acknowledgements are made to Dr John Hayman, Pathology Department, University of Melbourne, and Dr John Williamson, Director of the Hyperbaric Medicine Unit, Royal Adelaide Hospital for their assistance in revising this chapter.

## Recommended reading

EDMONDS, C., LOWRY, C. and PENNEFATHER, J. (1976). *Diving and Subaquatic Medicine*, 1st edn. Sydney: Diving Medical Centre.

FINDLEY, T.P. (1977). An autopsy protocol for skin and scuba-diving deaths. *American Journal of Clinical Pathology* **67**, 440–443.

HAYMAN, J.A. (1987). *Post mortem technique in fatal diving accidents*. Broadsheet No. 27. The Royal College of Pathologists of Australasia

KRATZ, P. and HOLTAS, S.P. (1983). Postmortem computed tomography in a diving fatality. *Journal of Computer Assisted Tomography* **7**, 132–134.

PALMER, A.C. (1986). The neuropathology of decompression sickness. In: *Recent Advances in Neuropathology*, edited by J.B. Cavanagh, pp. 141–162. Edinburgh: Churchill Livingstone.

PEARN, J. (1986). Pathophysiology of drowning. *Medical Journal of Australia* **142**, 586–588.

WILLIAMSON, J.A., KING, G.K., CALLANAN, V. et al. (1990). Fatal arterial gas embolism: Detection by post mortem, pre autopsy chest radiography and/or head and chest imaging. *Medical Journal of Australia* **153**, 97–100.

# 35

# Medical standards

## Introduction

To certify that a person is fit to be taught diving ideally implies that he is physically fit, medically healthy and psychologically stable. Many physicians limit their assessment to the exclusion of diseases. This may be inadequate, because the diving instructor needs more expert advice to guide him. A physician must at least be familiar with the diving environment, the equipment to be used and the skills required for the diver's safety. This implies knowledge that is not possessed by the usual medical graduate.

The imposition of **medical standards** for any occupational activity is, to a large extent, both presumptive and arbitrary. Although divers and hyperbaric personnel share some hazards, others are peculiar to one or the other. Within the diving environment, there may be considerably different medical requirements for the occasional, shallow water, recreation diver and the professional, deep or experimental diver.

The caisson worker is basically a labourer who is exposed to extended periods of pressure, and males tend to predominate. Hyperbaric oxygen therapists are often higher skilled staff, frequently being female nursing personnel in the reproductive periods of their life.

The medical standards which are applied to divers will be mainly considered in this chapter.

Reports of **diver selection** criteria are mainly anecdotal. These infer that the diver should have a psychologically stable or even phlegmatic personality, be able to endure physical and emotional stress, be free of all serious disease and also of minor illnesses of the respiratory tract. In appreciating the importance of selection criteria, it is necessary to consider three main aspects of diving: one is the high failure rate on professional diving courses and the characteristics necessary for success in these courses. The second is the hazardous nature of the marine environment and the sudden unexpected demands it is likely to make on the diver. The third is the variety of occupational diseases to which the diver is subjected. These aspects are discussed elsewhere.

The **professional diver** candidate is perhaps the easiest to assess. He may be a military diver, in which case there is considerable difference between the 'occasional' diver and the 'specialist'. He may be employed in civilian diving work in which he could be a shallow air diver working around harbours and in ship's repair and maintenance. Alternatively, he could be a deep helium diver employed on the offshore oil rigs.

The professional is required to reach higher standards of psychological stability, physical fitness and freedom from disease than his amateur counterpart. The main reasons for this relate to the sometimes demanding conditions under which he must work. The professional diver is often only one part of a team. He must be able to replace, and be replaced by, other members as the task demands. Most deviations from the norm make for complications. A diver less physically strong than the others will sooner or later be exposed to conditions which he will be unable to handle. He must be able to perform all the diving tasks expected of the team as a whole, and not have any specific restrictions or limitations imposed on him or his diving practice.

Successful diving candidates need to have a realistic attitude towards diving as a profession, a good general academic aptitude, encompassing mathematics and science, a basic seamanship background fitting in with the 'waterman' concept, and experience and skills of a mechanical nature. A higher school or college degree or its equivalent is a good indicator, although performance criteria are accepted in preference to academic knowledge.

In assessing the capabilities of a professional diver, the physician often finds himself acting on behalf of a commercial company or a government and not, as in the case of the recreational diver, in the more traditional doctor–patient relationship. It is in this activity that the physician is likely to represent an inflexible authority, to insist upon rigorous standards being achieved and maintained, and to be involved in legal considerations as well as safety.

Medical standards for **recreational diving** candidates leave greater room for flexibility and are harder to define in absolute terms. The recreational diver has the choice of depth and duration, he can avoid adverse environmental conditions and he can usually avoid strenuous exercise. It is therefore possible to consider voluntary restrictions both on the exposure to different diving environments and his diving practices (depth limits, equipment used etc.). Nevertheless, the physician should not forget that barotrauma can develop in very shallow depths and that unexpected emergencies may demand maximal physical performance.

The relationship between diving groups and physicians is sometimes strained. The diving instructor is stereotyped as the physical genius who can teach anyone to dive anywhere, and the physician is not uncommonly seen as the devil's advocate. This is unfortunate, but is partly valid if he applies the rigid criteria of professional diving medical standards to the recreational divers' needs. It is in this 'grey' area that a familiarity with diving and a good knowledge of diving physiology is essential. Nevertheless, there are certain hazardous activities which are common to all types of diving, and these will prevent certain candidates from being given medical approval to dive.

It is important that the **physician** does not act in an authoritarian manner when performing the diving medical examination. Extreme comments result in less respect from the diving community, and invoke ridicule. Such statements as 'you cannot dive while on drugs' and 'you can never dive again' are often recognized to be inaccurate by most divers. The 'thou-shalt-not-dive' syndrome is far more frequent among non-diving doctors than among those who dive themselves or who have some understanding of the sport.

Many countries have stringent medical standards for professional divers, but not even minimal requirements for recreational divers.

An argument against regulation frequently proposed is the protection of the rights of the individual. Most people accept the need for medical exclusions for driving or flying licence applicants. The rights of the individual are certainly not protected if he is allowed to dive in ignorance of risk superimposed by his medical condition.

In a democratic society, physicians can make recommendations, but not demand obedience from their patients. People do have a right to dive, as long as they do not involve or endanger others. If some candidates are forced into deciding 'to dive or not to dive', it is possible that they will ignore the advice and prove the physician incorrect. Diving candidates also have the right to seek alternative opinions from other diving physicians, and sometimes these hard lines are not shared by medical colleagues. The candidate seeks advice, and if this is given he will be able to make his own decision. It can be greatly facilitated by the use of reasonable explanations of the physician's recommendation.

A great deal of diving medical practice involves reviewing divers after they have been told by their local physician that they cannot dive again. Alternatively, a great deal of energy is required to convince a candidate with a potentially life-threatening disability not to dive if he has been 'passed' by another doctor.

Medical regulations must be explained rationally. Stating that diving should not be allowed while on drugs epitomizes the opposite attitude. There is no evidence available to suggest that anyone who is taking allopurinol for gout should not dive. Similarly with antibiotics for acne, or even chloroquine for malaria prophylaxis.

Stating that a patient with chronic sinusitis must not dive is not necessarily true. Some of these patients are said to be relieved considerably by the 'air washout' that they obtain from the diving, as long as the sinus ostia are not blocked. If the airways and the eustachian tubes are patent, there is also no reason why a person with a deviated nasal septum should not be allowed to dive. Commonly, patients who have been told they cannot dive because of otitis externa or a perforated tympanic membrane are reviewed. These are appropriate indications for treatment, and do not necessarily constitute permanent restrictions from diving.

Medical fitness to dive recreationally should be related to the environmental situation. In some environmental circumstances, no one is fit to dive, whereas in other circumstances, diving is safe for most people. It is often possible to tailor the type of diving to the person being examined.

> *Medical standards come in black and white, people come in shades of grey.*

In many cases, it can be stated that the recreational diver is fit in accordance with specific standards such as the Australian Standards Association, CIRIA, NOAA etc. In other cases, it has to be stated that the candidate is fit to dive, but under specific conditions and with specific recommended limitations. These limitations may be due to such conditions as physical disability, obesity, migraine, age, otological problems, visual impairment etc. Concessions can be more often made for the experienced diver, as compared to the novice.

Another pitfall for the physician is involvement with the setting of medical and diving standards which may be used or interpreted for political and administrative purposes. The physician should remain impartial. It is better for him not to affiliate with specific diving instructor organizations. If he does, competitive groups may doubt his impartiality. Absolute and unswerving professional integrity and the giving of advice that is limited to the medical aspects of any matter will ensure credibility and respect for the physician. If he advises truthfully and logically but does not impose, he eventually obtains more credence. There are so many people in the diving scene who are already on personal ego trips, in search of bureaucratic power and over-enthusiastic to impose views, that a similar approach by our profession is readily recognized.

The following discussion on various aspects of a diving medical evaluation is loosely based on a history and examination form devised by the authors to fill their needs (Figures 35.1–35.3).

# DIVING MEDICAL CENTRE

(MEDICAL HISTORY) TO BE FILLED IN BY CANDIDATE

| | |
|---|---|
| 1. SURNAME    OTHER NAMES | 2. DATE OF BIRTH |

3. ADDRESS     PHONE

4. SEX: MALE/FEMALE
5. MARITAL STATUS:   SINGLE ☐   DIVORCED ☐   MARRIED ☐

6. DIVING SCHOOL:

7. OCCUPATION

8. HAVE YOU ANY DISEASE OR DISABILITY AT PRESENT?   ☐ NO   ☐ YES   NAME OF CONDITION:

9. ARE YOU TAKING ANY TABLETS, MEDICINES OR OTHER DRUGS?   ☐ NO   ☐ YES   TYPE OF DRUG:

HAVE YOU EVER HAD OR DO YOU NOW HAVE ANY OF THE FOLLOWING:

| | | NO | YES | NOTES ON HISTORY |
|---|---|---|---|---|
| 10. | DO YOU WEAR GLASSES | | | |
| 11. | DO YOU WEAR CONTACT LENSES | | | |
| 12. | ANY HEART DISEASE OR BLOOD DISORDER | | | |
| 13. | HIGH BLOOD PRESSURE | | | |
| 14. | ABNORMAL SHORTNESS OF BREATH | | | |
| 15. | BRONCHITIS OR PNEUMONIA | | | |
| 16. | PLEURISY OR SEVERE CHEST PAINS | | | |
| 17. | COUGHING UP BLOOD | | | |
| 18. | T'B' (CONSUMPTION) | | | |
| 19. | CHRONIC OR PERSISTENT COUGH | | | |
| 20. | PNEUMOTHORAX (COLLAPSED LUNG) | | | |
| 21. | ASTHMA OR WHEEZING | | | |
| 22. | ANY OTHER CHEST COMPLAINT OR CHEST INJURY OR OPERATION ON CHEST, LUNGS OR HEART | | | |
| 23. | HAY FEVER | | | |
| 24. | SINUSITIS | | | |
| 25. | ANY OTHER NOSE OR THROAT TROUBLE | | | |
| 26. | DEAFNESS OR RINGING NOISES IN EAR | | | |
| 27. | DISCHARGING EARS OR OTHER INFECTION | | | |
| 28. | OPERATIONS ON EARS | | | |
| 29. | EYE OR VISUAL PROBLEMS | | | |
| 30. | DENTAL PROCEDURES (OVER LAST MONTH) | | | |
| 31. | FAINTING, BLACKOUTS, FITS OR EPILEPSY | | | |
| 32. | SEVERE HEADACHES OR MIGRAINE | | | |
| 33. | SLEEPWALKING OR SLEEP DISTURBANCES | | | |
| 34. | SEVERE DEPRESSION | | | |
| 35. | CLAUSTROPHOBIA | | | |
| 36. | ANY PSYCHIATRIC ILLNESS | | | |
| 37. | KIDNEY OR BLADDER DISEASE | | | |
| 38. | DIABETES | | | |
| 39. | INDIGESTION OR PEPTIC ULCER | | | |

**Figure 35.1** Medical history

MEDICAL HISTORY CONTINUED                                      NOTES ON HISTORY

| | NO | YES |
|---|---|---|
| 40. VOMITING BLOOD OR RECTAL BLEEDING | | |
| 41. RECURRENT VOMITING OR DIARRHOEA | | |
| 42. JAUNDICE OR HEPATITIS | | |
| 43. MALARIA OR OTHER TROPICAL DISEASE | | |
| 44. SEVERE LOSS OF WEIGHT | | |
| 45. VENEREAL DISEASE | | |
| 46. AIDS OR HIV POSITIVE | | |
| 47. HERNIA, RUPTURE OR PILES | | |
| 48. ANY SKIN DISEASE | | |
| 49. ANY REACTION TO DRUGS OR MEDICINES | | |
| 50. ANY OTHER ALLERGIES | | |
| 51. UNCONSCIOUSNESS | | |
| 52. CONCUSSION OR HEAD INJURY | | |
| 53. ANY MAJOR JOINT OR BACK INJURY | | |
| 54. ANY FRACTURES (BROKEN BONES) | | |
| 55. ANY PARALYSIS OR MUSCULAR WEAKNESS | | |
| 56. DENTURES | | |
| 57. MOTION SICKNESS (CAR, PLANE, SEA) | | |
| 58. DO YOU SMOKE | | |
| 59. APPROX. NUMBER OF CIGARETTES A DAY | | |
| 60. HAVE YOU EVER BEEN REJECTED FOR INSURANCE | | |
| 61. HAVE YOU EVER BEEN UNABLE TO WORK FOR MEDICAL REASONS | | |
| 62. HAVE YOU EVER BEEN ON A PENSION | | |
| 63. HAVE YOU ANY EAR PROBLEMS OR DISABILITY WHEN FLYING IN AN AIRCRAFT | | |
| 64. HAVE YOU ANY INCAPACITY DURING PERIODS | | |
| 65. ARE YOU NOW PREGNANT | | |
| 66. HAVE YOU BEEN IN HOSPITAL FOR ANY REASON | | |
| 67. HAVE YOU HAD ANY OPERATIONS | | |
| 68. HAVE YOU ANY OTHER ILLNESS OR INJURY NOT MENTIONED IN THIS LIST | | |
| 69. APPROX. DATE OF LAST CHEST XRAY: | NORMAL/ABNORMAL | |

} FEMALES ONLY (for items 64 and 65)

Additional History (taken by physician).
   Family history of cardiac disease.
   Personal history of lipid/cholesterol abnormality.
   Routine exercise exposure.

DIVING MEDICAL HISTORY (TO BE COMPLETED BY CANDIDATE)

| | | | |
|---|---|---|---|
| 1. | CAN YOU SNORKEL (FREE DIVE) | | |
| 2. | APPROX. DATE OF FIRST SCUBA DIVE | | |
| 3. | APPROX. NUMBER OF SCUBA DIVES | | |
| 4. | GREATEST DEPTH OF ANY DIVE | | |
| 5. | LONGEST DURATION OF ANY DIVE | | |

HAVE YOU EVER HAD ANY OF THE FOLLOWING
DISORDERS, DURING OR AFTER DIVING (DIVERS ONLY)

| | | NO | YES |
|---|---|---|---|
| 6. | SEVERE EAR SQUEEZE | | |
| 7. | RUPTURE OF EARDRUM | | |
| 8. | DEAFNESS | | |
| 9. | GIDDINESS OR DIZZINESS | | |
| 10. | SEVERE SINUS SQUEEZE | | |
| 11. | SEVERE LUNG SQUEEZE | | |
| 12. | RUPTURED LUNG (BURST LUNG) | | |
| 13. | EMPHYSEMA | | |
| 14. | PNEUMOTHORAX | | |
| 15. | AIR EMBOLISM | | |
| 16. | NITROGEN NARCOSIS | | |
| 17. | DECOMPRESSION SICKNESS (BENDS) | | |
| 18. | NEAR DROWNING | | |
| 19. | SEVERE MARINE ANIMAL INJURY | | |
| 20. | OXYGEN TOXICITY | | |
| 21. | CARBONDIOXIDE TOXICITY | | |
| 22. | CARBON MONOXIDE TOXICITY | | |
| 23. | DYSBARIC OSTEONECROSIS (BONES) | | |
| 24. | ANY OTHER DIVING ACCIDENTS | | |

I CERTIFY THAT THE ABOVE INFORMATION IS TRUE AND COMPLETE TO THE BEST OF MY KNOWLEDGE

SIGNED: ................................................................................   DATE ..............................................

**Figure 35.2** Diving medical history

MEDICAL EXAMINATION TO BE COMPLETED BY MEDICAL PRACTITIONER

| 1. PHYSIQUE GOOD AVERAGE POOR | 2. HEIGHT ins. cm | 3. WEIGHT lbs kg | 4. VISION R6/  CORR 6/ L6/  CORR 6/ | 5. B/P | 6. URINALYSIS ALBUMEN GLUCOSE |
|---|---|---|---|---|---|
| 7. CHEST X RAY, IF INDICATED DATE ................................... PLACE .................................. RESULT ................................. | | *8. RESPIRATORY FUNCTION TEST VITAL CAPACITY ...................... F.E.V.1.0 ..................................... PERCENTAGE ........................... | | COMMENTS: | |

9.  AUDIOMETRY

FREQUENCY (Hz)

| | 500 | 1000 | 2000 | 4000 | 6000 | 8000 |
|---|---|---|---|---|---|---|
| LOSS IN dB (R.E.) | | | | | | |
| LOSS IN dB (L.E.) | | | | | | |

REMARKS:

| CLINICAL EXAMINATION | NORMAL | ABNORMAL | NOTES ON ABNORMALITIES |
|---|---|---|---|
| 10.  NEUROLOGICAL SYSTEM | | | |
| *11.  CARDIOVASCULAR SYSTEM | | | |
| 12.  E.C.G. (IF INDICATED) | | | |
| 13.  E.N.T. SYSTEM | | | |
| *14.  EUSTACHIAN TUBE FUNCTION (VERIFIED) | | | |
| *15.  RESPIRATORY SYSTEM (AUSCULTATION WITH HYPERVENTILATION) | | | |
| 16.  MUSCULO-SKELETAL | | | |
| 17.  ENDOCRINE SYSTEM | | | |
| 18.  PERIPH, VASCULAR/LYMPHATIC | | | |
| 19.  OTHER ABNORMALITIES | | | |

## FITNESS TO DIVE

| | |
|---|---|
| | YES. PROFESSIONAL DIVING |
| | YES. RECREATIONAL DIVING |
| | YES (QUALIFIED). RESTRICTIONS: |
| | TEMP. UNFIT. REASON: |
| | PERM. UNFIT. REASON: |

SIGNATURE OF PHYSICIAN ................................................  DATE .......................

NAME AND ADDRESS: .........................................................................................

FURTHER INVESTIGATIONS REQUIRED:

NEXT MEDICAL ASSESSMENT DUE:

**Figure 35.3** Physical examination

# Physical fitness

This subject is still a contentious one. So often we are faced with diving candidates who have demonstrated their physical prowess by excelling in specific sports, who are then informed that they are not medically fit to dive. Thus a champion swimmer, who has active asthma, may well feel that his physical fitness qualifies him for scuba diving. This illustrates a major maxim. Even though a candidate can be very physically fit in one sport, e.g. marathon running, this proves only his fitness for that sport; it does not imply fitness for diving.

Physical fitness is not yet routinely tested in recreational diver assessments, but may be of life-saving importance in the unplanned emergency situations produced by tides, currents and changing weather conditions. Some idea of the candidate's fitness may be assessed by enquiring into his normal daily physical and sporting activities.

> *Physical fitness does not imply fitness for scuba diving.*

A statistical correlation is found with the degree of physical fitness and success in diving training. Candidates who have a maximum oxygen uptake in excess of 3 litres/min are more likely to succeed in diving courses than those who have not. Those who can swim 200 metres without fins in 5 minutes or less are far more likely to succeed in diving than those who cannot achieve this standard.

Groups throughout the world have their own particular tests for physical fitness, but it is hoped that in future there will be more attention given to **aquatic** fitness, which includes such parameters as swim speed and breath-holding capacity, than many of the terrestrial tests. Perhaps the most inappropriate application of fitness tests for divers is seen in the European Flack test and the Test de Ruffier. These, quite apart from their lack of standardization, have not been shown to be either reliable or valid in the diving context. Even the more standardized Masters' step test is inappropriate, because it discriminates against the moderately obese – who do not have to support this excess weight in the water.

# Psychological and psychiatric considerations

A full psychiatric assessment is impossible to perform in the limited time of a routine diving medical examination but some clues can be gleaned. A personality characterized by a tendency to introversion, neuroticism and global mood disturbance is more likely to panic (37% of diving deaths are due to this diver error). The 'cowboy' is overconfident and impulsive and may be recognized by a history of motor vehicle and other accidents, multiple injuries, police arrests etc. Useful insight may be gained by direct questions regarding the motivation to dive, a history of claustrophobia, hydrophobia and previous water sports.

The diving instructor is in a better position to assess the candidate's psychological suitability for diving during the period of instruction.

Freedom from gross psychiatric disorders is essential. There should be no evidence of: anxiety states, depression, claustrophobia or agoraphobia, psychoses or any organic cerebral syndromes (see Chapter 29).

A history of antidepressant, tranquillizer or other psychotropic drug intake is important both as an indication of psychopathology and because of possible interactions with the diving environment (see Chapter 31). The candidate with a history of alcohol or other drug abuse should be assessed critically.

The ability to endure an isolated and enclosed environment is important in commercial diving and caisson work.

# Age

The age range for the initial training of professional naval divers varies from 17–20 years at one extreme, to 35 at the other. Age is of limited value in success prediction in achieving diving skills, but the most satisfactory age is in the early twenties. Most professional diving schools prefer to select divers 22–29 years of age, with a mean of 24 years. Beyond this range the candidate will have a more limited life as a working diver, whereas under the age of 22 they are usually not experienced enough in their basic work skills, and also perhaps are not as reliable or mature. Failure rates in training professional diving candidates below the age of 19 years makes this practice commercially unprofitable.

Beyond the age of 35, there is an appreciable increase in susceptibility to decompression sickness, as well as a probable reluctance to persevere with adverse environmental and social conditions. In an Australian survey, the incidence of medical disorders causing failure to meet the strict Australian Standards for Professional Divers was 45% in the over thirty-fives. This was compared to a 20% incidence in the candidates in their twenties – illustrating the high medical standards required as well as the adverse effects of age.

The age range of the training for recreational divers is much more variable. There are still the same factors involved as mentioned above, but as the diving activities can be tailored to the individual, greater laxity can be allowed.

As a general rule, it is recommended that diving in excess of 9 metres (30 feet) should not be allowed prior to a **child** reaching osteogenic maturity, i.e. when the epiphyses have fused. This is a very common statement, but there is very little evidence that decompression sickness has really influenced bone growth in young animals. Nevertheless, the possibility makes for hesitation, when recommending that children be allowed to dive in excess of this depth.

Children, although they may be trained in diving techniques, often do not have the physical strength or psychological stability to cope with the occasional unexpected hazards of diving. A child exposed to scuba training must be totally and completely under the control of a competent adult diver, of instructor standard. A salutary warning about allowing children to dive is given by reference to the age range in the fatality statistics. So far the youngest child to die while scuba diving was aged 7, but many were between the ages of 10 and 14 years.

Although 'physiological age' is more important than 'chronological age', for divers over 40 years it is recommended that regular re-examinations be carried out in order to detect medical abnormalities which may interfere with efficiency and safety in the diving environment. Electrocardiographic examinations during maximal exercise may be recommended as part of this medical, especially if cardiac risk factors are present. There is now a tendency for much older people, and especially those associated with yachting, to take up diving as part of their marine lifestyle. Thus we now have people commencing diving, having retired from their normal occupation. This puts an added burden on the medical examiner, but diving is often a valuable contribution to the quality of life of these people.

With increasing age, allowance must be made for a more conservative approach to diving activity as well as to restricting the decompression schedules. These authors arbitrarily recommend that older divers reduce their allowable bottom time by 10% for each decade after the age of 30 years.

Many divers have continued diving into their eighties, and the social aspect of diving is not to be forgotten. In Australia, there is even a Subaquatic Geriatric Association (SAGA), to which one of the authors has received (junior) membership.

# Weight

Weight should be less than 20% above the average ideal weight for age, height and build. Obesity is undesirable because it may increase decompression sickness, even though it may reduce the likelihood of hypothermia. For sport diving, it is permissible to allow diving with degrees of obesity that would not normally be accepted in professional or military diving. This is achieved by imposing an added safety margin in calculating the allowable duration of the dive. With divers who are obese, the bottom time is reduced by somewhere between 25% and 50%, depending on the degree of obesity.

One arbitrary standard, used for many years at the Australian Diving Medical Centres, has been to reduce the allowable bottom time for the dive according to the percentage that the candidate's weight exceeds that expected for height and build. Appropriate tables or an index such as Cotton's Index of Build (CIB) can be applied. Thus, if the CIB is exceeded by one-third the permissible bottom time for a given depth is reduced by one third, but the longer duration is used for decompression calculations. An 18-metre dive allowing 60 minutes in the tables would allow an actual bottom time of only 40 minutes in this example.

Other standards (e.g. UK Health and Safety Executive) suggest the use of anthropometric measurements such as elbow epicondylar breadth to determine weight limits for small, medium and large frames.

## Occupation

The candidate's occupation may give some indication of his physical fitness, but may also be important in increasing the relevance of diving hazards, e.g. aviators or air crew should be specifically advised of the flying restrictions imposed after diving. Sonar operators and musicians may not wish to be exposed to the possible otological complications of diving, which may prejudice their professional life.

## Drugs

The thorough drug history is important in that it may give a clue to the presence and/or severity of otherwise undetected but significant diseases, such as hypertension, cardiac arrhythmia, epilepsy, asthma or psychosis. Also the effects of drugs may influence diver safety and predispose to diving diseases. Both therapeutic and 'recreational' drugs should be considered. These possibilities are discussed more fully in Chapter 31.

## Cardiovascular system

The existence of serious cardiovascular disease disqualifies the candidate from diving because of the risk of sudden collapse or decreased exercise tolerance. These diseases are responsible for 12–23% of the deaths in recreational scuba diving. A history of chest pain, unusual breathlessness, palpitations or syncope, especially on exercise, is likely to be significant.

An annual electrocardiogram (ECG), as a baseline for legal and compensation reasons, is required for all professional divers. The exercise ECG is a valuable addition to the medical examination of all divers over the age of 45, and even those younger where significant coronary risk factors are prevent (see Chapter 26).

**Coronary artery disease** is a potentially lethal, but often asymptomatic, disease which may be present from the mid-thirties onwards. It needs to be detected prior to medical approval for diving. With coronary artery disease, the myocardium is susceptible to ischaemia whenever there is an excessive load placed upon it, from physical activity or stress. The latter may produce an elevation in blood pressure, and can be initiated by such factors as cold, anxiety, and real or imagined threats. In these individuals, physical activity or elevation of the blood pressure may be required before the disease becomes noticeable, and may be particularly hazardous in the underwater environment.

> *Significant coronary artery disease may be present despite normal physical examination.*

Risk factors for coronary disease, such as smoking, hypertension, family history, raised serum cholesterol or triglycerides, should be sought. If in doubt, a resting and exercise electrocardiogram should be performed, and should not show evidence of abnormal arrhythmias or ST depression.

Myocardial ischaemia may have several manifestations. Symptoms of chest pain or discomfort, dyspnoea or syncope on exercise should be actively sought. Angina pectoris associated with exercise may or may not be associated with a history of myocardial infarction, and is likely to proceed to this condition in the event of severe exercise. A large infarction may result in sudden death.

The ECG shows abnormalities only when there is interference with the conduction system, or when significant damage has already been caused to the cardiac tissue. Thus in individuals over the age of 45, a maximal stress test producing demands comparable to that which is likely to be experienced in the diving environment may be appropriate. During this stress test there may be several important findings:

1. The blood pressure response may be abnormal.

2. The cardiac rhythm may show exercise-induced abnormalities, with conduction disorders, premature ventricular or atrial beats.
3. The electrocardiogram may suggest the presence of myocardial ischaemia, with ST segment or T wave changes.

Although occasional false-positive results with such examinations may be found, it would be unrealistic to subject such a person to professional diving without ensuring that there was no demonstrable coronary artery disease. Those with a genuinely positive stress test should be advised against diving.

An occasional false-positive result to the exercise ECG is seen when there is ventricular hypertrophy associated with extreme athletic activity. Other false positives may be noted in other causes of left ventricular hypertrophy or the use of digitalis derivatives, although in both these cases there are adequate reasons for exclusion from diving. Beta-blocking drugs may render the exercise ECG unreliable. Occasional premature ventricular and atrial beats are found in the ECGs of many asymptomatic individuals with no known heart disease. These do not preclude diving. However, if the arrhythmia becomes predominant with exercise, it may have far more significance.

A cold pressor test has also been suggested, with ECG monitoring. This consists of immersing a hand in cold water and recording cardiac and blood pressure responses.

Serum cholersterol and triglycerides, serum enzyme levels, glucose estimations and other biochemical tests have been suggested by various authorities for professional diving and may also be useful in assessing the older recreational diver, especially if other coronary risk factors exist.

Some physicians allow experienced divers who have had a myocardial infarction to return to non-strenuous recreational diving after a year or more, if there were no sequelae and a normal exercise stress test without evidence of ischaemia or arrhythmia on maximal exercise. Other physicians believe that this is poor advice because this disease has a high incidence of recurrence and increased propensity to arrhythmias; still others would require further investigations (e.g. echocardiography or even coronary angiography). The reader is reminded that it is virtually impossible to make initial diver training non-stressful or non-strenuous.

An experienced diver who has undergone coronary artery revascularization and has a normal stress test causes problems because he has an increased risk of myocardial infarction and arrhythmias are more likely. Also, not all obstructions may be overcome and the restenosis rate is high. With internal mammary artery grafting, the pleural cavity is usually invaded leading to the possibility of adhesions, thus also precluding diving.

**Arrhythmias**, whether due to coronary artery or other disease, are another cause of sudden death. Especially ominous are the cardiac dysrhythmias resulting in ventricular tachycardia and a reduction of cardiac output. These individuals are in danger of sudden death with any severe stress or exercise. The stress may be either environmentally or emotionally precipitated.

Although the diving reflex is one of the treatments for supraventricular tachycardia, it can also precipitate it.

Patients with **paroxysmal atrial** or **supraventricular tachycardia** are susceptible to cardiac symptoms that cannot be tolerated in scuba diving (see Chapter 26). **Wolff–Parkinson--White syndrome**, with the short P–R interval, is associated with paroxysmal atrial tachycardia, and these individuals can rapidly move into a shock state, with severe hypotension.

**Sinus bradycardia**, with a rate of less than 60/min, must also be investigated. The bradycardia associated with athletes will respond to exercise with an appropriate increase in rate, and this differentiates it from the more serious bradycardias due to ischaemia or conduction defects affecting the sinoatrial node, which respond inadequately or inappropriately to exercise. The most common cause of bradycardia in a general population could be drugs such as beta-blockers.

**Conduction defects** need to be assessed. Isolated right bundle-branch block in an asymptomatic individual with no other heart disease evident is acceptable, although a small percentage have associated atrial septal defect and this should be excluded. The left bundle-branch block is also occasionally found in the normal population, but is more likely to be associated with coronary artery disease. If, following adequate cardiac assessment, there is no evidence to believe that the left bundle-branch block is other than benign, then the individual may be allowed to dive.

First-degree **atrioventricular (AV) block** is sometimes a normal finding. If there is no evidence either in history or examination for cardiac disease, and if there is a normal ECG response to exercise, the individual should be allowed to undertake diving.

Second-degree AV block is much less likely to be of benign nature and usually excludes diving activities. It is sometimes a normal finding in athletic young adults with a high vagal tone; during sleep or at rest, it is vagally induced. The second-degree block of Mobitz type 2 is especially ominous and often precedes the onset of complete heart block. If the conduction abnormality disappears with a mild degree of exercise, the heart rate response is appropriate and there is no underlying disease or drug causing the rhythm disturbance, then the individual can be approved for diving.

Complete AV block is a contraindication, because of the inability of the heart to respond appropriately to exercise stress.

Although implanted cardiac **pacemakers** are built to withstand a pressure of about 33 metres, their owners usually have underlying disease precluding diving. Newer AV sequential pacemakers provide some increase in rate with exercise but this is limited. There is also the possibility of scar tissue increasing bubble formation.

**Valvular heart disease** is usually a contraindication to diving. In many cases the abnormal valve will produce a chronic overload on the work of the heart, and this may be aggravated by the effects of stress with increased cardiac demand. Valvular regurgitation, as well as obstruction to forward flow, must influence the capacity of the heart to respond with an appropriate cardiac output to stress and exercise. Turbulence may also increase gas phase separation.

Some authorities feel that the asymptomatic patient with mild aortic or mitral valve regurgitation, which does not limit exercise tolerance, may be passed for recreational diving. The prospect that turbulence across the valve may increase gas phase separation has not been investigated. Nevertheless, patients with aortic or mitral stenotic lesions should never dive because of the reduced fixed output and the likelihood of central blood shifts precipitating pulmonary oedema. Patients with prosthetic valves and/or who are taking anticoagulant drugs should also be excluded.

Mitral valve prolapse is found in about 12% of the general population (females:males, 2:1), with clinical evidence (systolic auscultatory click) in 1 in 7. The prolapse itself is of no consequence but associated arrhythmias may be. Their presence may require Holter monitoring for detection. The totally asymptomatic diver with a normal ECG (normal Q–T interval) and no redundant valve leaflets on echocardiography may be permitted to dive.

**Congenital heart disease** should be carefully assessed. Atrial or ventricular septal defect, even though diagnosed as having left-to-right shunts, is usually bidirectional with a small right-to-left flow during diastole. This could allow bubbles returning to the right heart from the periphery to pass into the left heart and thus the systemic circulation, bypassing the normal pulmonary filter.

A recent report has suggested an unexpectedly high incidence of (previously undetected and, of course, asymptomatic) patent foramen ovale in a series of patients with neurological decompression sickness. The patent foramen ovale and the intermittent reversal of shunt sometimes produced by such manoeuvres as that of Valsalva, were demonstrated by bubble contrast echocardiography. Patent foramen ovale can apparently be demonstrated in 17% of the population and 30% at autopsy.

Any other congenital abnormality which interferes with the exercise capacity of the individual, or reduces the cardiac response to exercise, precludes diving activity. This would be the case with such disorders as coarctation of the aorta.

**Blood pressure**: it is generally stated that blood pressure should not exceed 140 mmHg systolic and 90 mmHg diastolic. This is certainly so for the younger people who are likely to become involved in diving. However, there is usually more flexibility when considering the increasing age of many of the candidates currently being attracted to this activity. For recreational divers, it is reasonable that the blood pressure should be within the normal range for the age of the candidate.

In assessing the hypertensive diver, the following should be considered: the aetiology (e.g. coarctation, endocrine disorders), severity (end-organ damage), drug therapy and the increased risk of coronary artery disease and stroke. Patients on salt-restriction and/or mild diuretic therapy may be allowed restricted recreational diving. With other drugs, such as beta-blockers, there should be an awareness of the effects of reduced exercise tolerance and autonomic nervous system blockade, and the added danger of cardiac deaths if diving is carried out while on these drugs. Beta-blockers may also have other side effects, such as bronchospasm.

It is unreasonable to condone diving if there are any end-organ manifestations of chronic hypertension, such as retinal changes, left ventricular hypertrophy or dysfunction, or abnormal renal function. These candidates usually have sustained blood pressure elevation, with diastolic values above 100–110 mmHg. These individuals should be advised not to dive, and should be referred for diagnosis and treatment.

The exercise ECG is useful in evaluating patients with borderline hypertension. The stress simulates the physical activity required in diving, and the recording of the blood pressure during the test will allow an assessment as to how the individual will respond to diving stresses. The hypertensive individual will show a marked elevation in the systolic pressure and a small rise in the diastolic. The normal individual shows a rise in systolic to a lesser degree and a slight fall in diastolic pressure. The stresses associated with diving, other than exercise, may aggravate this hypertensive response. Individuals with labile hypertension and marked elevations of systolic blood pressure during exercise must be considered with some reservation for diving.

Antihypertensive drugs alter the capability of the circulation to respond to stress, or alternatively affect the heart rate and blood pressure responses during exercise. Unless the blood pressure is controlled by diet, weight loss, exercise plus, perhaps, a thiazide diuretic, moderate and severe hypertensives should be advised against diving. For the mild hypertensive and the labile hypertensive, individual judgement must be exercised in each case, possibly permitting restricted recreational diving.

**Peripheral vascular disease** would limit aquatic exercise capability, delay wound healing and perhaps delay the elimination of inert gas during decompression. Cold water may precipitate Raynaud's phenomenon in susceptible individuals.

**Varicose veins** are hydrostatically supported in the water and the main problems would be trauma causing haemorrhage, or infection if skin changes are present.

## Respiratory system

### Lungs

Respiratory disease is the major cause for disqualification of diving candidates. Divers must not only be able to tolerate severe physical exertion, which requires good respiratory function, but also be able to tolerate rapid changes in lung volumes and pressures with equal compliance throughout the lung.

Any local airway restriction, fibrosis, cysts etc. may result in pulmonary barotrauma, with a tearing of lung tissue and subsequent complications, including air embolism (see Chapter 9).

A history of **spontaneous pneumothorax**, because of the high incidence of recurrence and the implications of other basic pulmonary pathology, precludes diving. The recurrence rate after one episode of spontaneous pneumothorax is approximately 33% over a 5-year period. In one large series of cases, 31 patients were explored surgically and all of these had generalized cystic disease of the lungs, even though preoperatively only 6 had been thus diagnosed. These cysts are especially noted at the apices, and are particularly likely to rupture with pulmonary barotrauma. Spontaneous pneumothorax is predominantly a disease of young males, with the peak incidence being between 16 and 25 years. It is not considered familial and is not fatal in most cases, except when its recurrence is provoked by such activities as scuba diving, with transformation into a tension pneumothorax.

Surgical pleurodesis to prevent recurrence does not render the patient fit to dive, as small blebs or bullae are still present, and air embolism is not prevented by this operation. In one case, hemiplegia from cerebral arterial gas embolism developed in the first dive after pleurodesis. The resultant adhesions and decreased distensibility of the lung from pleurodesis may also predispose to other pulmonary barotrauma.

A history of **asthma** is particularly important, because its occurrence will result in increased pulmonary airway resistance and also may require the use of adrenergic drugs. Neither is acceptable in any diving operations, recreational or professional. The reprehensible tendency of some physicians to recommend that an asthmatic takes a bronchodilator prior to his dive has nothing to commend it. It ignores the facts that:

1. The asthmatic is far more susceptible to pulmonary barotrauma.
2. The aerosol bronchodilator may relieve some, but not all, areas of airway resistance.
3. The aerosol will be very effective in allowing the person to descend while breathing relatively normally, but is less effective at the end of the dive when the emergency rapid ascent is far more likely.
4. Most sympathomimetic drugs do have arrhythmogenic effects, aggravating a small but appreciable hazard that already exists in the diving environment (see Chapter 26).

Exercise-incuded asthma is a specific problem, which can be verified by repeating respiratory function tests while the candidate undergoes a reasonably strenuous exercise such as bicycling at 900 kpm/min for 5–6 min. This is analogous to a 1-knot swim, which most divers encounter during their diving career. Subsequent detection of rhonchi on auscultation (more obvious with hyperventilation) or a progressive reduction in lung function should give sufficient indication that the candidate should not proceed with his diving course.

Sea water is a hypertonic saline solution, which provokes bronchospasm in some asthmatics. It is used as an asthma provocation test akin to histamine, methacholine or exercise challenge. The combination of a number of trigger factors in the scuba environment may explain the increased incidence (>9%) of asthma in the recreational diving death statistics (see Chapter 8). These factors include:

1. Extreme exercise.
2. Hypertonic saline (seawater) inhalation.
3. Breathing cold dry hyperbaric air, which increases dehydration of the airway.

4. Increased inspiratory effort, from regulator resistance or increased gas density.
5. Hyperventilation or increased respiration.

The tendency for asthmatics to suffer pulmonary barotrauma may also be aggravated by: the greater inspiratory reserve volumes utilized by them to keep their airways open, interference with the elastic properties of the lung, greater resistance to exhalation or the occasional association of cystic changes.

Quite apart from the increased death rate in the asthmatics who dive, the authors have experienced great difficulty in treating asthmatic scuba divers who are rescued and survive until recompression. They were suffering from a confusing clinical complex comprised of deep unconsciousness from near-drowning and probable cerebral gas embolism, and respiratory impairment from near-drowning and asthma.

The problems of combining respiratory support and recompression therapy (restricted to 18 metres because of the requirement for 100% oxygen in the presence of arterial hypoxia), the dangers from arrhythmias, and the possible arteriolization of trapped pulmonary air emboli with sympathomimetic drugs, all make these cases a nightmare. Deeper recompression, even though the patient is not responding, may well be a death sentence, and ultimate decompression is daunting with an arterial oxygen tension less than 50 mmHg! Some of our successes are doubtful achievements with residual hypoxic brain damage.

Cystic lung lesions, chronic bronchitis, chronic obstructive pulmonary disease and emphysema, and active respiratory infections, such as tuberculosis, histoplasmosis, mycotic infections and their sequelae, are all contraindications to diving. Sarcoidosis is also a contraindication because the pulmonary involvement is usually greater than suspected clinically and the mucous membranes are also often involved.

Penetrating chest injuries and chest surgery should be considered as disqualifying because the scar formed in the lung tissue during healing may lead to tethering of the pleura or air trapping. It is of interest that the intensive care literature reports increased pulmonary barotrauma in the opposite lung when one lung has scars or decreased compliance. Also, systemic gas embolism has been reported with the use of positive end-expiratory pressure (PEEP).

*In assessing the diving candidate with a past history of 'wheeze' or asthma and a normal chest X-ray, the following protocol may be of value.*

*History of asthma over the last 5 years* ------------------------------- FAIL

*Use of bronchodilators over the last 5 years* --------------------------------- FAIL

*Respiratory rhonchi or other abnormalities on ausculation* ------------------- FAIL

*High pitched expiratory rhonchi on hyperventilation* ----------------------- FAIL

*High pitched expiratory rhonchi 5–10 minutes after exercise stress* -------------- FAIL

*$FEV_1/VC$ < 80% of predicted value* ------------------------------- FAIL

*Expiratory flow rates of < 70% of predicted value (basic spirometry MMEF, $MEF_{25,50,75}$* ----------------------------- FAIL

*Asthma provocation producing >10% reduction of expiratory flow rates after either conventional histamine or chest X-ray is normal, hypertonic saline, with or without dehumidified cold ventilation* ----------------------------------------- FAIL

*If all the above are clear, permit limited diving to a maximum depth of 18 metres without any free ascent practice* ---- PASS

The history of respiratory disorders is complemented by the **physical examination** and **simple respiratory function tests**. High pitched expiratory rhonchi, which may only be elicited during hyperventilation, indicate airway obstruction and preclude diving prior to further investigation. Thus auscultation should be performed during hyperventilation through a wide-open mouth.

Most standards for divers require that the forced vital capacity (FVC) should be more than 4 litres in males, 3 litres in females, and the forced expiratory volume in 1 second ($FEV_1$) should be more than 75% of the FVC. Any candidate with a result below 80% of the predicted values based on population norms for age, height and sex should be suspect. Forced expiratory flow (FEF, MEF) measurements have been found more useful by some investigators. Since the introduction of respiratory standards, there has been an apparent reduction in the incidence of pulmonary barotrauma.

Whenever it is decided to allow a candidate to continue diving, despite not meeting respiratory standards as described above, it is essential that the diver be made aware of the increased danger to himself, and the likelihood of serious consequences during rapid ascents. As a result of the morbidity and mortality from pulmonary barotrauma, we are less lenient in dealing with minor degrees of respiratory impairment than with other abnormalities in the diving medical examination. A burst lung may not allow for adequate resuscitation, whereas if a diver trainee ruptures an eardrum, or even loses hearing in one ear, or suffers dental barotrauma, then these events are not usually life threatening.

It would seem reasonable, if a person was perfectly normal in every other respect, but had reduced spirometry, to apply restrictions to his diving activities. These may include:

1. Slower than normal ascent. (This can be achieved by leaving the bottom earlier – perhaps coming up at the slower rate of 8 m/min or 25 feet/min, instead of 18 m/min or 60 feet/min.)
2. No 'free' or assisted swimming ascent or buoyant ascent practice. These are especially dangerous because of the involuntary tendency of the trainee to inhale deeply prior to the ascent, and therefore increase the likelihood of pulmonary barotrauma. In the event of a genuine emergency free ascent, it is more common for the diver to commence the ascent without a large lung volume because he is no longer able to inhale, either deep or shallow!
3. Restricted depth: it could also be suggested that the diver does not exceed 30 metres (100 feet), as beyond this the likelihood of exhausting the air supply is much greater – due to both the narcotic effect reducing his alertness and the increased consumption of air at greater depth.

---

## CASE REPORT 35.1

MB aged 25 was a very fit, mildly asthmatic, sportsman. He had been diving for 4 months when he went to 18 metres for 20 minutes. Without an obvious reason, he performed a rapid ascent, developing dyspnoea and confusion on the surface and left-sided hemiplegia within a few minutes. He was taken by helicopter to the Navy RCC. He was initially compressed to 18 metres on oxygen, but as he did not regain consciousness he was then taken to 50 metres.

After a 3-day vigil in which the patient was subjected to various procedures in an attempt to surface him, he died, still under pressure. During that time he was treated conscientiously for his asthma, which was evident on auscultation, and CAGE. He was given steroids and anticonvulsants (for his repeated epileptic episodes), measures to counter possible cerebral and pulmonary oedema, and maintenance of his electrolyte and pH levels.

The autopsy revealed mild cerebral oedema, congestion of the meningeal vessels and ischaemic cell damage in the right frontal lobe and the right thalamus. There was a tear on the posterior section of the upper lobe of the right lung, with intra-alveolar haemorrhages and rupture of alveolar septae. The basal membranes were thickened and muscles showed hypertrophy, consistent with asthma.

*Diagnosis:* asthma, pulmonary barotrauma, CAGE.

Courtesy of Royal Australian Navy School of Underwater Medicine

---

It would not usually be feasible to apply such restrictions to professional divers.

The full plate posteroanterior **chest X-ray** may be taken in inspiration and expiration, in an attempt to demonstrate air trapping. Combined with a lateral view, the yield may be increased but it certainly does not exclude significant degrees of air trapping. As for other aspects of the respiratory assessment, the X-ray must be considered in conjunction with the history, the clinical signs and respiratory function tests. Tomograms may be required to clarify doubtful radiological lesions.

The actual benefit of a chest X-ray is debatable. If there is no history of respiratory disorders, with a normal physical examination and acceptable lung function tests, the return from radiography is low. More conservative physicians would still require an X-ray to exclude cysts, bullae, fibrotic lesions and other abnormalities.

There is no need for routine follow-up annual chest X-rays unless there is a clinical indication.

In cases where the clinical history is equivocal or spirometry yields unexpected or borderline results, further sophisticated **pulmonary function testing** may be valuable, such as saline and histamine bronchial provocation testing, chest CT scanning, static lung volumes, compliance testing, CO diffusion coefficient determination and $CO_2$ tolerance. These tests may also be of value in further assessing the veteran diver (e.g. after obviously provoked pulmonary barotrauma).

The most common dilemma is to establish whether **bronchial hyperreactivity** is present in the diving candidate. We have found pulmonary function testing before and after both histamine and ultrasonically nebulized hypertonic saline inhalation very useful (as well as being a dramatic demonstration to the previously doubting candidate). Others have used distilled water, methacholine, hypercapnic hyperventilation and exercise provocation.

A 20% reduction in peak expiratory flow rate or forced expiratory volume after 15 ml 4.5% saline or after 4.0 mg/ml histamine, would verify clinically significant asthma, and a reduction of 10% would be considered sufficient to advise against scuba diving. Neither would indicate that treatment is required. Auscultation

## CASE REPORT 35.2

WD, aged 33, was a qualified diver for 4 years, despite being a known, but very mild, asthmatic. He was classified as fit by a doctor who alleged experience in diving medicine. The doctor also gave a prescription for salbutamol, and advised him to take it prior to diving. He followed this advice. He even had a pocket included in his wet suit to hold the inhaler.

He descended to 9 metres for 20 minutes, prior to an ascent to get his bearings. On returning to his companion, he appeared distressed and then did a further rapid ascent to the surface. There he appeared to be confused and removed the regulator from his mouth. He inhaled some sea water and then lost consciousness and had an epileptic convulsion.

He was rescued by his companion, and within 30 minutes reached the navy RCC by helicopter. He was comatose with brain-stem spasms and with a very inadequate air entry bilaterally. He was compressed to 18 metres on oxygen. Despite endotracheal intubation and 100% oxygen at 18 metres, with positive pressure respiration, the $Pa_{O_2}$ level remained at 50–70 mmHg. The $Pa_{CO_2}$ levels were usually above 100 mmHg and the pH remained below 7.0.

Mainly because of the death of an almost identical asthmatic diver, just previously, after a descent to a much greater depth, it was decided to surface this patient over a period of approximately 5 hours, while attempting to maintain as high an oxygen pressure as possible. The problem was in the combination of diagnoses, including cerebral gas embolism (the initial incident), asthma (as detected by the significant bronchospasm) and drowning (caused during the surface difficulties and rescue of the patient).

A decision to go deeper, to overcome the effects of the air embolism, would be complicated by prejudicing the $Pa_{O_2}$ level. The greater depth and increased density of the gases would probably interfere with adequate ventilation, $CO_2$ exchange and acidosis. Aminophylline could cause arterialization of pulmonary emboli. The coincidental hypothermia (33–35°C) was not considered a definite problem, and could even be advantageous – if it was not for the effect that sympathomimetics, required for asthma, could have on cardiac arrhythmias. Steroids were given for rather indefinite but multiple reasons, as given above (asthma, cerebral damage, drowning etc.).

Initially the chest X-rays verified gross pulmonary oedema, consistent with the combined effects of asthma and drowning. Subsequent chest X-rays revealed a persistent right lower lobe opacity, clearing up over the next month.

With attention to the respiratory status, the brain damage, fluid and electrolyte status, the patient gradually improved over the next few weeks and regained consciousness. The result was a severely brain-damaged young man, continually incapacitated by myoclonic spasms, almost certainly post-hypoxic but possibly contributed to by CAGE. There was a residual dysarthria, a left hemiparaesthesia, an ataxic gait and myoclonic jerks. The EEG was consistent with hypoxia and the CT scan was normal.

*Diagnosis:* asthma, CAGE, near drowning

## CASE REPORT 35.3

AB, aged 43, was a very experienced diver who previously had had asthma as a child, and who still had high pitched rhonchi on auscultation during hyperventilation.

A professor of respiratory physiology informed him that his lungs had quite adequate function for scuba diving. This advice was refuted by members of the Diving Medical Centre but academic brilliance won out.

At a depth of 27–18 metres while exploring a wreck, he suddenly became aware, as he floated up over the deck, of a pain in the left side of his chest. He then attempted to ascend, but took over half an hour to reach the surface. During this time there was a continual pain in the chest, aggravated if he tried to ascend rapidly. With extreme courage, and commendable control over his breathing gas consumption, despite the terrifying circumstances, he did reach the surface – although in great discomfort. He was then given oxygen and transferred to hospital.

The clinical and X-ray evidence verified the presumptive diagnosis of left pneumothorax, and a thoracocentesis was performed. He returned to the professor of respiratory physiology, to be reassured that it was unlikely to happen again. The Diving Medical Centre physicians assured him that not only would it happen again but that, with the lung damage and the treatment received, it was more likely to happen again and that it should not have been allowed to happen in the first place. He decided, this time, to take our advice.

*Diagnosis:* pneumothorax with minimal provocation, asthma.

## CASE REPORT 35.4

NZ, aged 20, had been certified fit to dive despite an asthma history. Prior to the dive there were no symptoms, but he still took a salbutamol inhalation.

In his first deep water dive, after 8 minutes at 30 metres, he took 23 minutes to reach 15 metres. A burning pain in his chest then caused him to make a rapid ascent. He was pulled out semi-conscious and apnoeic. He had four grand mal seizures and was given $O_2$. There were no neurological defects, other than disorientation, on examination. After 6 hours, during which time he had another three seizures, he was recompressed to 18 m on $O_2$ and treated with anticonvulsants. There was no evidence of pneumothorax, and he was eventually treated on an air table at 50 metres, having continued to convulse while on $O_2$ at 18 metres. He survived, but has subsequently stopped scuba diving.

*Diagnosis:* asthma, pulmonary barotrauma, CAGE.

Summarized from *SPUMS Journal*, courtesy of Dr David Clinton-Baker

## CASE REPORT 35.5

DMcM, age 23, was a very fit and courageous athlete, who had mild asthma and was advised against scuba diving. Unfortunately his father, who was a professor of medicine, succumbed to family pressure and wrote a fit-for-diving certificate.

This patient suffered two episodes of a very similar nature. In neither case had he had any evidence of active asthma prior to the dive, and with the second episode he had actually taken a salbutamol spray prior to the dive. They were in similar areas, at depths less than 10 metres. After 20–30 minutes he had developed dyspnoea and attempted to return to shore. On the first occasion, he had informed his buddy that he was returning to shore to take get another salbutamol spray but he appeared to panic and inhaled sea water. He was then rescued in a comatose state and eventually recovered after a week in intensive care.

The second episode was of a very similar nature, except that he did not recover. The autopsy revealed evidence of drowning, with mild asthma.

*Diagnosis:* asthma, panic, near drowning.

## CASE REPORT 35.6

DW, age 20 was a fit young diver who carried out 30 scuba dives to a maximum of 130 feet, without incident, prior to being examined by an experienced diving physician. There was a past history of asthma for which he had used steroid inhalers. On examination there was no evidence of bronchospasm and the $FEV_1/VC$ was 3.9/4.5 without bronchodilators. The chest X-ray was normal. He was advised that he would be medically fit to dive providing he was free of asthma and that he had taken an inhalation of Berotec prior to each dive.

While undertaking in-water rescue and resuscitation exercises, to a maximum of 15 feet, he developed dyspnoea on the surface. He informed the instructor that he was suffering from asthma and was towed 30 metres back to shore. By then he was cyanosed with wheezing on inspiration and expiration. He then lost consciousness and required expired air resuscitation (by two novice divers but experienced internists). He suffered a grand mal seizure and then gradually improved following oxygen inhalation. He responded to treatment of his asthma, over the next few days, with aminophylline.

There was no evidence of CAGE, and the seizure was considered to be due to cerebral hypoxia. In retrospect, a history of an asthmatic episode 4 days previously was elicited. It was presumed that the asthma, which developed on the surface, was triggered by the aspiration of sea water, exertion or cold exposure.

*Diagnosis:* asthma, near drowning.

---

**CASE REPORT 35.7**

JJM, age unknown. This reply, from a physician, was published in the *British Medical Journal* in response to a dubious suggestion that asthmatics could be allowed to scuba dive.

'I have extremely mild asthma, which manifests perhaps once every three years for a brief time during a respiratory tract infection. As I did not encounter any asthmatic symptoms during strenuous high altitude mountaineering I thought it would be reasonable to try scuba diving. I learnt to dive in a warm shallow swimming pool and experienced no difficulties during this or my first sea dive. During my first deep sea dive, however, I had an extremely severe and sudden attack of bronchospasm at a depth of 30 metres. I barely made it to the surface, where my obvious distress and lack of speech caused my partner to inflate my life jacket, thus compromising my respiration further. It was a frightening experience and I have not dived since.'

J.J. Martindale

---

tion with hyperventilation often demonstrates the expiratory restriction more than spirometry – especially if it is in a localized area. Sometimes the positive response to inhaled salbutamol is used to support the asthma diagnosis.

### Upper respiratory tract

Disorders of this system comprise the largest cause of occupational morbidity in divers. A history or physical signs of chronic or recurrent pharyngitis, tonsillitis or sinusitis may lead to problems with diving. Allergic rhinitis may affect sinus aeration or eustachian tube function as well as arousing the suspicion of bronchial hyperreactivity. Acute disorders of the ears, nose or throat may temporarily disqualify the diving candidate.

Sinus and nasal polyps may produce obstructions during ascent or descent, resulting in barotrauma. A deviated nasal septum may also result in abnormal air flow and nasal mucosa, influencing patency of sinus ostia and the eustachian tube. Whenever obstruction or restriction of the upper respiratory airways occurs, barotrauma is likely. If infection is present, it may be aggravated and spread by diving. Hyperbaria is thought to accentuate viral infections.

A break in the skin or mucosal lining of gas-filled spaces is a danger in diving, allowing access of gas into the deeper body tissues, resulting in barotrauma or surgical emphy-sema. This break is commonly produced by trauma (nasal injuries, dental extractions etc.).

The larynx is vital in protecting the airways and any significant pathology in this region precludes diving.

## Ear

### External ear

It is commonly stated that the external ear should be free of **cerumen**. The basis for this statement is that, if cerumen does block the external ear, then it may lead to either external-ear barotrauma or caloric-induced vertigo. Unfortunately, this attitude has led to many divers having the cerumen syringed from the external ear, and a consequent predisposition to otitis externa. The cerumen is of considerable value in preventing external-ear infections and, unless it is completely occluding the canal, should be left alone. Subjects who spend a considerable period of time in and under the water (without the use of hoods) have very little cerumen, and this is one way to refute fanciful reports of frequent and recent underwater activity.

Inspection should be made for the presence of **exostoses**, and these should not be of such a size as to block the external auditory canal, or lead to occlusion by superimposed cerumen or infection. Exostoses are particularly common in subjects who spend time in colder sea water.

A diver is rendered temporarily unfit by the presence of **acute** or **chronic otitis externa**. These disorders are discussed in Chapters 23 and 27.

## Middle ear

A healthy **tympanic membrane**, intact and mobile, is a prerequisite for diving. Current evidence of otitis media, however mild, should preclude diving until fully recovered. Chronic otitis media or cholesteatoma should be cured before diving. Candidates with a tympanic membrane **perforation** or ventilation tubes should not dive. Obviously it would be unwise to submit a tympanic membrane, which has been weakened by a thin atrophic scar, to pressure changes involved in diving. However, a healed perforation which left the tympanic membrane normal in strength and mobility would be quite acceptable. A tympanoplasty is not necessarily a contraindication to diving, if healing has been completed. A retracted and immobile tympanic membrane is unacceptable.

The middle-ear car cavity should be free of fluid and normally aerated. This is demonstrated during otoscopy by the appearance of the tympanic membrane and its mobility on autoinflation.

Otosclerosis **surgery**, with the use of an ossicle prosthesis, or stapedectomy, predisposes to spontaneous or provoked oval window rupture and therefore precludes diving. Patients who have undergone extensive mastoid surgery may experience a strong caloric response and severe vertigo.

> *Observation of tympanic membrane movement is an essential part of the medical examination.*

The eustachian tube must function normally, i.e. autoinflation must be accomplished voluntarily and without excessive force. The tympanic membrane is observed through the otoscope to move outward as the subject performs the **Valsalva manoeuvre**. It should be noted that the ability to autoinflate at any one point in time does not preclude the possibility of intermittent eustachian tube obstruction at another time. The function of the eustachian tube is dependent upon normal nasal function, and this requires careful assessment, especially in candidates with such conditions as allergic or vasomotor rhinitis, cleft palate or bifid uvula (see Chapter 27).

## Inner ear

### Cochlear function

Ideally, divers should have normal cochlear and vestibular function, but moderate changes in auditory acuity may be acceptable.

Loss of cochlear function may be associated with loss of vestibular function. If the vestibular portions of the inner ear respond to stimuli unequally, then vertigo might result, especially when visual fixation is poor, as frequently occurs in diving (see Chapter 27).

Threshold **hearing** for divers should ideally be 20 decibels at the frequencies between 500 and 4000 Hz using audiometers calibrated to ISO standard. This is the level classified as 'Standard 1' in most armed forces and it would seem to be appropriate to expect this standard to be reached by individuals who wish to participate in professional diving. Frequencies should extend to 6000 and 8000 cycles/s, in both initial baseline and annual examinations, even though these may be affected by noise damage. They are also the frequencies most commonly affected by diving.

This may be thought to be too harsh a standard, but it must be pointed out that it is a 'safe' level. Some individuals may have 'normal' ears which do not withstand stresses as well as others. A previously damaged inner ear is more susceptible to further damage.

Bone conduction is usually only tested if air condition is abnormal.

> *Audiometry is part of the routine diving medical examination.*

All divers should have an annual audiogram as part of a hearing conservation programme. The permissible duration of exposure to loud noise of different intensities is well documented and should be adhered to when exposing divers to such noise in helmets, compression chambers or near compressors.

## Vestibular function

It has been shown that vertigo can be induced by cold water entering one ear but not the other ear, owing to one external auditory meatus being occluded by cerumen. Similarly, vertigo can be expected to occur when diving, if one labyrinth is not functioning and the other normal ear is stimulated by the caloric effect of cold water.

The significance or importance of less-marked changes in vestibular function is not fully understood, but there is ample evidence to suggest that abnormal vestibular function may play a part in disorientation. It is wise to exclude from diving those individuals whose vestibular function is not normal and equal on each side. Divers who have inner-ear damage from decompression sickness or barotrauma fall into this category.

The sharpened Romberg test may detect vestibular abnormality, as may the use of Frenzel glasses and electronystagmography if indicated (see Chapter 27).

A history of Menière's disease or other chronic vestibular disorders should bar diving.

## Eye

Good **vision** is needed both under water to avoid dangerous situations and, after surfacing, when the diver may have to identify landmarks, floats, boats etc. Distant vision should not be less than 6/18 for both eyes, or 6/24 for the worse eye (corrected or uncorrected).

Presbyopia may lead to problems reading gauges and watches. Myopia is the most common deficiency requiring correction. The use of a corrected lens in the face mask is of value in reducing the danger of reduced visual acuity, but the technique of buddy diving (diving while attached by a line to a visually fit diver) is also important. Hypermetropia should be corrected by a convex lens added to the face mask.

Colour vision may be important in ship watch-keeping duties, colour coding of gases and explosives. It is not a requirement for diving.

During the physical examination, the visual fields and pupillary reactions should be tested, the retina examined fundoscopically and any abnormalities investigated.

In **ocular surgery**, the cornea is slow to heal. In radical keratotomy, it is thought that the cornea never attains full strength if the operation is successful. Mask squeeze or blunt trauma may lead to corneal rupture, usually along the surgical incisions. Patients who have undergone radial keratotomy are usually advised to avoid contact sports thereafter. Ophthalmic surgeons may be unaware of the pressure imbalance that develops between the mask and the eye surface, especially in novice divers. Experienced divers might be permitted to continue diving with special precautions to avoid pressure imbalance in the face mask.

Similar considerations apply to the person who has undergone corneal grafting. In addition, the risk of corneal abrasive trauma must be considered because the cornea has no sensory nerve supply for at least 3 months postoperatively and then only partially recovers.

Hyperbaric exposure has been said to cause deterioration of myopia and optic neuritis. Retinal artery spasm has been reported breathing hyperbaric oxygen. Retinal lesions (microaneurysm, pigmentary changes) have also been recorded in divers.

Hard corneal lenses, unless fenestrated, should not be worn when diving.

Ocular problems are discussed further in Chapter 30.

## Nervous system

Many neurological abnormalities will add danger to the diver, as well as complicating the management of neurological disorders due to diving, such as cerebral or spinal decompression sickness, air embolus from pulmonary barotrauma, oxygen toxicity etc.

**Cerebrovascular disease**, such as intracranial aneurysm and arteriovenous malformation, carry the risk of sudden death or coma. Subjects with a history of any form of intracranial haemorrhage should be discouraged from diving even if there are no apparent sequelae. Patients who have undergone craniotomy are at an increased risk of epilepsy (see below).

**Migraine** occurs commonly in the general population. Few see a doctor and even fewer are disabled, although may take drugs which may be relevant. In diving, migraine may be precipitated by: elevated arterial carbon dioxide tension (see Chapter 19); cold water exposure; psychological stress of diving; glare; intra-arterial bubbles (decompression sickness, cerebral arterial gas embolism); and possibly increased oxygen pressure (hyperbaric oxygen therapy).

Those with a history of migraine should either be advised against diving or advised of depth/duration limits so as to reduce the diagnostic dilemma of possible cerebral arterial gas embolus or neurological decompression sickness. Such advice might be a maximum depth of 18 metres, duration well within 'no decompression' limits, a slow ascent rate and avoidance of cold exposure to the head. Migraine sufferers with neurological features should not dive at all, and those with a history of associated vomiting are also at greater risk.

**Epilepsy** is an absolute contraindication to diving. Apart from the risk of drowning there is also the risk of pulmonary barotrauma if the diver is returned to the surface during the tonic–clonic phase. A diver's safety may be impaired under water by the sudden development of sensory disturbance, nausea, vertigo or severe headache. Vomiting under water can be disastrous.

Epilepsy, which may be defined as two or more definite seizures, occurs in 0.5% of the population. Salient points in history include the facts that: 34% of childhood epileptics recur after withdrawal of medication; 50% of people who have had one seizure will have another; 'controlled' epileptics are 2.5 times more likely to be involved in motor vehicle accidents.

In the diving environment, glare, sensory deprivation, narcosis, stress and hyperventilation may be possible 'triggering' factors. Some divers will have their first epileptic attack under water.

A history of **head injury** may be important because of both the risk of seizure and the effect on cognitive functioning. In assuming the severity of such an injury, the following points indicate a high risk of post-traumatic epilepsy within 6 months:

1. Duration of loss of consciousness greater than 10 minutes.
2. Seizure in the immediate post-trauma period.

3. Neurological deficit (e.g. post-traumatic amnesia for 24 hours, transient hemiparesis).
4. Disruption of cortex (depressed skull fracture, intracranial haematoma).

Where there is no loss of consciousness (i.e. subconcussive), there are generally no sequelae, but post-traumatic amnesia indicates a concussive injury which should be carefully assessed. A normal electroencephalogram in the immediate post-trauma period does not preclude the later development of post-traumatic epilepsy. Candidates with any of the above features should be free of seizures, should not require drug therapy and should be functioning normally in their daily lives. Those with a history of penetrating head injury (e.g. missile), post-traumatic amnesia greater than 24 hours, depressed skull fracture or acute haematoma should not dive for at least 5 years because of the risk of later post-traumatic epilepsy.

**Spinal cord injury or disease** is important because, in addition to the limitation exposed by the primary neurological deficit, there may also be an increased vulnerability to spinal decompression sickness and/or further injury. The vulnerability may be due to the exhaustion of spinal cord redundancy, e.g. in myelopathies due to decompression sickness or poliomyelitis. Candidates with trauma or disease of the cord should not take up diving even if there is no clinically detectable residual deficit.

Certain spinal cord neurological handicaps (such as traumatic paraplegia, muscular dystrophy, multiple sclerosis) may be 'accepted' only for special diving circumstances, such as the specialized 'handicapped diver programme'. As well as the obvious limitations, the candidates may also exhibit poor heat and cold tolerance.

A more common problem is the candidate with a history of **herniated intervertebral disc**. If asymptomatic and with no neurological signs, restricted diving may be permitted. Diving may also be considered reasonable 4–6 months after successful, uncomplicated surgery, provided there is no residual deficit.

**Spinal stenosis** due to degenerative joint disease renders the cord more vulnerable to damage from any cause.

**Peripheral neuropathy** may cause diagnostic confusion in assessing possible DCS and sensory loss may lead to trauma and delayed

**Table 35.1 Some important medical contraindications to diving***

Risk of sudden death
  Asthma (CAGE)
  Coronary artery disease
  Intracranial aneurysm or AV malformation
  Other cerebrovascular disease
  Cardiac arrhythmia ± drugs
  Severe hypertension
  Congestive heart failure
  Causes of vomiting

Impaired consciousness
  Drugs
  Epilepsy
  Diabetes
  Cardiac arrhythmia
  Transient ischaemic attacks
  Unexplained syncope

Impaired judgement
  Drugs
  Psychosis
  Severe anxiety
  Severe depression
  Claustrophobia

Risk of disorientation
  Tympanic membrane perforation
  Inner-ear disease or surgery
  Uncorrected poor visual acuity

Impaired mobility
  Spinal column/cord disease or injury
  Neuromuscular disease (neuropathy, myopathy)
  Obesity
  Poor physical fitness
  Pregnancy

Risk of barotrauma
  Asthma
  Spontaneous pneumothorax
  Pulmonary cysts, fibrosis, scars, bronchitis, chronic airway disease etc.
  Blocked eustachian tubes or sinus ostia
  Acute or chronic respiratory infections
  Radial keratotomy

Risk of decompression sickness
  Obesity
  Acute physical injury
  Spinal cord disease or injury
  Intracardiac shunts (ASD, VSD, foramen ovale)
  Extremes of age
  Pregnancy

* This list includes some common absolute and relative contraindications. It is in no way complete nor does the order signify importance.

wound healing. The underlying cause, however, usually precludes diving.

## Endocrine system

**Diabetes mellitus** should be regarded as a disqualifying condition for a number of reasons. The most obvious is the risk of hypoglycaemic coma in an insulin-dependent diabetic or even in those taking oral hypoglycaemia drugs. The early warning signs of such a reaction may be masked by the underwater environment which itself interferes with taking remedial action. Insulin reactions are the rule rather than the exception where there are variable exercise loads, and severe reactions are quite common in insulin-treated diabetics. The unpredictable nature of diving with the possibility of sudden high metabolic demands adds to the likelihood.

The second cause for concern is the association with vascular disease and end-organ damage in relatively young people despite conscientious control of glucose levels. Vascular disease may increase susceptibility to decompression sickness. Associated peripheral neuropathy may add to difficulties with differential diagnosis of neurological diving disorders.

Other considerations include hyperventilation and panic reactions associated with both hypoglycaemia and ketoacidosis.

Left ventricular function in young asymptomatic diabetics is reported to be reduced after strenuous exercise. This may be relevant in sudden cardiac death (see Chapter 26).

Diabetics are at an increased risk of developing infections from the marine environment (see Chapter 23).

Well-intentioned endocrine physicians without diving experience may not be fully aware of some of these potential problems.

Despite the foregoing, there are grounds for allowing a diet-controlled diabetic without complications to dive after an exploration of risk factors and limitations to avoid the above potential problems.

**Thyroid disorders** may be missed clinically but are important because of the profound effects they may have on cardiac and neurological function, if untreated. With good control of hyper- or hypothyroidism, verified by thyroid function tests, recreational diving may be undertaken. Significant goitre would preclude diving until corrected because of possible airway compression.

Other severe endocrine disorders, such as Addison's disease, Cushing's syndrome, hyperparathyroidism etc., are also unacceptable in the diving environment.

## Gastrointestinal tract

The mouth should be inspected for signs of dental **caries** and **periodontal disease** severe enough to produce fragile or loose teeth which could be inhaled or cause difficulty retaining the scuba mouthpiece. Full or partial **dentures** should be assessed for stability in maintaining the mouthpiece. Some authorities believe that dentures should always be removed before diving.

Abdominal wall **herniae** (inguinal, femoral, umbilical, incisional) which potentially contain bowel may cause problems with the variation in gas volumes during changes of depth. As well as restricting the diver's physical capabilities, there is the potential for incarceration incurred by lifting heavy scuba equipment. Candidates may be passed fit after successful surgical repair.

The presence of a **hiatus hernia** may lead to underwater reflux or regurgitation, especially with the head-down position of descent. During ascent, reflux is also possible as is gastrointestinal barotrauma due to expansion of gas in the stomach (see page 134). This is especially so with the para-oesophageal hernia.

After surgical repair of hiatus hernia, the candidate should be able to eructate, indicating the ability of gastric gas to escape during ascent. Otherwise, gastric rupture is possible.

A history of **peptic ulcer** may be important because of the potential risk of perforation or bleeding. A past history of gastric surgery may have led to a 'dumping syndrome' with the risk of hypoglycaemia. Pyloric obstruction may also cause stomach over-expansion during ascent. **Inflammatory bowel diseases**, such as Crohn's disease or ulcerative colitis, are not necessarily a bar to recreational diving during periods when the condition is in remission, and drug therapy is not required. The possibility of flare-up at a remote diving location should be borne in mind. Ileostomy or colostomy (except the 'continent' ileostomy type) should present no great problem with diving.

## Miscellaneous considerations

Space prevents discussion of all possible disorders that diving candidates may present to the examining physician. An experience of diving and a sound knowledge of diving medicine are vital in arriving at a sensible assessment of fitness to dive.

The presence of severe **systemic disease** has the same harmful sequelae as neurological disorders – making the diver a potential invalid in an environment that does not lend itself to first aid or medical support. It also increases the risk of misdiagnosing diving accidents.

A **haematological** assessment (haematocrit, red cell studies, full blood count, film examination) is often required for professional divers. Haemoglobin should be above 12 g/dl. If anaemia is detected, the underlying problem must be ascertained.

**Bleeding disorders**, such as haemophilia and von Willebrand's disease. are grounds to reject both the professional diver and the recreational diver, because of the risk of trauma and the unknown effect of expanding intravascular or tissue bubbles. Dysbaric pathology, especially in the brain, spinal cord or inner ear, may be extended by haemorrhage.

A **sickle-cell** assessment may be needed because of the exposure to potentially hypoxic conditions. A sickle-cell crisis may be catastrophic in remote localities, or under hyperbaric conditions. It will also complicate the management of serious decompression sickness cases, and is another cause of aseptic necrosis of bone (see Chapter 14). The candidate with sickle-cell disease should be advised not to dive. Those with asymptomatic sickle-cell trait may also be at risk with severe hypoxia or with local tissue hypoxia secondary to decompression sickness. If diving is undertaken, the diver should be advised to keep shallow (18 metres maximum) and well within decompression limits.

**Polycythaemia**, which causes a cellular circulatory overload, may lead to occlusive vascular phenomena and is thus disqualifying. Haemochromatosis is associated with an increased risk of marine *Vibrio vulnificus* infection. Candidates with leukaemia in remission would require careful assessment.

**Contagious skin diseases**, such as scabies, impetigo, plantar warts etc., cause problems in habitats, and with diving teams, and if using communal gear.

The professional diver should not be suffering from any **communicable diseases**. Individual decisions may be required in recreational divers. Syphilis may involve the cardiovascular or central nervous systems.

Acquired immune deficiency syndrome (**AIDS**) should disqualify candidates because of risk both to the individual and to potential rescuers. Some professional divers have indicated that they would be unwilling to dive with HIV-positive colleagues. Problems with sharing of equipment, such as demand valves, and reluctance to undertake cardiopulmonary resuscitation were cited.

The AIDS sufferer has a greatly increased risk of infection, particularly of the lung and brain. Recent reports describe cerebral dysfunction (cognitive deficits) and other neurological disturbances (ataxia, confusion, aseptic meningitis, hemiplegia) in otherwise previously asymptomatic HIV seropositive patients. On this basis, asymptomatic subjects (even with normal immune function) should be regarded as unfit for diving.

Other reports have suggested that the passage of the AIDS virus into the brain may be aggravated by the disruption to the blood–brain barrier which may occur with decompression.

The possibility that hyperbaric exposure might depress the immune system and activate the disease in an asymptomatic person is uncertain.

A **musculoskeletal** problem of any severity will limit the diver's physical capabilities, and complicate decompression sickness assessment. A history of back injury or recurrent back pain is a strong contraindication to professional diving, although the recreational diver may be considered after appropriate advice, provided that there is no neurological deficit.

For divers who are employed professionally, who undergo many decompressions or recompression treatments, or who are exposed to experimental diving, periodic technetium bone scans or long bone X-rays for **dysbaric osteonecrosis** are indicated (see Chapter 14).

**Minor illnesses** may be of specific relevance to the professional diver assessment, where general medical facilities and services in remote areas may not match the standard of those available to the urban recreational diver. Oil rigs are not as well equipped as the local pharmacy or hospital casualty. A thrombosed haemorrhoid will not receive the same sympathetic attention, while on a clandestine naval operation, that it would receive under domestic conditions.

Thus minor injuries and ailments may assume considerable importance, both to the patient and to the diving operation as a whole, either because of the remoteness of the operation or because of financial and strategic implications. Minor infectious diseases may become a major problem in the enclosed, cramped environment of an oil rig. Most skin disorders will be aggravated by the conditions present during saturation diving. Otitis externa is also extremely common under those conditions. Treatment of these conditions, or temporary exclusion of professional diving candidates because of them, may be appropriate.

**Pregnancy** is a contraindication to diving and is discussed further in Chapter 6.

**Cold urticaria** precludes diving in susceptible individuals (see Chapter 30).

**Speech** disorders are unacceptable in many professional divers, as it may further impede communication at depth and with helium.

**Motion sickness** is a dangerous disorder to have while diving from boats or in rough water. Vomiting under water is a problem especially if the diver vomits into his regulator. The psychological manifestations of motion sickness may also result in injudicious decisions, e.g. to return without completing adequate decompression stops (see Chapter 30).

**Smoking** is detrimental, because of its specific effect on upper and lower respiratory function increasing the chance of ear, sinus and pulmonary barotrauma. There is also an increased risk of coronary artery and peripheral vascular disease. Other recreational or social drugs also need to be assessed (see Chapter 31).

drugs also need to be assessed (see Chapter 31).

> *Any acute illness is usually a temporary bar to diving.*

## Diving history

A knowledge of previous hypobaric, hyperbaric and aquatic accidents may be invaluable in assessing the likelihood of potential future problems. Specifically, a history of barotrauma, decompression sickness, dysbaric osteonecrosis, nitrogen narcosis, gas toxicities, unconsciousness or near drowning should be sought.

Divers who have suffered minor (type 1) **decompression sickness** (DCS) should undergo thorough follow-up (see Chapter 13) and, in any case, should not dive for at least 4 weeks following the episode. If there are no sequelae, diving may be recommended but a more conservative diving profile is recommended.

Neurological sequelae after DCS are not uncommon and infer a subsequent predisposition to more accidents of a similar nature. Divers with any persisting neurological deficit after DCS should certainly never dive again. Some would argue that divers who had DCS with any neurological feature, no matter how rapidly and completely resolved, should be advised against further diving.

Divers who have had **pulmonary barotrauma** are usually regarded as permanently unfit for further diving (see Chapter 9).

## Results of medical examination

Of over 5000 prospective recreational divers examined at the Sydney and Brisbane Diving Medical Centres, approximately 10% are advised not to dive, and a further 10% are given specific restrictions to their diving.

In a survey of 473 sport divers, it was found that 33.3% were classified as medically unfit (temporarily or permanently) on the first examination, by rigid professional diving standards. This fell to 20.1% after subsequent treatment and examinations. The failure rate increased with age, and reached 45.5% over the age of 35 years.

A recent survey of prospective divers from many countries visiting the Great Barrier Reef found the most common reason for failure was asthma, followed by ear, nose and throat disorders. Some of the latter group passed subsequent examination. This was a young group, with an average age of 25 years, and the permanent failure rate was 5.7%.

The principles of **diver selection**, i.e. choosing the more successful divers once they comply with the medical standards, are discussed in Chapter 5.

## Recommended reading and references

AS 2299 (1990). *Underwater Air Breathing.* Australian Standards Association, North Sydney.

BREW, B.J. et al. (1989). The neurological features of early and "latent" human immunodeficiency virus infection. *Australia and New Zealand Journal of Medicine* **19**, 700–705.

DAVIS, J.C. (Ed.) (1986). *Medical Examination of Sports Scuba Divers.* San Antonio, Texas: Medical Seminars Inc.

FIELD, M., KUNZE, H., TATE, J. and FRAZER, I.H. (1989). Cerebral dysfunction with evidence of cerebral HIV infection amongst asymptomatic HIV seropositive subjects. *Australia and New Zealand Journal of Medicine* **19**, 694–698.

HICKEY, D.D. (1984). Outline of medical standards for divers. *Undersea Biomedical Research* **11**, 407–432.

LINAWEAVER, P.G. and BIERSNER, R.J. (1984). Physical and psychological examination for diving. In: *The Physician's Guide to Diving Medicine*, edited by C.W. Shilling, C.B. Carlston and R.A. Mathias. New York: Plenum Press.

MOON, R.E., CAMPORESI, E.M. and KISSLO, J.A. (1989). Patent foramen ovale and decompression in divers. *The Lancet* **i**, 513–514.

MAI (1987). *The Medical Examination of Divers.* Information and Advice from the (UK) Health and Safety Executive's Medical Division (Revised).

PARKER, J. (1990). Review of 1000 sports diving medicals. *SPUMS Journal* **20**(2), 84–86.

SCHIAVON, R.M., OSTI, A., SCHIRALDI, C. and RUSCA, F. (1987). Bronchial provocation in finer selection of sports scuba divers. *Ninth International Symposium on Underwater and Hyperbaric Physiology.* Undersea and Hyperbaric Medical Society.

THOMAS, R.L. and LOWRY, C.J. (1974). Medical examinations for sports divers: A review of 478 candidates. *Twentieth World Congress in Sports Medicine*, Melbourne.

# 36

# Deep and saturation diving*

---

HISTORY
  Problems
  Solutions

PROCEDURES
  Environmental control
  Special medical requirements
  The compression phase

Problems at maximum depth
Problems during decompression

RESCUE
  Rescue of divers trapped in a bell
  Evacuation of divers from a deck
  decompression chamber
  Treatment of ill and injured saturation
  divers

RECOMMENDED READING

---

## History

There has been a continuing effort to dive to greater depths (see Chapter 1). Early in the nineteenth century the depth was limited by the capacity of the air pumps. After technological improvements, the depth was limited by decompression sickness. Another problem was that the limited air supply caused carbon dioxide accumulation in the helmet of the standard diver.

When decompression tables were introduced and compressors improved, human beings could reach depths of about 70 metres before being seriously affected by nitrogen narcosis, and therefore not capable of useful work.

### Problems

The introduction of helium as a diluting gas allowed the depth limit to be extended and in 1937 an American diver reached 128 metres (420 feet). Dives to these depths required a long decompression even for a short time at the working depths.

For example, a 70-metre air dive would require 100–150 minutes of decompression for a bottom time of 30 minutes. For the same bottom time at 100 metres, while breathing a mixture of 16% oxygen in helium, nearly 3 hours of decompression are required (about 100 minutes of this is spent breathing oxygen, with a risk of oxygen toxicity). Both these dives

* The knowledge and experience required to conduct a saturation dive is beyond the scope of this text. This chapter is intended to give the reader enough background to comprehend the problems. It may give the medical specialist, who is called in to advise on the treatment of a saturation diver, a better understanding of the environment.

would involve a significant risk of decompression sickness. Difficulties relating to the physical properties of helium and other breathing gases are referred to in Chapters 12 and 16.

Deep diving is associated with a more rapid consumption of the gas supply, increased respiratory resistance, thermal difficulties, voice distortion, sensory deprivation, inadequate information about decompression schedules and equipment problems. Other difficulties include a much greater risk of dysbaric osteonecrosis, inner-ear disorders and a greater than usual danger from coincidental medical disorders.

### Solutions

Three ways have been developed to cope with this problem of excessive decompression times. One is to avoid the excess pressure by operating from a submersible vehicle, or a pressure-resistant suit, at atmospheric pressure.

Hannes Keller demonstrated that decompression times could be reduced by **changing gas mixtures** in order to capitalize on maximum gas tension gradients. In 1962 his experiments culminated in a dive to 305 metres for 5 minutes' bottom time. The divers still required 270 minutes of decompression. Keller's companion died and this approach did not become popular because of the risk of severe decompression sickness.

The decompression requirements can be reduced by allowing the diver to stay at depth until his task is finished, and then decompress him slowly in a chamber. Thus, only one decompression is required. This is called **saturation diving** and the first demonstration is attributed to Dr George Bond of the US Navy. He explored a suggestion first made by Behnke in 1942, as a method of increasing the duration of exposure in caisson workers. Although these men were instrumental in applying the concept of saturation diving, they were predated by Dr Cunningham (Kansas City, USA in 1927) who used air under pressure for several days, followed by a slow decompression, as a form of hyperbaric therapy.

The main value of saturation diving is that a diver needs the same decompression time for a dive lasting one day or one month. Once the body has equilibrated with the gases in the environment at any pressure, it will not take up any more gas.

Bond tested this concept with animals and then with men in compression chambers. In 1964 he lead a group of four men in a cylindrical underwater house for 9 days at a depth of nearly 60 metres (*Sea Lab I*). Other early dives based on underwater houses, or habitats, were conducted by Link and Cousteau.

Instead of permanent underwater habitats, saturation dives can be achieved by the use of transportable chambers. The first commercial work in saturation dive was conducted by Westinghouse Inc. The men lived in a pressurized chamber on the surface and were lowered to work in a capsule called a **submersible decompression chamber** (SDC). This allowed their transfer in the chamber to the working depth without any alteration in pressure. In 1965 this procedure was used for a series of dives to repair a dam in the USA. Four men at a time were pressurized; they performed 800 hours of work in 12 weeks. With surface diving, the same men could have performed only about 160 hours of work in the same period.

The main need for saturation diving is in the offshore oil industry which relies on saturation divers to carry out many tasks under water. These include observations, welding joins in pipes, cleaning, anti-fouling and repairing damaged components. Military saturation dives have been conducted for a variety of purposes. Most have been for the recovery of valuable, dangerous or strategic items from the sea bed.

The recovery of the components from crashed aircraft is a common task. Salvage divers and treasure hunters have also used this technique. The recovery of a large amount of gold from the wreck of *HMS Edinburgh* in over 200 metres of water is one example. Oceanographers often find the submersible decompression chambers too expensive and restrictive. They have found fixed **underwater habitats**, with direct access to the surrounding terrain, to be a useful alternative – allowing direct observation and prolonged data collection.

## Procedures

Many skills are needed to conduct a saturation dive. The facilities include a diving tender, compression chambers, large quantities of compressed gas and technical staff. There are also many logistic problems in navigation and seamanship, necessary to support such an operation. The details are beyond the scope of this book.

The first biomedical problem in conducting a saturation dive is the choice and maintenance of a habitable environment for the divers.

## Environmental control

The area occupied by the divers needs to have a controlled atmosphere. The loss of pressure or temperature control can cause the death of divers. The environmental maintenance systems need to be reliable and to be supplemented by alternative systems. Power failure must be allowed for. Evacuation proceedings to be used if the ship or oil rig has to be abandoned need consideration.

Contamination of the atmosphere also needs to be considered. Gas purity standards are discussed in Chapter 20. Prevention of contamination, with monitoring systems to control oxygen and carbon dioxide levels, are needed. Alternative breathing gases must be supplied direct to the divers, if the chamber atmosphere becomes contaminated. For a deep dive this could involve an enormous reserve of gas.

In large compression complexes it may be possible to transfer the divers to another chamber. Most groups conducting saturation dives have their own specified procedures and prescribed limits for certain contaminants. The limits specified reflect the attitudes of various authorities as well as the operational performance of each diving system. Examples of such recommendations are the following.

## *Oxygen*

Partial pressures of 0.2–0.5 ATA have been used, the most common being about 0.4 ATA. This gives a safety margin between risks of hypoxia and pulmonary oxygen toxicity. Recently, there has been a tendency to increase the oxygen pressure to about 0.5 ATA during decompression. This results in fewer cases of decompression sickness. Because of the fire risk associated with high oxygen concentrations, the chamber oxygen is generally kept below 21%. During the last 14 metres of ascent, the reduction of oxygen pressure may require a slowing of the ascent rate. The alternative is to use periods of breathing high

oxygen mixtures, from a mask with an overboard dump system.

## *Carbon dioxide*

This is kept below a limit of 0.005 ATA, equivalent to 0.5% at 1 ATA. For shorter periods a higher limit, 0.015–0.02 ATA, is tolerable. A high carbon dioxide level will lead to hypercapnoea and a reduced work capacity.

## *Diluting gas*

This may be nitrogen for shallow dives, but for deeper dives helium, hydrogen and nitrogen mixtures with oxygen have been used. Each mixture requires a different decompression schedule. Addition of extra nitrogen to an oxygen/helium mixture is often used to reduce the high-pressure neurological syndrome, but it increases the risks from decompression sickness. If it cannot be avoided, it may be necessary to use a slower decompression than the standard oxygen/helium schedule.

## *Trace contaminants*

Authorities specify arbitrary limits for a variety of possible contaminants. The limits are extrapolations from occupational health advisory groups, adjusted for depth. Because the designated contaminant limits are not comprehensive, medical staff need to consider the toxicology of many preparations they prescribe, or wish to use, at depth. For example, solvents may pose a problem. Mercury thermometers or sphygmomanometers are preferably avoided because of the possible generation of mercury vapour and the possibility of the chamber being condemned due to amalgam formation. Other common sources of toxic products include paints, welding, refrigeration leaks and cooking fumes. Activated carbon or molecular sieve compounds may be needed to control contamination.

## *Temperatures*

The high termal conductivity of helium and hydrogen mixtures requires an increase in the optimal working temperature and narrows the range for thermal comfort. This may increase from about 25°C to 33°C, with greater depths. Deviations from this range can cause hypothermia or hyperthermia and need to be avoided. Hyperthermia may be rapid and not easily detected at an early stage.

### Humidity

Humidity levels need less strict control than the other parameters. When using soda lime to remove carbon dioxide, a relative humidity (r.h.) of over 75% gives better performance. Other absorbents may require different optimal percentages. Higher r.h. also reduces the risk of static sparks, a possible source of ignition in the fire risk zone. The problem with accepting a high r.h. is the increased risk from certain bacterial and fungal infections, which can be a problem in saturation dives – so the range chosen will be a compromise. With water from wet gear and showering, it is often difficult to keep humidity down to the 60–75% r.h. range recommended.

### Fire hazards

If the oxygen pressure is kept at 0.4–0.6 ATA there will be a fire hazard in the chamber at depths shallower than 56 metres. This is called the fire risk zone. To reduce the hazard, precautions are needed to limit the amount of combustible material. At greater depths there will be insufficient oxygen concentrations present to support combustion.

### Special medical requirements

There are two additional problems in selection of saturation divers, as compared to normal divers. Psychological and dermatological problems are common in saturation diving. Not all divers have the stable, phlegmatic personality needed for saturation diving. The chamber operators and other support staff need to be aware of the stress on the divers and make allowances for this.

Infections are also causes for concern. The diver should be free of acne, bacterial and fungal conditions. Any skin infection is likely to be aggravated in the warm, humid, oxygen-rich environment of the saturation complex. The environment is similar to an incubator with the diver as the culture medium.

Aluminium acetate ear drops after each dive and shower, and routinely during the day, are often used to prevent otitis externa. The risk of cross-infection is reduced by having separate containers for each diver, or even for each ear. The risk of skin infection is reduced by daily showers and the use of medicated soap, followed by clean clothing. Preventive measures are also needed to avoid tinea of the feet or groin. Maintaining a high standard of cleanliness in the pressure chambers and of diving gear also helps to prevent serious infection.

### The compression phase

It is common to commence an oxygen/helium saturation dive by compressing the subjects to about 2 ATA on air, allowing the oxygen sensors to be checked following conventional standardization. At that stage the divers and operators can test the system before further compression with helium.

Apart from descent barotrauma, the main physiological problems to be expected during descent are compression arthralgia and the high-pressure neurological syndrome (HPNS). They may be minimized by using an established compression regime and are treated by suspending compression until symptoms abate. The HPNS has been reduced in deep dives by the use of nitrogen and/or hydrogen as part of breathing gas mixture.

Several problems of a mechanical nature can occur during compression. In chambers with poor gas mixing, the lighter diluting gases can float over the heavier nitrogen and oxygen, giving a hypoxic layer and an oxygen-rich layer. Sensors which are influenced by pressure can also give misleading indications of gas concentrations. A rapid compression can cause overheating and hyperthermia.

### Problems at maximum depth

Decompression sickness is usually expected during the decompression phase of a saturation dive. However, changes in the composition of the breathing gases, as well as excursions from the saturation depth, can both cause decompression sickness. A saturation diver can move through a range of depths with little risk of decompression sickness, for example from 100 metres to 129 metres and return. Situations in which a diver breathes one gas while he is surrounded by another can cause isobaric counterdiffusion (see Chapter 11).

The more common problems encountered at depth are related to the diving tasks. These include burns from the hot water used for heating the in-water diver. Hypothermia will occur quickly if the heating fails, either in the water, the bell or the habitat. Breathlessness, associated with exertion, is a common consequence of the density of the breathing gases at depth. Difficulties have been encountered by the attendant bringing an unconscious diver back into the submersible decompression chamber. One method is partially to flood the chamber so that the diver floats up into it. Then the attendant shuts the hatch and blows the water out.

Infections are also more likely with increased time at depth.

## Problems during decompression

Boredom in the divers and chamber operators, with subsequent loss of concentration, may develop during the protracted decompression from a saturation dive. If the decompression schedule used is a proven one, then decompression sickness should be uncommon. When it occurs it will usually be mild and develop close to the surface or after surfacing. If it develops during decompression it should respond to a pressure increase of 30 metres or less, with periods of breathing oxygen-rich mixtures, at an oxygen pressure of 1.5–2.5 ATA. Six periods of 20–30 minutes with 5-minute breaks are commonly used. Decompression can be continued after a 'hold' at the increased pressure, often with a reduced ascent rate. Cases which appear after surfacing are usually treated on a conventional oxygen therapy table.

Uncontrolled and rapid decompression is likely to result in a severe type of decompression sickness, such as when the habitat diver becomes buoyant and ascends to the surface, or when the pressurization within the decompression chamber is reduced too rapidly. Under these conditions the treatment may need to be vigorous, with a rapid return to the previous pressure.

# Rescue

## Rescue of divers trapped in a bell

Disconnection of a diving bell from its surface support can lead to divers being trapped on the sea bed. The other potential problem is a winch failure or fouling of the bell or cable. These incidents are rare and are usually preventable. Rescue procedures should be available. They include both emergency environmental control systems and salvage.

A rebreathing system can protect the diver from carbon dioxide accumulation in the bell. It may also give thermal support by reclaiming the heat in the exhaled gas and from carbon dioxide reacting with its absorbent. The outer surface of the rebreather should be insulated to avoid losing this heat. A supplementary oxygen, mixed gas or air supply may be needed, together with a means of monitoring the gas pressures.

Thermal protection may be active or passive. An active system incorporates a heating unit, usually an electrical or hot water supply from the surface. In deep dives and in cold water, active heating within the bell may be considered, such as from chemical or electrical energy. Both systems have a limited duration. Passive systems are simpler and rely on insulation to protect the diver from excessive heat loss. The general consensus is that a rebreathing system (exothermic) and thermal protective clothing are adequate for most diving situations.

These precautions, to prolong the life of divers trapped in a bell, need to be linked to a rescue procedure. For example, British regulations require each bell to be fitted with an acoustic beacon. This is to help rescuers locate it. Divers from a second bell may free the trapped bell or release its ballast weights. The other possible method is for the divers to transfer to the second bell. Freeing the trapped bell would normally be the preferred option.

## Evacuation of divers from a deck decompression chamber

There are several circumstances that may necessitate the evacuation of divers from a deck decompression chamber. It may be necessary to leave the diving platform because of fire, explosion or collision damage. Other factors may require abandoning the deck chamber. It may be uninhabitable, for example from contamination. Oil field diver operators are often well prepared for these incidents.

**Hyperbaric lifeboats** have been designed to allow divers to escape in a pressurized chamber. This consists of a lifeboat with a chamber in its hull. A connection to the deck chamber allows the divers to transfer under pressure to the lifeboat. The boat would proceed to another chamber where the divers would be transferred to a less restricted facility. The lifeboat itself has all the potential hazards associated with both watercraft and decompression chambers.

## Treatment of ill and injured divers

A saturation diver at depth is one of the most isolated people on earth. For example, it may take several days for a doctor to be transported and pressurized to reach him. An accident or illness may make it desirable to move a diver to a more appropriate facility, while he remains under pressure.

**Hyperbaric rescue chambers** have been developed to allow the evacuation of a sick or injured diver to a chamber connected to hospital facilities. The diver is moved into a portable chamber, called the transfer chamber, and taken by helicopter. After a flight to shore

the procedure is reversed to transfer the diver to a hospital-based chamber. The North Sea field system allows the transfer of a diver at a pressure of up to 23 ATA. This system is complex, takes time to set into operation and is weather dependent.

**Medical care on site** is the common approach to caring for sick or injured divers. To expedite this, several divers in each group need comprehensive paramedic training. The Royal Navy training, for example, includes suturing, catheterization and insertion of intravenous infusions. People with this type of training can then initiate treatment and obey expert advice without delay.

**Use of drugs under pressure** is a field or pharmacology where experience is very limited. Drugs may have different effects under high pressures (see Chapter 31).

## Recommended reading

DAVIS, R.H. (1962). *Deep Diving and Submarine Operations*, 7th edn. Surrey; Siebe Gorman & Company.

HAUX, G. (1982). *Subsea Manned Engineering*. London: Baillière Tindall.

SISMAN, D. (Ed.) (1982). *The Professional Diver's Handbook*. London: Submex.

*US Navy Diving Manual*, Vol. 2 (1989). NAVSHIPS 0994–001–9010. US Government Printing Office.

# Hyperbaric medicine

## Introduction

Certain diseases are eminently suitable for treatment by hyperbaric oxygen. The value in decompression sickness and air embolism is well established, and is described elsewhere. There are other medical and surgical diseases which respond very well to this form of therapy, and which are not particularly related to the diving or aquatic environment.

The subject of hyperbaric oxygenation in the treatment of medical and surgical disorders is of general interest to diving physicians. It is for this reason that this chapter has been included in a book on diving medicine. It is not the intention to provide a text on hyperbaric medicine, but merely to give an overview of this subject, and encourage any interested physicians into reading any of the major texts on hyperbaric medicine. These may be complemented by the proceedings of the ten International Conferences on Hyperbaric Medicine.

Because of their access to recompression chambers, diving physicians may be called on to advise and assist in the management of a wide variety of diseases which may be helped by hyperbaric medicine.

## Historical review

The first attempt to use a hyperbaric chamber in medicine was made by the British physician, Henshaw, in 1662. This chamber was fitted with a large pair of organ bellows, with valves placed so that air could either be compressed into the chamber, or extracted from it. Henslaw used increased pressures for treatment of acute diseases and reduced pressures for treatment of chronic diseases. Even this was not enough to satisfy his enthusiasm.

In time of good health this domicilium is proposed as a good expedient to help digestion, to promote insensible respiration, to facilitate breathing and expectoration, and consequently, of excellent use for prevention of most affections of the lungs.

In 1775, Priestley discovered oxygen, and his classic description is still pertinent.

From the greater strength and vivacity of the flame of a candle in this pure air, it may be conjectured, that it might be peculiarly salutary to the lungs in certain morbid cases . . . But, perhaps, we may also infer from these experiments, that though pure dephlogisticated air might be very useful as a medicine, it might not be so proper for us in the usual healthy state of the body; for as a candle burns out much faster in dephlogisticated than in common air, so we might, as may be said, live out too fast, and the animal powers be too soon exhausted in this pure kind of air. A moralist, at least, may say that the air which nature has provided for us is as good as we deserve . . . The feeling of it to my lungs was not sensibly different from that of common air; but I fancied that my breast felt peculiarly light and easy for some time afterwards. Who can tell but that, in time, this pure air may become a fashionable article of luxury. Hitherto only two mice and myself have had the privilege of breathing it.

In the Netherlands, the Dutch Academy of Sciences sponsored a prize in 1782 and subsequent years, for the design of an apparatus to study the effects of higher pressures in biology. There were no contenders, nor any recipients of the prize. It is ironic that the recent advances in hyperbaric medicine are based heavily on the work of the Dutch, almost two centuries later.

In the 1830s, France led the new fashion in hyperbaric medicine. Pressure chamber exposures of between 2 and 4 atmospheres absolute were stated to increase the circulation of the internal organs, improve the cerebral blood flow, and produce a feeling of well-being. Junod (1834) first made these observations, and they were taken up avidly by his colleagues, Taberie and Pravaz. The chambers were specially used for pulmonary diseases, including tuberculosis, laryngitis, tracheitis, pertussis etc., as well as apparently unrelated diseases such as deafness, cholera, rickets, menorrhagia, conjunctivitis etc.

Hypebaric technology advanced with the employment of compressed air for caisson work. Triger, in 1841, reported an experience with the first caisson for excavating the bed of the Loire River. This caisson was sunk to a depth of 20 metres (65 feet), and it was during this experience that many of the modern dysbaric problems were first described.

During the 1850s many hyperbaric chambers were in use throughout Europe. 'Pneumatic institutes' flourished and mobile hyperbaric facilities were introduced. In 1879, a mobile hyperbaric operating room was completed, so that surgery could be performed in hospitals, sanitaria and private homes. It was claimed that patients recovered from anaesthetics more rapidly when in the chamber (an observation of interest, in that the interaction of hyperbaria, gas elimination, inert gas narcosis and the high-pressure neurological syndrome are being actively studied). Cyanosis and asphyxia were less, or absent. Postanaesthetic excitement and vomiting were markedly decreased. The chamber was recommended to facilitate the reduction of hernia and for patients with asthma, emphysema, chronic bronchitis and anaemia. Twenty-seven operations were performed within a 3-month period in this chamber.

Success was so great that a large hyperbaric surgical amphitheatre, which would hold 300 people, was planned, but fortunately never reached fruition. Fontein had an accident in the Pneumatic Institute which resulted in his death, the first physician martyr to hyperbaric therapy.

Dr C.E. Williams, in the *British Medical Journal* of 1885, wrote a comment which would be thought by many to be applicable today:

The use of atmospheric air under different degrees of atmospheric pressure, in the treatment of disease, is one of the most important advances in modern medicine, and when we consider the simplicity of the agent, the exact methods by which it may be applied, and the precision with which it can be regulated to the requirements of each individual, we are astonished that in England this method of treatment has been so little used.

In the early twentieth century, the North American continent achieved dominance in the grandiose hyperbaric stakes. In 1927, Dr Orval J. Cunningham constructed a chamber in Kansas City measuring 10 feet in diameter and 88 feet long. It had individual rooms and many of these were provided with luxuries such as radios, phonographs, pianos, telephones and bathrooms. The treatments given were for hypertension, diabetes mellitus, syphilis and cancer. The reason for selecting these diseases for treatment was apparently that they were thought to have an associated anaerobic infection.

The American Medical Association investigated these claims, together with the stock transactions and the fees charged to patients, but their subsequent denunciation did not dissuade Cunningham and others from building the largest chamber ever – five storeys high and with a diameter of 20 metres (64 feet). Each storey had 12 bedrooms and the amenities of a good hotel. The American Medical Association's article included this statement.

Under the circumstances, is it to be wondered at if the medical profession looks askance at the 'tank treatment', and intimates that it seems tinctured much more strongly with economics than with scientific medicine. It is the mark of the scientist that he is ready to make available the evidence on which his claims are based. Dr Cunningham has been given repeated opportunities to present such evidence.

As we move into the 1990s, an almost untenable position has been taken by the health care insurance companies in the USA, despite the availability of much more impersonal research data.

The history of hyperbaric medicine is not entirely dishonourable. Brilliant workers such as Paul Bert and J. Lorrain Smith, around the turn of the century, demonstrated the toxicity problems associated with oxygen. Triger described accurately the problems that hyperbaric personnel would face. The observations by physicians on divers and caisson workers prepared the ground for our knowledge of hyperbaric physiology and the subsequent hyperbaric oxygen developments by a team in Amsterdam. Boerema, Brummelkamp and Meijne, in the early 1960s heralded the present-day investigations into hyperbaric oxygen therapy and their impressive work on the treatment of gas gangrene made at least one application of hyperbaric oxygenation more reputable. They also applied this technique as an adjunct to cardiac surgery, especially for hypoxic cases. This application allowed greater duration of temporary circulatory arrest, permitting cardiac surgery to be conducted. Massive chamber complexes were built to take the cardiac surgery teams, but this application of hyperbaric oxygen was made redundant by the development of effective cardiopulmonary bypass technology.

Despite the establishment of a rational and scientific basis for hyperbaric oxygen in certain diseases, the controversy surrounding hyperbaric oxygen persists.

# General principles

Oxygen's therapeutic use was predicted by Priestley, and has probably been used more widely than any other therapeutic agent. Oxygen is carried in the blood both in physical solution, and in combination with haemoglobin in arterial blood. Normally, at atmospheric pressure the haemoglobin in arterial blood is almost fully saturated with oxygen, carrying 20 ml $O_2$ per 100 ml blood. Increasing the inspired oxygen percentage or pressure does not significantly affect this.

When breathing air at 1 ATA, the arterial oxygen content is approximately 20 ml/100 ml of arterial blood. The mixed venous blood has 14 ml, and therefore 6 ml have been extracted by the tissues in the conversion of arterial to venous blood. There is, however, a considerable variation between the different tissues' oxygen requirements, e.g. myocardium typically has an extraction rate of 10 ml $O_2$/100 ml blood.

Dissolved oxygen rises in direct proportion to the rise of oxygen partial pressure in the inspired gas. When the subject breathes air or oxygen, the following amount of oxygen is transported in physical solution: at 1 ATA, 0.3 ml and 2 ml respectively; at 2 ATA, 0.8 ml and 4 ml; at 3 ATA, 1.3 ml and 6 ml. These figures are approximate and the volumes are expressed as surface values. They are less than the theoretical volume, because of the effects of ventilation–perfusion inequality, anatomical shunts and barriers to diffusion of gas.

Breathing oxygen at 3 ATA may supply almost all of the body's oxygen requirements from the oxygen dissolved in physical solution. At this pressure and breathing 100% oxygen, haemoglobin is not necessary for oxygen transport alone. This has been used therapeutically in the treatment of anaemic patients who have religious objections to the use of blood transfusions, or in whom red blood cell transfusions are not possible or must be delayed. Haemoglobin has many other functions as well, such as carbon dioxide transport and in acid–base buffering.

The effects of hyperbaric oxygen (HBO) on the cardiovascular system are very marked. There is a 10–20% reduction in cardiac output, mainly due to bradycardia. The arterial pressure remains reasonably constant, although there is a generalized vasoconstriction which may have beneficial effects in some illnesses.

Under some conditions when the venous blood haemoglobin remains saturated with oxygen, i.e. when the oxygen is supplied to the tissues mostly from that dissolved in physical solution, there may be a rise in the blood carbon dioxide tension, and a subsequent acid shift in pH. This is because the haemoglobin is no longer available for the transport of carbon dioxide (oxygenated haemoglobin, unlike reduced haemoglobin, cannot transport carbon dioxide). Although these effects are of interest, they present no significant problems.

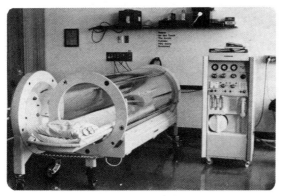

**Figure 37.1** One-person hyperbaric oxygen therapy chamber: maximum therapeutic pressure of 3 ATA

Hyperbaric medicine involves the use of a raised ambient pressure, usually incorporating hyperbaric oxygen (HBO), either directly to affect a disease or injury (e.g. reducing bubble volumes in decompression sickness, reducing toxicity of certain anaerobic organisms) or to enhance host resistance (e.g. restoration of polymorphonuclear leucocyte function in hypoxic wounds).

Although the mechanisms of hyperbaric therapy are well understood and the potential applications are numerous, and despite both the widespread use and advocacy, hyperbaric therapy is only established as a treatment of decompression sickness, arterial gas embolism, carbon monoxide poisoning, gas gangrene and osteoradionecrosis. The confusing literature for other applications such as wound healing are largely due to the inattention by HBO protagonists to the importance of oxygen dose (intensity, duration and frequency) and effect.

**Table 37.1 Indications**

Established mode of therapy
   Decompression sickness
   Arterial gas embolism
   Gas gangrene
   Carbon monoxide poisoning
   Osteoradionecrosis
   Chronic osteomyelitis

Possible role
   Radiotherapy
   Burns injury
   Cyanide poisoning
   Hydrogen sulphide poisoning
   Liver toxins (carbon tetrachloride, chloroform)
   Hypoxic wounds
   Diabetic ulcers
   Ischaemic vascular disorders

HBO at appropriate tissue levels will encourage fibroblast proliferation and collagen formation. HBO may also be of benefit by acting against anaerobic organisms, which lack enzymes to reduce toxic oxygen free radicals (see Chapter 12), deactivating bacterial toxins and enhancing polymorphonuclear leucocyte activity.

Other possible beneficial effects of HBO involve the effect on the microcirculation. HBO decreases interstitial fluid pressure and extracellular oedema. It also increases red cell elasticity and these effects combine to decrease viscosity. Platelet aggregation is also inhibited.

The sceptics of hyperbaric medicine point to its lack of prospective, controlled and randomized clinical data; but in this regard, the discipline is limited ethically in areas where reduction of mortality and morbidity is significant and is not essentially different from any other area of medicine.

## Gas gangrene (Plate 14)

This is a serious disease, with a high incidence of both morbidity and mortality. It is especially associated with trauma – 12% of combat injury wounds in World War I were infected by gas gangrene organisms. This dropped to 0.5% in World War II, and less than 0.1% in the Korean War. This significant reduction in the incidence of gas gangrene was due to delayed wound closure and good débridement. During the Vietnam War there were only 20 cases reported, 6 of which were treated by hyperbaric oxygen.

Unfortunately, civilian experience shows a trend in the opposite direction. Because most wounds in civilian practice are subjected to primary closure, and because of the use of occlusive dressings and/or plaster over compound fractures, there has been an increase in the incidence of civilian cases of gas gangrene. The USA have approximately 1000 such cases per year.

The main organism incriminated is *Clostridium perfringens (welchii)*. It is commonly found in soil, in the gastrointestinal tract and in the gall bladder. It is a partial anaerobe, growing freely if the oxygen pressure is less than 30 mmHg, and growing slowly if the oxygen pressure is 30–37 mmHg. It is a Gram-positive organism identified as a spore-bearing rod. The damage is due to an alpha-toxin, an exotoxin, lecithinase C, which destroys cell walls and thereby produces damage to the blood supply of tissues, resulting in gangrene. When this occurs oxygen tension falls, the organisms can proliferate, further reducing the blood supply to the area, and thereby produce a vicious circle.

The disease develops especially in association with impaired vascular supply, and this may be seen with neoplasia, diabetes mellitus, any form of ischaemia and other debilitating diseases. It is an ever-present risk in limb amputation surgery (especially above the knee) for peripheral vascular disease. It may also occur after bowel surgery as clostridia are part of the normal flora in some individuals.

Clinically, the gas gangrene can be divided into myonecrosis, either localized or generalized, and a cellulitis either with or without toxicity. The degree of infection will not only depend on the susceptibility of the tissue, but also on the degree of the infestation with the organisms. The incubation may take from hours to weeks and there is usually a low-grade fever, but with a disproportionately higher pulse rate, in excess of that expected from the injury. The tissue may be tense and pale with either gas blebs, haemorrhagic blebs or crepitations on palpation. Severe pain in the affected area is exacerbated by even slight movement. The conscious state is often impaired, and in serious cases develops into delirium and coma. Other systemic manifestations of the generalized muscle necrosis include a state of shock, with electrolyte and metabolic implications. Haemolysis may also be present, and can be important both in its own right, and because of its effect on potassium elevation and impaired renal function. The X-ray may demonstrate the existence of gas within the tissues.

---

*Diagnosis of gas gangrene:*
*Suspicion*
*Myonecrosis ($\pm$ gas formation)*
*Toxicity (tachycardia, low fever, haemolysis)*
*Gram-positive rods on microscopy of wound specimens*

---

Gas gangrene is often lethal; a mortality of about 15% is experienced even if appropriate antibiotics (penicillin) are administered and radical surgery is performed within 24 hours of the disease becoming apparent. This mortality is reduced to less than 5% if HBO (3 ATA) is also utilized and, importantly, far more conservative surgery is possible.

The only controlled study attempted in humans was abandoned when the mortality in the patients not receiving HBO was found to be twice that of the patients receiving HBO. A risk–benefit analysis of available clinical data shows that, even if the risk of gas gangrene is only 7%, the administration of HBO will save more lives.

HBO is toxic to anaerobic organisms (which lack enzymes to reduce oxygen free radicals). It also decreases interstitial pressure and increases oxygenation, and thus viability of ischaemic tissues.

Even if tissue oxygen tension cannot be increased to bactericidal levels, lower levels will still inhibit toxin production. In dogs with gas gangrene, survival is significantly improved if surgical débridement, antibiotics and HBO are given together, in comparison to any one or combination of two of these modalities.

Most units have adopted the Amsterdam protocol for treating gas gangrene. This involves at least daily surgery (with conservative débridement of obviously necrotic tissue and decompression of hypertensive compartments), high-dose penicillin (20–40 g daily) and HBO (2.8–3 ATA for 1–2 hours, three times in the first day and then twice daily). Hyperbaric oxygen therapy should be continued until the patient is no longer toxic and the local muscle is microscopically normal.

There are still many complications encountered with gas gangrene patients, and hyperbaric oxygen is not the only answer. Tetanus toxoid may be required. Management of the acute respiratory distress syndrome and/or disseminated intravascular coagulation can be very difficult. The haemolysis may require infusion of packed red blood cells, and the electrolyte and renal disorders have to be coped with on their own merits. Nevertheless, hyperbaric oxygen is a major asset in the treatment of this disease.

Available data are far less conclusive about HBO for both superficial bacterial gangrenes and necrotizing fasciitis, and it appears that adequate surgery and adjunctive antibiotics remain the cornerstone of treatment of these diseases.

# Carbon monoxide poisoning

Carbon monoxide is a colourless, odourless and non-irritating gas produced by incomplete combustion. Although it has been removed from most domestic gas supplies, it remains the most common fatal poison in all age groups world wide. Exposures to this gas in Western communities are often deliberate (i.e. suicide attempts), but can also result from domestic and industrial accidents. Car exhausts may contain 7% carbon monoxide. Carbon monoxide is the most common cause of death of victims in building fires. Such fires also often involve concurrent exposure to cyanide and, for as yet unknown reasons, the toxicities of carbon monoxide and cyanide appear to be synergistic.

Carbon monoxide binds to haemoproteins, such as haemoglobin, forming carboxyhaemoglobin, myoglobin, reduced cytochromes of the $P_{450}$ type, reduced cytochrome oxidase and tryptophan dioxygenase, sufficiently well to inhibit their function. The relative contributions of these inhibitions to clinical poisonings is not quantified, although it is well established that carbon monoxide has a significant toxicity which is not related to either haemoglobin or tissue oxygen delivery. Carbon monoxide could also exert its toxic effects by causing lipid peroxidation or by being absorbed onto biological surfaces. The brain (with extensive demyelination in fatal poisonings) and heart are the commonly affected organs, although severely poisoned patients can occasionally display pulmonary oedema.

The clinical presentations of carbon monoxide poisoning vary from headache to a progressive acute brain syndrome, and from asymptomatic ECG changes to myocardial infarction. A cardiac arrest is an obvious and poor prognostic sign. Removal of the victim from the source of carbon monoxide is often accompanied by rapid recovery and dissociation of carbon monoxide from haemoglobin, especially when 100% oxygen is administered. However, the natural history of this poisoning is characterized by subsequent deteriorations in brain function. These deteriorations can occur within days of the original poisoning or be delayed for several weeks. They may be due to carbon monoxide redistributing from slowly releasing tissue stores, such as myoglobin, a consequence of lipid peroxidation which appears to occur after removal from the carbon monoxide source, or may be part of the delayed encephalopathy common to many other hypoxic brain injuries. The most common long-term sequelae of carbon monoxide poisoning are neuropsychiatric, such as personality deteriorations and loss of memory functions.

The clinical and biochemical assessment of carbon monoxide poisoned patients on admission to hospital can be totally misleading. Patients can develop severe sequelae despite being neurologically normal, and having normal arterial blood gas tensions and carboxyhaemoglobin levels of less than 10%. The measurement of carboxyhaemoglobin concentrations at the time of admission cannot identify those patients who will develop sequelae; indeed, it cannot distinguish survivors from non-survivors. This is due, in part, to the significant carbon monoxide toxicity that is not related to haemoglobin and to the rapid dissociation of carboxyhaemoglobin (the half-life decreases from between 320 and 480 minutes in a subject breathing room air, to between 60 and 80 minutes when breathing 100% oxygen at atmospheric pressure, and to between 8 and 23 minutes under conditions of HBO). When treatment of carbon monoxide poisoning has been titrated against the level of carboxyhaemoglobin (e.g. oxygen administration until the level is less than 5%), a considerable number of patients will still develop sequelae. Also, even when carboxyhaemoglobin levels have returned to normal (less than 1% in non-smokers), patients who have been exposed to carbon monoxide will continue to excrete increased amounts of this gas under conditions of HBO and, to a lesser extent, while breathing 100% oxygen at atmospheric pressure. It follows then that any person who has a convincing history of both an exposure to carbon monoxide and intoxication should be offered treatment, regardless of their condition or biochemistry on admission to hospital.

In the absence of any treatment, up to 30% of exposed individuals will die. Of the survivors, more than 10% and up to 40% will be left with sequelae. Of these survivors with sequelae, at least half will have experienced an initial recovery, only to relapse or deteriorate later.

In contrast, in patients poisoned with carbon monoxide who are treated with HBO (at either 2.5 or 3 ATA for 1–2 hours) on admission, and then either 100% oxygen is continued or HBO is repeated daily for several weeks or as necessary from the patient's clinical condition, the outcome is significantly better. In these patients, those who do not have a cardiac arrest live and the long-term morbidity varies between 0% and 2.5%. More importantly, rarely does a patient treated in this way develop long-term sequelae as a result of a late deterioration. It is also noteworthy that repeated HBO is a highly effective treatment of these deteriorations when they do occur.

It is clear then that administration of HBO to patients poisoned with carbon monoxide on admission to hospital, and repeated either daily or as made necessary by the patient's condition, is the only adequate treatment yet assessed. This is particularly true with regard to preventing the late deteriorations typical of this poison. Because the permanent patient morbidity caused by HBO itself in this context

is very low, the current problem in the treatment of carbon monoxide poisonings is not treatment regime selection, but rather patient selection.

Despite the foregoing, carboxyhaemoglobin levels have been roughly correlated with the degree of symptoms during or immediately after exposure, as follows: (1) <7% recorded in heavy cigarette smokers and truck drivers; (2) 15%, no symptoms; (3) 15–25%, nausea, vomiting, headache, occasional, breathlessness and angina or myocardial infarction if there was previously marginal coronary blood flow; (4) 25%, ECG changes with a depressed ST segment, especially in leads 2, V5 and V6; and (5) >25%, significant weakness, may be unable to move although conscious, cortical blindness in children, stupor.

## Osteomyelitis

The mechanisms by which HBO acts in bone infection are well established. It appears that bone becomes hypoxic within a day of infection becoming established. In various animal models, HBO is an effective treatment of all forms of osteomyelitis. In humans, however, conventional antibiotic and surgical treatment of acute and chronic osteomyelitis is relatively cheap and highly effective, such that a role for HBO has not been demonstrated. Only when chronic osteomyelitis becomes refractory to conventional therapy (about 10% of all cases of chronic osteomyelitis) is there possibly a cost-effective role for HBO. Studies using patients as their own controls show that a combined approach of extensive and repeated surgical débridement, antibiotic therapy dictated by deep bone cultures and HBO (2.4–2.8 ATA) will cause more than 90% of these 'refractory' cases to enter a prolonged remission. Additional mechanisms by which HBO may be beneficial include increased antibiotic activity (aminoglycosides, sulphonamides and increased osteoclastic activity). This success rate is less if *Pseudomonas aeruginosa* is the causative organism rather than the far more common *Staphylococcus aureus*.

# Osteoradionecrosis and other hypoxic wounds

Oxyen administration should be pivotal to the treatment of hypoxic wounds. Prospective, properly controlled, clinical data for HBO therapy exist only for osteoradionecrosis, diabetic ulcers (a single study) and perhaps thermal burn injuries. Lack of attention to the effects of the varying oxygen dose negates many studies.

Not only will each patient require an individualized dose of oxygen (which will vary from 40% oxygen at atmospheric pressure to HBO at 3 ATA) in order to maintain the tissue oxygen tensions, adjacent to the hypoxic wound, in the optimal range for fibroblast proliferation and collagen formation, but also this dose will have to be continually adjusted down over a course of therapy as the wound is progressively revascularized.

Delivery of increased oxygen to a hypoxic wound raises the oxygen gradient across the wound and this stimulates the release of growth factor and angiogenesis factor by macrophages. Thus, not only does the oxygen therapy stimulate new vessel formation, but by stimulating the hydroxylation of proline and hence the formation and maturation of collagen and collagen cross-linking, it also provides a framework for blood vessels to invade the hypoxic wound and for re-epithelialization.

Other mechanisms by which oxygen can accelerate the healing of hypoxic wounds include reduced interstitial fluid pressure, reduced blood viscosity, reduced platelet aggregation and increased red blood cell elasticity (all of which improve the microcirculation), and increased polymorphonuclear leucocyte and osteoclast function.

## Osteonecrosis

Irradiation of tissues, usually as a form of cancer therapy, causes a predictable response which includes a local vasculitis and often the tissue becomes avascular. This is particularly true for bone and is a special problem in the facial skeleton after irradiation of head and neck cancers.

HBO has been shown, in a series of well-controlled prospective studies, to be the single most useful adjunct to surgery in the treatment of patients with irradiated bone. In particular, prophylactic HBO (2.4 ATA) is significantly better than penicillin in irradiated bone after tooth removal and increases the success rate of hemimandibular jaw reconstructions in irradiated tissues. A combined regime of surgery and HBO increases the success rate of treating osteoradionecrosis and the cost to the patient is less than a surgical regime without HBO. Importantly, HBO does not increase the local recurrence rate of the original cancer.

## Thermal burn injuries

Thermal burn injuries have a high mortality and morbidity. The frequent concurrence of thermal burn injury and carbon monoxide poisoning by itself demonstrates the need for a close liaison between hyperbaric units and burns units. In animal models of thermal burns, HBO (2 ATA) reduces both the progression of partial thickness burns to full thickness and plasma losses, and hence reduces the mortality, reduces the frequency of burn wound infection and increases the rate of burn wound revascularization and re-epithelialization. Clinical studies have been, with one exception, poorly controlled but do support these animal model findings. As such, the HBO treatment of thermal burns is not yet proven, but is an area of active interest.

# Other conditions

The use of hyperbaric oxygen has also been extended to many other diseases, some of which may be very valid. Unfortunately, at this stage it is necessary to classify them as areas for future research, more than established medical treatment. These include the use of hyperbaric oxygen for the treatment of cerebral oedema, dysbaric osteonecrosis, sickle-cell crises, liver toxins, peripheral vascular disease, spinal cord contusion and pneumatosis cystoides intestinalis. These and other potential applications of HBO await careful dose–response studies.

Some of the more controversial applications include myocardial infarction, multiple sclerosis and senility, leading to excessive optimism in the commercial literature. HBO currently has no established place for these conditions.

# Anaesthesia and medical support

## Equipment considerations

Under hyperbaric conditions, bobbin-type **rotameters** tend to read higher than the actual flow rate at higher settings. Ball-type **flowmeters** are largely unaffected up to 3 ATA. **Gas volume meters**, such as the Wright respirometer and the Drager volumeter, overestimate volumes at higher densities and should be recalibrated for the working pressure, as should pneumotachygraph flow transducers. Vaporizers for agents, such as halothane, deliver, at a constant setting, a slightly increased partial pressure with increasing ambient pressure. This effect is greater the higher the setting. Of course, the actual inspired concentration falls with increased ambient pressure. Thus, a modern vaporizer set at 1% would deliver 0.5–0.6% at 2 ATA. Anaesthesia is dependent on vapour pressure, not concentration. The vaporizer can be used as if under normobaric conditions, with allowance for the slightly increased partial pressure, especially above the 2% setting and/or greater than 3 ATA.

Gas flow through anaesthetic circuits, especially endotracheal tubes and connections, is affected by the increased gas density at pressure. The resultant increase in flow resistance is maximal with high flow and narrow tubes.

## Inhalational agents

The use of gaseous or volatile anaesthetics in hyperbaric environments can pose problems. **Nitrous oxide** was first considered under these conditions by Paul Bert. As its potency is low, large quantities of gas are dissolved in the organism, and this may make decompression very difficult. It will exacerbate decompression sickness and gas embolism. It has been thought to precipitate decompression sickness when administered post-dive, at normobaria. Being combustible under pressure, its use as a carrier for other anaesthetic vapours is not recommended. It also extends the flammability of halothane.

**Halothane** does not cause many problems at pressures up to 3 ATA. It is neither inflammable nor explosive in pure oxygen from 1 to 4 ATA. Its stability is apparently not affected by conventional hyperbaric pressures; however, it may increase reactivity with certain materials, e.g. rubber, plastics, copper etc. **Enflurane** and **isoflurane** would also probably be suitable.

**Other gases**, such as argon and xenon, have been considered. At 1 ATA, 80% xenon provides rapid but very mild anaesthesia with minimal side effects. Nevertheless, they are not considered suitable for anaesthesia under these conditions. There are problems with increased hypoxia by diffusion during the recovery phase. There is also the increased likelihood following ascent of precipitating bubble formation and decompression sickness. The problem of counterdiffusion occurs with inhalation of xenon while exposed to a nitrogen or helium environment. It is likely to result in gas-phase separation and isobaric decompression sickness (i.e. even without changing the ambient pressure, see page 149).

## Intravenous agents

With an ambient pressure of up to 19.2 ATA, and with oxygen at 0.2 ATA, the acute toxicity of thiopentone (Pentothal), ethanol, lignocaine and morphine does not change.

In practice, at up to 3–4 ATA, the action of most drugs used intravenously for anaesthesia does not seem to be changed in any way which is clinically detectable. Most opiates, tranquillizers, neuroleptics, analgesics and muscle relaxants have been used without significant adverse effects.

The antagonism of anaesthesia by very high pressure is discussed in Chapters 15 and 16. It has been confirmed in the case of most anaesthetic drugs in animals. However, anaesthesia will counteract certain deleterious effects of pressure, enabling animals to survive at far greater depths and reducing the manifestations of the high-pressure nervous syndrome. It is not a problem at the much lower pressures used for treatment.

## Barotrauma effects (see Chapters 9 and 10)

In some cases it is necessary to compress a patient who may be anaesthetized. Under these conditions bilateral myringotomy may be required.

During decompression, a painful dilatation of gastrointestinal gas may be noted. This is especially so if the patient has swallowed gas or if it has been introduced into his stomach during artificial respiration. This is one of the reasons why a nasogastric tube is recommended, although it cannot remove gas from the lower gastrointestinal tract.

The risk of air embolism from expansion of trapped gas in patients with chronic lung disease (e.g. in emphysematous bullae) may be reduced by the use of a very slow decompression schedule.

Gas expansion may be noted after the closure of a surgical wound, in the mediastinum, the pleura or the peritoneal cavities, and therefore these tissues should be examined carefully prior to their closure.

### Respiratory effects

An increase in the effort required for breathing, especially related to the increased density of respiratory gases, and a fall in lung compliance, may be poorly tolerated in the hyperbaric patient. There is evidence that disturbances in carbon dioxide and oxygen transfer occur at great depths (31 ATA). A degree of hypercapnia and resultant acidosis is common under hyperbaric conditions, and especially with hyperbaric oxygen at 2–3 ATA. There is also an increase in the heat loss through the upper airways, related to the increased density of gas.

For these reasons, controlled ventilation seems to be particularly advisable for general anaesthesia in hyperbaric environments.

### Oxygen toxicity

Strict attention must be paid to the partial pressure in the gases inhaled through artificial respirators. Several anaesthetic drugs can mask the external symptoms of oxygen toxicity, and this does not necessarily mean that the toxic effect has been prevented, merely that it is camouflaged (see Chapter 18).

### Effects of inert gas

At pressure, inert gases are able to depress the central nervous system (see Chapter 15). This calls for a careful choice of mixtures to be inhaled by the medical team, as well as by the patient. The narcosis may be of value in the anaesthesia, but it is not a significant factor. The high-pressure neurological syndrome (see Chapter 16) occurs in excess of 200 metres and can become hazardous. The problems of speeding up the descent of a medical team which may be called in to treat an injured diver, without impairing its efficiency from this disorder, are problems which beset deep diving operations. It can be reduced by titrating nitrogen with the helium so that each counteracts the untowards effects of the other. Nitrogen also relieves other problems such as voice communication and heat loss, which are especially associated with helium under pressure.

### Problems of compression and decompression

The existence of bubbles produces a number of pathological phenomena, anomalies of coagulation associated with the formation of platelet aggregates, fat embolism etc. These cause various circulatory and haematological disorders, the consequence of which may be serious in a patient who is already under an anaesthetic and subject to the vasomotor effects of anaesthetic drugs. It may also aggravate the patient's state of exhaustion and shock. Haemodynamic disorders resulting from shock hinder the movement of bubbles or delay the elimination of gas in solution from the body. The lung's capacity to filter circulating bubbles may be affected by artificial respiration and intermittent positive pressure. During inflation there is a drop in the instantaneous pulmonary blood flow, which is no longer matched to alveolar ventilation. Inflation at higher positive pressures raises the alveolar pressure and compresses the capillaries, producing an obstacle to the pulmonary circulation which could adversely affect the lung's capacity to discharge the circulating bubbles.

The effect of hyperbaric conditions on hepatic enzyme systems may interfere with the catabolism of drugs but are not well understood at this stage (see Chapter 31).

Anaesthesia in a moderate hyperbaric atmosphere, up to 4 ATA, poses problems which are mainly of a technical nature and relatively easy to solve. Beyond this level, the situation is different and is only just beginning to be explored.

Problems with equipment with changes in ambient pressure also have to be kept in mind. Endotracheal cuffs need to be deflated or filled with fluid. Intravenous fluid administration sets need to be observed as blood may be drawn back into the cannula (and clot, causing obstruction) during compression. During ascent, drugs or gas may be inadvertently infused. A similar situation may develop with an underwater drain from the thoracic cavity.

# Acknowledgement

This significant contribution of Dr D.F. Gorman, Director, Hyperbaric Unit, Royal Adelaide Hospital, Australia, and Director, Diving Medicine Unit, Royal New Zealand Navy, to this chapter is gratefully acknowledged.

# Recommended reading

## General

DAVIS, J.C. and HUNT, T.K. (Eds) (1977). *Hyperbaric Oxygen Therapy*. Bethesda: Undersea Medical Society.*

DAVIS, J.C. and HUNT, T.K. (Eds) (1988). *Problem Wounds. The Role of Oxygen*. New York: Elsevier.

FISCHER, B., JAIN, K.K., BRAUN, E. and LEHRL, S. (1988). *Handbook of Hyperbaric Oxygen Therapy*. Berlin: Springer-Verlag.*

JACOBSON, I.H. II, MORSCH, J.H.C. and RENDELL-BAKER, L. (1965). The historical perspective of hyperbaric therapy. *First International Congress on Hyperbaric Oxygenation*.

KERMORGANT, Y. (1978). *Anaesthesia in Hyperbaric Atmosphere*. 3733/78. Congress on Medical Aspects of Diving Accidents. EUBS publication.

KINDWALL, E.D. and GOLDMANN, R.W. (1984). *Hypebaric Medicine Procedures*. St Lukes Hospital, Milwaukee.*

* Textbooks on hyperbaric medicine.

## Carbon monoxide

GORMAN, D.F. (1991). Problems and pitfalls in the use of hyperbaric oxygen for the treatment of poisoned patients. *Medical Toxicology and Adverse Drug Experience* (in press).

MATHIEU, D., NOLF, M., DUROCHER, A. et al. (1985). Acute carbon monoxide poisoning. Risk of late sequelae and treatment by hyperbaric oxygen. *Clinical Toxicology* 23, 315–324.

MEREDITH, T. and VALE, A. (1988). Carbon monoxide poisoning. *British Medical Journal* 296, 77–79.

MYERS, R.A.M. SNYDER, S.K. and EMHOFF, T.A. (1985). Subacute sequelae of carbon monoxide poisoning. *Annals of Emergency Medicine* 14, 1163–1167.

## Gas gangrene and other infections

BAKKER, D.J. (1984). *Hyperbaric Oxygen and Infectious Diseases*. Wageningen: Drukkerij Veenman BV.

BRUMMELKAMP, W.H., HOOGENDIJK, L. and BOEREMA, I. (1961). Treatment of anaerobic infections by drenching the tissue with oxygen under high atmospheric pressure. *Surgery* 49, 229–302.

HITCHCOCK, C.R., DEMELLO, F.J. and HAGLIN, J.J. (1975). Gangrene infection. *Surgical Clinics of North America* 55, 1403–1410.

## Osteoradionecrosis and other hypoxic wounds

BARONI, G., PORRO, T., FAGLIA, E. et al. (1987). Hyperbaric oxygen in diabetic gangrene treatment. *Diabetes Care* 10, 81–86.

MEHM, W.J., PINSLER, M., BECKER, R.L. and LISSNER, C.R. (1988). Effect of oxygen on in-vitro fibroblast cell proliferation and collagen biosynthesis. *Journal of Hyperbaric Medicine* 3, 227–234.

NIU, A.K.C., YANG, C., LEE, H.C. and CHEN, L.P. (1987). Burns treated with adjunctive hyperbaric oxygen therapy: a comparative study in humans. *Journal of Hyperbaric Medicine* 2, 75–86.

## Controversy corner

GABB, G. and ROBIN, E.D. (1987). Hyperbaric oxygen. A therapy in search of disease. *Chest* 92, 1074–1082.

KINDWELL, E.P., GOLDMAN, R.W., BURTON, G.G. et al. (1988). Some defendents of hyperbaric oxygen. *Chest* 94, 414–419.

ROBIN, E.D., JAMES, P.B., KRIGBAUM, E.M. et al. (1988). Differing opinions on hyperbaric oxygen therapy. *Chest* 94, 667–674.

# 38

# Hyperbaric equipment

## Introduction

There are two main types of environmental pressure vessel used in medicine and research:

1. **Hyperbaric chambers** where the ambient pressure can be increased from 1 ATA to many times atmospheric pressure depending on the structural capabilities of the vessel concerned. These chambers are used for diving, and hyperbaric medicine and research, and are built to withstand an explosive force.
2. **Hypobaric chambers** where the ambient pressure can be decreased from 1 ATA to subatmospheric pressure levels. These chambers are used for aviation, space medicine and research, and are built to resist an implosive force.

Some chambers are capable of performing both functions, but these are not common and are mostly found in research centres.

The hyperbaric chamber is subject to differing nomenclature depending on its primary use. Terms used for chambers used in diving include the following: the **recompression chamber** where the major use of the hyperbaric chamber is for compressing a caisson worker or diver, usually as part of a therapeutic regime; it may also be used in the training of divers, so that they may experience the effects of hyperbaria; the **decompression chamber** where the major use is to decompress a subject already exposed to increased pressure. A **submersible decompression chamber** (SDC) which is used to transport divers under pressure to and from the working depth, usually allows transfer under pressure to a surface or **deck decompression chamber** (DDC). The DDC allows for the definitive decompression under controlled conditions. The diving bell, which is open at the bottom, and therefore is exposed to ambient sea pressure, was the forerunner of the SDC.

Only the hyperbaric or recompression chamber is discussed in this section, as this is the main structure of particular importance to diving medicine. The chamber consists of a strengthened vessel or hull which can be pressurized by compressed gas. This may be supplied direct from a gas cylinder or from a compressor. Decompression is achieved by allowing the gas to escape.

Since the 1920s, numerous hyperbaric chambers have been designed for the treatment of divers and caisson workers. Some are inefficient for this use, and may be dangerous. With the progress of hyperbaric and diving medicine, chambers are becoming increasingly complex. The design of these structures now follows the guidelines of a multitude of experienced personnel ranging from the specialist diving physician and the diver to the design and construction engineer.

For a description of the recompression facilities and transport needed for treatment of dysbaric accidents, see Chapters 13 and 33.

## Recompression chamber classification

The initial consideration in designing a hyperbaric chamber concerns its expected use. There are several main types of recompression chambers namely:

1. Large multicompartment chambers used for research as well as treatment of divers and caisson workers and capable of compression to many atmospheres (greater than 5 ATA). These may even incorporate wet and dry chambers where underwater pressure environments can be simulated for research activities.
2. Large multicompartment chambers capable only of low pressures (2–4 ATA) used for treatment with hyperbaric oxygen regimes.
3. Portable high pressure multi-person chambers for treating divers and caisson workers.
4. Portable one-person, high or low pressure chambers used for surface decompression of divers. Similar chambers are widely used in hyperbaric medicine units. Unfortunately these sometimes have to be used for treatment of divers and caisson workers requiring recompression therapy.

The low pressure units may be inadequate for the treatment of an emergency such as cerebral air embolism which may arise during their use. Any properly designed high-pressure complex should be capable of treatment of both diving accidents and hyperbaric medicine patients.

Fashionable jargon is often used to describe the numbers of places available in chambers. Thus 'multi-place' and 'mono-place' are meant to indicate the numbers of patients that can be accommodated. These terms also infer fixed and portable chambers respectively. The implication is not always accurate, and also the numbers of places available in a chamber may need to be modified, depending on the clinical circumstances.

## Large multicompartment recompression chamber

This is a high-pressure chamber capable of accommodating several persons in each lock. It should be suitable for treating divers, caisson workers and patients requiring hyperbaric oxygen.

The recompression chamber may be composed of the following elements, the principles of which have medical implications. The finer technical details will not be discussed.

### Hull

This should consist of two or more interconnecting chambers or locks some of which can be separately compressed or decompressed. The number of compartments depends on the use of the unit, but the usual system consists of a large inner lock and a smaller outer lock. The inner lock is used for therapy and the outer lock for transfer of personnel.

The inner lock should include a medical lock of sufficient dimensions to allow passage of items such as food, excreta, drugs and equipment.

The diameter should be sufficient for an adult to stand erect in both locks, especially the inner lock where most treatment is conducted. This requires an inner diameter of at least 2 metres. The length of the inner lock should exceed 3 metres in order to accommodate a prone patient on a stretcher and allow free movement of attendants around the patient.

Pressurization capabilities of such a chamber will depend on the anticipated requirements but should be as great as possible to allow for all eventualities. It is likely that a pressure capability of 150–200 metres will suffice for nearly all cases.

Pressure-sealed doors should be fitted to openings of the outer lock. In order to occupy minimal space within the outer lock during transfer, entry or exit pivoting hinges can be utilized. A similar pressure-sealed pivoting door should be fitted to the opening into the inner lock. Doorway dimensions and locations should allow easy entry and removal of persons and stretchers.

Large observation ports should be fitted to both or all locks so that the entire compartment can be easily observed. Hinged internal metal sealing covers should be fitted which can be used to seal the port should a leak occur. X-rays may be taken through the ports.

All interior surfaces should be painted with light, easily cleaned, non-reflective, fire retardant paint. The coating should also minimize noise and static electricity.

Removable floor boards in both locks must give a flat non-skid surface.

## Furniture and fittings

Comfortable seating should be available for the anticipated number of occupants because decompression may be prolonged. Fold-away seating allows maximum use of available space for different requirements.

Both locks should have metal storage shelves or lockers for storage of medical instruments etc.

Lighting of both locks can be either direct interior pressure-sealed and fire-safe lights, through-hull fibreoptic lighting, or external lights separated from ceiling ports by heat filters or air flow cooling systems. Both locks should have shadow-free lighting.

Facilities should exist for one or two stretchers or trolleys to be used, at least in the inner lock. The trolley should be 1 metre high with adjustable head and foot elevations, and fitted with antistatic straps and lockable wheels. Due to the confined chamber space and door design, the trolley system may not be appropriate. In such cases removable rails may be utilized to facilitate entry of a stretcher into the chamber's inner lock.

## Chamber plumbing

Intake openings into both locks should be muffled to keep sound levels below 90 dB at maximum compression rate. The inlets should be distant from the outlets to promote gas circulation, and not adjacent to personnel or movable objects. Outlets should be placed in inaccessible positions on the ceilings and covered by grids. Exhaust lines should be far removed from the control panel so as not to constitute a noise hazard. They should not be near heating or electrical apparatus due to the danger of fire from possible high oxygen partial pressures in the exhaust gases.

Equalization valves, able to be opened from both sides of bulkhead or door, should be fitted to the outer lock, medical lock and the wall between the inner lock and the outer lock. This will permit independent operation by personnel in either lock or for transfer under pressure purposes.

## Breathing gas supply

Pressurization of both locks should be under the direct control of the panel supervisor. Fine and coarse controlling valves should be fitted. The chamber should be capable of a pressurization rate at least equal to that of diving and therapeutic tables. High-pressure air should be ducted into both locks from a large storage bank after having passed through a filtration bank from an electrically driven compressor. A standby diesel or gasoline compressor may be needed. An auxiliary electrical power source is needed for compressor, lighting and all ancillary equipment.

An alternative gas supply using liquid oxygen and nitrogen may be available in some hospitals.

Provision for breathing helium/oxygen or other gas mixtures by staff is required if used in excess of 60 metres.

A second storage bank for oxygen, oxygen/nitrogen and oxygen/helium mixtures is connected to the chamber mask breathing system so that the inspired oxygen and inert gas concentration can be varied.

High-pressure oxygen, or gas mixtures for breathing by patients or attendants, should be ducted directly from external control valves into both locks where internal control valves are situated. From these a series of standard gas thread outlets should be provided to enable two systems of oxygen or mixture supply to patients, namely:

1. An automatic reducer, flowmeter, and an oronasal mask and bag.
2. A demand valve and regulator analogous to surface supply breathing apparatus, or scuba.

After exhalation, both should be fed into an overboard dump system to prevent high oxygen levels developing in the chamber.

Another technique for producing a variety of gas mixtures is by having two separate intakes attached to flowmeters, and varying the flows according to the concentrations required.

## Communications

Communication facilities should include sound-powered, electrically insulated telephones within both locks and on the control panel – all being interlinked. A secondary intercom or two-way transmit/receive unit should also be provided between both compartments and the control panel.

Closed circuit television coverage may be needed for both locks so that all inhabitants can be monitored from the control panel. The camera may be located either inside the lock or outside on an observation port.

## Transfer under pressure

The other opening of the outer lock should be fitted with some system enabling a transfer under pressure using a transfer sleeve. Such manoeuvres may require a sling and gantry or rails to support the mobile chamber. A stable system is needed to avoid pivoting at the connection between the chambers.

## Fire

The authors are aware of 9 fires in pressure chambers, which caused 29 deaths as well as other incidents involving experimental animals. The severity of these fires is indicated by the fact that in this series there were only 7 survivors, all badly burnt.

Any fire has three prerequisites: a source to ignite it, fuel and oxygen. Fire can be prevented by removing any of these elements. In a chamber the hair on the diver's skin can provide fuel to spread the fire and, if the oxygen partial pressure is greater than about 1 ATA, hairless skin will burn. Oxygen must be available for the diver to breathe and is often present at high partial pressures, so two elements of fire are always present.

Further aggravating factors are the increased ease of ignition and combustibility that exist in some hyperbaric conditions. Substances that do not burn in air can burn if the oxygen partial pressure is elevated. This includes some substances treated with fire-retarding chemicals. Even static sparks generated by clothing could cause a fire because of the increased ease of ignition.

An apparent contradiction to these facts is that it is impossible to sustain a fire in some of the gas mixtures used in deep diving because of the low oxygen concentration. This cannot be used as an excuse to avoid precautions against fire because in these conditions there may be pockets of gas that can sustain combustion and periods of high fire risk will be encountered during compression and decompression.

The safety of the chamber occupants depends on everyone involved being aware of the fire hazards and their continuing vigilance to prevent any action that could increase the risk of fire. Risks can be minimized and firefighting systems installed.

Both locks should be fitted with fire-fighting facilities using water as the extinguishing medium. A system of spray nozzles should be capable of wetting all surfaces thoroughly with a fine spray or mist within 2–3 seconds of the onset of any fire. Continuous spraying requires a compensatory air loss to avoid an increase in pressure as the locks flood to half their height. Activation of this system can occur automatically via ultraviolet, infrared and/or carbon dioxide sensors. Manual switches should be placed inside the locks and on the control panel. A secondary system of hand-operated hoses fitted with spray nozzles should be fitted in each lock so that an attendant can direct water on to any source of fire or heat.

An oxygen elimination or exhaust dump system is a mandatory requirement for modern chambers, when the subjects breathe from masks. It enables expired gases containing elevated oxygen and carbon dioxide pressures to be exhausted to the exterior. Techniques used include extraction from a reservoir bag using a Venturi system connected to the exhaust, or non-return valves.

Emergency air supplies (built-in breathing system – BIBS) should be fitted for all personnel in both compartments. These consist of demand valves connected by short high-pressure hoses to spring-loaded bayonet mountings on a bulkhead. All hoses should be fire resistant. The breathing gas supply should bypass the main supply, from emergency bottles. This system will ensure an oxygen supply and prevent toxic fumes caused by burning contents from overcoming the chamber occupants.

Any padding allowed on stretchers or seats is best constructed of material which is not only fire resistant or non-combustible but which will not, if exposed to extreme temperatures, produce toxic fumes. The same applies to all clothing and bedclothes within the chamber, and this should be specially treated to minimize the risk of static electricity build-up. High partial pressures and concentrations of oxygen increase the fire risk in a hyperbaric chamber.

## Instrumentation and operation

Emphasis should be placed on obtaining rugged reliable equipment in preference to highly sophisticated but delicate instruments. Some essential features are discussed.

Control panels should always be fitted with large easily read instruments. They must be located in such a manner as to prevent confusion as to which lock they refer. Colour codes are useful, each lock using different coloured instruments. The control operator and supervisor should be able to view all inhabitants in both locks simultaneously.

Pressure/depth gauges should be sited in both locks and on the control panel. Two gauges may be coupled, one covering the low pressure range and the other the high pressures. An independent pressure transducer connected to a linear chart recorder is useful in providing a permanent dive profile record.

Ambient oxygen concentrations should be measured in both locks and recorded on gauges or chart recorders on the control panel. A warning system can be incorporated, activated by deviation of oxygen concentration outside certain pre-set values. A similar system can be used to warn of a dangerous rise in carbon dioxide tension.

Clocks should be fitted so that total elapsed time and individual compression/decompression times are easily recorded.

Flowmeters should measure the ventilation rates on the exhaust lines from both locks so that adequate ventilation rates can be achieved.

Temperature and humidity should be controlled and monitored.

Electrodiagnostic monitoring should be possible in each lock. Physiological parameters which may need recording include the electrocardiogram, the electroencephalogram and the electronystagmogram.

A broad guide as to suitable design for a large treatment chamber has been discussed. Ideally, such facilities should be situated near major hospital complexes to ensure optimal medical control as well as expert maintenance. Ground level locations are preferable because of transfer under pressure requirements with mobile chambers. In view of the high noise levels associated with their function, soundproofing from the hospital is desirable.

## Portable recompression chamber

These treatment chambers should be capable of being transported by air; therefore size and weight problems are relevant. The gas pressurization systems accompanying such units must be included in overall size and weight estimations.

Most of these chambers are designed to accommodate a maximum of two or three persons in the single or main lock. Apparatus is best kept to a minimum, providing only the essential requisites. These chambers are principally used in the initial first aid to a diver suffering from decompression sickness or air embolism. Once compression is achieved, a larger recompression chamber should be sought, to which the patient can be transferred while still under pressure for subsequent therapeutic decompression. Occasionally, such a transfer is not feasible; therefore certain minimum requirements are essential to allow definitive treatment. If two portable chambers are available, providing compatible transfer-under-pressure facilities exist, they may be mated to facilitate access to the patient with equipment and personnel.

The minimum requirements for these chambers are as follows.

The hull should be of appropriate weight and dimensions to be loaded onto the transport aircraft. A maximum size would be about 2–3 metres in length, 1–1.5 metres in diameter, and less than 600 kilograms in weight. Trolley or pallet mounting of the unit will assist with later transport.

The door surround should have a transfer-under-pressure flange compatible with other systems.

A medical lock is valuable, as are observation ports. Adequate lighting and communication should be incorporated.

A roll-in stretcher may be of considerable advantage.

Soundproofing of inlets and protection of exhaust outlets similar to the large recompression chambers is essential. Temperature control may be needed, especially in extreme climates and with rebreathing systems.

Oxygen or other breathing gas should be supplied independently of the chamber gas. An oxygen elimination system would be advantageous. Rebreathing systems with carbon dioxide scrubbers may be used to reduce the air consumption.

Compressed air supplies and compression facilities should be sufficient to provide for maximum pressurization and adequate ventilation of the chamber (main lock) for two occupants for a period during which transportation will occur.

Control panels for these types of chambers are usually located on the hull structure and include clocks, pressure gauges, communication facilities, flowmeters, control valves and ancillary aids. Provisions for connection of pressure/time chart recorders is an advantage.

Electrophysiological monitoring connection plugs are advisable.

## Medical supplies

An emergency kit comprising examination and treatment instruments, drugs and dressings, should be available on site for both small and large recompression chambers. Some instruments and equipment which may be required by the chamber personnel include:

Stethoscope
Anaeroid sphygmomanometer
Percussion hammer, pin, tuning forks
Urinary catheter, introducers, collecting bag
Sterile syringes and needles
Sterile intravenous cannulae and catheters
Intravenous transfusion sets, 'cut down' and suture sets
Intravenous fluids, e.g. Hartmann's solution, physiological saline, plasma expanders
Thoracic trocar and cannula with sterile plastic tubing and underwater drain system or Heimlich valve
Endotracheal tubes and connections
Adhesive tape
Antiseptic solution and swabs
Sterile dressings
Automatic ventilator and connections
Ophthalmoscope, otoscope, laryngoscope (not to be taken into the chamber unless needed)
Drugs which should be immediately available include: steroids; frusemide; digoxin; lignocaine; aminophyline; phenytoin; diazepam; morphine; pethidine; prochlorperazine; promethazine; atropine; adrenaline; thiopentone; suxamethonium; a non-depolarizing muscle relaxant.

## Conclusion

This section has been included to familiarize readers with some of the requirements of recompression chambers so that, if possible, future designs of these units will be improved due to collaboration between doctor and engineer. One-person chambers have not been discussed as these are only used for treatment in the most dire circumstances. If fitted with transfer-under-pressure facilities, there is a chance of transporting the patient to a better unit; if not, then the patient is committed to whatever treatment is available. Unfortunately, should an emergency arise within the recompression chamber no help is possible directly to the occupant and it is for this reason that treatment in a one-person chamber should be avoided if possible.

Sophisticated 'one-person' chambers, such as the Sechrist Monoplace Hyperbaric Systems, have been developed and overcome many of these limitations and allow for positioning of the patient, intravenous infusions, cardiopulmonary resuscitation and surgical procedures. Electrodiagnostic monitoring, serum biochemistry and haematology, arterial gas measurements, as well as radiological assessments, are all available with these facilities.

Despite the excellent facilities which are available in most large chamber complexes, the majority of diving accidents are treated under primitive conditions in remote localities. Flexibility and improvisation are necessary and valuable qualities in the diving physician.

# Recommended reading

*Design Manual – Hyperbaric Facilities* (1972). US NAVFAC DM–39.

DORR, V.A. and SCHREINER, H.R. (1969). Region of non-combustion, flammability limits of hydrogen-mixtures, full scale combustion and extinguishing tests and flame-resistant materials. *Report by Ocean Systems Incorporated*, New York.

HAUX, G. (1970). *Tauchtechnik*. Band II. Berlin: Springer-Verlag.

HAUX, G. (1982). *Subsea Manned Engineering*. London: Baillière Tindall.

*Hyperbaric Facilities – General Requirements for Material Certification* (1970). US NAV-SHIPS 0994-007-7010; NAVFAC P422.

JACONSON, J.H. II, MORSCH, J.H.C. and RENDELL-BAKER, L. (1965). The historical perspective of hyperbaric therapy. *Annals of the New York Academy of Science*, 117.

PENZIAS, W. and GOODMAN, M.W. (1973). *Man Beneath the Sea*. New York: Wiley-Interscience.

*US Navy Diving Manual* (1979). NAVSEA 0994-LP-001-9010.

# 39

# Submarine medicine

Dale Molé MD*
Submarine Medical Officer
United States Navy

So they took up Jonah, and cast him forth into the sea: and the sea ceased from raging . . . Now the Lord had prepared a great fish to swallow up Jonah. And Jonah was in the belly of the fish three days and three nights . . . And the Lord spake unto the fish, and it vomited out Jonah upon the dry land.

Jonah, 1 and 2, *King James Version*

## Submarine development

In the eighth century BC, **Jonah** became a reluctant diver, then the world's first submariner, and finally the first submarine escaper, all in a remarkably short period of time. Although highly advanced hydrodynamically, his craft left much to be desired in terms of habitability.

**William Bourne**, an English innkeeper, designed a somewhat more practical method of undersea transportation in 1578. Published but never built, Bourne's design consisted of an air-tight wooden hull fitted with internal cylindrical air chambers, each similar to a giant syringe. To submerge, screw-driven plungers would be withdrawn allowing water to fill the cylinders. The reverse procedure forced the water out, surfacing the craft. A hollow mast would provide fresh air for the submerged boat, predating the German snorkel by some 360 years.

The first submarine actually constructed, an all-wooden craft covered in greased leather,

* Although Dr Dale Molé contributed to this chapter, the views are his personal ones and do not necessarily reflect the views of the US Navy.

was built about 1620. Its builder, a Dutchman named **Cornelis Drebbel**, migrated to England and impressed scholarly King James I to the point of receiving royal patronage. It is speculated that the King was a passenger on at least one underwater excursion. Powered by twelve oarsmen, this prototype submarine had a test depth (maximum depth capability) of 15 feet. A rudimentary atmosphere control system, consisting of lime water to remove carbon dioxide, was thought to have been used. Glass viewports provided enough light when submerged to allow the submariners 'to read the Bible without the aid of candlelight'.

The first practical military submarine was designed and constructed by **David Bushnell**, an American, during his summer break at Yale in 1775; 2.5 metres long and 2 metres high, the oak-timbered craft resembled two gigantic tortoise shells joined together, hence the name **The American Turtle**. Entry was gained through a brass hatch in a small protrusion on top of what formed the conning tower. Glass portholes in the conning tower, some of which could be opened, supplied fresh air and allowed the operator to navigate to his target prior to submersion. A hand crank attached to a four-blade propeller provided propulsion. The rudder, connected to an internal tiller, was used for steering as well as sculling forward. Nine hundred pounds of lead ballast allowed the boat to float in the water with the conning tower almost awash. Two hundred pounds of ballast could be dropped to provide emergency buoyancy, a practice still used by modern submersibles. A valve in the keel admitted water to submerge; forcing pumps ejected it to ascend.

The first operational mission of *The Turtle* was to have occurred during the winter of 1775 in an effort to break the British blockade of Boston Harbor. However, winter frost destroyed the phosphorescent properties of the fox fire wood used to illuminate the compass and the closed tube manometer depth gauge when the vessel was submerged. Use of a candle would consume far too much oxygen as well as compromise the submarine's stealth.

The following year the British fleet left Boston and arrived at New York, strategically located at the mouth of the Hudson River, causing much concern for General Washington. Bombardment of the fleet from shore proved embarrassingly ineffective; *The Turtle* seemed the ideal solution.

On the night of September 6 1776, Sergeant Ezra Lee squeezed into *The Turtle*. He was an inexperienced, hastily trained replacement for Bushnell's brother who contracted the Fever just days previously – not the first nor the last time illness would change the course of military history. His target was the British flagship, *HMS Eagle*, with Admiral Lord Richard 'Black Dick' Howe aboard.

A detachable mine containing 150 pounds of powder was placed aft of the conning tower and two whale boats towed *The Turtle* out into the bay. Lee miscalculated the pull of the tide and was swept past his target. Two and one-half hours later, with the tide slacked, he finally made his way alongside *HMS Eagle*. After making fast the portholes, he operated the foot valve allowing water to flow in and commenced his descent.

Once submerged, the submarine's atmosphere was good for only 30–45 minutes, depending upon the operator's metabolic rate. The task was now to place a detachable screw, secured to the mine by a short lanyard, into the hull of the target. When the submarine backed away, the screw and the mine remained attached to the unwary victim. A 60-minute clockwork delay mechanism allowed the attacker to retire to safety.

When Lee attempted to set the screw, he struck an iron bar connecting the rudder hinge to the stern of the *Eagle*. He now had to reposition a few inches in order to find wood or copper sheathing, which the screw was designed to penetrate. Again his inexperience was almost his undoing. *The Turtle* rapidly shot to the surface out of control, 2 or 3 feet from the hull of *HMS Eagle*, exposed to the spreading light of dawn. Quickly opening the flood valve, he submerged and made a hasty retreat. During his flight he released the mine, which blew up harmlessly one hour later, sending a column of water high into the sky. The explosion caused great alarm and confusion aboard the *Eagle* and the other ships of the British fleet. They instantly cut their cables and drifted in great disarray down the bay with the ebbing tide. Thus ended the first submarine attack in history. (In the interest of historical accuracy, it should be noted that the British account of the incident differs from the one just described.)

After the American War of Independence, the public came to detest submarines and exploding mines as dirty weapons not in keeping with the current standards of fair play. These sentiments were soon extended to designers of such weapons. David Bushnell dropped out of sight, only to reappear in Georgia as Dr David Bush, where he practised medicine as a country doctor until his death in 1826.

Another American inventor, **Robert Fulton**, became interested in submarines. On a visit to France he persuaded Napoleon to part with 10 000 francs for the construction of a submarine to destroy the British fleet. In the summer of 18000, the 21-foot-long, copper-clad, cigar-shaped *Nautilus* made her maiden voyage in the Seine River. Fulton and his propulsion unit (two brawny sailors) successfully reached the surface after a submerged run of 45 minutes. Later Fulton added a compressed air tank to increase the breathing supply.

On her single mission to destroy British warships, the *Nautilus* was unable to reach her objective because of adverse tide conditions. The following summer Fulton tested his submarine by placing a mine against a sloop provided by the French government. The explosion was so violent ' . . . that a Column of Water Smoak and the fibres of the Sloop was cast from 80 to 100 feet in the Air'. Upon observing the demonstration, Admiral de Pelley was horrified. He wrote a report stating the use of submarines was morally indefensible and successfully persuaded colleagues no civilized nation would use such a detestable weapon.

In an effort to obtain British backing, the apolitical Fulton then appealed to British Prime Minister Pitt. The PM enthusiastically referred him to the First Sea Lord, Admiral Sir Earl St Vincent, who candidly stated 'Pitt was the greatest fool that ever existed to encourage a mode of warfare which those who commanded the seas did not want, and which, if successful, would deprive them of it'.

In 1848, war erupted between Denmark and Germany. Danish warships blockaded the north German coast. A Bavarian cavalry corporal, Wilhelm Bauer, decided to build a submarine to break the blockade. He designed a sheet iron craft with a large square porthole on each side and powered by two sailors turning flywheels geared to a propeller. Christened *Brandtaucher*, meaning Surf Diver, it used a heavy weight which ran along a threaded rod to determine the up or down angle (pitch) of the submarine.

Early in 1851, while on a mission in Kiel harbour, Bauer gave the order to submerge. The heavy weight was sent too far forward, creating a steep diving angle. The boat plunged nose first, striking the bottom in 60 feet of water. Water began leaking in at an alarming rate. Bauer correctly reasoned he must flood the submarine to equalize the internal and external pressures before the upper hatch would open. His crew, failing to appreciate the physics involved, not only refused his orders but began to abuse him. As with all good submarine commanders, he abused them to an even greater degree and finally convinced them his way was the only means of salvation. His coercion was aided by men on the surface who, in an attempt to locate the submarine, dropped anchors and grapples which threatened to destroy the portholes. After being entombed some 5 hours, the pressure equalized and the hatch flew open. Bauer and his companions shot up to the surface, becoming the first to make a free ascent from a sunken submarine.

About 10 years later, during the American Civil War, the Union Navy placed a blockade along the Southern coast of the USA to prevent the exchange of goods between the Confederate Estates and Europe. Unable to break the Union stranglehold by conventional means, the Confederate Navy turned to submarines.

The best-known Confederate submarine was the *Hunley*, named after Horace L. Hunley, a wealthy New Orleans cotton merchant who designed and provided financial backing for construction of the boat. The slim, cigar-shaped, 25-foot-long craft, powered by eight men cranking a propeller, ran along on the surface until the last possible moment, then submerged close to the enemy. The torpedo, attached to a long spar protruding from the bow, was to be rammed into place by the full momentum of the submarine. A time delay mechanism allowed the attacker to retreat to safety.

The *Hunley*, badly designed and poorly built, failed to surface while conducting trials in Mobile Bay. Divers found her, but not in time to save the suffocated crew. Despite this setback, the submarine went by rail to Charleston, South Carolina. On 29 August 1863, while cruising on the surface, the *Hunley* passed too near a paddle steamer and swamped, drowning all hands. The submarine was raised, but another crew soon died when the craft's nose became stuck in mud at the bottom of the harbour. After salvaging the submarine a third time, it was decided one last trial was needed. The *Hunley* made a training attack on the Confederate ship, *Indian Chief*. The submarine struck the ship's anchor chain, which came away sending the *Hunley* to the bottom. The entire crew perished, including designer Horace Hunley aboard for the test.

When an opportunity for combat finally arrived, the *Hunley*, affectionately known as 'the coffin', put to sea shorthanded because a crew of eight experienced volunteers could not be found. Under the command of an inexperienced infantry lieutenant, she attacked the Union corvette *Housatonic* on a moonlit night in February 1864. Because the crew feared drowning, the *Hunley* made her final dash to the target just barely awash. Ramming the hull of the *Housatonic* and planting the torpedo, the submarine was preparing to back away when a faulty time delay fired prematurely. The explosion blew a large hole in the *Housatonic* and she sank upright in the bay with the loss of two officers and three crewmen. The *Hunley*, carried partially inside her victim by the rush of water through the recently made hole, sank for the last time, taking her entire crew with her. This marked the end of the Confederate submarine campaign and the first sinking of an enemy warship by a submarine.

By 1870, development of the **self-propelled torpedo** promised a new era in submarine warfare. Alternative forms of energy had to be found to replace human muscle power if the submarine was to become an effective weapon against targets other than nearby ships at anchor. Steam power, an obvious first choice, had the undesirable habit of turning the submarine into an underwater oven when submerged. Electric power was also considered because it was clean, cool and quiet. Its range, limited by the amount of electricity stored in the batteries, proved to be a significant disadvantage.

Another major problem was the lack of **longitudinal stability** when submerged. This is best illustrated by the following account of a steam-powered submarine demonstration conducted for prospective buyers by Thorsten Nordenfelt, a Swedish arms manufacturer, in the harbour at Constantinople, Turkey.

No sooner did one of the crew take two steps forward in the engine room than down went the bow, whereas the hot water in the steam boilers and the cold water in the ballast tanks all ran downhill, increasing the slant still further. English engineers, Turkish engineers, monkey wrenches, hot ashes from the boiler fires, Whitehead torpedos, and other moveables came tumbling after, till the submarine was nearly standing on her head, with everything inside packed into the bow like toys in the toe of a Christmas stocking.

The crew pulled themselves out of this mess and clawed their way aft, till suddenly up came the bow, down went the stern, and everything went gurgling and clattering to the end.

The submarine was a perpetual seesaw, and no mortal power could keep her on an even keel. Once they succeeded in steadying her long enough to fire a torpedo. Where it went no man could tell, but the sudden lightening of the bow and the recoil of the discharge made the submarine rear up and sit down so hard that she began to sink stern foremost, whereupon to correct this condition the water was blown out of her ballast tanks by steam pressure, and the main engine started full speed ahead, till she shot up to the surface like a flying fish.

The Turkish naval authorities, watching the trial from the shores of the Golden Horn, were so impressed by these antics that they bought the boat. But it was impossible to keep a crew on her, for every native engineer or seaman who was sent aboard prudently deserted on the first dark night.

The invention of the **internal combustion engine** (first gasoline, then diesel fuelled), combined with electric power for submerged operation, made the submarine a significant threat in time of war. Submarine design and construction during the late 1800s was dominated by two men – John Holland and Simon Lake.

**John P. Holland**, born in Ireland in 1841, viewed the submarine as a means to crush England's sea power. Holland emigrated to America in 1873 and began experimenting with small submarine designs. He received funds from the notorious Sinn Fein to build the three-man *Fenian Ram* in 1881. The submarine relied on compressed air from air tanks to supply oxygen to the petroleum-powered engine while submerged. Horizontal diving planes controlled depth and subdivided water ballast tanks ensured stability when the hull was at an angle. Factional strife within the Fenian Brotherhood resulted in the *Ram* being stolen and lost at sea. After 10 lean years, Holland formed the Holland Torpedo Boat Company and successfully competed for a US Navy contract to build submarines. The *USS Holland* became the Navy's first submarine. A group of lawyers and businessmen invested in Holland's company and eventually forced him out as manager. Renamed the Electric Boat Company, it is still building submarines for the US Navy today.

**Simon Lake** was born in Pleasantville, New Jersey in 1866. Inspired by his boyhood reading of Jules Verne's *Twenty Thousand Leagues Under the Sea*, he viewed the submarine as a means of **oceanographic exploration**. After losing out to Holland as contractor for the Navy's submarines, he built a crude home-made prototype of his underwater salvage boat, *Argonaut Jr*, as a demonstration for New York businessmen. It resembled a flatiron on wheels. Two large hand-powered wooden wheels on the bow allowed it to crawl along the bottom and a smaller rear wheel provided steering. Composed of water-proof canvas sandwiched between two layers of pitch pine and covered with an outer layer of tar, the submarine used an old carbon dioxide tank purchased from a bankrupt soda fountain owner as a compressed air tank. By exiting through an air lock, Lake could explore the ocean floor attired in a diving suit fashioned from sheet iron and painted canvas. Window-sash weights tied to his legs kept him on the bottom. Lake quickly gained the attention of the press. The public made sufficient contributions to allow him to construct the *Argonaut I*. This gasoline-powered submarine made a 1000-mile voyage, 200 of which were submerged, down the coast of the USA.

Holland and Lake both sold submarines to belligerents in the Russo–Japanese War. The German arms manufacturing firm of Krupp offered Lake a contract. Although never signed, it provided them time to copy his designs. On September 22 1914, a single German U-boat sank three British cruisers in just over an hour, sending 1400 sailors to a watery grave. The age of modern submarine warfare had arrived.

The submarine continued to be refined throughout two world wars. In 1955, the launching of the nuclear-powered *USS Nautilus* ushered in the era of the true submarine, i.e. a vessel able to operate completely independently of the surface. The Fleet Ballistic Missile Submarine, capable of not only sinking ships but destroying entire countries, soon followed.

## Submarine habitability

Advances in submarine technology resulted in submarine crews spending more time at sea and enduring longer periods of submergence. Improvements in submarine habitability were mandated by the need to maintain the physical and mental health of the submariner.

One of the most important aspects of submarine habitability is being able to maintain a **breathable atmosphere** when submerged. By design, most nuclear submarines are required to do this for 90 days without surfacing, while some conventionally powered European submarines are now able to run submerged for up to 2 weeks. Two important aspects of the submarine air quality are atmosphere control and monitoring.

Submarine atmosphere control systems are designed to provide oxygen to replenish that used by the crew and to remove waste gases and contaminants which would otherwise increase to physiologically undesirable concentrations. Assuming normal submarine activities, about 30 litres of oxygen is consumed per man hour. Using a respiratory quotient of 0.85, this results in the production of about 25 litres of carbon dioxide per man per hour. Major sources of air contamination include cigarette smoking (up to 50% of the particulates and most of the carbon monoxide), the human body (carbon dioxide and methane) and cooking (volatile decomposition products from deep-fat friers). Other sources include fluorinated hydrocarbons from refrigeration and air-conditioning systems, vapours from cleaning solvents, hydrocarbons from lubricants and bacteriological aerosols from sanitary tanks.

A breathable atmosphere is maintained by exchanging shipboard air with outdoor air,

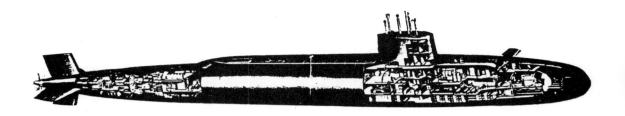

**Figure 39.1** *HMS Resolution*, an example of a modern nuclear-powered ballistic missile submarine. With a displacement of 8000 tons, she is 130 metres long and has a crew of 157

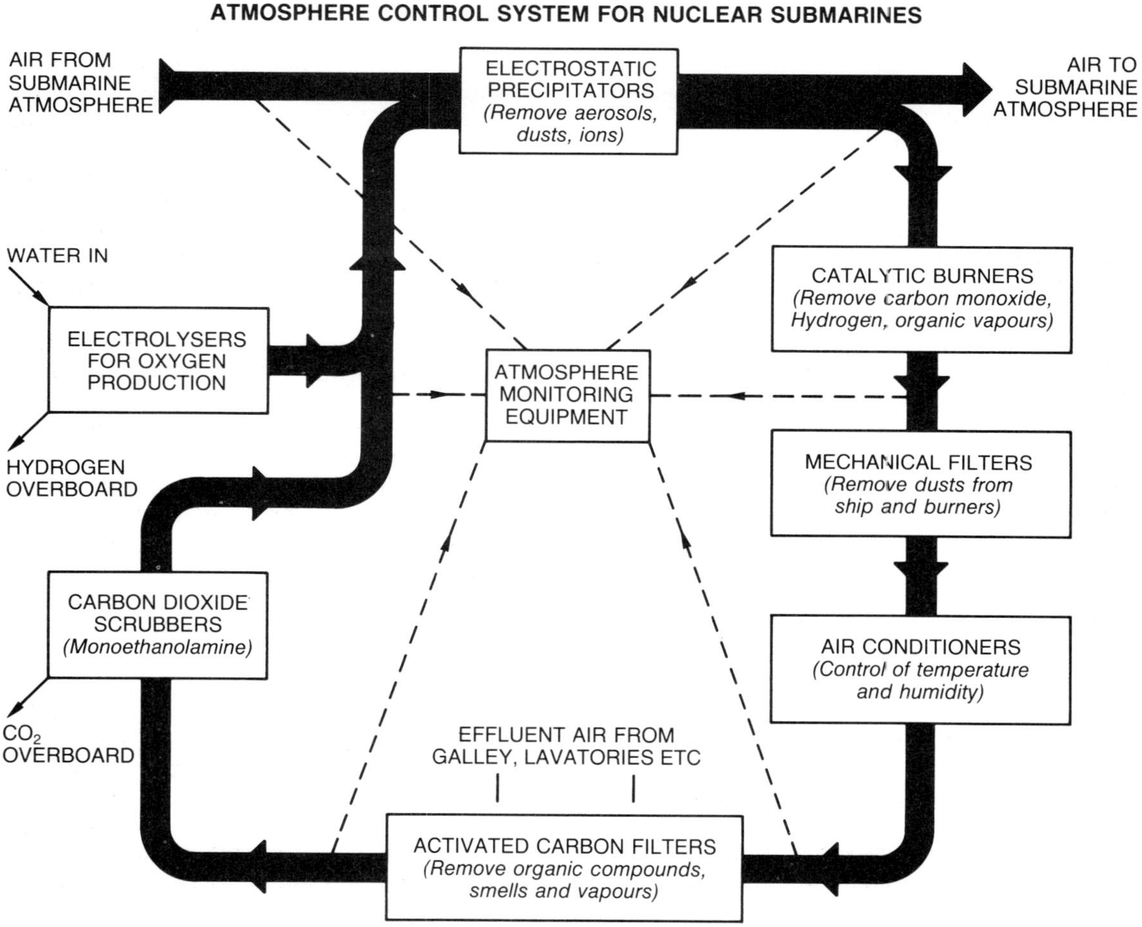

## ATMOSPHERE CONTROL SYSTEM FOR NUCLEAR SUBMARINES

AIR FROM SUBMARINE ATMOSPHERE

AIR TO SUBMARINE ATMOSPHERE

ELECTROSTATIC PRECIPITATORS
*(Remove aerosols, dusts, ions)*

WATER IN

ELECTROLYSERS FOR OXYGEN PRODUCTION

HYDROGEN OVERBOARD

ATMOSPHERE MONITORING EQUIPMENT

CATALYTIC BURNERS
*(Remove carbon monoxide, Hydrogen, organic vapours)*

MECHANICAL FILTERS
*(Remove dusts from ship and burners)*

CARBON DIOXIDE SCRUBBERS
*(Monoethanolamine)*

$CO_2$ OVERBOARD

AIR CONDITIONERS
*(Control of temperature and humidity)*

EFFLUENT AIR FROM GALLEY, LAVATORIES ETC

ACTIVATED CARBON FILTERS
*(Remove organic compounds, smells and vapours)*

**Figure 39.2** Diagram of one type of integrated atmosphere control system employed in nuclear submarines

restricting materials and activities permitted on board, and providing equipment to generate oxygen as well as remove contaminants.

**Ventilating**, the exchange of shipboard air with outdoor air, is simple, efficient and the least costly method of atmosphere control. It ensures that the concentrations of all contaminants are uniformly low, including those which cannot be removed by air purification equipment. Submerged submarines accomplish this by snorting, i.e. ventilating through the snorkel. The snorting time required to remove the contaminants is directly proportional to the internal (floodable) volume of the submarine and inversely proportional to the ventilation air flow rate.

Restricting the use or presence of certain materials on board minimizes the risk of particular air contaminants. Materials are usually classified as 'Permitted' (items with no use restrictions), 'Limited' (items which might be toxic, but for which there is no non-toxic substitute), 'Restricted' (items containing substantial amounts of toxic substances which are not allowed on board while a submarine is under way), and 'Prohibited' (items not allowed on submarines, except by special exemption). Restricted activities include welding, brazing and painting while the submarine is under way.

Atmosphere control equipment may include oxygen-generating apparatus, carbon dioxide scrubbers, carbon monoxide and hydrogen burners, activated charcoal filters and electrostatic precipitators.

Submarines with oxygen generators obtain oxygen through the electrolysis of water. The oxygen is then stored in high-pressure flasks for later use. Hydrogen formed during this process is discharged overboard. In an emergency, or for those submarines without oxygen generators, oxygen can be produced by burning sodium chlorate candles. Each candle burns for about 45 minutes and produces 115 cubic feet of oxygen. Small quantities of chlorine and carbon monoxide are also produced, 10 and 25 parts per million respectively.

Carbon dioxide can be removed by passing the submarine atmosphere through a regenerative scrubber which uses monoethanolamine (MEA) as the working fluid. MEA absorbs carbon dioxide when cold and releases it when heated. The liberated carbon dioxide is dumped overboard. Disadvantages include the production of small amounts of ammonia and other contaminants and the scrubber's inability always to maintain the desired low level of atmospheric carbon dioxide. In emergency situations or aboard submarines without MEA scrubbers, carbon dioxide is removed by chemically combining it with lithium hydroxide (US) or soda-lime (UK).

Catalytic oxidation, in a bed of copper oxide and manganese dioxide, converts carbon monoxide from burning cigarettes and human metabolism into carbon dioxide. It also converts hydrogen resulting from battery charging operations into water. Proper operation requires the catalytic bed temperature to be maintained at 600°F which can convert atmospheric flurocarbons into acidic contaminants. High-molecular-weight hydrocarbons and odours are removed by beds of activated charcoal. The main bed is located by the main circulating fan, with other beds in the galley, washrooms and above sanitary tanks. Electrostatic precipitators are installed in the ventilation system to remove solid and liquid aerosols. The precipitators produce ozone and nitrous oxide contaminants in small quantities.

Submarine atmosphere monitoring has made tremendous advances since the days when white mice were carried on submarines as biological monitors and entered on the payroll as part of the crew. Submariners spent many enjoyable hours debating whether the mouse alarm behaviour (first squeaking, then supinating their little feet) indicated the presence of carbon monoxide from exhaust gases or gasoline leaking from the injectors.

Many submarines now use a **central atmosphere monitoring system (CAMS)**. This system includes a dual isotope, fluorescence, nondispersive, infrared spectrophotometer to measure carbon monoxide and a fixed collector mass spectrometer to monitor oxygen, nitrogen, carbon dioxide, hydrogen, water vapour and several fluorocarbons. The CAMS monitors air samples from throughout the submarine and activates an alarm if out-of-tolerance conditions exist. For substances not measured by the CAMS, or on submarines which do not use a CAMS, other detection methods are available – Draeger tubes (see page 273.

# Deep submersibles

The term 'submersible' is commonly used to refer to normobaric underwater vehicles having an operating time of the order of hours and requiring a support vessel. A convenient starting place for the history of the **deep submergence vehicle (DSV)** is the bathysphere of **Dr William Beebe**.

Dr Beebe, an ornithologist for the New York Zoological Society, became interested in studying marine life. While diving off the coast of Bermuda, he became aware of the limitations of using existing techniques to study deep ocean life. He interested a wealthy engineer, Otis Barton, in the idea of constructing a deep sea observation chamber. The bathysphere was constructed of 1.25-inch steel and had three round observation windows of 3-inch thick fused quartz. An external diameter of only 57 inches made the sphere quite cramped considering it must hold Beebe, Barton, two oxygen cylinders, trays of calcium chloride to absorb moisture and soda lime to absorb carbon dioxide. A steel cable 3500 feet long and slightly less than 1 inch in diameter was all that prevented the 5400 pound bathysphere and its occupants from plunging to the ocean floor. In August of 1934, with only a dozen turns of the cable remaining on the winch drum, Beebe and Barton reached a depth of 3028 feet. A full and fascinating account may be read in Beebe's (1951) book, *Half Mile Down*.

A Swiss physics professor, **Auguste Piccard**, famous for his balloon ascents into the stratosphere, decided he also wanted to explore the deep ocean. Not trusting a steel cable to support his submersible, he adapted the principle of the aerial balloon to undersea exploration. An underwater balloon of thin sheet metal filled with gasoline, having a lower specific gravity than sea water, provided buoyancy for a heavy steel sphere suspended beneath. A heavy load of ballast allowed him to descend. By releasing part of the ballast, he could stop his descent upon reaching the desired depth. Piccard's work, which began in 1937, reached its culmination on January 23, 1960, when his son Jacques and US Navy Lieutenant Don Walsh descended 35 800 feet into the Challenger Deep of the Mariana Trench off the coast of Guam.

Modern submersibles do not require large gasoline-filled floats. Buoyancy is achieved by using light-weight, high-strength materials. The designer's goal is maximum buoyancy with minimum weight.

The heart of the submersible is the pressure hull. Its characteristics determine the ultimate safe diving depth. Most pressure hulls are either spherical or cylindrical. The sphere offers the most favourable weight to displacement ratio and evenly distributes the external pressure over its entire surface. The cylinder offers easy fabrication and low drag, but requires internal stiffeners for deeper depth capability. Hull materials commonly used are high yield strength (HY) steel or titanium. The **deep submergence rescue vehicle (DSRV)** pressure hull, with an operating depth of 5000 feet, uses HY-140 steel, i.e. the yield strength is 140 000 pounds per square inch.

In most designs, additional buoyancy is provided by syntactic foam. Composed of millions of tiny glass microspheres embedded in an epoxy resin, syntactic foam can withstand tremendous pressure without being crushed. It can be cut into many shapes, filling any void between the pressure hull and the glass-fibre reinforced plastic fairing which provides the vehicle with hydrodynamic streamlining.

Viewports are generally made of acrylic plastic. The plastic exhibits certain flow characteristics allowing redistribution of stresses and providing warning of impending failure in time to terminate the dive. Glass viewports can fail catastrophically without warning.

Life-support systems aboard a DSV generally consist of an oxygen source and a method of removing carbon dioxide. High-pressure gaseous oxygen is more commonly used, and is manually or automatically added or 'bled' into the cabin to maintain the partial pressure of oxygen at around 160 mmHg.

Other methods of providing oxygen include burning chlorate candles, using superoxides which absorb carbon dioxide and release oxygen, and cryogenic storage. An emergency oxygen system is also available should the cabin atmosphere become contaminated. Carbon dioxide is usually removed by fan-driven scrubbers which circulate the cabin atmosphere through canisters containing a granular chemical absorbent similar to that used in closed circuit diving rigs, i.e. lithium hydroxide or soda lime.

The major limitation for small submersibles is lack of an adequate power supply. Lead acid batteries have traditionally been used as a source of electric power, but are being replaced in some applications by zinc–silver cells offering a much greater power density. Most batteries, with the exception of some cells powering emergency equipment, are mounted outside the pressure hull and could be jettisoned if emergency buoyance is required.

Submersible propulsion is provided by electric or hydraulic motors driving propellers. The DSV *Sea Cliff* uses two hydraulic power units to power the stern propulsion units. Manoeuvrability is more important than absolute speed because most deep submergence work is performed near the ocean floor.

Submersibles are usually equipped with external lights, video cameras and recorders, and still cameras. Apart from making observations, DSVs can be equipped with manipulator arms allowing them to perform mechanical work at great depths. The *Sea Cliff*, with a 20 000 foot capability, has two electrohydraulic manipulators which can be fitted with a variety of tools, including a drill, a cable cutter, scissors and parallel jaws for retrieving small objects from the sea floor. Small shallower diving submersibles have provision for diver lockout.

# Submarine escape and rescue

Submarines operate in a hostile, unforgiving environment and on occasion disaster befalls them. Fortunately, this happens with much less frequency than was the case in the early days of submarine history. Since the turn of the century well over 100 non-combat-related subsunk incidents have occurred with the loss of almost 3000 submariners, most in water shallower than 100 metres. These incidents are more likely to occur over the continental shelf because of the increased risks associated with sea trials, submerging and surfacing evolutions, and transiting in areas with high sea traffic density, such as near major seaports. Subsunk mishaps in deep water often result in the submarine sinking beyond hull crush depth

and, because there are no survivors requiring treatment, are of less interest to the diving medical officer.

There are basically three methods by which submarine or submersible crews can be saved: salvage, escape or rescue.

## Submarine salvage

Prior to the twentieth century, submarines were still in their infancy and the possibility of being drowned was considered an occupational hazard. Submariners were viewed as 'pirates' by the majority of the world's navies and, if a few were to die in their unproven craft, little attention was paid.

Due to the fact that submarines were relatively small, they could often be grappled and hoisted to the surface following an accident. In 1904 the British submarine *A1* sank and was rapidly located by divers. Lines were attached to lift her, but the weather worsened and it took 5 weeks before she was raised. The following year the French submarine *Farfadet* sank with 14 crewmen known to be still alive. Salvage ships prepared to raise her, but heavy weather intervened for 3 days. Upon returning to the scene, divers tapping on the hull received no reply.

Rescue salvage does occasionally work. In 1917, the British submarine *K13* sank in Gareloch off the north bank of the Clyde just below Dumbarton, after boiler room ventilators were mistakenly left open. All her after compartments were flooded, but 47 survivors remained alive in the forends. Salvors were able to raise the bow clear of the water and cut through the hull with oxyacetylene torches. After being trapped for 54 hours, all the survivors were able to climb out through the opening to freedom.

About this same time the Danish submarine *Dykkeren* sank in the Skagerrak after being struck by a merchant ship. Some of the crew escaped, but five remained trapped in the bow. Salvage ships were able to raise the forward hatch clear of the water. All five scrambled to safety just as the lifting wires parted and the submarine sank back to the bottom.

Rescue by salvage is much more difficult today given the size of modern submarines. Success depends on being fortunate enough to sink in close proximity to a seaport with major salvage capabilities. It is still a feasible method of rescuing small submersibles, assuming another submersible or **remotely operated vehicle** (ROV) can attach a lifting line or cut through entangling wires to free the trapped craft.

In November 1989, the submersible *Turtle* became fouled in some lines on the ocean floor in 1300 feet of water off the coast of San Diego. A remotely operated vehicle provided topside observers with real-time video. They were able to give rudder orders to the trapped submersible, allowing her to manoeuvre free from the entangling cables. Fortunately, the *Turtle* has a life-support system duration of 72 hours for her three-person crew and a survival kit containing food, water and space blankets. The crew also minimized any unnecessary activity.

## Submarine escape

In North America, soon after the *A1* sinking, experiments were conducted on methods of individual escape. The only escape technique officially sanctioned was **compartment escape**. This technique entails deliberately flooding the compartment to equalize pressures. Each person then dons a life jacket, 'looks his companions steadfastly in the eyes', takes a deep breath and ducks under the steel skirt permanently fitted to the hatch. With luck he will float to the surface. Unfortunately, this method exposes the fellow survivors to ambient seawater pressure and temperature while awaiting their turn to escape, reducing the odds for survival. For this reason, individual escape became an attractive alternative. Although submarine escape trunks had yet to be developed, torpedo tubes provided a natural air-lock.

In 1940, two large dogs were ejected out of the torpedo tube of the *USS Shark*. They were later discovered swimming happily around on the surface. Five years later, Ensign Kenneth Whiting made the first successful human escape from a torpedo tube and performed the first deliberately planned experiment involving human escape from a submarine. This apparently developed into a sport within the US Submarine Service, as soon not only were others escaping, but also swimming down from the surface and entering the submarine through the torpedo tube at depths of as great as 40 feet.

In August 1916, Stoker Petty Officer Brown found himself alone in the engine room of His Majesty's Submarine *E41*, after she had been rammed and sunk by her sister ship in 45 feet of water. Brown began flooding his compartment to equalize the pressure across the after-hatch. The rising water shorted some of the energized circuits, shocking him severely whenever he touched metal. The battery compartment, flooded with sea water, began producing chlorine gas. As the pressure equalized, the hatch would pop open, release an air bubble and slam shut. This process repeated several times and, on one occasion, much to the dismay of Stoker Brown, the hatch slammed shut on his hand, crushing his fingers. Exercising great tenacity, he finally managed to effect his escape just as the small air pocket remaining in the engine room had all but disappeared.

The British were the first to develop and adopt a submarine escape appliance for fleet use. The hope was to increase the escaper's chance for survival by providing a means of breathing as well as flotation. The Germans and the Americans followed with their own variations. The US Navy soon realized their escape apparatus, the '**Momsen Lung**', was dangerous in the hands of untrained submariners. In 1920 the first submarine escape training tower was constructed in New London, followed 2 years later by another in Pearl Harbor. While in operation, each 135 foot tall tank allowed thousands of submariners to practise submarine escape in a controlled environment.

Shortly after World War II, the British formed the Ruck–Keene Committee to investigate survival from British, German and American submarine disasters. It concluded that the odds of successful escape were greatest when the escaper made a free ascent unencumbered by the presently available escape apparatus. Continued research and development in submarine escape resulted in the three methods recognized today: free ascent, blowing buoyant ascent and free breathing buoyant ascent.

For **free ascent** (escape without apparatus), the escaper relies upon the natural buoyancy of air in his lungs to carry him towards the surface. Exhaling too slowly risks pulmonary barotrauma and air embolism; exhaling too quickly results in loss of buoyancy and the unfortunate escaper sinks.

**Blowing buoyant ascent** involves additional flotation, usually an inflatable vest. The escaper exhales continuously until reaching the surface. This technique provides faster ascent rates and requires much less training than free ascent. Dr George Bond (1963) conducted alveolar gas exchange studies during buoyant ascent. He demonstrated alveolar carbon dioxide partial pressures were approximately the same prior to and immediately following buoyant ascent and arterial oxygen saturation remained almost normal. This held true as long as the escaper kept the volume of air in his lungs between resting lung volume and total lung capacity during ascent. The result is little or no desire to breathe even when ascending from relatively great depths.

**Free breathing buoyant ascent** requires an apparatus which provides buoyancy and an air pocket around the escaper's head, allowing him to breathe during ascent. The US Navy has been using the Steinke Hood since 1963. It consists of an inflatable vest with a hood to cover the escaper's head. After equalizing the escape trunk to ambient ocean pressure, the escaper inflates the vest and hood from a charging valve and then exits the submarine. During ascent, expanding air from the vest is vented into the hood, ensuring a continuous supply of fresh air. The escaper is instructed to breathe normally throughout the ascent. Unfortunately, the apparatus gives little thermal protection, making prolonged survival immersed in cold water unlikely.

The British have developed an individual escape system which not only provides thermal protection but allows successful ascents from depths as great as 180 metres. It has proved so successful that many other navies have adopted it for use. It consists of a **submarine escape immersion suit** (SEIS), which completely encloses the escaper in a water-tight exposure suit, and a one-person or two-person escape tower.

The rubberized cotton suit has a double-walled insulating layer which is inflated upon reaching the surface and is designed to provide sufficient thermal protection to allow survival in cold water for up to 24 hours.

The **escape towers** are located in the forward and aft compartments and are just large enough for two escapers to stand erect. Egress is from a top hatch which can be set to an open, shut or idle position from inside the submarine. The escaper enters the tower from below and plugs his hood and stole inflation hose into a spring loaded receptacle supplied by the **hood inflation system** (HIS) valve. This provides air at between 1 and 2 pounds per square inch over ambient pressure. While the trunk is being flooded, a vent located 27 inches below the upper hatch allows air to be displaced into the submarine, preventing pressurization of the tower. When the proper flood level is reached, the tenders close the vent valve and pressurize the tower. The average time to compress from sea level to 180 metres is 21 seconds. Once equalization occurs, the upper hatch opens and the escaper ascends to the surface at a rate of 2–3 metres per second.

The rapid compression rates are necessary to 'out run' the physiologically disastrous effects of breathing air under high pressure, i.e. central nervous system oxygen toxicity, nitrogen narcosis and decompression sickness. The primary physiological consequence of this rapid change in pressure is the possibility of barotrauma to the tympanic membranes or sinuses (see Chapter 10); the lungs are equalized by simply inhaling. Most escapers will not be able to equalize quickly enough to prevent tympanic membrane rupture; however with such rapid compression rates, it is reported to be relatively painless. In fact, during a recent British escape exercise, one escaper was unaware he had ruptured an eardrum until he experienced vertigo while relaxing in a swimming pool the following day.

Escape from small submersibles is possible, but highly unlikely from all but the shallowest of depths. A remarkable story of escape from a two-person submersible occurred in 1970 off the California coast. Dr Richard Slater and another man were in a submersible attempting to raise a speed boat sunk in 225 feet of water. After securing lift lines, the speed boat was hoisted by a large ship on the surface. As the boat was raised, it slipped its liners and dropped back down through the sea. It landed on the submersible, smashing the porthole beside Dr Slater's face. Knocked unconscious by the blow, he was soon revived by the flood of cold water. Taking one last breath before the craft completely flooded, he opened the hatch and pushed off. Being an experienced diver, Slater blew out air as he floated up. The last thing he remembers thinking was 'It's a long way up, it's a long way to go'. He arrived at the surface unconscious, but fortunately he bobbed up near two men in a dinghy. He regained consciousness several hours later. Unfortunately, his companion did not reach the surface alive.

## Submarine rescue

When a submarine in distress sinks beyond a depth that precludes successful escape, the only option remaining is to await rescue. Despite the extreme psychological and physiological stresses they have experienced, the survivors must take immediate action to alert search and rescue forces as to their fate and remain alive until assistance arrives.

Submarines in distress have a number of methods of signalling. Many carry emergency radio-transmitting buoys, either external to the hull or released through the signal ejector. The radio signals are then received by aircraft or search and rescue satellites. The main sonar system, if still operative, or specially designed emergency sonar homing beacons, may be used. Submarines have underwater telephones which can be heard for several miles under water and could provide valuable information concerning the number, condition and location of survivors, and the status of life-support stores. Tapping on the hull is a well-proven method of communication which has been used as long as submarines have been sinking. Unfortunately, it results in greatly increased oxygen consumption and carbon dioxide production by the sender. Submarines may also release signal flares, dye, oil, debris or air into the water to assist rescue forces in their location efforts.

Staying alive until rescue can be effected is the primary objective of the survivors. This is complicated by the reality that most modern submarines do not sink unless they experience significant flooding, either from collision or failure of main seawater systems. Because the submarine is a closed system, flooding will compress the internal atmosphere and trans-form the submariners into reluctant air saturation divers. The effects of elevated partial pressures of oxygen, nitrogen and any contaminant gases will not only reduce the submariners' chances for survival, but also make rescue efforts more difficult. Internal pressurization may also result from the use of emergency air breathing (EAB) apparatus by the crew if the submarine atmosphere is contaminated.

The physiological consequences of breathing oxygen at elevated partial pressures is well explained in Chapter 18. Of most concern is pulmonary oxygen toxicity. It has been demonstrated that healthy experimental subjects exposed to 5 ATA air for 48 hours will suffer significant symptoms of pulmonary oxygen toxicity, but will recover without sequelae. It is doubtful if this holds true for longer exposures. One mitigating factor is the decrease in oxygen partial pressure as the survivors 'breathe down' or metabolize oxygen. The rate of reduction depends upon the size of the compartment, and the number and metabolic rate of the submariners.

Elevated nitrogen partial pressures not only hamper survival but complicate rescue. Nitrogen produces narcosis in a dose-dependent fashion causing cognitive and psychomotor disturbances (see Chapter 15). This can significantly impair the abilities of the crew to take the necessary steps to ensure survival. Nitrogen is also absorbed by body tissues until equilibrium is achieved with the new partial pressure. This requires that extensive arrangements be made for an on-site saturation decompression of the survivors once they are rescued. Direct ascent to one atmosphere without symptoms of decompression sickness has been shown to be possible if the air saturation occurs at pressures of less than 1.7 ATA.

Perhaps the greatest threat to survival is the production of carbon dioxide. In most rescue scenarios this will be the limiting factor. Chapter 19 provides an account of the signs and symptoms of carbon dioxide toxicity.

Carbon monoxide, a lethal contaminant (see Chapter 20), results from incomplete combustion and is produced in great quantities by fires occurring aboard submarines. Small quantities are produced by human metabolic processes at a rate of 0.3–1.0 ml/h and may be enough to cause concern when a large number of people are crowded into a small enclosed space.

Hypothermia is a significant problem and is the result of direct exposure to flooding water and the increased conductive properties of pressurized air. In all but the most tropical waters, the internal submarine temperature will begin to fall until an equilibrium is reached with the ambient ocean temperature. The rate of cooling depends upon the compartment size, number of survivors, the amount of hull insulation, the temperature of any machinery in the compartment prior to the mishap and the water temperature. Shivering thermogenesis, while maintaining body temperature, is accompanied by a three- to four-fold increase in oxygen consumption and an equivalent rise in carbon dioxide production.

Several types of rescue devices are presently available to save trapped submariners. They can be conveniently divided into rescue chambers and rescue vehicles.

The **submarine rescue chamber (SRC)** concept was proposed by Sir Robert H. Davis in 1917. The idea was to lower the SRC down to the submarine and secure it to the escape hatch using divers. This allows the survivors to leave the disabled submarine without exposure to ambient sea pressure. Lieutenant Charles Momsen, of 'Momsen Lung' fame, made a similar suggestion following the loss of the American submarine *S-4*. Together with Allen McCann, he developed the US version of the SRC which, unveiled in 1931, successfully rescued submariners from the *USS Squalus*.

On 24 May 1939, the *USS Squalus* was conducting sea trials when a malfunction of the main air-induction valve caused massive flooding, sending her to the bottom in 243 feet of water. Twenty-six of her crew trapped aft died immediately; however, 33 remained alive in the forward compartments. Divers attached a downhaul cable to the forward hatch and the SRC winched down into position. After being trapped for 40 hours, the first survivors left the submarine cocooned in the SRC. Three additional trips were required to rescue the remaining crew.

The SRC is still in service today, relatively unchanged. It consists of two chambers separated by a pressure-tight hatch and is capable of performing rescues at depths as deep as 850 feet. The upper chamber is designed to house two operators and six rescuees per trip. The lower chamber is open to the sea at the bottom and contains a flat matting surface fitted with a rubber gasket which makes a water-tight seal over the submarine hatch. An umbilical from the support ship provides air, electricity and telephone. Because the SRC maintains a positive buoyancy of 1000 pounds, an air-powered downhaul winch is used to haul it into place over the hatch. Once in position, the lower chamber is dewatered using high-pressure air, four hold-down turnbuckle rods are attached and the submarine hatch is then opened. Once back on the surface, the SRC remains in the water and rescuees exit through the upper hatch.

Rescue vehicles have been constructed by many nations including the United Kingdom, Sweden, Japan, Italy, the Soviet Union and the United States of America. The **American deep submergence rescue vehicle** (DSRV) is representative of this type of rescue system.

The DSRV is an air-transportable rescue vehicle designed to operate from a mother submarine or specially constructed surface support ships. It consists of three interconnected 90-inch diameter HY-140 steel spheres which form the pressure hull and provide an operational depth of 5000 feet of sea water. The forward sphere is the control sphere where the pilot and co-pilot reside. The mid and aft spheres are designed to accommodate one operator and 12 rescuees each. There are water-tight hatches between each sphere. A free-flooding, glass-reinforced, plastic fairing covers the pressure hull and external equipment such as batteries, hydraulic and ballast systems. A framework of titanium and aluminium forms the principal load-bearing structure and syntactic form sections provide additional buoyancy. Silver–zinc batteries supply enough electric power for two or three round trips from the support vessel to the disabled submarine. A three-bladed shrouded propeller provides main propulsion at speeds of up to 4.1 knots as well as control of both pitch and yaw. There are also four ducted thrusters which provide low speed manoeuvrability. A mercury trim and list system controls roll and can be used to set and hold pitch angles of up to 45 degrees. Navigation and sensor systems provide long- and short-range search, position keeping and obstacle avoidance capability. In addition to sonar, there are pan and tilt video cameras, periscopes, a mechanical optics column and viewports.

During a rescue operation, the mating system allows the transfer of rescuees from the disabled submarine to the midsphere of the DSRV via the transfer skirt which is rated to 2000 feet. After the skirt and escape hatch mating surfaces are approximated, the skirt is dewatered and the submarine upper hatch opened. Up to 24 rescuees are embarked, the skirt flooded, and the DSRV returns to the mother submarine or surface support ship to unload the survivors. Life-support systems are designed to operate for up to 12 hours with a full load of rescuees aboard.

If the disabled submarine is pressurized, the DSRV is designed to withstand internal pressures as high as 5 ATA. When operating with British mother submarines, the DSRV is able to mate with the forward hatch and transfer rescuees under pressure to the bow compartment pressurized up to 2 ATA. The US Navy maintains two specially designed surface support ships that have decompression facilities which would allow decompression of saturated rescuees.

During a recent Anglo-American submarine rescue exercise, the British submersible, *LR5*, performed the first pressurized transfer of personnel from a simulated disabled submarine to a mother submarine. The 'rescuees' were then afforded controlled decompression in the bow compartment.

## Recommended reading

ADKISSION, G. and RAFFAELLI, P. (1988). *SUBSUNK: Notes for Medical Officers*. Alverstoke: Institute of Naval Medicine.

BEEBE, W. (1951). *Half Mile Down*. New York: Duell, Sloan and Pierce.

COMPTON-HALL, R. (1988). *Submarine vs Submarine*. London: Grub Street.

FRIEDMAN, N. (1984). *Submarine Design and Development*. Annapolis: Naval Institute Press.

LIMBURG, P.R. and SWEENEY, J.B. (1973). *Vessels for Underwater Exploration*. New York: Crown Publishers.

MOLE, D. (1990). *Submarine Escape and Rescue: An Overview*. San Diego: Commander Submarine Development Group One.

NATIONAL RESEARCH COUNCIL (1988). *Submarine Air Quality*. Washington: National Academy Press.

PICCARD, J. and DIETZ, R.S. (1961). *Seven Miles Down: The Story of the Bathyscaph TRIESTE*. New York: Putnam.

SHELFORD, W. (1960). *SUBSUNK: The Story of Submarine Escape*. New York: Doubleday & Company.

# Appendices

**Caution**: the reader is advised to consult the original source of any table used. The authors have no way of transferring any changes to the reader or of correcting any errors discovered after publication. Also some tables have been condensed and information that may be important to a user omitted.

## Appendix I British Sub-Aqua Club (BSAC) decompression tables

The complete version of the 1988 BSAC tables consist of seven tables for diving in the altitude range from sea level to 250 metres. The first three are printed here with the permission of the BSAC and Dr Tom Hennessy who developed them. It should be noted that the tables are a copyright document. The information presented here is to assist the reader in assessing if a diver has followed the tables. The complete tables are available in a waterproof booklet from the BSAC (16 Upper Woburn Place, London).

For his first dive, the diver uses Table A; the table is entered on the left-hand side with the depth, the deepest depth reached during the dive. The diver then looks across to find the dive time. This is the time from leaving the surface to reaching 6 metres on the return to the surface (or reaching 9 metres if a 9-metre decompression stop is required). The time used should be the next longer tabulated if the exact time of the dive is not listed.

If the dive is to the left of the line that separates No-stop from Decompression stops the diver can surface at a rate of 15 metres/min to 6 metres and 6 metres/min for the last 6 metres.

If the dive is on the decompression side of the table then the decompression stop(s) listed below the time are to be taken. The diver may then ascend to the surface at the stipulated rate.

At the foot of each table is a series of letters in a row entitled surfacing code. This is an estimate of the nitrogen load at the end of the dive. To allow for any nitrogen remaining from previous dives the diver uses the Surface Interval Table (page 517) and enters on the line that starts wih his surfacing code. For example if his surfacing code was F he goes to line F. The surface interval till the next dive is found and another letter found called the current tissue code. For example, a diver who surfaced in group F and then spends between 90 min and 4 hours on the surface is in group C. This means he should use Table C for the next dive.

For example, a diver wishes to make two dives to 18 metres with a surface interval of 2 hours. How long can each dive be without having to make decompression stops? What decompression stops are needed if the dive time for the second dive is to be 50 min?

Table A is used for the first dive. It will be found that the longest time allowed before decompression is required is 51 min. It should be noted that the diver has to be back at 6 metres by that time. To get there it would be necessary to leave the bottom 50 min after leaving the surface. On returning to the surface the diver is in surface code F. In the surface interval table for a diver that surfaces in group F it will be found that the diver is in group C after 2 hours.

Table C is used for the second dive. It will be found that the second dive can be for no longer than 15 minutes if decompression stops are to be avoided. If the dive time for the second dive is to be 50 min the decompression required is 21 min at 6 metres.

The complete BSAC tables also contain altitude tables and rules for flying after diving.

## Table A

| Depth (metres) | Ascent time (min) | Dive time (minutes) | | | | | | | | | | | | |
|---|---|---|---|---|---|---|---|---|---|---|---|---|---|---|
| | | No-stop dives | | | | | Decompression stop dives | | | | | | | |
| **3** | (1) | – | 166 | ∞ | | | | | | | | | | |
| **6** | (1) | – | 36 | 166 | 593 | ∞ | | | | | | | | |
| **9** | 1 | – | 17 | 67 | 167 | 203 | 243 | 311 | 328 | 336 | 348 | 356 | 363 | 370 | 376 |
| **12** | 1 | – | 10 | 37 | 87 | 104 | 122 | 156 | 169 | 177 | 183 | 188 | 192 | 197 | 201 |
| **15** | 1 | – | 6 | 24 | 54 | 64 | 74 | 98 | 109 | 116 | 121 | 125 | 129 | 133 | 136 |
| **18** | 1 | | – | 17 | 37 | 44 | 51 | 68 | 78 | 84 | 88 | 92 | 95 | 98 | 101 |
| Decompression stop (minutes) at **6 metres** | | | | | | | | 1 | 3 | 6 | 9 | 12 | 15 | 18 | 21 |
| Surfacing code | | **B** | **C** | **D** | **E** | **F** | **G** | **G** | **G** | **G** | **G** | **G** | **G** | **G** |

| Depth (metres) | Ascent time (min) | Dive time (minutes) | | | | | | | | | | | | |
|---|---|---|---|---|---|---|---|---|---|---|---|---|---|---|
| **21** | 1 | – | 13 | 28 | 32 | 37 | 51 | 59 | 65 | 68 | 72 | 75 | 77 | |
| **24** | 2 | – | 11 | 22 | 26 | 30 | 41 | 49 | 53 | 56 | 59 | 62 | 64 | |
| **27** | 2 | – | 8 | 18 | 21 | 24 | 34 | 41 | 45 | 47 | 50 | 52 | 55 | |
| **30** | 2 | – | 7 | 15 | 17 | 20 | 29 | 35 | 39 | 41 | 43 | 45 | 47 | |
| **33** | 2 | – | 13 | 15 | 17 | 25 | 30 | 34 | 36 | 38 | 40 | 42 | | |
| **36** | 2 | – | 11 | 12 | 14 | 22 | 27 | 30 | 32 | 34 | 36 | 37 | | |
| **39** | 3 | – | 10 | 12 | 13 | 20 | 25 | 29 | 30 | 32 | 33 | 35 | | |
| Decompression stops (minutes) at **9 metres** | | | | | | | | | 1 | 1 | 1 | 1 | 2 | |
| at **6 metres** | | | | | | | 1 | 3 | 6 | 9 | 12 | 15 | 18 | |
| Surfacing code | | **B** | **C** | **D** | **E** | **F** | **G** | **G** | **G** | **G** | **G** | **G** | **G** | |

| Depth (metres) | Ascent time (min) | Dive time (minutes) | | | | | | | | | | | |
|---|---|---|---|---|---|---|---|---|---|---|---|---|---|
| **42** | 3 | – | 9 | 10 | 12 | 21 | 23 | 26 | 28 | 29 | 31 | 32 |
| **45** | 3 | – | 8 | 9 | 10 | 19 | 22 | 24 | 26 | 27 | 28 | 30 |
| **48** | 3 | – | 8 | 9 | 18 | 21 | 23 | 24 | 25 | 26 | 28 | |
| **51** | 3 | – | 8 | 17 | 19 | 21 | 22 | 24 | 25 | 26 | | |
| Decompression stops (minutes) at **9 metres** | | | | | | 1 | 1 | 1 | 2 | 2 | 3 | |
| at **6 metres** | | | | | 2 | 3 | 6 | 9 | 12 | 15 | 18 | |
| Surfacing code | | **B** | **C** | **D** | **E** | **F** | **G** | **G** | **G** | **G** | **G** | **G** | **G** |

**Table B**

| Depth (metres) | Ascent time (min) | Dive time (minutes) | | | | | | | | | | | | |
|---|---|---|---|---|---|---|---|---|---|---|---|---|---|---|
| | | No-stop dives | | | | | Decompression stop dives | | | | | | | |
| **3** | (1) | – | ∞ | | | | | | | | | | | |
| **6** | (1) | – | 80 | 504 | ∞ | | | | | | | | | |
| **9** | 1 | – | 27 | 113 | 148 | 188 | 255 | 272 | 284 | 292 | 300 | 307 | 314 | 321 |
| **12** | 1 | – | 14 | 52 | 67 | 84 | 116 | 129 | 137 | 143 | 148 | 152 | 156 | 160 |
| **15** | 1 | – | 8 | 31 | 40 | 48 | 69 | 79 | 86 | 90 | 94 | 98 | 101 | 105 |
| **18** | 1 | | – | 21 | 27 | 32 | 47 | 55 | 61 | 64 | 68 | 71 | 74 | 76 |
| Decompression stop (minutes) at **6 metres** | | | | | | | 1 | 3 | 6 | 9 | 12 | 15 | 18 | 21 |
| Surfacing code | | **B** | **C** | **D** | **E** | **F** | **G** | **G** | **G** | **G** | **G** | **G** | **G** | **G** |

| Depth (metres) | Ascent time (min) | No-stop dives | | | | | Decompression stop dives | | | | | | | |
|---|---|---|---|---|---|---|---|---|---|---|---|---|---|
| **21** | 1 | | – | 15 | 19 | 23 | 35 | 42 | 47 | 50 | 52 | 55 | 57 |
| **24** | 2 | | – | 12 | 15 | 19 | 28 | 35 | 39 | 41 | 43 | 45 | 47 |
| **27** | 2 | | – | 10 | 12 | 15 | 23 | 29 | 33 | 35 | 36 | 38 | 40 |
| **30** | 2 | | – | 8 | 10 | 12 | 20 | 25 | 28 | 30 | 32 | 33 | 35 |
| **33** | 2 | | | – | 8 | 10 | 17 | 22 | 25 | 26 | 28 | 29 | 31 |
| **36** | 2 | | | – | 7 | 8 | 15 | 20 | 22 | 24 | 25 | 26 | 28 |
| **39** | 3 | | | | – | 8 | 14 | 19 | 21 | 23 | 24 | 25 | 26 |
| Decompression stops (minutes) at **9 metres** | | | | | | | | | 1 | 1 | 1 | 1 | 2 |
| at **6 metres** | | | | | | | 1 | 3 | 6 | 9 | 12 | 15 | 18 |
| Surfacing code | | **B** | **C** | **D** | **E** | **F** | **G** | **G** | **G** | **G** | **G** | **G** | **G** |

| Depth (metres) | Ascent time (min) | No-stop dives | | | | | Decompression stop dives | | | | | | | |
|---|---|---|---|---|---|---|---|---|---|---|---|---|---|
| **42** | 3 | | | | | – | 15 | 17 | 20 | 21 | 22 | 23 | 24 |
| **45** | 3 | | | | | – | 14 | 17 | 18 | 19 | 20 | 21 | 22 |
| **48** | 3 | | | | | – | 13 | 16 | 17 | 18 | 19 | 20 | 21 |
| **51** | 3 | | | | | – | 12 | 15 | 16 | 17 | 18 | 19 | |
| Decompression stops (minutes) at **9 metres** | | | | | | | | 1 | 1 | 1 | 2 | 2 | 3 |
| at **6 metres** | | | | | | | 2 | 3 | 6 | 9 | 12 | 15 | 18 |
| Surfacing code | | **B** | **C** | **D** | **E** | **F** | **G** | **G** | **G** | **G** | **G** | **G** | **G** |

**Table C**

| Depth (metres) | Ascent time (min) | Dive time (minutes) | | | | | | | | | | | |
|---|---|---|---|---|---|---|---|---|---|---|---|---|---|
| | | No-stop dives | | | | Decompression stop dives | | | | | | | |
| **3** | (1) | – | ∞ | | | | | | | | | | |
| **6** | (1) | – | 359 | ∞ | | | | | | | | | |
| **9** | 1 | – | 49 | 79 | 116 | 182 | 199 | 211 | 220 | 227 | 234 | 241 | 248 |
| **12** | 1 | – | 20 | 31 | 44 | 71 | 83 | 90 | 95 | 100 | 104 | 108 | 112 |
| **15** | 1 | – | 11 | 17 | 24 | 40 | 48 | 54 | 57 | 61 | 64 | 67 | 70 |
| **18** | 1 | – | 7 | 11 | 15 | 27 | 34 | 38 | 40 | 43 | 45 | 47 | 50 |
| Decompression stop (minutes) at **6 metres** | | | | | | 1 | 3 | 6 | 9 | 12 | 15 | 18 | 21 |
| Surfacing code | | **B** | **C** | **D** | **E** | **F** | **G** | **G** | **G** | **G** | **G** | **G** | **G** | **G** |

| **21** | 1 | | – | 7 | 10 | 20 | 26 | 29 | 31 | 33 | 35 | 37 |
|---|---|---|---|---|---|---|---|---|---|---|---|---|
| **24** | 2 | | | – | 8 | 16 | 22 | 25 | 26 | 28 | 29 | 31 |
| **27** | 2 | | | | – | 13 | 18 | 21 | 22 | 24 | 25 | 26 |
| **30** | 2 | | | | – | 11 | 16 | 18 | 19 | 20 | 22 | 23 |
| **33** | 2 | | | | – | 10 | 14 | 16 | 17 | 18 | 19 | 20 |
| **36** | 2 | | | | – | 8 | 12 | 14 | 15 | 16 | 17 | 18 |
| **39** | 3 | | | | – | 8 | 12 | 14 | 15 | 16 | 17 | 18 |
| Decompression stops (minutes) at **9 metres** | | | | | | | | 1 | 1 | 1 | 1 | 2 |
| at **6 metres** | | | | | | 1 | 3 | 6 | 9 | 12 | 15 | 18 |
| Surfacing code | | **B** | **C** | **D** | **E** | **F** | **G** | **G** | **G** | **G** | **G** | **G** |

| **42** | 3 | | | | – | 10 | ● | 13 | 14 | 15 | 16 |
|---|---|---|---|---|---|---|---|---|---|---|---|
| **45** | 3 | | | | – | 9 | ● | 12 | ● | 14 | ● | 15 |
| **48** | 3 | | | | – | 8 | ● | 12 | ● | 13 | 14 |
| **51** | 3 | | | | – | 8 | 10 | 11 | 12 | ● | 13 |
| Decompression stops (minutes) at **9 metres** | | | | | | | 1 | 1 | 1 | 2 | 2 | 3 |
| at **6 metres** | | | | | | 2 | 3 | 6 | 9 | 12 | 15 | 18 |
| Surfacing code | | **B** | **C** | **D** | **E** | **F** | **G** | **G** | **G** | **G** | **G** | **G** |

| Surface interval table | | | | | | | | | | | | | |
|---|---|---|---|---|---|---|---|---|---|---|---|---|---|
| Last dive code | Minutes | | | | Hours | | | | | | | | |
| | 15 | 30 | 60 | 90 | 2 | 3 | 4 | 6 | 10 | 12 | 14 | 15 | 16 |
| **G** | **G** | **F** | **E** | **D** | | **C** | | | **B** | | | | **A** |
| **F** | **F** | **E** | **D** | | **C** | | | **B** | | | **A** | | |
| **E** | **E** | **D** | | **C** | | | **B** | | | **A** | | | |
| **D** | **D** | | **C** | | | **B** | | | **A** | | | | |
| **C** | **C** | | | | **B** | | | **A** | | | | | |
| **B** | **B** | | | | | **A** | | | | | | | |
| **A** | **A** | | | | | | | | | | | | |

ALL TABLES COPYRIGHT, BS-AC 1988.©

# Appendix II Decompression procedures and tables from *US Navy Diving Manual*

## Repetitive dive procedure

A dive performed within 12 hours of surfacing from a previous dive is a repetitive dive. The period between dives is the surface interval. Excess nitrogen requires 12 hours to be effectively lost from the body. These tables are designed to protect the diver from the effects of this residual nitrogen. Allow a minimum surface interval of 10 minutes between all dives. For any interval under 10 minutes, add the bottom time of the previous dives to that of the repetitive dive and choose the decompression schedule for the total bottom time and the deepest dive. Specific instructions are given for the use of each table in the following order:

1. The *No-decompression Table* or the *Navy Standard Air Decompression Table* gives the repetitive group designation for all schedules which may precede a repetitive dive.
2. The *Surface Interval Credit Table* gives credit for the desaturation occurring during the surface interval.
3. The *Repetitive Dive Timetable* gives the number of minutes of residual nitrogen time to add to the actual bottom time of the repetitive dive to obtain decompression for the residual nitrogen.
4. The *No-decompression Table* or the *Navy Standard Air Decompression Table* gives the decompression required for the repetitive dive.

## US Navy standard air decompression table

### Instructions for use

Time of decompression stops in the table is in minutes.

Enter the table at the exact or the next greater depth than the maximum depth attained during the dive. Select the listed bottom time that is exactly equal to or is next greater than the bottom time of the dive. Maintain the diver's chest as close as possible to each decompression depth for the number of minutes listed. The rate of ascent *between* stops is not critical for stops of 50 feet or less. Commence timing each stop on arrival at the decompression depth and resume ascent when the specified time has lapsed.

Example 1: a dive to 82 feet for 36 minutes. To determine the proper decompression procedure: the next greater depth listed in this table is 90 feet. The next greater bottom time listed opposite 90 feet is 40. Stop 7 minutes at 10 feet in accordance with the 90/40 schedule.

Example 2: a dive to 110 feet for 30 minutes. It is known that the depth did not exceed 110 feet. To determine the proper decompression schedule: the exact depth of 110 feet is listed the exact bottom time of 30 minutes is listed opposite 110 feet. Decompress according to the 110/30 schedule unless the dive was particularly cold or arduous. In that case, go to the schedule for the next deeper and longer dive, i.e. 120/40.

## US Navy standard air decompression

| Depth (feet) | Bottom time (min) | Time to first stop (min:s) | Decompression stops (feet) | | | | | Total ascent (min:s) | Repetitive group |
|---|---|---|---|---|---|---|---|---|---|
| | | | 50 | 40 | 30 | 20 | 10 | | |
| 40 | 200 | – | – | – | – | – | 0 | 0:40 | (*) |
| | 210 | 0:30 | – | – | – | – | 2 | 2:40 | N |
| | 230 | 0:30 | – | – | – | – | 7 | 7:40 | N |
| | 250 | 0:30 | – | – | – | – | 11 | 11:40 | O |
| | 270 | 0:30 | – | – | – | – | 15 | 15:40 | O |
| | 300 | 0:30 | – | – | – | – | 19 | 19:40 | Z |
| 50 | 100 | – | – | – | – | – | 0 | 0:50 | (*) |
| | 110 | 0:40 | – | – | – | – | 3 | 3:50 | L |
| | 120 | 0:40 | – | – | – | – | 5 | 5:50 | M |
| | 140 | 0:40 | – | – | – | – | 10 | 10:50 | M |
| | 160 | 0:40 | – | – | – | – | 21 | 21:50 | N |
| | 180 | 0:40 | – | – | – | – | 29 | 29:50 | O |
| | 200 | 0:40 | – | – | – | – | 35 | 35:50 | O |
| | 220 | 0:40 | – | – | – | – | 40 | 40:50 | Z |
| | 240 | 0:40 | – | – | – | – | 47 | 47:50 | Z |
| 60 | 60 | – | – | – | – | – | 0 | 1:00 | (*) |
| | 70 | 0:50 | – | – | – | – | 2 | 3:00 | K |
| | 80 | 0:50 | – | – | – | – | 7 | 8:00 | L |
| | 100 | 0:50 | – | – | – | – | 14 | 15:00 | M |
| | 120 | 0:50 | – | – | – | – | 26 | 27:00 | N |
| | 140 | 0:50 | – | – | – | – | 39 | 40:00 | O |
| | 160 | 0:50 | – | – | – | – | 48 | 49:00 | Z |
| | 180 | 0:50 | – | – | – | – | 56 | 57:00 | Z |
| | 200 | 0:40 | – | – | – | 1 | 69 | 71:00 | Z |
| 70 | 50 | – | – | – | – | – | 0 | 1:10 | (*) |
| | 60 | 1:00 | – | – | – | – | 8 | 9:10 | K |
| | 70 | 1:00 | – | – | – | – | 14 | 15:10 | L |
| | 80 | 1:00 | – | – | – | – | 18 | 19:10 | M |
| | 90 | 1:00 | – | – | – | – | 23 | 24:10 | N |
| | 100 | 1:00 | – | – | – | – | 33 | 34:10 | N |
| | 110 | 0:50 | – | – | – | 2 | 41 | 44:10 | O |
| | 120 | 0:50 | – | – | – | 4 | 47 | 52:10 | O |
| | 130 | 0:50 | – | – | – | 6 | 52 | 59:10 | O |
| | 140 | 0:50 | – | – | – | 8 | 56 | 65:10 | Z |
| | 150 | 0:50 | – | – | – | 9 | 61 | 71:10 | Z |
| | 160 | 0:50 | – | – | – | 13 | 72 | 86:10 | Z |
| | 170 | 0:50 | – | – | – | 19 | 79 | 99:10 | Z |
| 80 | 40 | – | – | – | – | – | 0 | 1:20 | (*) |
| | 50 | 1:10 | – | – | – | – | 10 | 11:20 | K |
| | 60 | 1:10 | – | – | – | – | 17 | 18:20 | L |
| | 70 | 1:10 | – | – | – | – | 23 | 24:20 | M |
| | 80 | 1:00 | – | – | – | 2 | 31 | 34:20 | N |
| | 90 | 1:00 | – | – | – | 7 | 39 | 47:20 | N |
| | 100 | 1:00 | – | – | – | 11 | 46 | 58:20 | O |
| | 110 | 1:00 | – | – | – | 13 | 53 | 67:20 | O |
| | 120 | 1:00 | – | – | – | 17 | 56 | 74:20 | Z |
| | 130 | 1:00 | – | – | – | 19 | 63 | 83:20 | Z |
| | 140 | 1:00 | – | – | – | 26 | 69 | 96:20 | Z |
| | 150 | 1:00 | – | – | – | 32 | 77 | 110:20 | Z |
| 90 | 30 | – | – | – | – | – | 0 | 1:30 | (*) |
| | 40 | 1:20 | – | – | – | – | 7 | 8:30 | J |
| | 50 | 1:20 | – | – | – | – | 18 | 19:30 | L |
| | 60 | 1:20 | – | – | – | – | 25 | 26:30 | M |
| | 70 | 1:10 | – | – | – | 7 | 30 | 38:30 | N |
| | 80 | 1:10 | – | – | – | 13 | 40 | 54:30 | N |
| | 90 | 1:10 | – | – | – | 18 | 48 | 67:30 | O |
| | 100 | 1:10 | – | – | – | 21 | 54 | 76:30 | Z |
| | 110 | 1:10 | – | – | – | 24 | 61 | 86:30 | Z |
| | 120 | 1:10 | – | – | – | 32 | 68 | 101:30 | Z |
| | 130 | 1:00 | – | – | 5 | 36 | 74 | 116:30 | Z |
| 100 | 25 | – | – | – | – | – | 0 | 1:40 | (*) |
| | 30 | 1:30 | – | – | – | – | 3 | 4:40 | I |
| | 40 | 1:30 | – | – | – | – | 15 | 16:40 | K |
| | 50 | 1:20 | – | – | – | 2 | 24 | 27:40 | L |
| | 60 | 1:20 | – | – | – | 9 | 28 | 38:40 | N |
| | 70 | 1:20 | – | – | – | 17 | 39 | 57:40 | O |
| | 80 | 1:20 | – | – | – | 23 | 48 | 72:40 | O |
| | 90 | 1:10 | – | – | 3 | 23 | 57 | 84:40 | Z |
| | 100 | 1:10 | – | – | 7 | 23 | 66 | 97:40 | Z |
| | 110 | 1:10 | – | – | 10 | 34 | 72 | 117:40 | Z |
| | 120 | 1:10 | – | – | 12 | 41 | 78 | 132:40 | Z |

**Table (*contd*)**

| Depth (feet) | Bottom time (min) | Time to first stop (min:s) | Decompression stops (feet) | | | | | Total ascent (min:s) | Repeti-tive group |
|---|---|---|---|---|---|---|---|---|---|
| | | | 50 | 40 | 30 | 20 | 10 | | |
| 110 | 20 | – | – | – | – | – | 0 | 1.50 | (*) |
| | 25 | 1:40 | – | – | – | – | 3 | 4.50 | H |
| | 30 | 1:40 | – | – | – | – | 7 | 8.50 | J |
| | 40 | 1:30 | – | – | – | 2 | 21 | 24.50 | L |
| | 50 | 1:30 | – | – | – | 8 | 26 | 35.50 | M |
| | 60 | 1:30 | – | – | – | 18 | 36 | 55.50 | N |
| | 70 | 1:20 | – | – | 1 | 23 | 48 | 73.50 | O |
| | 80 | 1:20 | – | – | 7 | 23 | 57 | 88.50 | Z |
| | 90 | 1:20 | – | – | 12 | 30 | 64 | 107.50 | Z |
| | 100 | 1:20 | – | – | 15 | 37 | 72 | 125.50 | Z |
| 120 | 15 | – | – | – | – | – | 0 | 2:00 | (*) |
| | 20 | 1:50 | – | – | – | – | 2 | 4:00 | H |
| | 25 | 1:50 | – | – | – | – | 6 | 8:00 | I |
| | 30 | 1:50 | – | – | – | – | 14 | 16:00 | J |
| | 40 | 1:40 | – | – | – | 5 | 25 | 32:00 | L |
| | 50 | 1:40 | – | – | – | 15 | 31 | 48:00 | N |
| | 60 | 1:30 | – | – | 2 | 22 | 45 | 71:00 | O |
| | 70 | 1:30 | – | – | 9 | 23 | 55 | 89:00 | O |
| | 80 | 1:30 | – | – | 15 | 27 | 63 | 107:00 | Z |
| | 90 | 1:30 | – | – | 19 | 37 | 74 | 132:00 | Z |
| | 100 | 1:30 | – | – | 23 | 45 | 80 | 150:00 | Z |
| 130 | 10 | – | – | – | – | – | 0 | 2:10 | (*) |
| | 15 | 2:00 | – | – | – | – | 1 | 3:10 | F |
| | 20 | 2:00 | – | – | – | – | 4 | 6:10 | H |
| | 25 | 2:00 | – | – | – | – | 10 | 12:10 | J |
| | 30 | 1:50 | – | – | – | 3 | 18 | 23:10 | M |
| | 40 | 1:50 | – | – | – | 10 | 25 | 37:10 | N |
| | 50 | 1:40 | – | – | 3 | 21 | 37 | 63:10 | O |
| | 60 | 1:40 | – | – | 9 | 23 | 52 | 86:10 | Z |
| | 70 | 1:40 | – | – | 16 | 24 | 61 | 103:10 | Z |
| | 80 | 1:30 | – | 3 | 19 | 35 | 72 | 131:10 | Z |
| | 90 | 1:30 | – | 8 | 19 | 45 | 80 | 154:10 | Z |
| 140 | 10 | – | – | – | – | – | 0 | 2:20 | (*) |
| | 15 | 2:10 | – | – | – | – | 2 | 4:20 | G |
| | 20 | 2:10 | – | – | – | – | 6 | 8:20 | I |
| | 25 | 2:00 | – | – | – | 2 | 14 | 18:20 | J |
| | 30 | 2:00 | – | – | – | 5 | 21 | 28:20 | K |
| | 40 | 1:50 | – | – | 2 | 16 | 26 | 46:20 | N |
| | 50 | 1:50 | – | – | 6 | 24 | 44 | 76:20 | O |
| | 60 | 1:50 | – | – | 16 | 23 | 56 | 97:20 | Z |
| | 70 | 1:40 | – | 4 | 19 | 32 | 68 | 125:20 | Z |
| | 80 | 1:40 | – | 10 | 23 | 41 · | 79 | 155:20 | Z |
| 150 | 5 | – | – | – | – | – | 0 | 2:50 | C |
| | 10 | 2:20 | – | – | – | – | 1 | 3:50 | E |
| | 15 | 2:20 | – | – | – | – | 3 | 5:50 | G |
| | 20 | 2:10 | – | – | – | 2 | 7 | 11:50 | H |
| | 25 | 2:10 | – | – | – | 4 | 17 | 23:50 | K |
| | 30 | 2:10 | – | – | – | 8 | 24 | 34:50 | L |
| | 40 | 2:00 | – | – | 5 | 19 | 33 | 59:50 | N |
| | 50 | 2:00 | – | – | 12 | 23 | 51 | 88:50 | O |
| | 60 | 1:50 | – | 3 | 19 | 26 | 62 | 112:50 | Z |
| | 70 | 1:50 | – | 11 | 19 | 39 | 75 | 146:50 | Z |
| | 80 | 1:40 | 1 | 17 | 19 | 50 | 84 | 173:50 | Z |
| 160 | 5 | – | – | – | – | – | 0 | 2:40 | D |
| | 10 | 2:30 | – | – | – | – | 1 | 3:40 | F |
| | 15 | 2:20 | – | – | – | 1 | 4 | 7:40 | H |
| | 20 | 2:20 | – | – | – | 3 | 11 | 16:40 | J |
| | 25 | 2:20 | – | – | – | 7 | 20 | 29:40 | K |
| | 30 | 2:10 | – | – | 2 | 11 | 25 | 40:40 | M |
| | 40 | 2:10 | – | – | 7 | 23 | 39 | 71:40 | N |
| | 50 | 2:00 | – | 2 | 16 | 23 | 55 | 98:40 | Z |
| | 60 | 2:00 | – | 9 | 19 | 33 | 69 | 132:40 | Z |
| 170 | 5 | – | – | – | – | – | 0 | 2:50 | D |
| | 10 | 2:40 | – | – | – | – | 2 | 4:50 | F |
| | 15 | 2:30 | – | – | – | 2 | 5 | 9:50 | H |
| | 20 | 2:30 | – | – | – | 4 | 15 | 21:50 | J |
| | 25 | 2:20 | – | – | 2 | 7 | 23 | 34:50 | L |
| | 30 | 2:20 | – | – | 4 | 13 | 26 | 45:50 | M |
| | 40 | 2:10 | – | 1 | 10 | 23 | 45 | 81:50 | O |
| | 50 | 2:10 | – | 5 | 18 | 23 | 61 | 109:50 | Z |
| | 60 | 2:00 | 2 | 15 | 22 | 37 | 74 | 152:50 | Z |

**Table** (*contd*)

| Depth (feet) | Bottom time (min) | Time to first stop (min:s) | Decompression stops (feet) | | | | | Total ascent (min:s) | Repetitive group |
|---|---|---|---|---|---|---|---|---|---|
| | | | 50 | 40 | 30 | 20 | 10 | | |
| 180 | 5 | – | – | – | – | – | 0 | 3:00 | D |
| | 10 | 2:50 | – | – | – | – | 3 | 6:00 | F |
| | 15 | 2:40 | – | – | – | 3 | 6 | 12:00 | I |
| | 20 | 2:30 | – | – | 1 | 5 | 17 | 26:00 | K |
| | 25 | 2:30 | – | – | 3 | 10 | 24 | 40:00 | L |
| | 30 | 2:30 | – | – | 6 | 17 | 27 | 53:00 | N |
| | 40 | 2:20 | – | 3 | 14 | 23 | 50 | 93:00 | O |
| | 50 | 2:10 | 2 | 9 | 19 | 30 | 65 | 128:00 | Z |
| | 60 | 2:10 | 5 | 16 | 19 | 44 | 81 | 168:00 | Z |
| 190 | 5 | – | – | – | – | – | 0 | 3:10 | D |
| | 10 | 2:50 | – | – | – | 1 | 3 | 7:10 | G |
| | 15 | 2:50 | – | – | – | 4 | 7 | 14:10 | I |
| | 20 | 2:40 | – | – | 2 | 6 | 20 | 31:10 | K |
| | 25 | 2:40 | – | – | 5 | 11 | 25 | 44:10 | M |
| | 30 | 2:30 | – | 1 | 8 | 19 | 32 | 63:10 | N |
| | 40 | 2:30 | – | 8 | 14 | 23 | 55 | 103:10 | O |
| | | | | 19 | | | | | |

\* See Table II.2 for repetitive groups in no-decompression dives.

**No-decompression limits and repetitive group designation table for no-decompression air dives**

| Depth (feet) | No-decompression limits (min) | Repetitive groups (air dives) | | | | | | | | | | | | | | |
|---|---|---|---|---|---|---|---|---|---|---|---|---|---|---|---|---|
| | | A | B | C | D | E | F | G | H | I | J | K | L | M | N | O |
| 10 | – | 60 | 120 | 210 | 300 | – | – | – | – | – | – | – | – | – | – | – |
| 15 | – | 35 | 70 | 110 | 160 | 225 | 350 | – | – | – | – | – | – | – | – | – |
| 20 | – | 25 | 50 | 75 | 100 | 135 | 180 | 240 | 325 | – | – | – | – | – | – | – |
| 25 | – | 20 | 35 | 55 | 75 | 100 | 125 | 160 | 195 | 245 | 315 | – | – | – | – | – |
| 30 | – | 15 | 30 | 45 | 60 | 75 | 95 | 120 | 145 | 170 | 205 | 250 | 310 | – | – | – |
| 35 | 310 | 5 | 15 | 25 | 40 | 50 | 60 | 80 | 100 | 120 | 140 | 160 | 190 | 220 | 270 | 310 |
| 40 | 200 | 5 | 15 | 25 | 30 | 40 | 50 | 70 | 80 | 100 | 110 | 130 | 150 | 170 | 200 | – |
| 50 | 100 | – | 10 | 15 | 25 | 30 | 40 | 50 | 60 | 70 | 80 | 90 | 100 | – | – | – |
| 60 | 60 | – | 10 | 15 | 20 | 25 | 30 | 40 | 50 | 55 | 60 | – | – | – | – | – |
| 70 | 50 | – | 5 | 10 | 15 | 20 | 30 | 35 | 40 | 45 | 50 | – | – | – | – | – |
| 80 | 40 | – | 5 | 10 | 15 | 20 | 25 | 30 | 35 | 40 | – | – | – | – | – | – |
| 90 | 30 | – | 5 | 10 | 12 | 15 | 20 | 25 | 30 | – | – | – | – | – | – | – |
| 100 | 25 | – | 5 | 7 | 10 | 15 | 20 | 22 | 25 | – | – | – | – | – | – | – |
| 110 | 20 | – | – | 5 | 10 | 13 | 15 | 20 | – | – | – | – | – | – | – | – |
| 120 | 15 | – | – | 5 | 10 | 12 | 15 | – | – | – | – | – | – | – | – | – |
| 130 | 10 | – | – | 5 | 8 | 10 | – | – | – | – | – | – | – | – | – | – |
| 140 | 10 | – | – | 5 | 7 | 10 | – | – | – | – | – | – | – | – | – | – |
| 150 | 5 | – | – | 5 | – | – | – | – | – | – | – | – | – | – | – | – |
| 160 | 5 | – | – | – | 5 | – | – | – | – | – | – | – | – | – | – | – |
| 170 | 5 | – | – | – | 5 | – | – | – | – | – | – | – | – | – | – | – |
| 180 | 5 | – | – | – | 5 | – | – | – | – | – | – | – | – | – | – | – |
| 190 | 5 | – | – | – | 5 | – | – | – | – | – | – | – | – | – | – | – |

## Instructions for use

### No-decompression limits

This column shows at various depths greater than 30 feet the allowable diving times (in minutes) which permit surfacing directly at 60 feet/min with no decompression stops. Longer exposure times require the use of the Standard Air Decompression Table.

### Repetitive group designation table

The tabulated exposure times (or bottom times) are in minutes. The times at the various depths in each vertical column are the maximum exposures during which a diver will remain within the group listed at the head of the column.

To find the repetitive group designation at surfacing for dives involving exposures up to and including the no-decompression limits: enter the table on the *exact* or *next greater depth* than that to which exposed and select the listed exposure time *exact* or *next greater* than the actual exposure time. The repetitive group designation is indicated by the letter at the head of the vertical column where the selected exposure time is listed.

Example: a dive was to 32 feet for 45 minutes. Enter the table along the 35-foot-depth line since it is next greater than 32 feet. The table shows that since group D is left after 40 minutes' exposure and group E after 50 minutes, group E (at the head of the column where the 50-minute exposure is listed) is the proper selection.

Exposure times for depths less than 40 feet are listed only up to approximately 5 hours since this is considered to be beyond field requirements for this table.

**Surface interval credit table for air decompression dives [repetitive group at the end of the surface interval (air dive)**

New group designation

| | Z | O | N | M | L | K | J | I | H | G | F | E | D | C | B | A |
|---|---|---|---|---|---|---|---|---|---|---|---|---|---|---|---|---|
| Z | 0:10 0:22 | 0:23 0:34 | 0:35 0:48 | 0:49 1:02 | 1:03 1:18 | 1:19 1:36 | 1:37 1:55 | 1:56 2:17 | 2:18 2:42 | 2:43 3:10 | 3:11 3:45 | 3:46 4:29 | 4:30 5:27 | 5:28 6:56 | 6:57 10:05 | 10:06 12:00 |
| O | | 0:10 0:23 | 0:24 0:36 | 0:37 0:51 | 0:52 1:07 | 1:08 1:24 | 1:25 1:43 | 1:44 2:04 | 2:05 2:29 | 2:30 2:59 | 3:00 3:33 | 3:34 4:17 | 4:18 5:16 | 5:17 6:44 | 6:45 9:54 | 9:55 12:00 |
| N | | | 0:10 0:24 | 0:25 0:39 | 0:40 0:54 | 0:55 1:11 | 1:12 1:30 | 1:31 1:53 | 1:54 2:18 | 2:19 2:47 | 2:48 3:22 | 3:23 4:04 | 4:05 5:03 | 5:04 6:32 | 6:33 9:43 | 9:44 12:00 |
| M | | | | 0:10 0:25 | 0:26 0:42 | 0:43 0:59 | 1:00 1:18 | 1:19 1:39 | 1:40 2:05 | 2:06 2:34 | 2:35 3:08 | 3:09 3:52 | 3:53 4:49 | 4:50 6:18 | 6:19 9:28 | 9:29 12:00 |
| L | | | | | 0:10 0:26 | 0:27 0:45 | 0:46 1:04 | 1:05 1:25 | 1:26 1:49 | 1:50 2:19 | 2:20 2:53 | 2:54 3:36 | 3:37 4:35 | 4:36 6:02 | 6:03 9:12 | 9:13 12:00 |
| K | | | | | | 0:10 0:28 | 0:29 0:49 | 0:50 1:11 | 1:12 1:35 | 1:36 2:03 | 2:04 2:38 | 2:39 3:21 | 3:22 4:19 | 4:20 5:48 | 5:49 8:58 | 8:59 12:00 |
| J | | | | | | | 0:10 0:31 | 0:32 0:54 | 0:55 1:19 | 1:20 1:47 | 1:48 2:20 | 2:21 3:04 | 3:05 4:02 | 4:03 5:40 | 5:41 8:40 | 8:41 12:00 |
| I | | | | | | | | 0:10 0:33 | 0:34 0:59 | 1:00 1:29 | 1:30 2:02 | 2:03 2:44 | 2:45 3:43 | 3:44 5:12 | 5:13 8:21 | 8:22 12:00 |
| H | | | | | | | | | 0:10 0:36 | 0:37 1:06 | 1:07 1:41 | 1:42 2:23 | 2:24 3:20 | 3:21 4:49 | 4:50 7:59 | 8:00 12:00 |
| G | | | | | | | | | | 0:10 0:40 | 0:41 1:15 | 1:16 1:59 | 2:00 2:58 | 2:59 4:25 | 4:26 7:35 | 7:36 12:00 |
| F | | | | | | | | | | | 0:10 0:45 | 0:46 1:29 | 1:30 2:28 | 2:29 3:57 | 3:58 7:05 | 7:06 12:00 |
| E | | | | | | | | | | | | 0:10 0:54 | 0:55 1:57 | 1:58 3:22 | 3:23 6:32 | 6:33 12:00 |
| D | | | | | | | | | | | | | 0:10 1:09 | 1:10 2:38 | 2:39 5:48 | 5:49 12:00 |
| C | | | | | | | | | | | | | | 0:10 1:39 | 1:40 2:49 | 2:50 12:00 |
| B | | | | | | | | | | | | | | | 0:10 2:10 | 2:11 12:00 |
| A | | | | | | | | | | | | | | | | 0:10 12:00 |

*Repetitive group at the beginning of the surface interval from previous dive*

ENTER HERE

## Instructions for use

Surface interval time in the table is *in hours* and *minutes* (7:59 means 7 hours and 59 minutes.) The surface interval must be at least 10 minutes.

Find the *repetitive group designation letter* (from the previous dive schedule) on the diagonal slope. Enter the table horizontally to select the surface interval time that is exactly between the actual surface interval times shown. The repetitve group designation for the *end* of the surface interval is at the head of the vertical column where the selected surface interval time is listed. For example, a previous dive was to 110 feet for 30 minutes. The diver remains on the surface 1 hour and 30 minutes and wishes to find the new repetitive group designation. The repetitive group from the last column of the 110/30 schedule in the Standard Air Decompression Tables is 'J'. Enter the surface interval credit table along the horizontal line labelled 'J'. The 1-hour-and-30-minute surface interval lies between the times 1:20 and 1:47.

Therefore, the diver has lost sufficient inert gas to place him in group 'G' (at the head of the vertical column selected).

*Note:* dives following surface intervals of more than 12 hours are not considered repetitive dives. *Actual* bottom times in the Standard Air Decompression Tables may be used in computing decompression for such dives.

**Repetitive dive timetable for air dives**

Residual nitrogen times (minutes)

| Repetitive groups | Repetitive | | dive | | | | depth | | | (ft) | | (air | | | | dives) | |
|---|---|---|---|---|---|---|---|---|---|---|---|---|---|---|---|---|---|
| | 40 | 50 | 60 | 70 | 80 | 90 | 100 | 110 | 120 | 130 | 140 | 150 | 160 | 170 | 180 | 190 |
| A | 7 | 6 | 5 | 4 | 4 | 3 | 3 | 3 | 3 | 3 | 2 | 2 | 2 | 2 | 2 | 2 |
| B | 17 | 13 | 11 | 9 | 8 | 7 | 7 | 6 | 6 | 6 | 5 | 5 | 4 | 4 | 4 | 4 |
| C | 25 | 21 | 17 | 15 | 13 | 11 | 10 | 10 | 9 | 8 | 7 | 7 | 6 | 6 | 6 | 6 |
| D | 37 | 29 | 24 | 20 | 18 | 16 | 14 | 13 | 12 | 11 | 10 | 9 | 8 | 8 | 8 | 8 |
| E | 49 | 38 | 30 | 26 | 23 | 20 | 18 | 16 | 15 | 13 | 12 | 12 | 11 | 10 | 10 | 10 |
| F | 61 | 47 | 36 | 31 | 28 | 24 | 22 | 20 | 18 | 16 | 15 | 14 | 13 | 13 | 12 | 11 |
| G | 73 | 56 | 44 | 37 | 32 | 29 | 26 | 24 | 21 | 19 | 18 | 17 | 16 | 15 | 14 | 13 |
| H | 87 | 66 | 52 | 43 | 38 | 33 | 30 | 27 | 25 | 22 | 20 | 19 | 18 | 17 | 16 | 15 |
| I | 101 | 76 | 61 | 50 | 43 | 38 | 34 | 31 | 28 | 25 | 23 | 22 | 20 | 19 | 18 | 17 |
| J | 116 | 87 | 70 | 57 | 48 | 43 | 38 | 34 | 32 | 28 | 26 | 24 | 23 | 22 | 20 | 19 |
| K | 138 | 99 | 79 | 64 | 54 | 47 | 43 | 38 | 35 | 31 | 29 | 27 | 26 | 24 | 22 | 21 |
| L | 161 | 111 | 88 | 72 | 61 | 53 | 48 | 42 | 39 | 35 | 32 | 30 | 28 | 26 | 25 | 24 |
| M | 187 | 124 | 97 | 80 | 68 | 58 | 52 | 47 | 43 | 38 | 35 | 32 | 31 | 29 | 27 | 26 |
| N | 213 | 142 | 107 | 87 | 73 | 64 | 57 | 51 | 46 | 40 | 38 | 35 | 33 | 31 | 29 | 28 |
| O | 241 | 160 | 117 | 96 | 80 | 70 | 62 | 55 | 50 | 44 | 40 | 38 | 36 | 34 | 31 | 30 |
| Z | 257 | 169 | 122 | 100 | 84 | 73 | 64 | 57 | 52 | 46 | 42 | 40 | 37 | 35 | 32 | 31 |

## Instructions for use

The bottom times listed in this table are called 'residual nitrogen times' and are the times a diver is to consider he has *already* spent on bottom when he *starts* a repetitive dive to a specific depth. They are in minutes.

Enter the table horizontally with the repetitive group designation from the Surface Interval Credit Table. The time in each vertical column is the number of minutes that would be required (at the depth listed at the head of the column) to saturate to the particular group.

Example: the final group designation from the Surface Interval Credit Table, on the basis of a previous dive and surface interval, is 'H'. To plan a dive to 110 feet, determine the residual nitrogen time for this depth required by the repetitive group designation: enter this table along the horizontal line labelled 'H'. The table shows that one must *start* a dive to 110 feet as though he had already been on the bottom for 27 minutes. This information can then be applied to the Standard Air Decompression Table or No-decompression Table in a number of ways:

1. Assuming a diver is going to finish a job and take whatever decompression is required, he must add 27 minutes to his actual bottom time and be prepared to take decompression according to the 110-foot schedules for the sum or equivalent single dive time.

2. Assuming one wishes to make a quick inspection dive for the minimum decompression, he will decompress according to the 110/30 schedule for a dive of 3 minutes or less (27 + 3 = 30). For a dive of over 3 minutes but less than 13, he will decompress according to the 110/40 schedule (27 + 13 = 40).

3. Assuming that one does not want to exceed the 110/50 schedule and the amount of decompression it requires, he will have to start ascent before 23 minutes of actual bottom time (50 − 27 = 23).

4. Assuming that a diver has air for approximately 45 minutes bottom time and decompression stops, the possible dives can be computed: a dive of 13 minutes will require 23 minutes of decompression (110/40 schedule), for a total submerged time of 36 minutes. A dive of 13 to 23 minutes will require 34 minutes of decompression (110/50 schedule), for a total submerged time of 47 to 57 minutes. Therefore, to be safe, the diver will have to start ascent before 13 minutes or a standby air source will have to be provided.

# Appendix III French decompression tables: Instructions for use of French Navy '90 Air Decompression Table*

## Restriction for use

The use of French Navy '90 Air Decompression Table (FN 90 Table) is reserved for scuba diving, for dives requiring no physical effort greater than swimming at a speed of 0.5 knot. Surface supplied decompression is also applicable (air or oxygen supply).

French Ministry of Labour regulations do not allow the use of this table for professional purposes.

## Diving conditions

- The table gives the depth and duration of the stops as a function of maximum depth and bottom line.
- The ascent rate from the bottom to the first decompression stop must be between 15 and 17 msw/min. It must not, under any circumstances, be greater than 17 msw/min.
- The bottom time is counted in full minutes (any fraction of a minute is considered as an elapsed minute) from leaving the surface to leaving the bottom.
- The depth of the dive is the maximum depth reached during the dive.
- If bottom time or depth values for the dive are not in the table, the value immediately above must be chosen. Interpolation of bottom times or depths is forbidden.
- The table gives, for each combined time–depth, the depth and duration of decompression stops, the total ascent time rounded to the nearest minute, and the repetitive dive group for computing repetitive dives.
- Diving to 62 and 65 msw is not allowed. The table is given for this depth as a rescue table to be used if maximum depth of 60 msw is overstepped. In such a case, it is forbidden to dive again within 8 hours 30 min.

* These FN 90 air decompression tables are published by special authorization of the French Government (Ministry of Defence). As they were established for the use of the French Navy, no guarantee can be given in any other field of use; the French Government waive all responsibility for the use of these tables and procedures by anyone not specifically authorized to do so.

## Decompression stops with oxygen inhalation

When divers are allowed to breathe pure oxygen during decompression stops, the duration of each decompression stop is reduced by one-third: 2 minutes' breathing pure oxygen are equivalent to 3 minutes' breathing air.

Breathing pure oxygen during decompression stops reduces the duration of decompression stops but does not modify the repetitive dive group of the achieved dive.

## Repetitive dives

- Two dives separated by a surface interval less than or equal to 8 hours 30 min are called repetitive dives. In this case, when beginning the second dive, the dissolved nitrogen is not totally eliminated from the diver's organism.
- To take this gas burden into account (the residual nitrogen), an overestimation of bottom time is computed, as the time spent at the second dive depth which would dissolve the same residual nitrogen amount. This extra time is called residual nitrogen time.
- Table I of French tables (page 533) allows the determination of residual nitrogen in the diver's body as a function of repetitive dive group and surface interval. If the exact surface interval is not in the table, the value immediately below must be taken.
- The intersection of the repetitive dive group line and the surface interval column gives the residual nitrogen value, which is to be carried into the first column of Table II (page 534).
- If this value is not here available, the value immediately above must be taken. Table II gives, at the intersection of the residual nitrogen line and second dive depth column, the residual nitrogen time in minutes. It must be added to the effective bottom time of the second dive to calculate a repetitive bottom time.
- Using the FN 90 Table, this repetitive bottom time allows the determination of the different decompression stops.
- If the depth of the second dive is not in Table II, take the depth immediately deeper, which will be chosen to determine the second dive decompression stops.
- If the surface interval is less than 15 minutes, the two dives are considered as the same dive. To determine the second dive decompression stops, use the FN 90 Table with a repetitive bottom time equal to the sum of both the bottom times, and a depth equal to the maximum depth reached during the two dives.

- The calculation of repetitive dives is valid for surface intervals up to 8 hours 30 min; between 8 hours and 8 hours 30 min, the residual nitrogen time must be computed for an 8-hour interval.
- FN 90 Table does not permit carrying out of more than two repetitive dives a day.

## Surface oxygen breathing

During the surface interval, breathing pure oxygen leads to a faster decrease of the residual nitrogen burden.

Table III of the FN tables gives the residual nitrogen values after different durations of breathing pure oxygen, either from surfacing (enter the table by the repetitive dive group) or from any residual nitrogen value (enter the table by the column: 'Residual nitrogen equivalent'). The new residual nitrogen found is used to go into Table II to determine the residual nitrogen time.

When the exact period spent breathing pure oxygen at surface is not in Table III, take the value immediately below.

## Table adjustment for altitude diving

To use the FN 90 Table in altitude, it is necessary to know the barometric pressure $H$ at the location of the dive.

A fictitious depth $P'$ is computed:

$$P' = P \times 1013/H$$

which $P$ is the actually reached depth (in metres) and $H$ the local barometric pressure (in millibars or hectopascals).

Enter the FN 90 Table with $P'$ instead of $P$.

The decompression stops will be done at the actual depth $p'$:

$$p' = p \times H/1013$$

where $p$ is the depth of the decompression stop given by the FN 90 Table (i.e. 3, 6, 9 or 12 msw).

**French Navy '90 Air Decompression Table (FN 90 Table)**

| Depth (m) | Bottom time (min) | Duration of decompression stops at | | | | | Total ascent time | Repetitive dive group |
|---|---|---|---|---|---|---|---|---|
| | | 15 m | 12 m | 9 m | 6 m | 3 m | | |
| 65 | 5 | | | | | 3 | 7 | * |
| | 10 | | | | 3 | 8 | 15 | * |
| | 15 | | | 2 | 5 | 24 | 35 | * |
| 62 | 5 | | | | | 2 | 6 | * |
| | 10 | | | | 2 | 7 | 13 | * |
| | 15 | | | 1 | 5 | 21 | 31 | * |
| 60 | 5 | | | | | 2 | 6 | D |
| | 10 | | | | 2 | 6 | 12 | G |
| | 15 | | | 1 | 4 | 19 | 28 | J |
| | 20 | | | 3 | 8 | 32 | 47 | L |
| | 25 | | | 5 | 15 | 41 | 65 | M |
| | 30 | | 1 | 8 | 22 | 48 | 83 | O |
| | 35 | | 4 | 11 | 28 | 54 | 101 | P |
| | 40 | | 6 | 17 | 30 | 62 | 119 | P |
| 58 | 5 | | | | | 2 | 5 | D |
| | 10 | | | | 2 | 5 | 10 | G |
| | 15 | | | 1 | 4 | 16 | 24 | J |
| | 20 | | | 2 | 7 | 30 | 42 | K |
| | 25 | | | 4 | 13 | 40 | 60 | M |
| | 30 | | 1 | 7 | 21 | 46 | 78 | N |
| | 35 | | 2 | 11 | 26 | 52 | 94 | O |
| | 40 | | 5 | 15 | 30 | 59 | 112 | P |
| 55 | 5 | | | | | 1 | 4 | D |
| | 10 | | | | 1 | 5 | 9 | G |
| | 15 | | | | 4 | 13 | 20 | I |
| | 20 | | | 1 | 6 | 27 | 37 | K |
| | 25 | | | 3 | 11 | 37 | 54 | M |
| | 30 | | | 6 | 18 | 44 | 71 | N |
| | 35 | | 1 | 9 | 23 | 50 | 86 | O |
| | 40 | | 3 | 12 | 29 | 55 | 102 | P |
| 52 | 5 | | | | | 1 | 4 | D |
| | 10 | | | | 1 | 4 | 8 | F |
| | 15 | | | | 3 | 10 | 16 | I |
| | 20 | | | 1 | 5 | 23 | 32 | K |
| | 25 | | | 2 | 9 | 34 | 48 | L |
| | 30 | | | 4 | 15 | 41 | 63 | M |
| | 35 | | | 6 | 22 | 47 | 78 | O |
| | 40 | | 1 | 10 | 26 | 52 | 92 | O |

Ascent rate: 15–17 m/min.

**FN 90 Table** (*contd*)

| Depth (m) | Bottom time (min) | Duration of decompression stops at | | | | | Total ascent time | Repetitive dive group |
|---|---|---|---|---|---|---|---|---|
| | | *15 m* | *12 m* | *9 m* | *6 m* | *3 m* | | |
| 50 | 5 | | | | | 1 | 4 | D |
| | 10 | | | | | 4 | 7 | F |
| | 15 | | | | 2 | 9 | 14 | H |
| | 20 | | | | 4 | 22 | 29 | J |
| | 25 | | | 1 | 8 | 32 | 44 | L |
| | 30 | | | 2 | 14 | 39 | 58 | M |
| | 35 | | | 5 | 20 | 45 | 73 | N |
| | 40 | | | 9 | 24 | 50 | 86 | O |
| 48 | 5 | | | | | | 3 | D |
| | 10 | | | | | 4 | 7 | F |
| | 15 | | | | 2 | 7 | 12 | H |
| | 20 | | | | 4 | 19 | 26 | J |
| | 25 | | | | 7 | 30 | 40 | K |
| | 30 | | | 1 | 12 | 37 | 53 | M |
| | 35 | | | 3 | 18 | 44 | 68 | N |
| | 40 | | | 6 | 23 | 48 | 80 | O |
| 45 | 5 | | | | | | 3 | C |
| | 10 | | | | | 3 | 6 | F |
| | 15 | | | | 1 | 6 | 10 | H |
| | 20 | | | | 3 | 15 | 21 | I |
| | 25 | | | | 5 | 25 | 33 | K |
| | 30 | | | | 9 | 35 | 47 | L |
| | 35 | | | 1 | 15 | 40 | 59 | M |
| | 40 | | | 3 | 20 | 46 | 72 | N |
| 42 | 5 | | | | | | 3 | C |
| | 10 | | | | | 2 | 5 | E |
| | 15 | | | | | 5 | 8 | G |
| | 20 | | | | 1 | 12 | 15 | I |
| | 25 | | | | 3 | 22 | 27 | J |
| | 30 | | | | 6 | 31 | 39 | L |
| | 35 | | | | 11 | 37 | 50 | M |
| | 40 | | | 1 | 16 | 43 | 62 | N |
| 40 | 5 | | | | | | 3 | C |
| | 10 | | | | | 2 | 5 | E |
| | 15 | | | | | 4 | 7 | G |
| | 20 | | | | 1 | 9 | 12 | H |
| | 25 | | | | 2 | 19 | 23 | J |
| | 30 | | | | 4 | 28 | 34 | K |
| | 35 | | | | 8 | 35 | 45 | L |
| | 40 | | | | 13 | 40 | 55 | M |
| | 45 | | | 1 | 18 | 45 | 66 | N |
| | 50 | | | 2 | 23 | 48 | 75 | O |
| | 55 | | | 5 | 26 | 52 | 85 | O |
| | 1 h | | | 8 | 29 | 57 | 96 | P |

Ascent rate: 15–17 m/min.

**FN 90 Table** (*contd*)

| Depth (m) | Bottom time (min) | Duration of decompression stops at | | | | | Total ascent time | Repetitive dive group |
|---|---|---|---|---|---|---|---|---|
| | | 15 m | 12 m | 9 m | 6 m | 3 m | | |
| 38 | 5 | | | | | | 2 | C |
| | 10 | | | | | 1 | 3 | E |
| | 15 | | | | | 4 | 6 | F |
| | 20 | | | | | 8 | 10 | H |
| | 25 | | | | 1 | 16 | 19 | J |
| | 30 | | | | 3 | 24 | 29 | K |
| | 35 | | | | 5 | 33 | 40 | L |
| | 40 | | | | 10 | 38 | 50 | M |
| | 45 | | | | 15 | 43 | 60 | N |
| | 50 | | | | 20 | 47 | 69 | N |
| | 55 | | | 2 | 23 | 50 | 77 | O |
| | 1 h | | | 5 | 27 | 53 | 87 | P |
| 35 | 5 | | | | | | 2 | C |
| | 10 | | | | | | 2 | D |
| | 15 | | | | | 2 | 4 | F |
| | 20 | | | | | 5 | 7 | H |
| | 25 | | | | | 11 | 13 | I |
| | 30 | | | | 1 | 20 | 23 | J |
| | 35 | | | | 2 | 27 | 31 | K |
| | 40 | | | | 5 | 34 | 41 | L |
| | 45 | | | | 9 | 39 | 50 | M |
| | 50 | | | | 14 | 43 | 59 | N |
| | 55 | | | | 18 | 47 | 67 | N |
| | 1 h | | | | 22 | 50 | 74 | O |
| 32 | 5 | | | | | | 2 | B |
| | 10 | | | | | | 2 | D |
| | 15 | | | | | 1 | 3 | E |
| | 20 | | | | | 3 | 5 | G |
| | 25 | | | | | 6 | 8 | H |
| | 30 | | | | | 14 | 16 | I |
| | 35 | | | | | 22 | 24 | K |
| | 40 | | | | 1 | 29 | 32 | K |
| | 45 | | | | 4 | 34 | 40 | L |
| | 50 | | | | 7 | 39 | 48 | M |
| | 55 | | | | 11 | 43 | 56 | N |
| | 1 h | | | | 15 | 46 | 63 | N |
| | 1 h 05 | | | | 19 | 48 | 69 | O |
| | 1 h 10 | | | | 23 | 50 | 75 | O |

Ascent rate: 15–17 m/min.

**FN 90 Table** (*contd*)

| Depth (m) | Bottom time (min) | Duration of decompression stops at | | | | | Total ascent time | Repetitive dive group |
|---|---|---|---|---|---|---|---|---|
| | | 15 m | 12 m | 9 m | 6 m | 3 m | | |
| 30 | 5 | | | | | | 2 | B |
| | 10 | | | | | | 2 | D |
| | 15 | | | | | 1 | 3 | E |
| | 20 | | | | | 2 | 4 | F |
| | 25 | | | | | 4 | 6 | H |
| | 30 | | | | | 9 | 11 | I |
| | 35 | | | | | 17 | 19 | J |
| | 40 | | | | | 24 | 26 | K |
| | 45 | | | | 1 | 31 | 34 | L |
| | 50 | | | | 3 | 36 | 41 | M |
| | 55 | | | | 6 | 39 | 47 | M |
| | 1h | | | | 10 | 43 | 55 | N |
| | 1 h 05 | | | | 14 | 46 | 62 | N |
| | 1 h 10 | | | | 17 | 48 | 67 | O |
| 28 | 5 | | | | | | 2 | B |
| | 10 | | | | | | 2 | D |
| | 15 | | | | | | 2 | E |
| | 20 | | | | | 1 | 3 | F |
| | 25 | | | | | 2 | 4 | G |
| | 30 | | | | | 6 | 8 | H |
| | 35 | | | | | 12 | 14 | I |
| | 40 | | | | | 19 | 21 | J |
| | 45 | | | | | 25 | 27 | K |
| | 50 | | | | | 32 | 34 | L |
| | 55 | | | | 2 | 36 | 40 | M |
| | 1 h | | | | 4 | 40 | 46 | M |
| | 1 h 05 | | | | 8 | 43 | 53 | N |
| | 1 h 10 | | | | 11 | 46 | 59 | N |
| | 1 h 15 | | | | 14 | 48 | 64 | O |
| | 1 h 20 | | | | 17 | 50 | 69 | O |
| | 1 h 25 | | | | 20 | 53 | 75 | O |
| | 1 h 30 | | | | 23 | 56 | 81 | P |
| 25 | 5 | | | | | | 2 | B |
| | 10 | | | | | | 2 | C |
| | 15 | | | | | | 2 | D |
| | 20 | | | | | | 2 | E |
| | 25 | | | | | 1 | 3 | F |
| | 30 | | | | | 2 | 4 | H |
| | 35 | | | | | 5 | 7 | I |
| | 40 | | | | | 10 | 11 | J |
| | 45 | | | | | 16 | 17 | J |
| | 50 | | | | | 21 | 22 | K |
| | 55 | | | | | 27 | 28 | L |
| | 1 h | | | | | 32 | 33 | L |
| | 1 h 05 | | | | | 37 | 38 | M |
| | 1 h 10 | | | | 1 | 41 | 43 | M |
| | 1 h 15 | | | | 4 | 43 | 48 | N |
| | 1 h 20 | | | | 7 | 45 | 53 | N |
| | 1 h 25 | | | | 9 | 48 | 58 | O |
| | 1 h 30 | | | | 11 | 50 | 62 | O |

Ascent rate: 15–17 m/min.

**FN 90 Table** (*contd*)

| Depth (m) | Bottom time (min) | Duration of decompression stops at 15 m | 12 m | 9 m | 6 m | 3 m | Total ascent time | Repetitive dive group |
|---|---|---|---|---|---|---|---|---|
| 22 | 5 | | | | | | 2 | B |
| | 10 | | | | | | 2 | C |
| | 15 | | | | | | 2 | D |
| | 20 | | | | | | 2 | E |
| | 25 | | | | | | 2 | F |
| | 30 | | | | | | 2 | G |
| | 35 | | | | | | 2 | H |
| | 40 | | | | | 2 | 4 | I |
| | 45 | | | | | 7 | 9 | I |
| | 50 | | | | | 12 | 13 | J |
| | 55 | | | | | 16 | 17 | K |
| | 1 h | | | | | 20 | 21 | K |
| | 1 h 05 | | | | | 25 | 26 | L |
| | 1 h 10 | | | | | 29 | 30 | L |
| | 1 h 15 | | | | | 33 | 34 | M |
| | 1 h 20 | | | | | 37 | 38 | M |
| | 1 h 25 | | | | | 41 | 42 | N |
| | 1 h 30 | | | | | 44 | 45 | N |
| 20 | 5 | | | | | | 1.2 | B |
| | 10 | | | | | | 1.2 | B |
| | 15 | | | | | | 1.2 | D |
| | 20 | | | | | | 1.2 | D |
| | 25 | | | | | | 1.2 | E |
| | 30 | | | | | | 1.2 | F |
| | 35 | | | | | | 1.2 | G |
| | 40 | | | | | | 1.2 | H |
| | 45 | | | | | 1 | 2 | J |
| | 50 | | | | | 4 | 5 | K |
| | 55 | | | | | 9 | 10 | K |
| | 1 h | | | | | 13 | 14 | L |
| | 1 h 05 | | | | | 16 | 17 | M |
| | 1 h 10 | | | | | 20 | 21 | M |
| | 1 h 15 | | | | | 24 | 25 | N |
| | 1 h 20 | | | | | 27 | 28 | N |
| | 1 h 25 | | | | | 30 | 31 | N |
| | 1 h 30 | | | | | 34 | 35 | O |

Ascent rate: 15–17 m/min.

**FN 90 Table (*contd*)**

| Depth (m) | Bottom time (min) | Duration of decompression stops at | | | | | Total ascent time | Repetitive dive group |
|---|---|---|---|---|---|---|---|---|
| | | 15 m | 12 m | 9 m | 6 m | 3 m | | |
| 18 | 5 | | | | | | 1 | B |
| | 10 | | | | | | 1 | B |
| | 15 | | | | | | 1 | C |
| | 20 | | | | | | 1 | D |
| | 25 | | | | | | 1 | E |
| | 30 | | | | | | 1 | F |
| | 35 | | | | | | 1 | F |
| | 40 | | | | | | 1 | G |
| | 45 | | | | | | 1 | H |
| | 50 | | | | | | 1 | H |
| | 55 | | | | | 1 | 2 | I |
| | 1 h | | | | | 5 | 6 | J |
| | 1 h 05 | | | | | 8 | 9 | J |
| | 1 h 10 | | | | | 11 | 12 | K |
| | 1 h 15 | | | | | 14 | 15 | K |
| | 1 h 20 | | | | | 17 | 18 | L |
| | 1 h 25 | | | | | 21 | 22 | L |
| | 1 h 30 | | | | | 23 | 24 | M |
| | 1 h 35 | | | | | 26 | 27 | M |
| | 1 h 40 | | | | | 28 | 29 | M |
| | 1 h 45 | | | | | 31 | 32 | N |
| | 1 h 50 | | | | | 34 | 35 | N |
| | 1 h 55 | | | | | 36 | 37 | N |
| | 2 h | | | | | 38 | 39 | O |
| 15 | 5 | | | | | | 1 | A |
| | 10 | | | | | | 1 | B |
| | 15 | | | | | | 1 | C |
| | 20 | | | | | | 1 | C |
| | 25 | | | | | | 1 | D |
| | 30 | | | | | | 1 | E |
| | 35 | | | | | | 1 | E |
| | 40 | | | | | | 1 | F |
| | 45 | | | | | | 1 | G |
| | 50 | | | | | | 1 | G |
| | 55 | | | | | | 1 | H |
| | 1 h | | | | | | 1 | H |
| | 1 h 05 | | | | | | 1 | I |
| | 1 h 10 | | | | | | 1 | I |
| | 1 h 15 | | | | | | 1 | J |
| | 1 h 20 | | | | | 2 | 3 | J |
| | 1 h 25 | | | | | 4 | 5 | K |
| | 1 h 30 | | | | | 6 | 7 | K |
| | 1 h 35 | | | | | 8 | 9 | L |
| | 1 h 40 | | | | | 11 | 12 | L |
| | 1 h 45 | | | | | 13 | 14 | L |
| | 1 h 50 | | | | | 15 | 16 | M |
| | 1 h 55 | | | | | 17 | 18 | M |
| | 2 h | | | | | 18 | 19 | M |

Ascent rate: 15–17 m/min.

**FN 90 Table (***contd***)**

| Depth (m) | Bottom time (min) | Duration of decompression stops at | | | | | Total ascent time | Repetitive dive group |
|---|---|---|---|---|---|---|---|---|
| | | 15 m | 12 m | 9 m | 6 m | 3 m | | |
| 12 | 5 | | | | | | 1 | A |
| | 15 | | | | | | 1 | B |
| | 25 | | | | | | 1 | C |
| | 35 | | | | | | 1 | D |
| | 45 | | | | | | 1 | E |
| | 55 | | | | | | 1 | F |
| | 1 h 05 | | | | | | 1 | G |
| | 1 h 20 | | | | | | 1 | H |
| | 1 h 30 | | | | | | 1 | I |
| | 1 h 45 | | | | | | 1 | J |
| | 2 h | | | | | | 1 | K |
| | 2 h 15 | | | | | | 1 | L |
| | 2 h 20 | | | | | 2 | 3 | L |
| | 2 h 30 | | | | | 4 | 5 | M |
| | 2 h 40 | | | | | 6 | 7 | M |
| | 2 h 50 | | | | | 7 | 8 | N |
| | 3 h | | | | | 9 | 10 | N |
| | 3 h10 | | | | | 11 | 12 | N |
| | 3 h 20 | | | | | 13 | 14 | O |
| | 3 h 30 | | | | | 14 | 15 | O |
| | 3 h 40 | | | | | 15 | 16 | O |
| | 3 h 50 | | | | | 16 | 17 | O |
| | 4 h | | | | | 17 | 18 | O |
| | 4 h 10 | | | | | 18 | 19 | P |
| | 4 h 15 | | | | | 19 | 20 | P |
| | 4 h 30 | | | | | 22 | 23 | P |
| | 4 h 45 | | | | | 24 | 25 | P |
| | 5 h | | | | | 26 | 27 | P |
| 10 | 15 | | | | | | 0.6 | B |
| | 30 | | | | | | 0.6 | C |
| | 45 | | | | | | 0.6 | D |
| | 1 h | | | | | | 0.6 | F |
| | 1 h 15 | | | | | | 0.6 | G |
| | 1 h 45 | | | | | | 0.6 | H |
| | 2 h | | | | | | 0.6 | I |
| | 2 h 15 | | | | | | 0.6 | J |
| | 2 h 45 | | | | | | 0.6 | K |
| | 3 h | | | | | | 0.6 | L |
| | 4 h | | | | | | 0.6 | M |
| | 4 h 15 | | | | | | 0.6 | N |
| | 5 h 15 | | | | | | 0.6 | O |
| | 5 h 30 | | | | | | 0.6 | P |
| | 6 h | | | | | 1 | 2 | P |

Ascent rate: 15–17 m/min.

**FN 90 Table** (*contd*)

| Depth (m) | Bottom time (min) | Duration of decompression stops at | | | | | Total ascent time | Repetitive dive group |
|---|---|---|---|---|---|---|---|---|
| | | 15 m | 12 m | 9 m | 6 m | 3 m | | |
| 8 | 15 | | | | | | 0.5 | B |
| | 30 | | | | | | 0.5 | C |
| | 45 | | | | | | 0.5 | D |
| | 1 h | | | | | | 0.5 | E |
| | 1 h 30 | | | | | | 0.5 | F |
| | 1 h 45 | | | | | | 0.5 | G |
| | 2 h 15 | | | | | | 0.5 | H |
| | 2 h 45 | | | | | | 0.5 | I |
| | 3 h 15 | | | | | | 0.5 | J |
| | 4 h 15 | | | | | | 0.5 | K |
| | 5 h | | | | | | 0.5 | L |
| | 6 h | | | | | | 0.5 | M |
| 6 | 15 | | | | | | 0.4 | A |
| | 30 | | | | | | 0.4 | B |
| | 45 | | | | | | 0.4 | C |
| | 1 h 15 | | | | | | 0.4 | D |
| | 1 h 45 | | | | | | 0.4 | E |
| | 2 h 15 | | | | | | 0.4 | F |
| | 3 h | | | | | | 0.4 | G |
| | 4 h | | | | | | 0.4 | H |
| | 5 h 15 | | | | | | 0.4 | I |
| | 6 h | | | | | | 0.4 | J |

Ascent rate: 15–17 m/min.

**Table I  Determination of residual nitrogen**

| Repetitive dive group | Surface intervals | | | | | | | | | | |
|---|---|---|---|---|---|---|---|---|---|---|---|
| | 15 | 30 | 45 | 1 h | 1 h 30 | 2 h | 2 h 30 | 3 h | 4 h | 6 h | 8 h |
| A | 0.84 | 0.83 | 0.83 | 0.83 | 0.82 | 0.82 | 0.82 | 0.81 | 0.81 | 0.81 | 0.80 |
| B | 0.88 | 0.88 | 0.87 | 0.86 | 0.85 | 0.85 | 0.84 | 0.83 | 0.82 | 0.81 | 0.81 |
| C | 0.92 | 0.91 | 0.90 | 0.89 | 0.88 | 0.87 | 0.85 | 0.85 | 0.83 | 0.82 | 0.81 |
| D | 0.97 | 0.95 | 0.94 | 0.93 | 0.91 | 0.89 | 0.88 | 0.86 | 0.85 | 0.82 | 0.81 |
| E | 1.00 | 0.98 | 0.97 | 0.96 | 0.93 | 0.91 | 0.89 | 0.88 | 0.86 | 0.83 | 0.81 |
| F | 1.05 | 1.03 | 1.01 | 0.99 | 0.96 | 0.94 | 0.91 | 0.90 | 0.87 | 0.83 | 0.82 |
| G | 1.08 | 1.06 | 1.04 | 1.02 | 0.98 | 0.96 | 0.93 | 0.91 | 0.88 | 0.84 | 0.82 |
| H | 1.13 | 1.10 | 1.08 | 1.05 | 1.01 | 0.98 | 0.95 | 0.93 | 0.89 | 0.85 | 0.82 |
| I | 1.17 | 1.14 | 1.11 | 1.08 | 1.04 | 1.00 | 0.97 | 0.94 | 0.90 | 0.85 | 0.83 |
| J | 1.20 | 1.17 | 1.14 | 1.11 | 1.06 | 1.02 | 0.98 | 0.96 | 0.91 | 0.86 | 0.83 |
| K | 1.25 | 1.21 | 1.18 | 1.15 | 1.09 | 1.04 | 1.01 | 0.97 | 0.92 | 0.86 | 0.83 |
| L | 1.29 | 1.25 | 1.21 | 1.17 | 1.12 | 1.07 | 1.02 | 0.99 | 0.93 | 0.87 | 0.83 |
| M | 1.33 | 1.29 | 1.25 | 1.21 | 1.14 | 1.09 | 1.04 | 1.01 | 0.94 | 0.87 | 0.84 |
| N | 1.37 | 1.32 | 1.28 | 1.24 | 1.17 | 1.11 | 1.06 | 1.02 | 0.95 | 0.88 | 0.84 |
| O | 1.41 | 1.36 | 1.32 | 1.27 | 1.20 | 1.13 | 1.08 | 1.04 | 0.97 | 0.88 | 0.84 |
| P | 1.45 | 1.40 | 1.35 | 1.30 | 1.22 | 1.15 | 1.10 | 1.05 | 0.98 | 0.89 | 0.84 |

**Table II  Residual nitrogen time**

| Residual nitrogen | Second dive depth | | | | | | | | | | | | | | | | | | | |
|---|---|---|---|---|---|---|---|---|---|---|---|---|---|---|---|---|---|---|---|---|
| | 12 | 15 | 18 | 20 | 22 | 25 | 28 | 30 | 32 | 35 | 38 | 40 | 42 | 45 | 48 | 50 | 52 | 55 | 58 | 60 |
| 0.82 | 4 | 3 | 2 | 2 | 2 | 2 | 2 | 1 | 1 | 1 | 1 | 1 | 1 | 1 | 1 | 1 | 1 | 1 | 1 | 1 |
| 0.84 | 7 | 6 | 5 | 4 | 4 | 3 | 3 | 3 | 3 | 2 | 2 | 2 | 2 | 2 | 2 | 2 | 2 | 2 | 1 | 1 |
| 0.86 | 11 | 9 | 7 | 7 | 6 | 5 | 5 | 4 | 4 | 4 | 3 | 3 | 3 | 3 | 3 | 3 | 3 | 2 | 2 | 2 |
| 0.89 | 17 | 13 | 11 | 10 | 9 | 8 | 7 | 7 | 6 | 6 | 5 | 5 | 5 | 4 | 4 | 4 | 4 | 4 | 3 | 3 |
| 0.92 | 23 | 18 | 15 | 13 | 12 | 11 | 10 | 9 | 8 | 8 | 7 | 7 | 6 | 6 | 5 | 5 | 5 | 5 | 5 | 4 |
| 0.95 | 29 | 23 | 19 | 17 | 15 | 13 | 12 | 11 | 10 | 10 | 9 | 8 | 8 | 7 | 7 | 7 | 6 | 6 | 6 | 5 |
| 0.99 | 38 | 30 | 24 | 22 | 20 | 17 | 15 | 14 | 13 | 12 | 11 | 11 | 10 | 9 | 9 | 8 | 8 | 8 | 7 | 7 |
| 1.03 | 47 | 37 | 30 | 27 | 24 | 21 | 19 | 17 | 16 | 15 | 14 | 13 | 12 | 11 | 11 | 10 | 10 | 9 | 9 | 9 |
| 1.07 | 57 | 44 | 36 | 32 | 29 | 25 | 22 | 21 | 19 | 18 | 16 | 15 | 15 | 13 | 13 | 12 | 12 | 11 | 10 | 10 |
| 1.11 | 68 | 52 | 42 | 37 | 34 | 29 | 26 | 24 | 22 | 20 | 19 | 18 | 17 | 16 | 15 | 14 | 13 | 13 | 12 | 12 |
| 1.16 | 81 | 62 | 50 | 44 | 40 | 34 | 30 | 28 | 26 | 24 | 22 | 21 | 20 | 18 | 17 | 16 | 16 | 15 | 14 | 13 |
| 1.20 | 93 | 70 | 56 | 50 | 45 | 39 | 34 | 32 | 29 | 27 | 24 | 23 | 22 | 20 | 19 | 18 | 18 | 17 | 16 | 15 |
| 1.24 | 106 | 79 | 63 | 56 | 50 | 43 | 38 | 35 | 33 | 30 | 27 | 26 | 24 | 23 | 21 | 20 | 19 | 18 | 17 | 17 |
| 1.29 | 124 | 91 | 72 | 63 | 56 | 49 | 43 | 40 | 37 | 33 | 30 | 29 | 27 | 25 | 24 | 23 | 22 | 20 | 19 | 19 |
| 1.33 | 139 | 101 | 79 | 70 | 62 | 53 | 47 | 43 | 40 | 36 | 33 | 31 | 30 | 28 | 26 | 25 | 24 | 22 | 21 | 20 |
| 1.38 | 160 | 114 | 89 | 78 | 69 | 59 | 52 | 48 | 44 | 40 | 37 | 35 | 33 | 30 | 28 | 27 | 26 | 24 | 23 | 22 |
| 1.42 | 180 | 126 | 97 | 85 | 75 | 64 | 56 | 52 | 48 | 43 | 39 | 37 | 35 | 33 | 30 | 29 | 28 | 26 | 25 | 24 |
| 1.45 | 196 | 135 | 104 | 90 | 80 | 68 | 59 | 55 | 51 | 46 | 42 | 39 | 37 | 34 | 32 | 31 | 29 | 28 | 26 | 25 |

**Table III  Residual nitrogen decrease by breathing pure oxygen at surface**

| Repetitive dive group | Residual nitrogen equivalent | Duration of oxygen breathing | | | | | | | | |
|---|---|---|---|---|---|---|---|---|---|---|
| | | 15 | 30 | 45 | 1 h | 1 h 30 | 2 h | 2 h 30 | 3 h | 3 h 30 |
| A | 0.84 | | | | | | | | | |
| B | 0.89 | 0.85 | 0.82 | | | | | | | |
| C | 0.93 | 0.89 | 0.85 | 0.82 | | | | | | |
| D | 0.98 | 0.94 | 0.90 | 0.86 | 0.82 | | | | | |
| E | 1.02 | 0.98 | 0.94 | 0.90 | 0.86 | | | | | |
| F | 1.07 | 1.02 | 0.98 | 0.94 | 0.90 | 0.83 | | | | |
| G | 1.11 | 1.06 | 1.02 | 0.97 | 0.93 | 0.86 | | | | |
| H | 1.16 | 1.11 | 1.06 | 1.02 | 0.98 | 0.89 | 0.82 | | | |
| I | 1.20 | 1.15 | 1.10 | 1.05 | 1.01 | 0.93 | 0.85 | | | |
| J | 1.24 | 1.19 | 1.14 | 1.09 | 1.04 | 0.96 | 0.88 | | | |
| K | 1.29 | 1.24 | 1.18 | 1.13 | 1.08 | 0.99 | 0.91 | 0.84 | | |
| L | 1.33 | 1.27 | 1.22 | 1.17 | 1.12 | 1.03 | 0.94 | 0.86 | | |
| M | 1.38 | 1.32 | 1.27 | 1.21 | 1.16 | 1.06 | 0.98 | 0.89 | 0.82 | |
| N | 1.42 | 1.36 | 1.30 | 1.25 | 1.19 | 1.09 | 1.00 | 0.92 | 0.84 | |
| O | 1.47 | 1.41 | 1.35 | 1.29 | 1.24 | 1.13 | 1.04 | 0.95 | 0.87 | |
| P | 1.51 | 1.45 | 1.38 | 1.33 | 1.27 | 1.16 | 1.07 | 0.98 | 0.90 | 0.82 |

# Appendix IV The DCIEM sport diving tables

The complete Canadian Defence and Civil Institute of Environmental Medicine, Toronto, Canada (DCIEM) decompression publication contains tables for in-water and surface decompression with the diver breathing oxygen as well as a wider selection of depths and times for in-water decompression with the diver breathing air. The information in this appendix is from a short version of the tables for the sports diver marketed by UDT Inc. and is presented with the permission of DCIEM and UDT. The tables, in a waterproof format, and an instruction book are available from UDT, 2691 Viscount Way, Richmond, BC, Canada. The complete DCIEM tables should be consulted for the other tables.

## Table A: Air Decompression

This gives no-decompression limits, repetitive group letters and decompression stops for dives that require stops. The group letters move from A through to M as the diver spends more time at depth. For example, for a dive to 60 feet (18 metres) for less than 14 min the diver is in group A and at the maximum dive without stops (50 min) he is group F. If he remains at depth for longer, he crosses onto the right-hand side of the tables and must make the decompression stops listed further down the tables. Note that there are two sets of decompression stops: the 3 metre (10 feet) stops for shallower dives and the schedules for dives deeper than 18 metres; these may require stops at 6 metres (20 feet)

## Table B: Surface Intervals

This is used to allow for the elimination of nitrogen during intervals on the surface. The user enters the table on the line corresponding to his repetitive dive group at the end of the last dive and finds the number that is in the column headed by his surface interval. This factor can then be transferred to Table C to find the no-decompression stops limit for a second dive. For example, a diver surfaces in group F and spends 2 hours 15 min on the surface. What is the longest dive he can make to 18 metres without stops? He enters Table B on row F. At the intersection of this row with the column from 2 hours to 2 hours 59 min he finds 1.4. This is transferred to Table C. At the intersection of 1.4 and 18 metres is the no-stops limit for the second dive, 29 min.

The factor from Table B can also be used to calculate stops. If the task in the second dive considered above took 50 min the diver multiplies this by the factor obtained from the surface interval table and uses this time in Table A to get the decompres-sion time. In this case the $1.4 \times 50 = 70$, so the stop(s) for the second dive are for a 70-minute dive to 18 metres (10 min at 3 metres). The resulting repetitive group letter (H) can be transferred to Tables B and C for any later dive. The diver can use Table A without allowance for a previous dive when he has been on the surface for enough time for the factor to fall to 1.0.

The depth, as in other tables, is the maximum depth reached during the dive. The bottom time is the time from leaving the surface till beginning the ascent to the stop or surface. The ascent rate should be $18 \pm 3$ metres/min ($60 \pm 10$ feet/min). The stops times are the times to be spent at the nominated depths.

## Table D

This is used to convert the depth of a dive at altitude to an effective depth that can be used in Table A and to find the correct depth for any decompression stops. The table is entered on the left-hand column in the row with the actual depth of the dive. A correction to be added to the depth obtained is obtained from the intersection of this row with the column that includes the altitude of the water surface at the dive site. For example, a diver intends to conduct a 50-foot dive in water where the surface is at 4500 feet. What is the effective depth to be used for decompression? At the intersection of the actual depth 50 feet row and the 4000–5000 feet column is found 10 feet. This is to be added, so the diver should decompress for a 60-foot dive. The foot of the column shows that any stops to be taken should be at 18 and 9 feet instead of 20 and 10 feet. A further increase of one depth should be added if the diver has been at a lower altitude less than 12 hours before the dive. This corrects for the additional nitrogen remaining in the diver's body.

For a diver to fly after a no-decompression-stops dive the DCIEM table instructions require that he should wait till his repetitive factor in Table B has decreased to 1. He should have a minimum surface interval of 24 hours after a decompression dive.*

---

* Flying after diving guidelines have recently been the subject of a workshop organized by the Undersea and Hyperbaric Medicine Society. It is reported (Sheffield, PJ, Abstract 20, Supplement to Undersea Biomedical Research, Vol 17, 1990) that the consensus was for more stringent rules than the DCIEM rules.

The workshop suggested a wait of 12 hours for divers who had less than 2 hours' diving (surface to surface) in the last 2 days. Divers should wait at least 24 hours before flying after multiday unlimited dives. A delay of at least 24 hours, and preferably 48 hours, was suggested affter any dives requiring decompression stops. It is not known if DCIEM will change their rules in line with these guidelines.

The complete instructions for the tables have much information that has been omitted here. This includes rules for omitted decompression and a multilevel dive decompression procedure as well as rules for adjustments for multiple repetitive dives.

## DCIEM sport diving tables

### A: AIR DECOMPRESSION

| Depth | No-decompression bottom times (minutes) | | | | Decompression required bottom times | | | |
|---|---|---|---|---|---|---|---|---|
| 20'  6 m | 30 A<br>60 B<br>90 C<br>120 D | 150 E<br>180 F<br>240 G<br>300 H | 360 I<br>420 J<br>480 K<br>600 L | 720 M<br>∞ | | | | |
| 30'  9 m | 30 A<br>45 B<br>60 C<br>90 D | 100 E<br>120 F<br>150 G<br>180 H | 190 I<br>210 J<br>240 K<br>270 L | 300 M | 360 | 400 | | |
| 40'  12 m | 22 A<br>30 B<br>40 C | 60 D<br>70 E<br>80 F | 90 G<br>120 H<br>130 I | 150 J | 160 K<br>170 L | 180 M<br>190 | 200 | 215 |
| 50'  15 m | 18 A<br>25 B | 30 C<br>40 D | 50 E<br>60 F | 75 G | 85 H<br>95 I | 105 J<br>115 K | 124 L | 132 M |
| 60'  18 m | 14 A<br>20 B | 25 C<br>30 D | 40 E | 50 F | 60 G | 70 H<br>80 I | 85 J | 92 K |
| **Decompression stops in minutes** | | | **at 10'   3 m** | | **5** | **10** | **15** | **20** |

| Depth | | | | | | | | |
|---|---|---|---|---|---|---|---|---|
| 70'  21 m | 12 A<br>15 B | 20 C | 25 D | 35 E | 40 F | 50 G | 60 H<br>63 I | 66 J |
| 80'  24 m | 10 A<br>13 B | 15 C | 20 D | 25 E | 29 F | 35 G | 48 H | 52 I |
| 90'  27 m | 9 A | 12 B | 15 C | 20 D | 23 E | 27 F | 35 G | 40 H<br>43 I |
| 100'  30 m | 7 A | 10 B | 12 C | 15 D | 18 D | 21 E | 25 F<br>29 G | 36 H |
| 110'  33 m | | 6 A | 10 B | 12 C | 15 D | 18 E | 22 F | 26 G<br>30 H |
| 120'  36 m | | 6 A | 8B | 10 C | 12 D | 15 E | 19 F | 25 G |
| 130'  39 m | | | 5 A | 8 B | 10 C | 13 D | 16 F | 21 G |
| 140'  42 m | | | 5 A | 7 B | 9 C | 11 D | 14 F | 18 G |
| 150'  45 m | | | 4 A | 6 B | 8 C | 10 D | 12 E | 15 F |
| **Decompression stops in minutes** | | | **at 20'   6m** | | – | – | **5** | **10** |
| | | | **at 10'   3m** | | **5** | **10** | **10** | **10** |

- ASCENT RATE is 60' (18 m) plus or minus 10' (3 m) per minute
  NO-DECOMPRESSION LIMITS are given for first dives
- DECOMPRESSION STOPS are taken at mid-chest level for the times indicated at the specified stop depths

→ Table B for **Minimum Surface Intervals** and Repetitive Factors
→ Table C for **Repetitive Dive No-Decompression Limits**
→ Table D for **Depth Corrections** required at Altitudes above 1000' (300 m)

**B: SURFACE INTERVALS**

| Rep. group | 0:15 0:29 | 0:30 0:59 | 1:00 1:29 | 1:30 1:59 | 2:00 2:59 | 3:00 3:59 | 4:00 5:59 | 6:00 8:59 | 9:00 11:59 | 12:00 14:59 | 15:00 18:00 |
|---|---|---|---|---|---|---|---|---|---|---|---|
| A | 1.4 | 1.2 | 1.1 | 1.1 | 1.1 | 1.1 | 1.1 | 1.1 | 1.0 | 1.0 | 1.0 |
| B | 1.5 | 1.3 | 1.2 | 1.2 | 1.2 | 1.1 | 1.1 | 1.1 | 1.1 | 1.0 | 1.0 |
| C | 1.6 | 1.4 | 1.3 | 1.2 | 1.2 | 1.2 | 1.1 | 1.1 | 1.1 | 1.0 | 1.0 |
| D | 1.8 | 1.5 | 1.4 | 1.3 | 1.3 | 1.2 | 1.2 | 1.1 | 1.1 | 1.0 | 1.0 |
| E | 1.9 | 1.6 | 1.5 | 1.4 | 1.3 | 1.3 | 1.2 | 1.2 | 1.1 | 1.1 | 1.0 |
| F | 2.0 | 1.7 | 1.6 | 1.5 | 1.4 | 1.3 | 1.3 | 1.2 | 1.1 | 1.1 | 1.0 |
| G | – | 1.9 | 1.7 | 1.6 | 1.5 | 1.4 | 1.3 | 1.2 | 1.1 | 1.1 | 1.0 |
| H | – | – | 1.9 | 1.7 | 1.6 | 1.5 | 1.4 | 1.3 | 1.1 | 1.1 | 1.1 |
| I | – | – | 2.0 | 1.8 | 1.7 | 1.5 | 1.4 | 1.3 | 1.1 | 1.1 | 1.1 |
| J | – | – | – | 1.9 | 1.8 | 1.6 | 1.5 | 1.3 | 1.2 | 1.1 | 1.1 |
| K | – | – | – | 2.0 | 1.9 | 1.7 | 1.5 | 1.3 | 1.2 | 1.1 | 1.1 |
| L | – | – | – | – | 2.0 | 1.7 | 1.6 | 1.4 | 1.2 | 1.1 | 1.1 |
| M | – | – | – | – | – | 1.8 | 1.6 | 1.4 | 1.2 | 1.1 | 1.1 |

Repetitive factors (RF) given for surface intervals (h:min)

**C: REPETITIVE DIVING**

| Depth | | 1.1 | 1.2 | 1.3 | 1.4 | 1.5 | 1.6 | 1.7 | 1.8 | 1.9 | 2.0 |
|---|---|---|---|---|---|---|---|---|---|---|---|
| 30' | 9m | 272 | 250 | 230 | 214 | 200 | 187 | 176 | 166 | 157 | 150 |
| 40' | 12m | 136 | 125 | 115 | 107 | 100 | 93 | 88 | 83 | 78 | 75 |
| 50' | 15m | 60 | 55 | 50 | 45 | 41 | 38 | 36 | 34 | 32 | 31 |
| 60' | 18m | 40 | 35 | 31 | 29 | 27 | 26 | 24 | 23 | 22 | 21 |
| 70' | 21m | 30 | 25 | 21 | 19 | 18 | 17 | 16 | 15 | 14 | 13 |
| 80' | 24m | 20 | 18 | 16 | 15 | 14 | 13 | 12 | 12 | 11 | 11 |
| 90' | 27m | 16 | 14 | 12 | 11 | 11 | 10 | 9 | 9 | 8 | 8 |
| 100' | 30m | 13 | 11 | 10 | 9 | 9 | 8 | 8 | 7 | 7 | 7 |
| 110' | 33m | 10 | 9 | 8 | 8 | 7 | 7 | 6 | 6 | 6 | 6 |
| 120' | 36m | 8 | 7 | 7 | 6 | 6 | 6 | 5 | 5 | 5 | 5 |
| 130' | 39m | 7 | 6 | 6 | 5 | 5 | 5 | 4 | 4 | 4 | 4 |
| 140' | 42m | 6 | 5 | 5 | 5 | 4 | 4 | 4 | 3 | 3 | 3 |
| 150' | 45m | 5 | 5 | 4 | 4 | 4 | 3 | 3 | 3 | 3 | 3 |

Repetitive factors no-D limits given in minutes according to depth and RF

## D: DEPTH CORRECTIONS

| Actual depth | | 1000' → 1999 / 300m → 599 | | 2000' → 2999 / 600m → 899 | | 3000' → 3999 / 900m → 1199 | | 4000' → 4999 / 1200m → 1499 | | 5000' → 5999 / 1500m → 1799 | | 6000' → 6999 / 1800m → 2099 | | 7000' → 7999 / 2100m → 2399 | | 8000' → 10 000 / 2400m → 3000 | |
|---|---|---|---|---|---|---|---|---|---|---|---|---|---|---|---|---|---|
| 30' | 9m | 10 | 3 | 10 | 3 | 10 | 3 | 10 | 3 | 10 | 3 | 10 | 3 | 20 | 6 | 20 | 6 |
| 40' | 12m | 10 | 3 | 10 | 3 | 10 | 3 | 10 | 3 | 10 | 3 | 20 | 6 | 20 | 6 | 20 | 6 |
| 50' | 15m | 10 | 3 | 10 | 3 | 10 | 3 | 10 | 3 | 20 | 6 | 20 | 6 | 20 | 6 | 20 | 6 |
| 60' | 18m | 10 | 3 | 10 | 3 | 10 | 3 | 20 | 6 | 20 | 6 | 20 | 6 | 20 | 6 | 30 | 9 |
| 70' | 21m | 10 | 3 | 10 | 3 | 10 | 3 | 20 | 6 | 20 | 6 | 20 | 6 | 30 | 9 | 30 | 9 |
| 80' | 24m | 10 | 3 | 10 | 3 | 20 | 6 | 20 | 6 | 20 | 6 | 30 | 9 | 30 | 9 | 40 | 12 |
| 90' | 27m | 10 | 3 | 10 | 3 | 20 | 6 | 20 | 6 | 20 | 6 | 30 | 9 | 30 | 9 | 40 | 12 |
| 100' | 30m | 10 | 3 | 10 | 3 | 20 | 6 | 20 | 6 | 30 | 9 | 30 | 9 | 30 | 9 | 40 | 12 |
| 110' | 33m | 10 | 3 | 20 | 6 | 20 | 6 | 20 | 6 | 30 | 9 | 30 | 9 | 40 | 12 | | |
| 120' | 36m | 10 | 3 | 20 | 6 | 20 | 6 | 30 | 9 | 30 | 9 | 30 | 9 | | | | |
| 130' | 39m | 10 | 3 | 20 | 6 | 20 | 6 | | | | | | | | | | |
| 140' | 42m | 10 | 3 | | | | | | | | | | | | | | |

Add depth correction to actual depth of altitude dive

| 10' | 3m | 10 | 3.0 | 10 | 3.0 | 9 | 3.0 | 9 | 3.0 | 9 | 3.0 | 8 | 2.5 | 8 | 2.5 | 8 | 2.5 |
| 20' | 6m | 20 | 6.0 | 19 | 6.0 | 18 | 5.5 | 18 | 5.5 | 17 | 5.0 | 16 | 15.0 | 16 | 5.0 | 15 | 4.5 |

Actual decompression stop depths (feet/*metres*) at altitude

# Appendix V  US Navy recompression therapy tables

To guide its users in the selection of a decompression therapy table the *US Navy Diving manual* contains four flow charts. These are reproduced below. After following the appropriate chart the reader is guided to selecting an appropriate table. These are also presented below.

It should be noted that it has been necessary to omit much of the text that contains advice on selecting and using the tables. Any person using these tables, or any other therapy table, should have the complete original document. This presentation is offered as a teaching aid, not as an official guide.

NOTES:

1. As an option, the on-site Diving Medical Officer, Diving Officer, or Master Diver may elect not to recompress the diver 10 feet in the water, but to remove the diver from the water when decompression risks are acceptable and treat the diver in the chamber.

2. No oxygen available.

3. If recompression goes deeper than the depth of the first stop in the decompression table use a stop time equal to $1\frac{1}{2}$ times the first stop time in the decompression table for the one or two stops deeper than the first stop. Always take a stop every 10 feet.

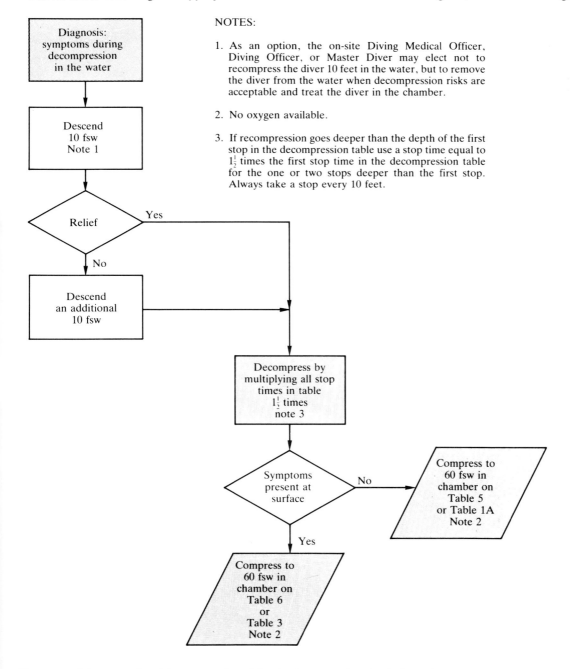

Treatment of decompression sickness occurring while at a decompression stop in the water

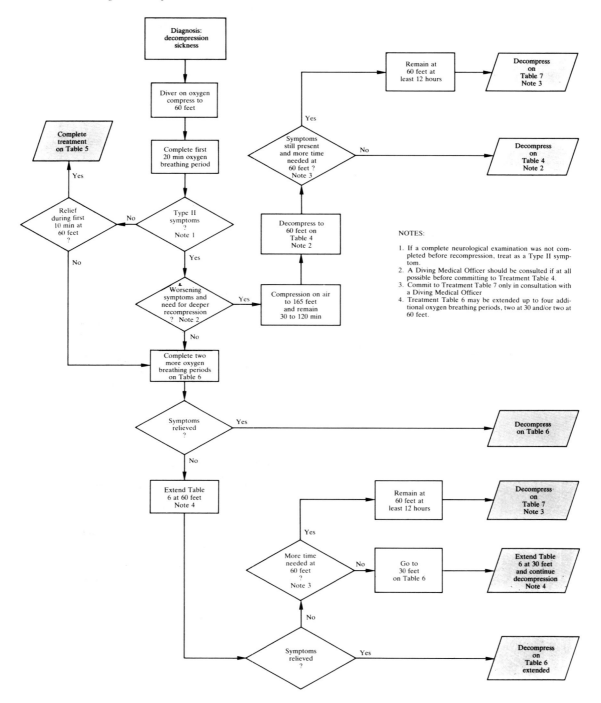

Decompression sickness treatment from diving or altitude exposures

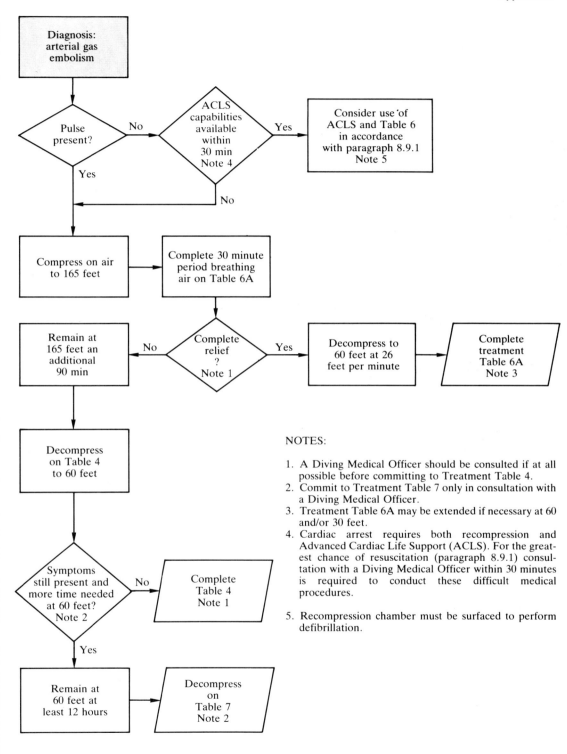

NOTES:

1. A Diving Medical Officer should be consulted if at all possible before committing to Treatment Table 4.
2. Commit to Treatment Table 7 only in consultation with a Diving Medical Officer.
3. Treatment Table 6A may be extended if necessary at 60 and/or 30 feet.
4. Cardiac arrest requires both recompression and Advanced Cardiac Life Support (ACLS). For the greatest chance of resuscitation (paragraph 8.9.1) consultation with a Diving Medical Officer within 30 minutes is required to conduct these difficult medical procedures.

5. Recompression chamber must be surfaced to perform defibrillation.

Treatment of arterial gas embolism

Recurrence during treatment

Recurrence following treatment

NOTES:

1. A Diving Medical Officer should be consulted if at all possible before committing to Treatment Table 4.
2. Commit to Treatment Table 7 only in consultation with a Diving Medical Officer.
3. Treatment Table 6 may be extended up to two additional oxygen breathing periods at 30 and/or 60 feet.

Treatment of symptom recurrence

**Treatment Table 5**: Oxygen treatment of type I decompression sickness

1. Treatment of type 1 decompression sickness when symptoms are relieved within 10 minutes at 60 feet and a complete neurological exam is normal.
2. Descent rate – 25 feet/min.
3. Ascent rate – 1 feet/min. Do not compensate for slower ascent rates. Compensate for faster rates by halting the ascent.
4. Time at 60 feet begins on arrival at 60 feet.
5. If oxygen breathing must be interrupted, allow 15 minutes after the reaction has entirely subsided and resume schedule at point of interruption.
6. If oxygen breathing must be interrupted at 60 feet, switch to Treatment Table 6 upon arrival at the 30-foot stop.
7. Tender breathes air throughout unless he has had a hyperbaric exposure within the past 12 hours, in which case he breathes oxygen at 30 feet in accordance with paragraph 8.13.5.7.

| Depth (feet) | Time (minutes) | Breathing media | Total elapsed time (h:min) |
|---|---|---|---|
| 60 | 20 | Oxygen | 0:20 |
| 60 | 5 | Air | 0:25 |
| 60 | 20 | Oxygen | 0:45 |
| 60–30 | 30 | Oxygen | 1:15 |
| 30 | 5 | Air | 1:20 |
| 30 | 20 | Oxygen | 1:40 |
| 30 | 5 | Air | 1:45 |
| 30–0 | 30 | Oxygen | 2:15 |

**Treatment Table 6**: Oxygen treatment of type II decompression sickness

1. Treatment of type II or type I decompression sickness when symptoms are not relieved within 10 minutes at 60 feet.
2. Descent rate – 25 feet/min.
3. Ascent rate – 1 foot/min. Do not compensate for slower ascent rates. Compensate for faster rates by halting the ascent.
4. Time at 60 feet begins on arrival at 60 feet.
5. If oxygen breathing must be interrupted, allow 15 minutes after the reaction has entirely subsided and resume schedule at point of interruption.
6. Tender breathes air throughout unless the tender has had a hyperbaric exposure within the last 12 hours, in which case oxygen is breathed at 30 feet in accordance with paragraph 8.13.5.7.
7. Table 6 can be lengthened up to two additional 25-minute periods at 60 feet (20 minutes on oxygen and 5 minutes on air), or up to two additional 75-minute periods at 30 feet (15 minutes on air and 60 minutes on

oxygen), or both. If Table 6 is extended only once at either 60 or 30 feet, the tender breathes oxygen during the ascent from 30 feet to the surface. If more than one extension is done, the tender begins oxygen breathing for the last hour at 30 feet and during ascent to the surface.

| Depth (feet) | Time (minutes) | Breathing media | Total elapsed time (h:min) |
|---|---|---|---|
| 60 | 20 | Oxygen | 0:20 |
| 60 | 5 | Air | 0:25 |
| 60 | 20 | Oxygen | 0:45 |
| 60 | 5 | Air | 0:50 |
| 60 | 20 | Oxygen | 1:10 |
| 60 | 5 | Air | 1:15 |
| 60–30 | 30 | Oxygen | 1:45 |
| 30 | 15 | Air | 2:00 |
| 30 | 60 | Oxygen | 3:00 |
| 30 | 15 | Air | 3:15 |
| 30 | 60 | Oxygen | 4:15 |
| 30–0 | 30 | Oxygen | 4:45 |

**Treatment Table 6A**: Initial air and oxygen treatment of arterial gas embolism

1. Treatment of arterial gas embolism where complete relief is obtained within 30 min at 165 feet. Use also when unable to determine whether symptoms are caused by gas embolism or severe decompression sickness.
2. Descent rate – as fast as possible.
3. Ascent rate – 1 foot/min. Do not compensate for slower ascent rates. Compensate for faster rates by halting the ascent.
4. Time at 165 feet – includes time from the surface.
5. If oxygen breathing must be interrupted, allow 15 minutes after the reaction has entirely subsided and resume schedule at point of interruption.
6. Tender breathes oxygen during ascent from 30 feet to the surface unless the tender has had a hyperbaric exposure within the last 12 hours, in which case oxygen is breathed at 30 feet in accordance with paragraph 8.13.5.7.
7. Table 6A can be lengthened up to two additional 25-minute periods at 60 feet (20 minutes on oxygen and 5 minutes on air), or up to two additional 75-minute periods at 30 feet (60 minutes on oxygen and 15 minutes on air), or both. If Table 6A is extended either at 60 or 30 feet, the tender breathes oxygen during the last 90 minutes of the treatment; 60 minutes at 30 feet and 30 minutes during ascent to the surface.
8. If complete relief is not obtained within 30 minutes at 165 feet, switch to Table 4. Consult with a Diving Medical Officer before switching if possible.

| Depth (feet) | Time (minutes) | Breathing media | Total elapsed time (h:min) |
|---|---|---|---|
| 165 | 30 | Air | 0:30 |
| 165 – 60 | 4 | Air | 0:34 |
| 60 | 20 | Oxygen | 0:54 |
| 60 | 5 | Air | 0:59 |
| 60 | 20 | Oxygen | 1:19 |
| 60 | 5 | Air | 1:29 |
| 60 | 20 | Oxygen | 1:44 |
| 60 | 5 | Air | 1:49 |
| 60 – 30 | 30 | Oxygen | 2:19 |
| 30 | 15 | Air | 2:34 |
| 30 | 60 | Oxygen | 3:34 |
| 30 | 15 | Air | 3:49 |
| 30 | 60 | Oxygen | 4:49 |
| 30 – 0 | 30 | Oxygen | 5:19 |

**Treatment Table 4**: Air or air and oxygen treatment of type II decompression sickness or arterial gas embolism

1. Treatment of worsening symptoms during the first 20-minute oxygen breathing period at 60 feet on Table 6, or when symptoms are not relieved within 30 minutes at 165 feet using air treatment Table 3 or 6A.
2. Descent rate – as fast as possible.
3. Ascent rate – 1 minute between stops.
4. Time at 165 feet – includes time from the surface.
5. If only air is available, decompress on air. If oxygen is available, patient begins oxygen breathing upon arrival at 60 feet with appropriate air breaks. Both tender and patient breathe oxygen beginning 2 hours before leaving 30 feet.
6. Ensure life support considerations can be met before committing to a Table 4. Internal chamber temperature should be below 85°F.
7. If oxygen breathing is interrupted, no compensatory lengthening of the table is required.
8. If switching from a Treatment Table 6A or 3 at 165 feet, stay the full 2 hours at 165 feet before decompressing.

| Depth (feet) | Time | Breathing media | Total elapsed time (h:min) |
|---|---|---|---|
| 165 | ½–2 h | | 2:00 |
| 140 | ½ h | | 2:31 |
| 120 | ½ h | Air | 3:02 |
| 100 | ½ h | | 3:33 |
| 80 | ½ h | | 4:04 |
| 60 | 6 h | | 10:05 |
| 50 | 6 h | | 16:06 |
| 40 | 6 h | | 22:07 |
| 30 | 12 h | Oxygen/Air | 34:08 |
| 20 | 2 h | | 36:09 |
| 10 | 2 h | | 38:10 |
| 0 | 1 min | | 38:11 |

**Treatment Table 7**: Oxygen/air treatment of unresolved or life-threatening symptoms of decompression sickness or arterial gas embolism

1. Used for treatment of unresolved and life-threatening symptoms after initial treatment on Table 6 or 4.
2. Use only under the direction of or in consultation with a Diving Medical Officer.
3. Table begins upon arrival at 60 feet. Arrival at 60 feet is accomplished by initial treatment on Table 6, 6A or 4. If initial treatment has progressed to a depth shallower than 60 feet, compress to 60 feet at 25 feet/min to begin Table 7.
4. Maximum duration at 60 feet is unlimited. Remain at 60 feet a minimum of 12 hours unless overriding circumstances dictate earlier decompression.
5. Patient begins oxygen breathing periods at 60 feet. Tender need breathe only chamber atmosphere throughout. If oxygen breathing is interrupted, no lengthening of the table is required.
6. Minimum chamber $O_2$ concentrations is 19%. Maximum $CO_2$ concentrations is 1.5% SEV (11.4 mmHg). Maximum chamber internal temperature is 85°F.
7. Decompression starts with a 2 foot upward excursion from 60 to 58 feet. Decompress with stops every 2 feet for times shown in profile below. Ascent time between stops is approximately 30 seconds. Stop time begins with ascent from deeper to next shallower step. Stop at 4 feet for 4 hours and then ascend to the surface at 1 foot/min.
8. Ensure chamber life support requirements can be met before committing to Treatment Table 7.
9. Chapter 8 of the *USN Manual* emphasizes that Table 7 is a table to be considered as 'a heroic measure for the treatment of life-threatening decompression sickness'. It is normally invoked at the end of the time at 60 feet on another table, e.g. Table 6, 6A or 4. The decision to change to Table 7 should only be made if the condition of the patient is such as to expect 'that marked residual impairment or loss of life may result if the currently prescribed decompression from 60 feet is undertaken'.
10. The manual suggests that the decision to commence ascent after the 12 hours at 60 should be made based on the patient's condition. A patient who has shown signs of improvement may benefit from further time at 60 feet; a patient who has not shown any signs of improvement probably will not.
11. Periods of breathing oxygen should be used if the patient can stand it. Because of the variable times that the patient may have spent on oxygen it is not possible to stipulate what these should be.
12. Further guidance on the use of this table is contained in Chapter 8 of the *USN Diving Manual*. This should be consulted, and it would be prudent to seek the advice of the USN (Medical Research Institute or Experimental Diving Unit) before using this table.

| Depth (feet) | Time (hours) from leaving 60 feet | Ascent rate (feet/hour) | Steps to get ascent rate |
|---|---|---|---|
| 60 | A minimum of 12 hours hold at 60 feet | | |
| 60 | 0 | 3 | 2 feet every 40 min |
| 40 | 6 | 2 | 2 feet every 60 min |
| 20 | 16 | 1 | 2 feet every 120 min |
| 4 | 32 | – | (4 hours hold and then surface 36 hours after leaving bottom) |

**Air Treatment Table 1A**: Air treatment of type I decompression sickness – 100-foot treatment

1. Treatment of type I decompression sickness when oxygen is unavailable and pain is relieved at a depth less than 66 feet.
2. Descent rate – 25 feet/min.
3. Ascent rate – 1 minute between stops.
4. Time at 100 feet – includes time from the surface.
5. If the piping configuration of the chamber does not allow it to return to atmospheric pressure from the 10-foot stop in the 1 minute specified, disregard the additional time required.

| Depth (feet) | Time (minutes) | Breathing media | Total elapsed time (h:min) |
|---|---|---|---|
| 100 | 30 | Air | 0:30 |
| 80 | 12 | Air | 0:43 |
| 60 | 30 | Air | 1:14 |
| 50 | 30 | Air | 1:45 |
| 40 | 30 | Air | 2:16 |
| 30 | 60 | Air | 3:17 |
| 20 | 60 | Air | 4:18 |
| 10 | 120 | Air | 6:19 |
| 0 | 1 | Air | 6:20 |

**Air Treatment Table 2A**: Air treatment of type I decompression sickness – 165-foot treatment

1. Treatment of type I decompression sickness when oxygen is unavailable and pain is relieved at a depth greater than 66 feet.
2. Descent rate – 25 feet/min.
3. Ascent rate – 1 minute between stops.
4. Time at 165 feet – includes time from the surface.

| Depth (feet) | Time (minutes) | Breathing media | Total elapsed time (h:min) |
|---|---|---|---|
| 165 | 30 | Air | 0:30 |
| 140 | 12 | Air | 0:43 |
| 120 | 12 | Air | 0:56 |
| 100 | 12 | Air | 1:09 |
| 80 | 12 | Air | 1:22 |
| 60 | 30 | Air | 1:53 |
| 50 | 30 | Air | 2:24 |
| 40 | 30 | Air | 2:55 |
| 30 | 120 | Air | 4:56 |
| 20 | 120 | Air | 6:57 |
| 10 | 240 | Air | 10:58 |
| 0 | 1 | Air | 10:59 |

**Air Treatment Table 3**: Air treatment of type II decompression sickness or arterial gas embolism

1. Treatment of type II symptoms or arterial gas embolism when oxygen is unavailable and symptoms are relieved within 30 minutes at 165 feet.
2. Descent rate – as rapidly as tolerated.
3. Ascent rate – 1 minute between stops.
4. Time at 165 feet – includes time from the surface.

| Depth (feet) | Time (minutes) | Breathing media | Total elapsed time (h:min) |
|---|---|---|---|
| 165 | 30 | Air | 0:30 |
| 140 | 12 | Air | 0:43 |
| 120 | 12 | Air | 0:56 |
| 100 | 12 | Air | 1:09 |
| 80 | 12 | Air | 1:22 |
| 60 | 30 | Air | 1:53 |
| 50 | 30 | Air | 2:24 |
| 40 | 30 | Air | 2:55 |
| 30 | 720 | Air | 14:56 |
| 20 | 120 | Air | 16:57 |
| 10 | 120 | AAAAir | 18:58 |
| 0 | 1 | Air | 18:59 |

# Appendix VI US Navy saturation therapy procedures and tables

Decompression sickness during saturation diving may result from excursion ascents or may be associated with the Standard Saturation Decompression. In the US Navy, decompression sickness manifesting during saturation decompression is common and has been characterized by musculoskeletal pain alone. The onset is usually gradual and generally occurs while the diver is still under pressure. However, decompression sickness resulting from excursion ascents may be more severe and may involve the cardiorespiratory system, the central nervous system and the organs of special sense.

Serious decompression sickness resulting from an excursion ascent should be treated by immediate recompression at 30 feet per minute to at least the depth from which the excursion ascent originated. If there is not complete relief at that depth, recompression should continue deeper until relief is accomplished.

Decompression sickness manifested only as musculoskeletal pain and occurring during Standard Saturation Decompression should be treated by recompression in increments of 10 feet at 5 feet per minute until distinct improvement is indicated by the diver. In most instances, improvement continues to complete resolution of the symptoms. Recompression of more than 30 feet is usually not necessary and causes increasing pain in some cases.

During recompression and at treatment depth, a treatment mixture may be given by mask to provide an oxygen partial pressure of 1.5–2.5 atmospheres. Pure oxygen may be used at treatment depths of 60 feet or less. The mask treatment should be interrupted every 20 minutes with 5 minutes of breathing the chamber atmosphere.

A stricken diver should remain at the treatment depth for a minimum of 12 hours in serious decompression sickness and a minimum of 2 hours in pain-only decompression sickness. The Standard Saturation Decompression Schedule can then resume from the treatment depth. However, excursion ascents must not be performed.

## Treatment gas mixtures

For treatment use, the following gas mixtures, having a range of oxygen partial pressure from 1.5 to 2.5 atmospheres (pure oxygen is used to the depth of 60 feet), should be available:

| Depth | Mix |
|---|---|
| 0–60 | 100% $O_2$ |
| 60–100 | 40/60 |
| 100–200 | 64/36 |
| 200–350 | 79/21 |
| 350–600 | 87/13 |
| 600–1000 | 92/8 |
| 1000–1600 | 95/5 |

# Appendix VII Comex therapy tables (1986)

Type I DCS

Recompress to 12 metres on O$_2$

| If relief within 15 min | If no re- |
| Use Cx12 | lief |
| | Use Cx18 |

Type 2 DCS

Recompress to 30 metres on Heliox 50/50

Use Cx30

## Cx12

| Depth (metres) | Duration (minutes) | Gas mixtures | | | Elapsed time |
| | | Patient | Attendant | Chamber | |
| --- | --- | --- | --- | --- | --- |
| 12 | 120 | Oxygen: four sessions (25 min on, 5 min off) | Ambient | Heliox 20/80 or air | 2 hours |
| 12 → 0 | 30 | Oxygen | Oxygen | | 2 h 30 min |

## Cx18

| Depth (metres) | Duration (minutes) | Gas mixtures | | | Elapsed time |
| | | Patient | Attendant | Chamber | |
| --- | --- | --- | --- | --- | --- |
| 18 | 90 | Oxygen: three sessions (25 min on, 5 min off) | Ambient | Heliox 20/80 or air | 1 h 30 min |
| 18 → 12 | 30 | Oxygen: one session (25 min on, 5 min off) | Ambient | | 2 hours |
| 12 | 150 | Oxygen: five sessions (25 min on, 5 min off) | 90 min ambient Then O$_2$, two sessions (25 min on, 5 min off | | 4 h 30 min |
| 12 → 0 | 30 | Oxygen | Oxygen | | 5 hours |

## Cx30

| Depth (metres) | Duration (minutes) | Gas mixtures | | | Elapsed time |
| --- | --- | --- | --- | --- | --- |
| | | *Patient* | *Attendant* | *Chamber* | |
| 30 | 60 | Heliox 50/50 | Ambient | Heliox 20/80 or air | 1 hour |
| 30 → 24 | 30 | Heliox 50/50: one session (25 min on, 5 min off) | Ambient | | 1 h 30 min |
| 24 | 30 | Heliox 50/50: one session (25 min on, 5 min off) | Ambient | | 2 hours |
| 24 → 18 | 30 | Heliox 50/50: one session (25 min on, 5 min off) | Ambient | | 2 h 30 min |
| 18 | 60 | Oxygen: two sessions (25 min on, 5 min off) | Ambient | | 3 h 30 min |
| 18 → 12 | 30 | Oxygen: one session (25 min on, 5 min off) | Ambient | | 4 hours |
| 12 | 180 | Oxygen: six sessions (25 min on, 5 min off) | Oxygen: six sessions (25 min on, 5 min off) | | 7 hours |
| 12 → 0 | 30 | Oxygen | Oxygen | | 7 h 30 min |

For failures, recurrences or worsening of symptoms, and for other than simple cases of DCS, refer to *Comex Medical Book*, 1986, for other procedures and tables.

# Appendix VIII Australian underwater oxygen table

## Notes

1. This technique may be useful in treating cases of decompression sickness in localities remote from recompression facilities. It may also be of use while suitable transport to such a centre is being arranged.
2. In planning, it should be realised that the therapy may take up to 3 hours. The risks of cold, immersion and other environmental factors should be balanced against the beneficial effects. The diver must be accompanied by an attendant.

## Equipment

The following equipment is essential before attempting this form of treatment:

1. Full face mask with demand valve and surface supply system *or* helmet with free flow.
2. Adequate supply of 100% oxygen for patient, and air for attendant.
3. Wet suit for thermal protection.
4. Shot with at least 10 metres of rope (a seat or harness may be rigged to the shot).
5. Some form of communication system between patient, attendant and surface.

## Method

1. The patient is lowered on the shot rope to 9 metres, breathing 100% oxygen.
2. Ascent is commenced after 30 minutes in mild cases, or 60 minutes in severe cases, if improvement has occurred. These times may be extended to 60 minutes and 90 minutes respectively if there is no improvement.
3. Ascent is at the rate of 1 metre every 12 minutes.
4. If symptoms recur remain at depth a further 30 minutes before continuing ascent.
5. If oxygen supply is exhausted, return to the surface, rather than breathe air.
6. After surfacing the patient should be given one hour on oxygen, one hour off, for a further 12 hours.

**Table Aust 9 (RAN 82)**: Short oxygen table

| Depth (metres) | Elapsed time Mild | Serious | Rate of ascent |
|---|---|---|---|
| 9 | 0030–0100 | 0100–0130 | |
| 8 | 0042–0112 | 0112–0142 | |
| 7 | 0054–0124 | 0124–0154 | 12 minutes |
| 6 | 0106–0136 | 0136–0206 | per metre |
| 5 | 0118–0148 | 0148–0218 | (4 min/foot) |
| 4 | 0130–0200 | 0200–0230 | |
| 3 | 0142–0212 | 0212–0242 | |
| 2 | 0154–0224 | 0224–0254 | |
| 1 | 0206–0236 | 0236–0306 | |

Total table time: 2 hours 6 min – 2 hours 36 min for mild cases
2 hours 36 min – 3 hours 6 min for serious cases.

# Appendix IX Duke University flow chart

## Guidelines for the treatment of decompression sickness

L. Fagaeus, J.N. Miller and P.B. Bennett
Department of Anesthesiology
Duke University Medical Center
Durham, NC

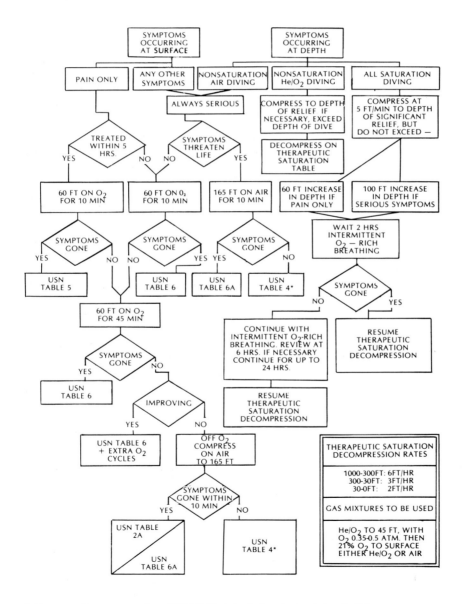

* Always use the oxygen version of USN Table 4, for both patient and attendant(s).

# Appendix X Diving medical information reading list

## Classics

*La Pression Barometric* (Barometric Pressure) by Paul Bert (1878). The Hitchcock translation has been reprinted for The Undersea Medical Society, Bethesda, MD.

*Caisson Sickness and the Physiology of Work in Compressed Air* (1912) by Sir Leonard Hill, Edward Arnold, London.

*Respiration* (1935) by J.S. Haldane and J.G. Priestley, Clarendon Press, Oxford.

*Decompression Sickness* (1951) edited by J.F. Fulton, Saunders, London.

*Deep Diving and Submarine Operations* (1955) by R.H. Davis, Siebe, Gorman and Co. Ltd, London.

*Key Documents of the Biomedical Aspects of Deep-Sea Diving* (1983) A selection from the world's literature 1608–1982. Published by The Undersea Medical Society, Bethesda, MD.

## Current medical texts

*Diving and Subaquatic Medicine*, 3rd edn (1991) by C. Edmonds, C. Lowry and J. Pennefather, Butterworth, London ISBN 0-7506-0259-7.

*Diving Medicine*, 2nd edn (1990) by A.A. Bove and J.C. Davis, Saunders, Philadelphia etc. ISBN 0-7216-2934-2.

*The Physician's Guide to Diving Medicine* (1984) edited by C.W. Shilling, C.B. Carlson and R.A. Mathias, Plenum Press, New York and London. ISBN 0-306-41428-7.

*Case Histories of Diving and Hyperbaric Accidents* (1988) edited by C. L. Waite for the Undersea and Hyperbaric Medical Society, Bethesda, MD.

*Medical Examination of Sports Scuba Divers* (1986) 2nd edn, edited by J.C. Davis, Best Publishers., San Pedro, CA.

## First aid

*Diver's Medical Manual* (1991) by C. Edmonds, R.L. Thomas and B.J. McKenzie, Diving Medical Centre, St Leonards 2065, Australia (in press).

*The DAN Emergency Handbook*, revised 2nd edn (1989) by J. Lippman and S. Bugg, JL Publications Carnegie, Victoria ISBN 0-9590306-1-1.

*SCUBA Diving Safety* (1978) by C.W. Dueker, World Publications, Mountain View, CA. ISBN 0-89037-135-0

*Field Guide for the Diver Medic* (1983) by C.G. Daugherty, distributed by the National Association of Diver Medical Technicians, Houston, TX.

## Specialist texts

*The Physiology and Medicine of Diving*, 3rd edition (1982), edited by P.B. Bennett and D.H. Elliott, Baillière Tindall and Cassell, London. ISBN 0-941 332-020. 4th edn in press.

*Hyperbaric Oxygen Therapy* (1977), edited by J.C. Davis and T.K. Hunt, Undersea Biomedical Society, Bethesda, MD. ISBN 0-930406-01-X.

*Decompression Sickness: The Biophysical Basis of Prevention and Treatment* by B.A. Hills, Wiley, New York. ISBN 0-471-99-457-X.

*Decompression–Recompression Sickness* (1981) by A.A. Buhlmann, Springer–Verlag, Berlin. ISBN 3-387-13308-9.

*Stress and Performance in Diving* (1987) by A.J. Bachrach and G.H. Egstrom, Best Publishers, San Pedro. ISBN 0-941332-06-3.

*Accidental Hypothermia* (1977) by D. Maclean and D. Emslie-Smith, Blackwell, Oxford. ISBN 0-632-00831-8.

*The Nature and Treatment of Hypothermia* (1983) edited by R.S. Pozos and L.E. Wittmers, University of Minnesota Press, Minneapolis. ISBN 0-8166-1154-8.

*Dangerous Marine Creatures* (1989) by C. Edmonds, Reid Books, Sydney. ISBN 0-7301-02149.

*Poisonous and Venomous Marine Animals of the World* (1978) by B.W. Halstead, Darwin Press, New Jersey.

*A Medical Guide to Hazardous Marine Life* (1987) P.S. Auerbach, Progressive Printing, Jacksonville, FA.

*Australian Animal Toxins* (1983) by S.K. Sutherland, Oxford University Press, Oxford. ISBN 0-19-55-4367X.

## Journals

*Undersea Biomedical Research*. Undersea and Hyperbaric Medical Society. ISSN 0093-5387.

*Journal of Hyperbaric Medicine* (first published as Hyperbaric Oxygen Review), Undersea and Hyperbaric Medical Society. ISSN 00884-1225.

*Pressure*, Undersea and Hyperbaric Medical Society, ISSN 0889–0242.

*Aviation, Space and Environmental Medicine*, Aerospace Medical Association ISSN 0095-6562.

*EUBS (European Undersea Biomedical Society)* Newsletter.

*SPUMS Journal*, South Pacific Underwater Medicine Society. ISSN 0813–1988.

### Indexes

*Underwater and Hyperbaric Medicine: Abstracts from the Literature*. Undersea and Hyperbaric Medical Society, ISSN 0886-3474.

*A Bibliographic Sourcebook of Compressed Air, Diving and Submarine* Medicine, E.C. Hoff and L.J. Greenbaum, 3 vols covering the period up to 1961, Dept of the Navy, Washington.

*An Annotated Bibliography of Diving and Submarine Medicine* (1971) C.W. Shilling and M.F. Wertz, covering the period 1962–69, Gordon and Breach, New York.

*Underwater Medicine and Related Sciences: A guide to the literature*. Five volumes covering the period 1967–79, C.W. Shilling et al. The Undersea Medical Society, Bethesda, MD.

### Divers Alert Network

This organisation is based in the USA, but has extensions in Europe, Australia and Japan. It collates data on diving accidents and analyses this in regular reports. It also supplies emergency and routine information to divers, diving physicians and others. It distributes diving safety texts and runs courses in diving medicine. It also assists in insurance and emergency transport for divers.

*Address*: DAN, Box 3823, Duke University Medical Center, Durham, North Carolina 27710, USA. Tel. (919) 684 8111.

### Conferences and proceedings

The Undersea and Hyperbaric Medical Society, The European Undersea Biomedical Society and the South Pacific Underwater Medicine Society host regular conferences. The proceedings of each are published in full or abstract form. The Undersea and Hyperbaric Medical Society also hosts workshops on specialized topics. Details of these may be obtained from the respective societies.

### Diving manuals

US Navy NAVSEA 0994-LP-001-9010.

Royal Navy BR2806. HMSO, London, UK.

NOAA (National Oceanographic and Atmospheric Administration), US Government Printing Office, Washington, USA.

BSAC (British Sub-Aqua Club), London, UK.

### Professional societies

The Undersea and Hyperbaric Medical Society, 9650 Rockville Pike, Bethesda, Maryland 20014, USA is probably the most important single organization. Their journals, newsletters and abstracts are required reading for an interested physician. It has a world-wide membership.

More local societies include:

- The European Undersea Biomedical Society, currently c/o National Hyperbaric Centre Aberdeen, AB2 5FA, UK.

- Diver's Alert Network, F.G. Hall Hyperbaric Center, Duke University Medical Center, Durham, NC 27710, USA (largely in the Americas, but expanding).

- Société Française de Médécine Subaquatique et Hyperbare (France).

- Società Italiana di Medicina Subacquea Iperbaeica (Italy).

- Barologia (South Africa).

- The South Pacific Underwater Medicine Society, membership mainly from South East Asia, Australia, New Zealand. c/o The Australian College of Occupational Medicine, PO Box 2090, St Kilda, West Victoria 3182, Australia.

### Diving medical training

The Royal Navy, the United States Navy and the Royal Australian Navy have regular courses for their officers; on occasion places are made available to members of other navies. The British and Australian courses have sometimes offered the course to civilian physicians who can demonstrate a need to attend.

Other courses are offered by the societies mentioned. Some hospitals with chambers offer courses, often combined with training in hyperbaric medicine. The courses are normally advertised in the Journal or newsletter of the appropriate Diving Medical society.

# Index

54-60

57, 84, 392-393 Panic

84-85, 284-285 Salt Water Aspiration
Syndrome

379 & 390 Vertigo (Sensory Deprivation)
Trouble Equalizing
(Dizziness)

456 - Children